FOUNDATIONS IN CRANIOSACRAL BIODYNAMICS

VOLUME TWO

FOUNDATIONS IN CRANIOSACRAL BIODYNAMICS

The Sentient Embryo, Tissue Intelligence, and Trauma Resolution

VOLUME TWO

FRANKLYN SILLS

Illustrations by Dominique Degranges

North Atlantic Books
Berkeley, California

Published by
North Atlantic Books
Berkeley, California

Cover photo ©iStockphoto.com/SABarton
Cover and book design by Jan Camp
Printed in the United States of America

MEDICAL DISCLAIMER: The following information is intended for general information purposes only. Individuals should always see their health care provider before administering any suggestions made in this book. Any application of the material set forth in the following pages is at the reader's discretion and is his or her sole responsibility.

Foundations in Craniosacral Biodynamics: The Sentient Embryo, Tissue Intelligence, and Trauma Resolution is sponsored and published by the Society for the Study of Native Arts and Sciences (dba North Atlantic Books), an educational nonprofit based in Berkeley, California, that collaborates with partners to develop cross-cultural perspectives, nurture holistic views of art, science, the humanities, and healing, and seed personal and global transformation by publishing work on the relationship of body, spirit, and nature.

North Atlantic Books' publications are available through most bookstores. For further information, visit our website at www.northatlanticbooks.com or call 800-733-3000.

ISBN for Volume Two: 978-1-58394-487-5

Library of Congress Cataloging-in-Publication Data

The first volume of this series was catalogued under the following information:

Sills, Franklyn, 1947–
    Foundations in craniosacral biodynamics / Franklyn Sills ; illustrations by Dominique Degranges.
        p. ; cm.
    Includes bibliographical references and index.
    Summary: "Biodynamic Craniosacral Therapy (BCST) is commonly seen as the spiritual approach to craniosacral therapy (CST); in fact, BCST as taught by Franklyn Sills, the pioneer in the field, is quite different from conventional CST. Biodynamic work is based on the development of perceptual skills where the practitioner learns to become sensitive to subtle respiratory motions called primary respiration and also to the power of spontaneous healing. Through the Breath of Life, which, Sills asserts, echoes the Holy Spirit in the Judeo-Christian tradition, bodhicitta in Buddhism, and the Tai Chi in Taoism, students of BCST learn to enter a state of presence oriented to the client's inherent ability to heal.In Foundations in Craniosacral Biodynamics, Sills offers students and practitioners an in-depth, step-by-step guide to the development of perceptual and clinical skills with specific clinical exercises and explorations to help students and practitioners learn the essentials of a biodynamic approach. Individual chapters cover such topics as holism and biodynamics; mid-tide, Long Tide, Dynamic Stillness and stillpoint process; the motility of tissues and the central nervous system; transference and the shadow; shamanistic resonances; and more"—Provided by publisher.
    ISBN-13: 978-1-55643-925-4 (pbk.)
    ISBN-10: 1-55643-925-3 (pbk.)
    1. Craniosacral therapy. I. Title.
    [DNLM: 1. Musculoskeletal Manipulations—methods. 2. Mind-Body Relations, Metaphysical. 3. Mind-Body Therapies—methods. 4.Sacrum—physiology. 5. Skull—physiology. 6. Spiritual Therapies—methods. WB 535]
    RZ399.C73S56 2011
    615.8'2—dc22

                                                            2011000210

4 5 6 7 8 9 SHERIDAN 21 20 19 18

North Atlantic Books is committed to the protection of our environment. We partner with FSC-certified printers using soy-based inks and print on recycled paper whenever possible.

ACKNOWLEDGMENTS

I would like to acknowledge the feedback given to me by tutors at Karuna on the wording of certain areas of description, including the augmentation visceral sections. I would like to also acknowledge the contribution of my wife, Cherionna Menzam-Sills, who wrote the important and formative second and third chapters in this volume. Cherionna is a senior biodynamic craniosacral teacher in the USA and Canada; she has her MA in somatic psychology and her PhD in pre- and perinatal psychology. She has worked deeply in these areas and her contributions in this volume on the sentient embryo and the importance of the pre- and perinatal period in our relational life and personality development point to key aspects of work in this field.

I would also like to acknowledge the wonderful work of Dominique Degranges in his illustrations for this volume. Dominique is director of a training center in Winterthur, Switzerland, is a senior tutor in craniosacral biodynamics, and runs courses and trainings in pre- and perinatal psychology and therapy. He is an old friend and colleague in this wonderful work we do.

I would also like to deeply acknowledge my former wife, Maura Sills. Maura and I are still co-directors of the Karuna Institute, which offers training both in craniosacral biodynamics and in core process psychotherapy, a truly integrated mindfulness-based psychotherapy form. Maura supports my work in many ways and we both are still involved in the running of the Institute and the raising of our younger daughter, Ella, a truly brave and lovely being. I also would like to acknowledge my older daughter, Laurel, who always reminds me of the goodness and joy in my life.

Finally I would like to appreciate North Atlantic Books for the support of my writings over the years. North Atlantic Books has become an important haven for writings in the cranial field, psychology, and the healing of trauma in our lives.

CONTENTS

ILLUSTRATIONS

INTRODUCTION

I believe osteopathy's orientation to health is unique in Western medicine. Andrew T. Still, the founder of osteopathy, consistently directed his students to listen for health as a starting point. Emphasizing health challenges our prevailing modern medical culture, which has a combative and aggressive preoccupation with disease. Still's words inspire a deep examination of what health is and how to hear its constant call. An orientation to health deeply shifts the clinician's intentions and clinical work and is something that must be developed and nurtured over time. In this process, it can be very hard to shift from our cultural conditioning. We tend to see disease as something to be conquered, thus polarizing our experience of health and illness. In a biodynamic context, health is perceived to be a deeper resource at work throughout life, centering the conditions present in the best possible fashion.

One role of the biodynamic practitioner is to orient to the expression of health via the presence and action of what the founder of the work, Dr. William Garner Sutherland, called the *Breath of Life* and its *unerring potency*. As I have oriented to this principle over many years, I have learned that the decisions about what has to occur in a person's healing process is not up to me to determine. The knowledge of the healing needs of the client—and the precise sequence of their unfoldment—is already present in the forces and conditions at work, which if oriented to, will lead the way.

This volume is a continuation of the approach outlined in Foundations Volume One. The underpinnings of this approach are practitioner presence, the ability to generate a negotiated relational field—to hold a wide perceptual field that is not intrusive or invasive—and to be able to orient to the conditions in a client's system in the context of what Sutherland called *primary respiration*. As we settle into a wide perceptual field oriented to primary respiration in relationship to a client's system, a wonderful process begins to unfold. Over a number of minutes—or in some cases a number of sessions—the client's system begins to settle out of the waveforms of history and conditions and deepens into what Sutherland called the *tide*. As this occurs, healing intentions begin to clarify that are not a function of practitioner analysis or technique. Dr. Rollin Becker, a disciple of Sutherland's, called this the unfolding of the *inherent treatment plan*. The healing forces of primary respiration come to the forefront, decisions are made beyond our human mentality, and the practitioner's role is to facilitate and support this process.

One important addition to this most fundamental ground is an awareness of personal and interpersonal process. Our understanding of the totality of human health and disease has moved on since Still and Sutherland developed their work in the osteopathic tradition. As a practitioner deepens into the nature of health and suffering, a realization emerges that the psycho-emotional and interpersonal nature of a person must be held along with the physical-physiological whole. Modern journeys into the human psyche taken by analysts and psychotherapists of many persuasions—along with a growing understanding of the neurology of stress and personality—have greatly enhanced our understanding of the human condition, and these must be held at least in awareness in the work we do. Please see my earlier book on personality formation (*Being and Becoming: Psychodynamics, Buddhism, and the oOrigin of Selfhood*). Likewise—given the stressed and traumatized condition of many of our clients in this tense human realm of ours—trauma skills, both in the cranial context and in the development of appropriate verbal skills, must all be part of a modern training in biodynamic craniosacral therapy. Helping clients develop their own skills in self-regulation—and in the regulation of stress cycling and traumatic activation—is very empowering for them.

These basics are the foundations of the topics discussed in this second volume. Its intention is to clarify and deepen our awareness of the territories that emerge in session work:

- The first five chapters add important explorations of the embryonic and pre- and perinatal period—including three chapters on the birth process and its unfolding in session work.

- Subsequent chapters explore important tissue relationships not covered in Volume One.

- The final four chapters look more deeply at the nature of trauma, its physiology and unfolding in session work, and the primary skills needed as traumatic history, central nervous system activation, and the cycling of the stress response emerge in session work. These include both cranial and mindfulness-based verbal skills.

I hope you find the following chapters useful in both your studies and in clinical practice.

CHAPTER 1

Starting Points

As a starting point in this second volume, I would like to review some basic concepts and to expand some areas introduced in Foundations Volume One. I will remind readers of the nature of primary respiration, briefly review the unfolding of the inherent treatment plan and deepen our appreciation of what I call the suspensory nature of the three bodies—the physical, fluid, and tidal bodies. I will try to describe this suspensory state in some detail, as the unfolding of the inherent treatment plan and its related healing processes is founded upon its field of action. I will also remind readers of the importance of the primal midline and of establishing clinical baselines.

Presence

Presence is a theme that takes us deeply into the nature of our work and to the heart of our human condition. In Volume One, we stressed the primacy of presence, the ability to settle into a still, receptive, and aware state. We emphasized that presence is natural—it is not about creating presence, but rather about letting go of what is in its way. As we deepen into stillness, we discover that presence is inherent and is found at the very core of our being, our core state.

We presented various meditative explorations in Volume One that help us deepen into this state. In one exercise, we suggested that you might find a comfortable sitting position and orient to your breath, following the sensation of breath in and out of your body. We then suggested that, once comfortably resting in breath, you might settle into a state of sensory awareness, oriented to sensations and feelings in your body. From here, we then introduced various contemplative exercises oriented to awareness of the fluid tide, Long Tide, and stillness, first in your own system and then oriented to the client's.

When a practitioner settles into a state of presence oriented both to the client's system and to the formative forces that support and maintain it, a resonance occurs within which the client can access new potential and possibility, beyond the suffering currently centered in the mind-body system. When one enters a state of presence attuned to another, it naturally resonates with the deeper core state. We called this resonance the *being-to-being* state—a mutually co-arising state of presence from which attunement and direct knowing arise. From here, we discussed the importance of generating a receptive and negotiated relational field.

The Relational Field

Life is deeply relational in nature, and the work we do is grounded in relationship, attunement, and compassionate resonance with the client's arising process. We form a relationship both to ourselves and to our clients—their joys and suffering—and to the deeper potential in us all for healing and resolution. As introduced above, the fundamental starting point in the generation of a secure relational environment is our ability to deepen into a still and receptive state—a being state—and to form a negotiated and appropriate relationship to our clients—a being-to-being attuned and empathetic holding field.

We emphasized this territory in the early chapters of Fundamentals Volume One, where much time was spent orienting the reader to meditative processes, entering a state of presence and the six-step relational orientation we called the *ritual of contact*—clearing space, moving toward, negotiating our distance of attention and physical touch, and settling into a still, receptive, and wide perceptual field, within which we holistically orient to the client's system, primary respiration, and the arising process. The key aspect of this was a growing ability to appropriately meet the client's system, to negotiate contact without crowding or invading it, and to orient to the arising process. From this ground we explored the nature of what Sutherland called primary respiration and the tide.

The Breath of Life and Primary Respiration

One fundamental orientation in a biodynamic context is practitioner awareness of primary respiration and the forces it generates in the human system. As discussed in Fundamentals Volume One, Sutherland—in his later work—oriented to the Breath of Life and its unerring potency. The Breath of Life is a sacred principle that is difficult to talk about or describe. It is a spiritual essence that mediates the creative impulse and connects all things to the ground of creation. It is experienced as heart-opening love and seems to arise out of a profound stillness called Dynamic Stillness. It generates organizing forces that orchestrate and maintain all form—from the vastness of galaxies, solar systems, stars, and planets, to the huge variety of life—from the simplest cell to the most complex tissue structure and living form. This is, at its root, not just an expression of physical evolution, but of consciousness itself. Thus life can be experienced as an interplay of consciousness manifesting creative impulses, driving life to generate new and more complex forms.

As discussed in Volume One, these creative forces manifest in a rhythmic phenomenon that Sutherland called *primary respiration,* or the tide. Rollin Becker DO called the most fundamental expression of primary respiration the *Long Tide*, which manifests at a constant rate of 50 seconds of inhalation and 50 seconds of exhalation.

Locally, the Long Tide generates an ordering matrix and midline—manifesting as a bioelectric-biomagnetic field—which orchestrates the morphology of the embryo and maintains tissue organization throughout life. In a biodynamic orientation, the bioelectric field that the Long Tide generates and the midline within it—which I call the *primal midline*—is sensed to be the primary organizing principle for cellular and tissue organization. This field and midline orchestrate the formation both of the primitive streak and notochord in the early embryo, around which embryonic folding and tissue organization develop. The primal midline is the midline that the notochord forms within and can be sensed as an uprising force through the vertebral and cranial base axis throughout life. An awareness of the dynamics of this midline is incredibly useful in clinical work, as the organization of the tissue field is in direct relationship to its presence.

In relatively recent research at Tufts University, shifts in the bioelectric field were discovered to orchestrate the folding of the frog embryo into its embryonic form. You can even see the rising of a quantum-bioelectric midline phenomenon in the video that the researchers produced. The bioelectric ordering field was found to be more primary in the generation of morphology than genes and genetic process (Jonathan 2011).

As you hold a wide perceptual field, with the client's midline in its center, the Long Tide may be perceived as a tidal phenomenon in stable 50-second cycles of streaming from the horizon toward and away from the client's midline in a vast torus-shaped form called the *tidal body*. As your awareness is widened toward the horizon, and resonates with a deeper stillness, you may even sense the Long Tide manifesting an even slower rate, with a sense of endless expansion—here you are very near to its arising from the Dynamic Stillness itself. The Long Tide can also be sensed as spaciousness, radiance, and spiral-like forces around the client's body. The Long Tide is totally stable and is never in shock. Indeed, awareness of its presence can help resolve CNS trauma and the cycling of stress states.

As the Long Tide generates the local bioelectric field, forces are introduced into the fluids of the body via a process that Sutherland called *transmutation*—a change in state and vibration from Long Tide to fluids. Sutherland called these embodied ordering forces *potency*—a similar ordering force is called *chi* (sometimes spelled *qi*) in Chinese philosophy and medicine. As this occurs, another rhythmic phenomenon called the *fluid tide* is also generated, which manifests at a rate of 1–3 cycles a minute, most commonly 2–2.5 cycles a minute. This more embodied tidal phenomenon is also called *mid-tide*, a term that acknowledges the interplay of potency, fluids, and tissues. Potency is the ordering and driving force, fluids are the medium of that force, and tissues are organized by its action. The potency in the fluids generates the fluid tide, organizes the form of the body, and orchestrates tissue motility.

- **Mid-tide**—The interplay in the fluid and physical bodies between potency, fluids, and tissues, manifesting at 1–3 cycles a minute. Fluids express it as the fluid tide, tissues as tissue motility.

- **Long Tide**—The ground of primary respiration, the fundamental ordering principle, manifesting at a stable rate of 50 seconds exhalation and 50 seconds inhalation. It generates a local bioelectric ordering field.

- **Dynamic Stillness**—The ground of emergence for the Breath of Life and primary respiration. All things arise and return to the stillness and the stillness holds the potential for the emergence of creativity, energy, and form.

The Inherent Treatment Plan

In biodynamics, the practitioner learns to hold a reciprocal awareness of primary respiration in his or her own system, along with its expression relative to the client's system and midline. In this framework, the practitioner also learns to hold the conditions and patterns sensed in the client's system in the context of primary respiration. As a client's system deepens into its relationship to primary respiration, healing processes naturally unfold in its own time and sequence. As we saw in Foundations Volume One, Rollin Becker called this the emergence of the *inherent treatment plan*.

The heart of biodynamic work orients to the unfolding of the inherent treatment plan. In Foundations Volume One, I used this concept to outline the development of a biodynamic mental set and clinical process. In this understanding, as the practitioner enters a state of presence oriented to the client's system in certain ways, the healing process unfolds in a precise and unique fashion that I, as practitioner, could not have analyzed, motion tested for, or anticipated. The central orientation is to primary respiration, the health that manifests as a primary ordering and healing principle in our mind-body system. The conditions of mind and body are held in this wider context until a dynamic equilibrium of the forces involved clarifies, and healing intentions emerge from a deeper source than our human mentality. This is the heart of a biodynamic approach, no matter how it is taught or oriented to.

In Volume One, I outlined ways to describe this unfolding process, which I would like to review here. The first and most primary intention is to settle out of one's conditioned mental states and ego processes, into a more basic state of presence. I call this state a *being-state.* From this state, we first orient to primary respiration relative to our own system. Sutherland stressed that knowledge of primary respiration in our own mind-body system will support our awareness of primary respiration relative to the client's system. We then negotiate our relationship to the client's system and tissues, and maintain a wide perceptual field, with the client's midline in the center of that field. We then hold the intention to orient to the deeper being-state of the client, which I called the *being-to-being holding field*, and to primary respiration relative to the client's system, which supports our incarnation in this body as a particular human being.

Very commonly, when a practitioner first contacts a client's system, a multitude of information is present. Various inertial fulcrums and patterns of experience and history are communicated and the more superficial rhythm—the *cranial rhythmic impulse* (CRI)—presents. The CRI, or cranial rhythm, is a variable manifestation of history, autonomic activation, and the unresolved conditional forces still active in the client's system. It is like waveforms of experience, which are expressed as a variable rhythm like conditional waves on top of the ocean. As practitioners deepen into their wide perceptual field oriented to stillness and primary respiration, they discover that the expression of history and conditions, and the waveforms of the CRI, settle over time as primary respiration and the wholeness of the human system comes to the forefront. I call this the *holistic shift*, a shift from history, conditions, and waveforms, to primary respiration, wholeness, and new potential. This territory is sometimes called the *patient's neutral* in osteopathic practice.

As the holistic shift deepens, particular healing intentions emerge, which I could not have analyzed or motion tested for. Indeed, analysis and practitioner intervention at this point only gets in the way of this process unfolding. As the system deepens into its relationship to primary respiration, we discover that healing decisions are made from within and our role is to facilitate and support this process. We also discover that our human system is truly suspended in the universe by the presence of primary respiration—within what Becker called the Long Tide—and everything is, in turn, suspended in stillness—stillness so deep and pervasive that it is called the Dynamic Stillness in biodynamics.

It is from this depth that healing processes clarify and the inherent treatment plan unfolds. We also discover that healing intentions may clarify from any level of primary respiration and stillness—the potency or ordering forces in the fluids of the system may initiate healing processes, the Long Tide may come to the forefront and initiate processes, and, likewise, the system may deepen into stillness from which healing intentions then emerge. We learn to trust the unfolding of this process, with the realization that appropriate expressions of healing may emerge from any level.

As the inherent treatment plan unfolds, a basic healing phenomenon that Becker described as a three-phase awareness also unfolds. In Foundations Volume One, we described these three phases—*seeking, settling,* and *reorganization and realignment*—largely in terms of physical and fluid bodies and mid-tide processes. However, the three phases manifest in some way in all healing processes and I would like to review and clarify this very basic understanding with a wider orientation.

As the system begins to access the holistic shift, the practitioner may perceive a quality of seeking. The system begins to settle out of the waveforms of history and CRI, and a seeking of equilibrium may be sensed. You may perceive the tissue field shifting, expressing various historical forms and beginning to seek a deeper stillness. You may sense the tissue field becoming suspended in fluid as a settling of waveforms and patterning occurs as potency, fluids, and tissues seek equilibrium. This is Becker's first phase of his three-phase healing awareness—the *seeking* phase.

As equilibrium deepens, a settling into the holistic shift is sensed and any level of healing process may then emerge. This is Becker's second phase of *settling* into a state of balance—a state where all forces and fields of expression enter dynamic equilibrium. This occurs over a number of minutes, or even a number of sessions, where the system may shift to one level of settling, clear some autonomic activation, deepen again, with more clearing occurring, until a much deeper state of equilibrium is accessed.

As the holistic shift deepens, the three bodies—the physical, fluid, and tidal bodies—express their suspensory nature and healing processes emerge from any level (see the next section). Basically the tissue field is now suspended in the fluid body, suspended in Long Tide, and the tissues orient to the biodynamic forces that have been organizing the body since embryological development occurred. In many ways, the tissues are returning to their embryological origins and entering a fluid state.

As this state deepens, healing processes are engaged in many ways. Commonly, a particular issue uncouples from all others and comes to the forefront as an inertial fulcrum clarifies. As discussed in detail in Volume One, an inertial fulcrum is a locus of forces, where the potency of the Breath of Life has become inertial in order to center and contain a conditional force of some kind. Conditional forces impinge on the mid-body system in some way and are myriad—the forces of trauma, genetics, accidents, birth, toxins, pathogens, etc.—indeed any force that affects the system in some way. If these could not be resolved at the time of the experience, then potency coalesces and becomes inertial in order to contain their effect on the system to as local an area as possible. Locally this generates tissue changes of various kinds, and will also have wider repercussions—lowering a person's energies and vitality, facilitating nervous system sensitivity and activation, and even initiating a stress response in the system.

As the system continues to settle around the inertial fulcrum, a further seeking process is initiated where the forces in the inertial fulcrum seek equilibrium, a *state of balance*, in the suspensory field of the three bodies. Commonly, as the state of balance deepens, the fluid tide may subside as potency shifts in the fluids and orients to specific inertial issues in the system. Healing intentions may then emerge from any level of action—from within the fluid body via the shifting of potency, from the Long Tide as it shifts through the client's midline and field, and/or from a deepening into the Dynamic Stillness. Commonly, healing may entail a number of interactive processes emerging—Long Tide initiating the action of potency in fluids, intentions emerging from Dynamic Stillness initiating Long Tide and fluid-body tidal potency healing territories, etc. As healing processes complete, the practitioner will sense potency, fluids, and tissues *reorganizing and realigning* to midline and natural fulcrums—Becker's third phase. Commonly, sessions complete with a surge in the fluid tide, or a deepening stillness (Figure 1.1).

The Inherent Treatment Plan Unfolds

The First Settling: The Relational Field

The practitioner orients to primary respiration and the relational field is negotiated and settles.

The Second Settling: The Holistic Shift

As the practitioner settles into a receptive state oriented to primary respiration and to the client's midline and biosphere, a holistic shift from conditional processes and CRI level of expressions to wholeness and primary respiration occurs and deepens. The three bodies manifest their suspensory nature— physical body suspended in fluid body, suspended in tidal body—and healing intentions may emerge from any level.

Holistic shift deepens and the Long Tide clarifies as healing intentions emerge as a direct expression of Long Tide phenomena.

Holistic shift deepens and healing intentions emerge at a mid-tide level mediated by the tidal potencies. Becker's phases of seeking and settling into dynamic equilibrium emerge.

Holistic shift deepens into the Dynamic Stillness and healing intentions emerge within and from a ground of emergence that is both dynamic and vibrantly alive.

Becker's third phase of reorganization and realignment to midline clarifies.

Figure 1.1. The unfolding of the inherent treatment plan.

The Suspensory Nature of the Three Bodies and the Holistic Shift

In Foundations Volume One, Chapters 3 and 10, we learned to orient to the human system by holding a wide perceptual field oriented to what we called the three bodies—the physical, fluid, and tidal bodies. The physical body is the tissue field as a whole, the fluid body is the body of fluid and the ordering forces—the potency—in the fluids, and the tidal body is the Long Tide as it moves toward and away from the client's midline. The boundary of the physical body is the skin, that of the fluid body is a fluid-energetic field that extends anywhere from 25–30 centimeters (10–12 inches) to 50 centimeters (20 inches) around the body, and that of the tidal body is the vast torus-shaped form of the Long Tide, which seems to move from the horizon toward and away from the client's midline, while the whole system seems to be suspended in its wider field.

As the holistic shift deepens, we may discover a fascinating process, which is also a key to understanding the emergence of healing forces and intentions in clinical work. As I settle into my relationship to the client's system, I set up a wide perceptual field with his or her midline in the center of my orientation. As I touch the client's body, I allow my hands to float on the tissues, suspended in fluid, as both the client and I are suspended in a wider tidal field. As I settle into this field while oriented to primary respiration, I begin to sense a wonderful phenomenon as the holistic shift clarifies.

The physical body seems to settle, soften, and deepen, and becomes suspended in the fluid body. It literally feels as though every cell and tissue is now suspended in a fluid field, while the client's body is also sensed to be unified and whole. It is as though the tissue field is returning to an earlier, more fluid embryonic state, as cells and tissues reorient to the forces of primary respiration, around which the embryo formed, and through which tissue organization is maintained throughout life.

As the holistic shift continues to settle, one can perceive that the physical and fluid bodies are suspended in the wider tidal body of Long Tide—field within field suspended in the wider universe! As this again deepens, one can also perceive that all three bodies are further suspended in stillness—the Dynamic Stillness that both Sutherland and Becker pointed to. It is from this suspensory system—physical body suspended in fluid body, suspended in tidal body, suspended in stillness—that healing processes emerge. All fields are interdependent, mutually supporting life in this form and containing, as Sutherland maintained, Intelligence beyond my human mentality.

Inertial Fulcrums and the Suspensory Nature of the Three Bodies

Another fascinating process may also be sensed as this suspensory system clarifies and deepens. Not only is the physical body perceived to be suspended in the fluid and tidal bodies, but all inertial fulcrums in the client's system are also now suspended in this wider field. As healing intentions clarify—and potency shifts in the fluids toward a specific fulcrum—the inertial fulcrum being attended to is uncoupled from all other fulcrums in the system and becomes suspended in the wider tissue field and fluid body. The tissues—now suspended in fluid—shift as a unified fluid-tissue field and organize around it. The inertial fulcrum literally becomes suspended in all fields and the body's tissues—suspended in the fluid and tidal bodies—will holistically organize around it for healing purposes.

As this occurs, all three bodies are now oriented to the inertial fulcrum being attended to and the forces in the fulcrum can enter equilibrium—the *state of balance*—and, as this suspensory state deepens, any level of healing process may emerge relative to the fulcrum being attended to. The state of balance is thus not just a local phenomenon. It is systemic and extends to all levels of action: tissues fluids, forces, and tidal fields—all oriented to the healing of the inertial issue that has clarified. As the state of balance deepens, the whole field of potency is now oriented to the inertial forces in the fulcrum, Long Tide phenomena may come to the forefront and the whole process may deepen into stillness and an interchange between the stillness, potency, and tissues may be perceived. Becker called this *balanced rhythmic interchange* (Figure 1.2).

One way to image this, if you have not yet perceived it, is to imagine that a wool blanket is a fluid-tissue field. Imagine that two friends are holding the blanket upright very tautly, suspended in space. Further imagine that you are standing behind the blanket and press a finger into it from behind. This is like potency in the fluids shifting to a specific fulcrum in the wider field. Notice how the entire blanket organizes around the place you are pressing. It is not really like this, but the image may help to conceptualize the process—the blanket, suspended in space, will naturally organize as a whole around the fulcrum you create as you press its fabric. Likewise, as an inertial fulcrum in the body uncouples and clarifies in the wider field, the tissue field—now suspended as a whole in the fluid and tidal bodies—will naturally organize around it. The whole healing process can then deepen.

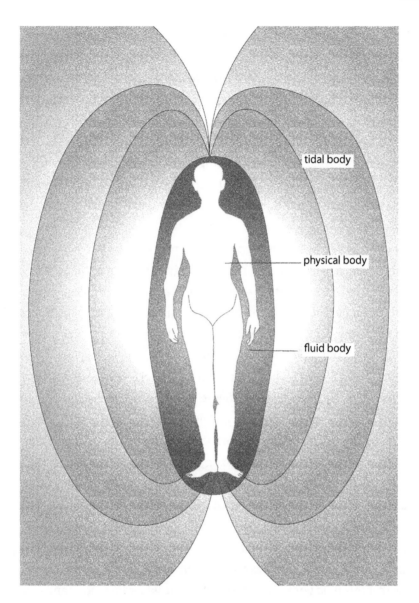

Figure 1.2. The three bodies.

Contemplative Exercise:
Three-Body Chi Kung _____

I would like to review the practice introduced in Foundations Volume One that I called three-body chi kung. It is a standing practice that helps the practitioner and student attune to the three bodies and primary respiration—first, relative to their own system, and then relative to the client's. As we commonly begin a session by standing at the side of the table, it is a very useful starting point. The following is an edited version of the contemplative exercise presented in Volume One.

Stand with your feet hip-width apart, knees gently bent. Sink your pelvis as you gently lift your occiput upward. Relax your shoulders and let your arms settle into a soft, circular form: elbows slightly outward, hands at the level of your hips, fingers gently raised, and palms facing the floor. Imagine that your arms and hands are suspended in a fluid field. This stance helps to subtly lengthen your vertebral-notochord midline and creates a more upright and fluent posture. Settle into this standing position.

Imagine-sense a midline through the center of your body and, through this midline, settle your awareness into your body. A good orientation is to sink your awareness into body sensation—settling your awareness caudal along the midline to a fulcrum behind your heart or navel. From this midline and inner fulcrum, widen your awareness to the whole of your body and the local field around it, your physical and fluid bodies or biosphere.

See if you can rest in a holistic awareness of sensations and feelings, allowing all sensation to be present at once. Sense your midline and biosphere as a unified, singular fluid-tissue-sensory-body. Now extend this awareness slowly outward in all directions, first to include the room you are standing in and then out into the environment, toward the horizon, as previously explored. Imagine-sense that you are suspended in this wider field around the centerline of a vast torus-shaped tidal body that has substance and presence. This is the tidal body of the Long Tide. Rest suspended in this field.

Now, in this wide perceptual field, orient to your fluid body, which extends from the midline 10–20 inches around your body (25–50 centimeters). Imagine-sense that this fluid body is a denser field in the wider tidal body and is suspended in it. Stay with this awareness for a while.

Now add an awareness of your physical body as a denser field suspended in the fluid body. Your skin is its boundary. Imagine-sense that your physical body is suspended in your fluid body. Rest in this awareness for a few moments. Then extend this awareness and imagine-sense that your physical and fluid bodies are both suspended in the wider tidal body. Again let yourself rest in this awareness.

Settle into an awareness of all three bodies as a suspensory system supporting and sustaining you in each and every moment of life. Let yourself be suspended and rest in this vast supportive field. As you settle into this awareness, you may also become aware of the respiratory phases of primary respiration clarifying relative to your own midline.

To end the exercise, move around the room or space you are standing in. As you do this, explore your senses—seeing, hearing, feeling, moving—and see if the sense of being in the world is a little different now.

Second Exercise:
Orienting to the Client's System with Awareness of the Three Bodies and Holistic Shift

This second perceptual exercise extends the contemplative standing form explored above and is oriented to the holistic shift. You will move from the side of the table to the client's feet and orient to the three bodies relative to the client's midline. This adds another level of discernment and clarity as you settle into a wide perceptual field.

With the client in the supine position, stand at the side of the table, establish your fulcrums and state of presence, and settle into the standing position outlined above. Orient to your midline and your sense of being suspended in a tidal body. As above, see if you can sense your fluid and physical bodies suspended in this wider field. Rest in this awareness and sense the presence of primary respiration around and in your own system. Settle into this awareness for a few moments. Then, still standing at the side of the table, orient to the client's midline, biosphere, and tidal body. Imagine-sense that the client is suspended in the tidal body of the Long Tide. Allow your shared relational field to settle.

When your relationship to the client's system is established, move to the foot of the treatment table. Settle into your midline and fulcrums, orient to client's midline, and again establish a wide perceptual field. Slowly make contact with the client's feet—you can be in the standing or sitting position to do this. Allow your hands to float on tissues, suspended in a wider fluid field. Really allow your hands to feel fluid and do not place too much attention in them. Orient to the client's midline and widen your perceptual field to include the whole of the biosphere—the client's physical and fluid bodies. Settle into this awareness for a few moments and then again slowly widen your perceptual field toward the horizon with the client's midline still in the center of your field of awareness. Do not widen your awareness from your head, but from your heart center or belly, so that you are still grounded in embodied awareness, and do not space-out or dissociate. As you do this, again imagine-sense that the client is suspended in the tidal body of the Long Tide. Sense that his or her fluid and physical bodies are denser forms in this wider field and are suspended in its presence. Locally, orient to the client's system as a unified fluid-tissue-sensory body. Settle and deepen into this awareness.

As you settle into this relationship, you will commonly sense potency, fluids, and tissues expressing and communicating historical patterns to you as motion and form. The CRI level of rhythm will also commonly be prevalent. After five to ten minutes of listening, you may notice that the conditioned motions and patterns and the CRI seem to settle. You may have the experience of the system settling, softening, and deepening. The tissue field may seem to soften and widen and, as this occurs, you may perceive that the system seems more fluidic, unified, and whole, with a clarification or intensification of primary respiration.

This commonly manifests as a series of deepenings—softening, settling, widening, and stilling—until it literally feels like you are holding a unified suspensory potency-fluid-tissue field. This heralds a shift in orientation from the conditions and patterns present, to primary respiration and its inherent potency and resources.

As the holistic shift deepens, it may be perceived that the physical and fluid bodies are literally suspended in action of the tidal body and that all three bodies enter equilibrium and coherency. Again, as the client's system settles into the holistic shift, notice the qualities present. One person's system may seem dense, another vibrant, another weak in its expression of potency, and so on.

As the holistic shift settles and deepens, you likewise deepen and maintain orientation to the client's midline and local biosphere in your wide perceptual field. Simply orient to the clarification of primary respiration and for healing decisions to emerge from any level of action.

The Primal Midline

As you may remember from Foundations Volume One, Chapter 19, the primal midline is the main ordering midline both for embryonic development and for cells and tissues throughout life. It is perceived as an uprising force through the notochord axis and is part of a wider bioelectric field. We discovered that awareness of this midline has important clinical consequences and discussed the importance of practitioner awareness of its presence, suggested some perceptual exercises that help you orient to it, and discussed the dynamics that emerge as inertial issues resolve and the tissue field reorganizes. I'd like to review some of these territories, as we will be discussing various tissue relationships in this volume.

In embryological development, a waveform arises through the center of the primitive disc. This midline phenomenon generates the primitive streak and notochord, around which differentiation and tissue organization occur. We call the energetic aspect of this waveform the primal midline, which can be sensed throughout life as an uprising force through the vertebral bodies and cranial base. Randolph Stone DO called this the *fountain spray of life*, stating that all healing processes must include an awareness of this midline, which he said has the "neuter essence" at its core (Stone 1999). (See Figures 1.3 and 1.4.)

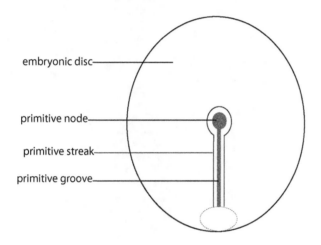

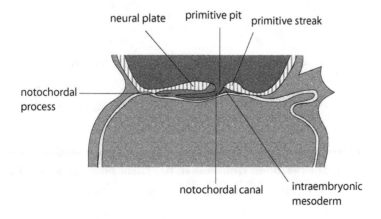

Figure 1.3. Primitive streak and notochord.

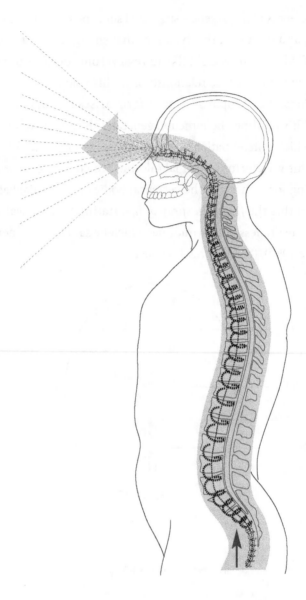

Figure 1.4. The primal midline—the fountain spray of life.

In Volume One we first sensitized readers to this uprising force in the standing position and then on the treatment table while holding the sacrum, and in side-lying via the sacral-ethmoid hold. In standing, both people faced forward, one standing behind the other. The person in front was in the client position, while the person behind was in the practitioner position. Both explorers oriented to the Long Tide and client's primal midline, without narrowing their perceptual field. The person in the practitioner position placed his or her hands lightly over the shoulders of the person in front, while oriented to that person's midline. Settling into that listening field, both waited to see if they sensed the uprising force in the client's system. In terms of whole-body awareness, the tissue field can sometimes feel like a kelp bed suspended in fluid being moved by the uprising force.

We then asked the participants to move to the table, where the person in the practitioner role, after the holistic shift at the feet, oriented to the client's primal midline first via the sacral hold, and then via the sacral-ethmoid hold. You might want to again explore this process with colleagues and also orient to it in client work. The importance of an awareness of the primal midline is essential in tissue work. The embryo formed in relationship to this midline and the tissue field is continually oriented to its presence. Awareness of tissue organization relative to the primal midline yields clear clinical information. Again, research at Tufts University on frog embryos showed that shifts in a local bioelectric field, with an uprising midline, generates the folding of the frog embryo (Jonathan 2011). Dr. Stone likewise stated that all tissue work must be oriented to the presence of the notochord midline, which he described as a spiraling uprising force through the vertebral axis (Stone 1999).

Augmentation Processes

I would also like to briefly touch upon the idea of augmentation processes, as many are described in this volume. I must admit that I find augmentation to be one of the most difficult areas to describe. It is a territory that has a true Taoist doing-not-doing quality to it. It is an area that is continually debated in biodynamics, as to its uses, approaches, whether practitioner intentions like these are useful at all, whether they undercut the natural unfolding of healing processes, and so on. Some practitioners do like the term *augmentation*, which is used in osteopathic practice; as with any term, please find your own words that resonate for you. Over many years of clinical practice, I find that in very inertial, dense, and historically entrenched situations, practitioner intentions, like the augmentation of space, can be of great help in deepening a process, and allowing potency to be expressed in deep-rooted conditions.

The intention in augmentation processes is to augment or amplify naturally occurring processes and, ideally, not to introduce new forces into the system. If we do, we may be experienced as an outside force—and potency will respond to our presence in some way—which may be to protect against our presence. I describe a general approach to augmentation of space below to initiate a discussion of these intentions.

In many ways, the term *augmentation of space* is not really helpful, in that space cannot be augmented—it is always present. But the *relationship* of potency, fluids, and tissues to the space they inhabit, *can* be augmented, and that is what occurs in this process. As we orient to the relationship of potency, fluids, and tissues in the cycles of fluid-tide/mid-tide, we discover that, at the height of inhalation, space is naturally augmented in the tissue field as a whole. Locally, this may be sensed as though tissues are taking a deeper "breath" at the height of inhalation and space is accessed within their relationships. We use this analogy and felt-sense in one of the descriptions below, where we orient to the augmentation of space in historically dense and entrenched conditions.

There are a number of instances when augmentation processes may be of clinical value. First, if the holistic shift cannot be expressed in a client's system, usually due to a depth of inertia, an activated stress response, autonomic activation, or dissociative processes, then the practitioner can facilitate a reconnection to resources and stillness. Commonly, the practitioner "augments" a shift to holism and primary respiration by deepening into stillness and into his or her own relationship to primary respiration—especially Long Tide—and by resourcing the client in awareness of felt-OK-ness and wellness, and via stillpoint processes. These are all augmentation processes in their own right.

When the system can access and deepen into the holistic shift, healing intentions emerge, and commonly particular inertial issues come to the forefront for healing purposes. Potency shifts in the fluid and physical bodies toward an inertial area and fulcrum. As this occurs, an inertial fulcrum clarifies and becomes suspended in all three bodies, as described above. Ideally as the inertial fulcrum clarifies, the seeking and settling phases of Becker's three-phase awareness occur, and there is a deepening into the state of balance, a systemic state of dynamic equilibrium at every level of action. Here, the tissue field accesses its inherent fluidity, where embryonic ordering forces come to the forefront. In many ways, it can be said that the physical body has returned to its embryonic fluid-tissue state—physical body suspended in fluid body—where potential for resolution and healing is foremost.

However, it is also not uncommon that the presence of very entrenched and dense inertial forces and their repercussions—such as intense local tissue compression, fluid congestion, and related nociceptive and autonomic activation—prevents a deepening into the state of balance. Here an augmentation of space may help the state of balance to clarify and deepen. One important aspect to consider here is whether the fluid tide is present at this stage. As the holistic shift deepens, and potency shifts in fluids to a particular site, it is not uncommon for the fluid tide to settle into stillness. Here the potency that drives the fluid tide is now oriented to a particular inertial fulcrum, the system is entering a deeper equilibrium, the fluid tide enters stillness, and the whole field of potency is now oriented to this particular healing intention. In the description below we will describe the augmentation of space in both circumstances—when the fluid tide is present and when it has settled into stillness.

Augmentation of Space

The most important aspect of any augmentation process is the nature of our own state as practitioner. Maintaining a state of interior stillness, and allowing this state to deepen, while maintaining orientation to the client's midline, three bodies, and arising process, is critical. If an inertial fulcrum cannot deepen into a state of balance, the first clinical orientation is for the practitioner to deepen further into stillness and spaciousness while oriented to the inertial issue being attended to. If this does not help the system to enter equilibrium, then an augmentation of space or fluid drive (the drive of potency in fluids) may be a useful practitioner inquiry.

In the following example, imagine that you are oriented to an inertial fulcrum whose forces have not been able to deepen into equilibrium—the state of balance. One clinical intention is oriented to the relationship of potency, fluid, and tissues both to the space they inhabit and to the space that is naturally expressed at the height of inhalation. As this clarifies, you will find that the inertial potency in the fulcrum expresses itself as its relationship to space is augmented, and the system will deepen into healing processes as the inherent treatment plan clarifies. We are assuming, in the description below, that the holistic shift has deepened, an inertial fulcrum has clarified, and that the forces within it cannot deepen into equilibrium.

General Example

Allow your hands to come into relationship to the tissue area involved. For instance, if it is a suture, place fingers on either side of it. If it is a joint, hold the joint in an appropriate manner—for instance, place your hands around a knee joint, or fingers on either side of an inertial connective tissue area, and so on.

Orient to the inertial fulcrum as though it is suspended in the wider fluid and tidal field. In your wide perceptual field, settle into awareness of the fluid tide and tissue motility in the physical and fluid bodies, and orient to the felt quality of the inhalation surge of primary respiration.

Allow your fingers and hands to float on tissue, suspended in fluid. As you truly allow this, it may feel like your hands and fingers are literally fluidic forms. As your fingers—suspended in fluid—are oriented to the motility of the tissues and moved by the tide, allow them to be "breathed" by the tide at the height of inhalation. Your fingers are literally moved/breathed by the tide's expression. This also has the quality of your fingers taking a deeper breath in the direction of tide and motility as the inhalation phase reaches its peak. I sometimes also take a deeper physical breath as I feel my hands and fingers "being breathed" at the height of inhalation.

A few other possibilities may also occur. The fluid tide may not be present or clear. As described above, as an inertial fulcrum clarifies—and potency shifts in fluids in order to orient to the inertial forces within it—the fluid tide may be sensed to enter stillness. Another scenario is that the inertial issue is so dense that tidal phenomenon cannot be clearly sensed. In these not uncommon circumstances, the practitioner can still augment potency and tissues' relationship to the space they inhabit.

With your hands in relationship to the inertial area, again allowing them to be suspended in fluid, sense the quality of space present—not the inertial issue or fulcrum, but the space these inhabit. Allow your hands and fingers to again breathe deeper in this space—as though the tide is present—by filling and widening subtly around the area. This is again as though they are being breathed, or moved by a wider tide. This intention orients the potencies and tissues in the area to the space they inhabit and augments their relationship to space in general.

Example in Vault Hold

A more specific example of this might be when you are holding the vault hold and a compressive fulcrum in the SBJ cannot settle, as the forces within it cannot enter equilibrium. While in the vault hold, at the height of an inhalation phase, allow your fingers to be suspended in fluid and moved by the expression of tidal, fluid potency. This is somewhat like kelp at the bottom of the ocean being moved by tidal forces. As your fingers are moved/breathed by fluid potency, they also take a deeper breath with the flower petals of the cranium as they open at the height of inhalation. As this occurs, your fingers will subtly spread apart in resonance with both tidal motion and tissue motility. Again, this has the feeling quality of your fingers and hands being breathed and breathing deeper. This doing-not-doing quality augments the natural expression of space in the inhalation phase of primary respiration in the SBJ and the cranial bowl as a whole.

Again, it is not uncommon for the tide to recede and enter stillness as an inertial fulcrum clarifies, or for a density of inertia to be present. In this case, as described above, orient to the space present, not the inertial force or compressive issue. Allow your hands, suspended in fluid, to take a deeper breath by filling and expanding around the area as though the tide is moving them. This again orients the tissues and potencies present to the space they inhabit.

When space is accessed, remember Becker's admonition to orient to a *change in state in the potency,* not just to emergent tissue patterns or motions. Potency may be sensed to build in the relationship as pulsation and heat are sensed, to shift in the fluids toward the inertial fulcrum involved, or to permeate the area in some way.

Alternatively, when space is accessed, you may sense a settling into a deepening state of equilibrium emerging—physical body suspended in fluid body, suspended in tidal body, suspended in Dynamic Stillness. As this suspensory system deepens, listen for the level of healing process that emerges from the deepening stillness and wait to sense an expression of potency in the compressive fulcrum. This may be sensed as pulsation, a driving force in the fluids, or as a deeper, softer welling up and permeation of potency in the area. As this occurs, you may sense the inertial forces being dissipated back to the environment in some way—commonly via heat and pulsation or as a vector-like streaming. The system may then again settle and enter its reorganization and realignment phase.

This is a process that may be oriented to whenever the system cannot deepen into the state of balance as an inertial fulcrum clarifies. I find that 90–95 percent of the time I am working via my orientation and resonance to stillness and primary respiration—and to the client's midline, three bodies, and unfolding process. Around 5–10 percent of the time I find that orienting to stillpoint process, or to the augmentation of space or fluid drive, can be very helpful. It is not of use to simply sit with inertial, freezing, or activated states. It can lead to a client's symptoms intensifying. Please also read the later chapters on trauma resolution, as this area is so common in everyday practice.

Clinical Baselines

In Volume One, we discussed the importance of establishing clinical baselines. It is always important to establish baselines so that you can judge how the system is responding to treatment. The intention described throughout Volume One was to be able to sense and relate to changes in the organization of tissues, the state of the

CNS, and the expression of potency and its fluid drive throughout the unfolding of a client's healing process.

The growing awareness of the primal midline is one such baseline, which yields important clinical information—both about how the tissue field is initially organized and how it shifts relative to the midline after inertial forces are resolved in Becker's third phase of reorganization and realignment. It thus helps to establish clinical baselines in terms of the initial organization of the tissue field and its new organization after inertial forces, traumatic impacts, and early pre- and perinatal and childhood issues are addressed. A few other important baselines to be aware of at the beginning and end of sessions are the quality of the fluid tide and how it manifests its drive, and how tissue motility and patterning orient to automatically shifting fulcrums, such as the SBJ and Sutherland's fulcrum. With these reminders, let's now move on to our next five chapters, oriented to embryonic, prenatal, and birthing dynamics.

CHAPTER 2

The Intelligent Embryo

By Cherionna Menzam-Sills PhD, OTR, RCST°

This chapter is about the miracle of our formation in the womb, particularly during the first few weeks after conception. It is also about the profound expression of sentience and intelligence long before our brains develop or we can speak in words. In biodynamics, we work with what Sutherland called Intelligence, with a capital I. We know the healing power of this intelligence, as we align ourselves with the Breath of Life.

One way of understanding the effects of biodynamic sessions is that the structures and patterns reinforced and hardened over a lifetime of experience melt. The body returns to a fluid state and is sensed to be unified. Tissues seem to become less differentiated, as in the early embryo. Similar to the little one forming in the womb, we orient to primary biodynamic forces and access their potential. It is as if the individual dissolves, returns to an embryonic state, and re-forms on our treatment table. Highly relevant to the Breath of Life and the potency we are familiar with in biodynamics are the remarkable developments following conception. The same biodynamic forces we orient to in therapy sessions are at play in the formation of the embryo.

It can be very helpful—as we orient to a client's system—to understand the forces involved in embryonic development, along with the somatic and psychological nature of this early experience. This helps us recognize emergent embryonic states in sessions. It also facilitates supporting our clients in their challenging moments, as we comprehend their possible experience in navigating this miraculous yet challenging time of life. It is also, of course, useful in holding pregnant women and their little ones, who are very present with us in prenatal sessions. In this vein, we explore relevant psychological processes in the sections below, drawn from the session work of many therapists over the last fifty years. This includes the work of Frank Lake, William Emerson, Raymond Castellino, and other leaders in the field of pre- and perinatal psychology. Although some of the following descriptions of the possible impact of prenatal trauma may seem speculative, they have been developed over many, many years of client session work, in the psychotherapy world and cranial field, and via a multitude of small group seminars.

In the Beginning

The embryonic period refers to the first eight weeks of life when the little person is called an embryo. It begins with conception when we are a unicellular being. By the end of this remarkably short time, all our parts are essentially in place. On a physical level, the main developmental work from this point on is about growing and filling in the details.

Let's begin by returning to our origins. The one cell we were at conception is really a combination of two—sperm and egg—in union. Once these two cells have found each other and merged, as if in honor of the long journey they have both just taken, they rest in stillness and unity, having become one. This resting phase lasts around twenty minutes. Here we digest and integrate our experience and rest in the primary intelligence that forms us and holds us in this moment and is present throughout our lives.

This pause is a time of reorganization and reorientation. Not only have polar opposite types of cells, sperm and egg, come together to form one cell, but two beings have come together to make possible the emergence of a third. A new individual is coming into being. As embryologist Jaap van der Wal points out: "Man is not reproducing himself. Two parents do not recreate themselves in their offspring and progeny. Every human conception is a matter of Three, of a Third one" (van der Wal 2007, p. 154). A being is incarnating. This being is sentient, directly experiencing the nature of its life.

While genetic material combines on a physical level, consciousness is also combining on a deeper level. Our psyches are affected by the history we bring with us to each moment. This moment of stillness after conception is no exception. It is as if during this quiet time, we stock the library of our psyches with material from our ancestors. The egg has been inside mother's body since she was a tiny fetus inside her own mother (the egg's grandmother). The sperm is derived from a tiny germ cell when the father was just a fetus. In other words, both egg and sperm have had direct experience of being inside their mother's *and* grandmother's fields. Having floated in parental fluids and bioelectric fields, they carry this ancestral influence.

The conception experience also seems to be informed by other incoming tendencies, perhaps from other lifetimes, or other dimensions, expressions of our own being. I have had clients describe experiences of entering this life as a sentient being—of bringing who they are to pre-conception and conception processes—which cover a whole spectrum of positive, negative, and traumatic experience. Thus we enter life as a sentient being, become a sentient embryo, and begin a long period of marinating in the unconscious of our parents (Emerson and Schorr-Kon 1993). Upon arrival, we may still be oriented to wherever we have come from, the cosmos, the divine, or creation. We may need some time to settle into this new life.

In the Stillness

In the twenty minutes or so of stillness after conception, it is as if Dynamic Stillness delivers instructions on how to form a human body. In this stillness, the human ordering matrix is laid down and carries a primal template that orders embryological development and coherency of function throughout life. In biodynamics, we value returning to the stillness, where we have the opportunity to reorient to this original blueprint.

In the Dynamic Stillness after conception, the Breath of Life ignites a spark of life in the conceptus and lays down a quantum field of light with an ordering midline. This is reminiscent of the research of Mae Won Ho (Ho 1998), which demonstrates that microscopic multicellular animals are organized in quantum fields of light with a shaft of light in the center. As this occurs, the Long Tide is drawn into the conceptus, generating a resonant local bioelectric field with its own ordering midline (see Foundations Volume One, Chapter 2). This midline can be sensed as an uprising, spiraling force through the center of vertebral bodies and the cranial base throughout life. Stone called this a "step-down" in intensity, from the light to bioelectrics (Stone 1999). The entire structure of the body arises and organizes in relationship to this spiraling midline laid down at conception. Embryonic development, and the form of our bodies throughout life, are organized in quantum level and bioelectric fields of action.

Exciting new research at Tufts University has captured the importance of bioelectric signaling in the formation of the frog embryo on film (Jonathan 2011). An amazing video, easily viewed on YouTube, shows a bioelectric midline, folding, and aspects of the face of the frog lighting up before these are actually present as embryo tissues. The Tufts scientists concluded that the signals cause the embryonic cells to form patterns indicated by membrane voltage and pH levels. Furthermore, if the bioelectric signaling is experimentally interrupted, development is abnormal. The little embryo might, for example, grow two brains instead of one. This research suggests that bioelectric influence is an essential aspect of embryonic formation and that the field is more primary than genetics. This may also imply previously unconsidered ethical implications to the rampant bioelectrical pollution on our planet via electrical fields, WiFi, microwaves, and much more.

The Pain of Coming into Being

Our journey into being is often not easy. According to Emerson, little ones as early as conception may have an experience of loss, of divine homesickness, of longing to return to spirit upon realizing that they have left it. Emerson believes that divine exile, or the experience of betrayal, are also possible—with a sense of having been sent away from, abandoned, or tricked by spirit (Emerson 1995). During the journey into incarnation and conception, there may be an experience of shock, confusion, disorientation, grief, denial, anger, resentment, depression, hopelessness, resignation, or acceptance at losing the divine oneness we may have come from. It is also possible to feel joy, excitement, or eagerness at having an opportunity to be in a body and the concurrent experience that we have tasks to accomplish in this life. Such feelings are frequently reported by regresses, as well as by toddlers too small to have learned that they should not express such things. They may arise in session work in relation to conception ignition or as dissociation and other habitual defensive patterns begin to melt and the client begins to embody more fully.

Inherent in these reactions is a sense of being carried along by powerful forces much larger than we are. In our more existential moments, we may feel like tiny pawns in a system too expansive to even imagine. The new being is carried into form, the Breath of Life acting regardless of how we may feel about it. At conception, as throughout life, we are exposed to both these formative ordering forces *and* to those of the conditions we meet.

Conditional forces include the nature of the parental field we incarnate into. Some parents strive for an ideal, conscious conception, preparing to invite and welcome their child into a field of love (Luminare-Rosen 2000; Parvati Baker and Baker 1986). Consider the impact of entering this welcoming field, compared to arriving as an unwanted or unplanned "accident." Likewise, conception may involve a struggle to survive in a relatively hostile field. Pregnancy may result from rape, with terror, rage, hatred, and confusion infusing the field. Conceptions frequently occur under the influence of alcohol or other drugs, where parental consciousness is cloudy and judgment impaired. One or both parents may wake up the next morning regretting the night before. The little one may bathe in guilt, shame, confusion, despair, anger, or fear. This is quite different from welcome. A less obvious obscuration of welcome may occur when the couple has planned and longed for a child, but has previously lost one to miscarriage or other misfortune. The conceptus may enter a field of unresolved feelings of grief, shame, and fear of loss, generating ambivalence and confusion.

In the womb, the prenate bathes in the biochemical and emotional field of the mother. If mom feels fear, the little one experiences a wash of fear, without knowing its context. Mom's shame becomes baby's. Little ones in the womb, and for the first two or three years after birth, cannot differentiate their own feelings and needs from those of others (Fairbairn 1994; Lake 1979). What is "out-there" is felt as "in-here."

Where we do not feel welcomed, our most basic needs to be recognized, acknowledged, and received are not met. Fully incarnating in the body then becomes difficult. How this affects relational dynamics will be discussed in the next chapter. For now, consider that even a little conceptus has needs and suffers when they are not met. Early traumatic experiences become major inertial fulcrums affecting development, function, and relationships throughout life.

Resonance, Fluid Awareness, and Cellular Memory

We might wonder how a little one at conception, being but a unicellular organism, can experience trauma, feelings, or consciousness. Remember that the single cell, and the embryo that forms from it, is a fluid-water being. The work of Masaru Emoto and others investigates the response of water to thoughts and intentions. Emoto has photographed water crystals, showing very different shapes depending on what words, prayers, or even thoughts they were exposed to (Emoto 2004). While Emoto's research has been difficult to replicate, William Tiller has clearly demonstrated that water responds to intention. In Tiller's research, experienced meditators concentrated on raising or lowering the pH of water. The water, even miles away, shifted according to the meditators' intentions (Tiller 2001) This research is very relevant to biodynamics, where we work primarily through presence and resonance, in relationship to the watery, fluid body. Our intentions as practitioners have a profound effect on the client's system, where there seems to be a fluid communication, a cellular resonance, between practitioner and client.

We are composed primarily of water, particularly as embryos. The fertilized egg is the largest human cell, containing more cytoplasm, or fluid, than any other cell. If a jar of water can respond to meditators' intentions to increase its pH value, why would a human conceptus not respond to intentions it is exposed to? A conceptus, however, is just one cell, so how can it remember?

That cells and unicellular organisms composed primarily of water have memory is actually well established. Candace Pert demonstrated that our immune system, stress response, and other bodily functions depend on cell receptor memory (Pert 1997). Other research has shown that simple unicellular and multicellular organisms demonstrate memory, even without a nervous system (Ginsburg and Jablonka 2009). The complexity of multicellular organisms is possible because cells specialize in response to conditions in and around the organism. Specialization is an expression of genes being turned on or off as needed (Alberts, Bray, and Lewis 1994). Cells remembering is key to survival. If they forget which genes to turn on or off, cancer may result (BBC News 2005).

Pre- and perinatal psychologists and others who work with early trauma are familiar with the concept of cellular memory, which may be explained by neuropeptide activity, membrane receptors, or other cellular events (Farrant and Larimore 1995; Farrant 1986; Hendricks and Hendricks 1991; Buchheimer 1987). Memory, however, may extend even beyond cellular functions. Young children, barely able to talk and lacking any known way to have this knowledge, spontaneously tell accurate stories of events occurring before their conception, or even other lifetimes they claim to have lived (Bowman 1997). Children apparently communicate with their parents before they have been conceived, and later recall the experience (Hallett 1995). Even as adults, perceptual experiences seem not to be confined to the physical body. For instance, people have been reported to perceive activities and conversations occurring at a significant distance from where their bodies lay unconscious (Lundahl 1982). Likewise, people who have nearly died may give accurate reports of conversations and activities of others occurring while they were technically dead (Audette 1982; Moody 1982; Osis and Haraldsson 1982; Sabom and Kreutziger 1982; Garfield 1982; Lundahl 1982; Grosso 1982).

Perception outside the body may even exceed more physical perception, as in the case of blind people who report accurately seeing during near-death or out-of-body experiences (Ring and Cooper 1997; Chamberlain 1990). We cannot explain these apparent nonphysical memories through cellular activity. In seeking understanding here, we may need to transcend biology, as memory apparently does. Indeed, some studies have concluded that memory is not located solely in the brain, but rather occurs as a wider holographic phenomenon informing our neurophysiology (Jibu and Yasue 1995; Talbot 1991; Wade 1996). This brings us full circle to the significance of bioelectric signaling. We might understand traumatic memory as an expression of bioelectric frequencies relating to unresolved conditional experience. Perhaps there is something important about the potential of the bioelectric field in and around our bodies for holding memory and even the response to present experience.

As mentioned in the chapter on ignition in Foundations Volume One, a traumatic beginning at conception may manifest as a dampening of ignition processes throughout life, profoundly affecting general health and wellbeing. Practitioners may perceive weak fluid drive, along with a sense of vacancy related to patterns of dissociation and disconnection. As we hold clients with challenging conception history, it can be helpful to remember that they actually survived this difficult entry into life. While we acknowledge the pain encountered back then, we can orient to the strength that supported them through it.

Journey to the Womb

The implantation journey of the new conceptus into the womb is often described in regressions as peaceful floating, like a continuation of the Dynamic Stillness preceding it. On a cellular level, there is much activity after ignition. Cells divide every twenty-four hours, as the fertilized egg moves down the fallopian tube and into the uterus. The cells of this new being respond intelligently to their environment, accessing nourishment and taking care of their metabolic needs. The cells on the periphery, in closest contact with maternal fluids, develop differently from those on the interior.

During this journey, the zona pellucida, a strong containing membrane, protects us from being attacked as foreign matter within our mother until day 5. Hatching out of this membrane exposes us directly to mom's inner ocean. It also enables us to begin to expand, take up more space, and reach out toward the uterine wall in order to implant. Entering the uterus may be experienced as a movement out of constriction into vast, open space. There may be a sense here of wholeness and connectedness, even of being reconnected with the divine, which can serve as a resourcing reference throughout the first trimester. Lake described clients who accessed this territory experiencing profoundly blissful states. He found that re-experiencing this *blastocyst bliss* potentially was extremely healing (Lake 1979).

Toward the end of this expansive journey, however, there may be a sense of urgency, as we must implant by the end of the first week after conception in order to survive. There may be a sense of disorientation, as the new being may be still oriented to its previous existence, whether it be a former lifetime or oneness with the greater cosmos. Again, a sense of loss, repulsion, homesickness, or longing may be associated with this time, affecting the person's sense of commitment to life, activities, or relationships later in life.

At this time, parents commonly do not yet know they have conceived. The little one may or may not look forward to being discovered, depending on circumstances. Questions may arise relating to being accepted and belonging. Anxiety associated with these issues may be rekindled at times of transition, arriving, or leaving later in life. Implantation issues may even arise as clients enter the treatment room.

Implantation

Once we hatch from the zona pellucida, we must implant into the uterine wall, where we can access a greater source of nourishment. This is a truly challenging time in the embryo's development. Implantation is a life-or-death experience. If we do not meet the challenge presented, we die. Many embryos, including twins, perish this early without anyone ever knowing they existed (Emerson 1996). We cannot survive without contacting and being received by mom.

Implantation is our first physical contact with mom. We may feel welcomed if her uterine wall is soft and easy to enter, or we may experience varying degrees of struggle and rejection. The mother's uterine wall responds to her feelings about being female, becoming pregnant, and her relationship with her partner. If she is challenged, uncomfortable, or rejecting of any of these, her uterus may become less hospitable both to her partner's sperm and to a little one trying to implant.

Our experience at implantation relates to feelings of finding a home and belonging. We may experience the uterine wall as inviting, welcoming, engulfing, suffocating, deficient, harsh, cold, or infertile. Implantation may be relatively easy, or we may need to work very hard to implant, trying several times before we succeed.

The embryo initiates implantation, sending out a small gelatinous "foot" to attach to the wall of the uterus. It is important to acknowledge that this new being is reaching out for contact and nourishment, similar to a baby reaching for mom's breast. The embryo is in active, intelligent, interactional relationship.

A dance occurs here, within which the little embryo is completely dependent and vulnerable. Embryo reaches out and mother responds. The reaching does not and cannot happen in a void. It is relational. Without mom, it would be meaning-less, and the embryo would die. Implantation experiences may be carried into later relationships affecting one's sense of being seen, received, and wanted, as well as feeling nurtured, protected, and safe. These relational qualities may arise in session work. As the practitioner's intimate contact and presence resonate with these early territories, areas of wounding become available for resolution and healing.

From implantation on, the little one has a profound impact on mother. Hor-mones from the tiny embryo affect mom's pituitary gland, influencing her entire physiology. The embryo becomes a major fulcrum for the mother's entire system. Mother and child become in many ways as one unit, two beings profoundly inter-twined. This can have far-reaching psychological effects for both.

Mother and child at this point both undergo a major shift in their indepen-dence. For the little one, transitioning from floating in spaciousness to implantation in the uterine tissue may be experienced as smothering or engulfing. This may reca-pitulate a similar experience of the sperm entering the ovum at conception. These experiences may then color one's perception of intimate relationships later in life. The life-or-death quality of both implantation and conception may be translated later in life as anxiety, ambivalence, avoidance of intimacy, or a sense of intense struggle when under stress or fear.

In clinical work, these very early feelings may be rekindled in the relational field of a session, or when negotiating contact with a client. Interestingly, implantation memories tend to be associated with the forehead or frontal area and may stir with contact there. Clients sometimes move their forehead around as if seeking contact and connection with another. I usually speak reassuring words here and offer the client the opportunity to both explore the sense of seeking and making contact, while verbally sharing the felt-sense of their immediate experience. If challeng-ing processes arise as this territory is accessed, it can be resourcing for clients to acknowledge that they have already made it through this formative process, sur-vived, and are now present to explore it and heal whatever wounding is present-ing. Many of us seem to have survived this time and carried on through our lives because of a strong desire or impulse to live. The next major development for the embryo is truly amazing and, in my opinion, worth surviving for!

Midline Dynamics: The Primitive Streak

Once we have established ourselves in the uterine wall through implantation, the next major embryological milestone is the appearance of a midline. This occurs as an uprising force, the centerline of the bioelectric field laid down by the Long Tide, emerges in the centerline of the primitive disc. We call this centering and orienting principle the *primal midline*. The primal midline is the organizing midline for the tissue field, both in embryonic development and throughout life. It is in relationship to this energetic principle that, at the end of the second week after conception, the primitive streak appears. Remembering that the quantum midline is established at conception—the primal midline, primitive streak, and the notochord following it—are like reflections of this original energetic shimmer, like the bioelectric midline seen in frog embryos.

It is fascinating to watch films of the primitive streak appearing in the embryonic clump of cells, as if from nowhere. This monumental event establishes the little one as a creature with a midline, head end, tail end, right side, left side, front, and back. This sets the stage for development of the nervous system and all the body tissues, which organize in relation to the midline. Before the primitive streak arises, the embryo is a two-layered form. With the appearance of the primitive streak, a third layer, the mesodermal layer, is created and the embryo begins actively building its inner body as it becomes a three-layered disc. The ectoderm develops into skin and nervous system. The endoderm gives rise to the gut tube and digestive organs. The third layer between them, the mesoderm, will become the connective tissues, bones, muscles, and blood of the embryo. As we develop a third mesoderm layer, we begin to have depth, a third dimension (van der Wal, 2005).

During the third week the notochord forms in response to the presence of the primal midline, rising up through the mesodermal layer from the primitive node, the end point of the primitive streak. The bodies of the vertebrae will form around the notochord. In biodynamics, we sense its energetic pathway throughout life arising as the primal midline running from the coccyx up through the vertebral bodies and the intervetebral discs, through the basilar part of the occiput, the body of the sphenoid, to the ethmoid bone. Awareness of this midline yields clear clinical insights into the organization of the tissue field and its reorganization after inertial forces are processed.

For the embryo, the notochord is of immense importance. It establishes a midline fulcrum influencing development of the nervous system. All the connective tissue of the body is also established in relation to the notochord, beginning as *somites,* or condensations of mesoderm, along either side of it. These eventually develop into the vertebrae, and distribute cells through the body to become other tissues. Cells destined to become the heart also begin alongside the midline. Orienting to this midline in session work supports the client's system in accessing the immense potential of this time.

At this point in our development, we are lengthening, stretching ourselves out. In the next week, we fold in on ourselves and become truly three-dimensional.

Discovery and the Heart

In the fourth week, a truly amazing event occurs in the human embryo. The heart starts beating! Just a few days earlier we did not even display a midline! The major developmental milestone of the fourth week is embryonic folding. The heart, which has been developing along with its anterior pericardium at the cranial end of the embryo, moves in toward the primitive node at the center, assuming the position we are accustomed to. Concurrently, the major systems of the body become established as tubes. The outer edges of the neural plate on the back of the body fold in toward the midline, creating a neural tube. The digestive tube arises at the front as the embryo folds in. In the process, the vast opening to the yolk sac narrows, creating what will become the umbilical cord. In session work, it is not uncommon to sense the client as a little fluid embryo folding, clearly accessing early formative forces. This commonly clarifies as deep inertial issues are resolved in the context of arising embryonic ordering forces in healing processes.

The embryo is starting to resemble something more familiar to us as a body. At its center is a massive heart. By day 18–22 after conception, the new heart begins to beat. It continues until the day we die. How it knows to do this is mysterious. It seems to express a basic life rhythm that has begun before the actual heart is formed.

Prior to folding, blood organizes into blood islands and then blood vessels in the extra-embryonic mesoderm of the outer body of the embryo. Some blood islands meet with the mother's blood, establishing an essential oscillating connection. By week 4, the blood vessels organize into two major heart tubes, one on each side of the embryo. As the embryo folds, these two tubes come together to merge in the midline. The heart that has been forming at the cranial end of the embryo, actually outside the main embryonic body, now spirals into the embryonic center, meeting the energetic heart center. This folding is revisited with each inhalation of the mid-tide, expressed through the motility of the heart and surrounding tissues.

Folding Into Form, Receiving Recognition

As we take more recognizable form through folding, those around us begin to have more opportunity to perceive our presence. The fourth week, when the heart starts beating, is also often the time when the mother misses her period and pregnancy is confirmed. Discovery of the pregnancy (and the baby's existence) may happen earlier these days, as early pregnancy tests can detect the telltale hormonal changes just after implantation. Some women (and men) are intuitively aware of the conception as soon as it happens. For many in the modern world, however, the pregnancy is not confirmed until around the fourth week, and often it is not suspected until the first period is missed.

Discovery of the pregnancy is a profound occurrence for not only the parents and family, but also for the sentient embryo, the youngest member of the family. Emerson describes discovery as an important prenatal stage of psychological development. He notes that how the news of the pregnancy is received can affect how the heart develops, as well as the child's sense of safety, welcome, and self-esteem. Accompanying influences on bonding and attachment will be discussed in the next chapter. According to Emerson, little ones need their arrival and existence to be acknowledged and celebrated. Anything less than celebration is shocking. Both their small bodies and their psyches are marked by their experience (Emerson 1995). This relates to a common embryological concept that certain developments need to occur within a critical period of time, with later developments being dependent on earlier ones. If interference occurs, development will be abnormal. For example, low maternal folic acid at the time of neural tube formation correlates with the tube not forming properly. Folding is incomplete, the ends of the tube don't close, and a condition called spina bifida results.

Similarly, when traumatic or shocking events occur during development, organs or parts due to change at that time may be affected. When discovery has been characterized by ambivalence, shock, rejection, denial, or other less-than-celebratory reactions, the little one grows with sensitivity or protectiveness in this area (Emerson 1995). Thus, the heart, being the major focus of embryonic attention at the time of discovery, may hold psycho-emotional scars from this time. In clinical work, pulling in, tension, aching, or hunching over in the chest area are often seen, as well as breathing difficulties and issues like asthma. Likewise, wounding during this formative time of heart formation and discovery may later manifest as cardiac dysfunction. Although there are many causes for these types of conditions, it is not uncommon for discovery issues to arise in session work, and for related chest and heart issues to resolve at least to some extent through addressing this sensitive, important developmental milestone. It is important when working with these areas to be aware that we may be approaching or activating very early fear, terror, or shock. Previous wounding related to discovery may be reinforced at birth or later if the child is again not welcomed and received. When we negotiate contact with respect and awareness, these early issues have an opportunity to surface and shift. Approaching without this awareness can recapitulate the client's early experience of not being received or recognized.

It can be illuminating to examine the statistics regarding how discovery of pregnancy is received. Approximately half of pregnancies are unplanned (Henshaw 1998). In this case, discovery is often characterized by ambivalence, at least initially. Many couples are caught unprepared. Even if they very much want to conceive, they may have feelings about not being ready, needing more time, and so on. Parental feelings of ambivalence, shock, surprise, or even dread and fear, may shift quite quickly to celebration, but the shock to the little embryo of the initial reaction may have already occurred.

Fortunately, embryos are remarkably aware, responsive, and resilient. Letting them know how much they are wanted can be extremely healing. Parents can counter the effects of their initial negative reaction with simple, straightforward repair work. For example, letting the little one know how sorry you are to have reacted negatively can be helpful. Little ones particularly respond if you explain that your reaction was not about them personally, but that it related to your own issues and needs. As with anyone of any age, such words are most effective when true and spoken from the heart. Little ones are even more sensitive than their elders to unspoken feelings. They sense their parents' deepest feelings. Like little children, they tend to conclude they are the cause of their parents' distress, and absorb these perceptions into their developing personality structure.

Little ones whose presence is not celebrated do not feel safe. This is an intelligent response on the part of the embryo. Survival at this stage depends on parental receptivity and protection. Parental rejection, particularly maternal, is dangerous. Little ones appropriately develop in ways to watch out for and protect themselves. Depending on the level of rejection perceived, the individual develops a heightened stress response. Where there have been abortion attempts or ideation (considering or planning for abortion), the child may grow up with a hypervigilant nervous system. The imprint from this experience includes having to be always on the lookout and prepared for danger. Thoughts about or plans for giving up the child for adoption can be extremely stressful and terrifying for the little one. This can lead to the child having a heightened stress response and less resilience throughout life.

While there are times when not keeping a child may be necessary, it is important for children's wellbeing to explain to them as much as possible about why this is happening, and, when possible, to let the prenate become familiar with the adoptive parents as early as is practical. It is also important to let little ones know that this is a necessary life situation, rather than being about who they are.

People develop life strategies based on their early experience. How their parents, particularly mom, feel about being pregnant affects the baby's way of being throughout life. Little ones are often sensitive to how mom may react to discovery before it occurs. Even before discovery, little ones may try to prevent anticipated rejection by shrinking in on themselves. They may later live their lives by holding themselves back, staying as small and unseen as possible, avoiding rejection by never fully expressing themselves or never revealing their authentic self. Such children may be painfully shy, hiding behind their mother's skirts and avoiding trying anything new.

We all need to be recognized, acknowledged, and received. Being unwanted at any age is painful, but for little ones in the womb, it is intolerable and dangerous. Children whose presence has been rejected may try to protect themselves by presenting a false self. They may try to be very good so as never to draw attention to themselves. This is common with adopted children until they hit adolescence, when they often begin acting out, seeking to find out who they truly are, or trying to test or prove they are as unworthy and unacceptable as they feel. Chamberlain writes, "To be born unwanted may be a baby's greatest peril" (Chamberlain 2011, p. 49). Severe emotional disturbance, suicide attempts, delinquency, hyperactivity, school problems, and criminal activity are all more likely for those met with rejection as little ones (Chamberlain 2011).

Lack of acknowledgment of the pregnancy may lead to doubts about the right to exist and a sense of worthlessness, inadequacy, or impotence. Little ones who perceive this before discovery often develop tension or holding just above the heart area in the chest. Some prenates are quite happily coming into life until they experience the shock of rejection at discovery. For some, the wounding happens a bit later when ambivalence or rejection occurs after discovery. For instance, a young mother may begin to feel inadequate later in pregnancy, or be told to have an abortion or give the child away for adoption, all leaving powerful imprints on the developing little one. Considering abortion or adoption is often characterized by grief, shock, and shame. These become part of the field the child marinates in. Children in this situation tend to incorporate shame into their identity. They cannot help but believe there is something wrong with them, they are unworthy of love, or can never be enough. In these painful situations, it can be profoundly helpful to let children know this is/was not about them personally. Little ones, even before birth, actually seem to understand what is explained to them. It may be as simple as differentiating for the child that "This isn't about you—it is mommy's and daddy's fear."

Little ones need to know that they are lovable and accepted. If they have not received this message early on in the womb, they can still benefit from being welcomed, acknowledged, and appreciated for who they are later. They can blossom in a field of love and acceptance. I find this is one of the most common themes I encounter with clients during biodynamic sessions. The receptive, respectful holding field in this work can have profound effects for clients who were not welcomed as little ones. The practitioner can be particularly supportive when meeting the client with awareness and appreciation for early prenatal and birth dynamics that may be at play.

Embodiment and the Heart

Folding in the fourth week is profoundly important in our early development. Our shape shifts significantly. No longer a relatively flat arrangement of tissues, we now have a body to settle into. Many traditions consider the new being to hover near or come in and out of the embryo until the fourth week. With establishment of the heart and a body with more depth, embodiment becomes possible. As described in Volume One, heart ignition occurs at this time, as the physical heart, the heart center, and the locus of being become aligned and connected with Source. As the heart folds into the center of the body, the incarnated being follows it into form to become more fully embodied.

As we have seen, the developmental events of this time may occur in a less-than-optimal field. When our existence is met with ambivalence, fear, hostility, or other unwelcoming reactions, embodiment becomes challenging or undesirable. We may then find ourselves struggling through our lives, never feeling quite at home in our bodies or fully present or alive in our relationships and other pursuits. Clients who have not fully embodied may present with dissociative tendencies. Practitioners may sense sluggishness, or low-potency fluid drive. Working with heart ignition as described in Volume One may be extremely helpful, and may activate deep feelings from the time of discovery.

It can be helpful in client work to remember the exquisite sensitivity of the prenate. One way to understand this is to consider how huge the heart is. Heart size to body size ratio in the embryo is many times greater than that of an adult or even an infant. The heart literally bulges out from the little one's body. When we access embryonic or fetal states of consciousness, we revisit that open-hearted vulnerability and sensitivity, along with any wounding that may have accompanied it.

Heart intelligence develops early, prior to brain intelligence. It continues to be important throughout our lives, with neural and other communications from heart to brain affecting perception, amygdala, and stress response (McCraty 2002; Childre and Martin 1999). The electromagnetic field of the heart is the largest in the body, suggesting the significance of the heart (Childre and Martin 1999). This may also be reminiscent of the heart's origins outside the body. Remember that the blood and blood vessels all originally form outside the main body of the embryo. The heart is both the first organ to form and function, and the only organ to form outside the body. It doesn't really enter the body until folding in the fourth week. The heart seems to bring with it a relational awareness of what is beyond our physical boundaries, enabling an innate ability to connect with other. It is through the blood and the original blood islands in the embryo's outer body that the embryo and mother meet and combine forces to form the placenta. The relational field between embryo and mother is thus embodied through the blood and the heart, providing a ground for our continuing development.

Falling into Our Parts

During the next four weeks, the basic layout for the new body is established. By eight weeks after conception, all of our parts are essentially there. The main job of the embryo, now officially termed a fetus, becomes growing and refining. How does this mass of mostly heart develop into a human form with arms, legs, and organs? Van der Wal notes that we begin in wholeness. As we form, we "fall apart into" our parts. The body is not built up from parts; rather, the parts fall out of the whole (van der Wal 2005). From our wholeness, our cells and tissues differentiate for specific tasks. Initially, our cells are totipotent, capable of becoming anything in the body. Through differentiation, they become lung cells, muscle cells, or bone cells, depending on context. Genes in the cells are turned on or off according to what surrounds them at critical periods of development. For example, if cells meant to become an eye are moved to the hip region, they become hip cells prior to six weeks. If moved after this, they develop into an eye on the hip (van der Wal 2005).

The relatively new field of epigenetics underlines the intelligence of cells in development. The old belief that genes determine development is challenged by an understanding that embryo development is relationally based, depending on context. The embryo does not develop in a vacuum. Babies growing in a field of fear and threat tend to develop a heightened stress response. Prenatal experience produces physiological programming (Nathanielsz 1999). For example, if the mother is excessively stressed, the placenta is unable to prevent stress hormones from reaching the baby. This can reset the fetal stress axis, sensitizing the child's later stress reactions, and may contribute to later conditions involving mood or anxiety. Cell biologist Bruce Lipton shows that genes are activated in response to the mother's perception of her environment as safe or threatening. This is passed on to the prenate as information signals in the form of neuropeptides and hormones, read by receptors on prenatal cells. The cells are then programmed for growth or protection, as a way to prepare for the perceived environment the baby will be born into (Lipton 1998).

Dr. Frank Lake (1979), one of the fathers of pre- and perinatal psychology, wrote of the intimate relationship between fetus, infant, and mother, and how resonances of umbilical experience can permeate the organs, as well as personality development. He discussed what he called *umbilical affect,* the fetus and infant's direct felt-experience of mother's emotional life and world. Lake believed that little ones directly sense mother's inner states via their umbilical connection and cannot differentiate these from their own state. The direct infusion of mother's inner states, and experience of her world via the umbilical cord, become theirs. Thus mother's emotions and inner feelings are also theirs. This will be revisited in the next chapter.

Sensing, Moving, Processing

Deep imprints are established during our time in the womb, as we are already sensitive to our environment. Before the heart folds, the nervous system begins forming around the midline. As mentioned above, the neural plate folds in the fourth week to become a neural tube, which will develop into the brain and spinal cord, with primitive brain waves recorded as early as the sixth week.

The senses begin developing very early. Our vestibular sense, involved with balance and orientation in space, begins as early as the fifth week, while the sense of touch begins as early as the third week after conception (Foster 2007). Our tiny limbs begin spontaneously and reflexively moving by the sixth week. Soon, we can bring our hands together, kick, and turn our head. Ultrasound has revealed that babies in the womb move with remarkable grace (de Vries 1992). Once out of the womb negotiating gravity, they apparently must relearn many of the movements previously mastered in the womb.

While the ears are not fully developed until mid-term, hearing apparently does not depend entirely on development of the ear, as babies have been found to respond to sound by sixteen weeks, eight weeks before the ear is structurally complete (Chamberlain and Arms 1999; Chamberlain 2011). Hearing may begin with the skin and skeletal systems, being amplified later by the vestibular and cochlear structures, as they develop (Chamberlain and Arms 1999). The senses of taste and smell develop by weeks 14 and 11, respectively. The fetus also responds to light shone on the mother's belly even when the eyelids are not yet open.

Van der Wal reminds us that the little embryo is not only human but also perfectly designed for its environment from the very first moment of life. At each stage of development the little one is whole and perfectly attuned to its own needs (van der Wal 2005). As we view the rather odd-looking embryo, we might consider this perfection.

The heart remains a central fulcrum throughout development. The face grows in direct contact with the heart, and continues to express the heart throughout life. Our arms, which begin as little buds in the fifth week, rest on the heart bulge, as if reaching around and embracing it. The legs, also beginning as buds lower down, grow around the huge umbilical cord, our roots into mother's source of nourishment. They continue throughout life to root us into the great mother earth as we walk upon her.

Beginning with translucent, ethereal bodies, we continue forming, becoming more substantial, but still extremely vulnerable and sensitive. Over time, our cells and tissues become more differentiated and more solid, a process that continues throughout life. As a fertilized egg, we are almost entirely composed of water. The percentage of water in our bodies decreases as we solidify. A newborn is less fluid than a conceptus but much more so than an adult. Elderly people often complain because their bodies have become too solid, too stiff, having lost much of their fluidity.

Little ones are representatives of the unknown, the mystery. They are sensitive, vulnerable, aware, sentient beings. We all have this within us. We have the intelligence of the embryo available to return to. When we hold a client and a major inertial fulcrum resolves, we can sense the embryological imperative re-establishing itself and the tissue field reorganizing in alignment with it. The fluidity of our origins flows again. In the flow, our exquisite sensitivity is rekindled. The little one is alive and well.

CHAPTER 3

The Pre- and Perinatal Paradigm and Attachment Dynamics

By Cherionna Menzam-Sills PhD, OTR, RCST

To be human
is to become visible
while carrying
what is hidden
as a gift to others.
(David Whyte, *What to Remember When Waking*)

As we saw in the previous chapter, the little one in the womb is a sentient being having and responding to experience. This chapter examines in more detail how our early experience before, during, and shortly after birth can profoundly affect our perceptions, experience, behaviors, and relationships throughout life. These formative experiences frequently clarify in biodynamic session work. Research in the field of pre- and perinatal psychology (the psychology of our experience before and around the time of birth) has oriented to not only how our early experience affects physical and psychological development, but also how it can affect behavior on a much grander scale. For example, Lloyd deMause proposes that historical events are expressions of unresolved prenatal and birth trauma (deMause 1982). Through the lens of such a far-reaching paradigm, we might expect to attain new understanding of psychological issues, such as relational development and attachment dynamics. These are of particular interest in biodynamics, where we carefully attend to the relational field between practitioner and client.

Attachment theory emerged from John Bowlby's observations of maternal deprivation in institutionalized children in the 1940s. It examines the affectional bonds, or attachment, between infant and mother, and attachment behavior, which keeps two people in close proximity to enhance safety. The mother, or primary caregiver, is recognized as a secure base from which the child can explore. *Attachment* is often used to refer to the child's behavior to maintain proximity, while *bonding* refers to the parents' feelings toward the child, with the terms sometimes used interchangeably. As even newly conceived prenates are sentient, I prefer to use the terms equally for parents and child. Both act to maintain attachment proximity and both have bonding feelings. Recent research in neuropsychology reveals that the nature of these earliest relationships organize our brains, affecting our perceptions and relationships throughout life, unless, through awareness, we transform them (Schore 2001a). Similar territories have been investigated by object relations theorists such as Ronald Fairbairn and Donald Winnicott (Sills 2008). These ideas have also been applied to prenatal parenting (Wirth 2001).

In that prenatal and birth experiences are preverbal, noncognitive, and grounded in the little one's felt-experience, they generally become part of our shadow consciousness, as described in Foundations Volume One. As with any shadow material, the more aware we can be of our own early histories, the less likely we are to perceive, relate, or act unconsciously from early imprints. As practitioners, we can benefit from knowing how this time of our own development may have affected our sense of self, and still be influencing our perceptions and relational experiences. Awareness enables us to meet and receive others, including our clients, differently from our history or theirs. It allows us to more clearly differentiate what is now from what was, and enables us to hold, and bring awareness to, the effects of the client's earliest experiences.

Not having a functional brain does not prevent us from having experience or learning as little ones. Quite the contrary, we know that early learning tends to establish particularly strong, deep imprints that can affect our perception and behavior throughout life. Most of these imprints are acquired before our brains are fully developed and functional. To put this in perspective, consider that our brains are not fully myelinated until adolescence or even the mid-fifties (Paus et al. 1999; Gudrais 2001). Personally, I sense my own brain and nervous system to be continuing to grow and develop even as I write this. Yours are too, as you read.

Considering prenatal and perinatal consciousness, memory, and learning, we might refer to the wisdom of Rupert Sheldrake. He questions as unproved many assumptions of scientific belief, such as that objects like the sun don't have consciousness (Sheldrake 2012). Developmental research in recent decades has challenged similar assumptions about preverbal babies. These untested beliefs led to well-meaning doctors performing surgery on babies without anesthesia, common practice until 1987! Babies were not supposed to feel pain or remember the experience! We now know that many such babies were highly traumatized due to this erroneous assumption.

We also know that newborns and babies in the womb are highly sensitive beings, who remember and are informed by this early experience. They are also relational beings, in relationship with mom and others even before birth. Appropriately, researchers in attachment theory are beginning to study how attachment styles may begin prenatally, affected by maternal attitudes and feelings and the little one's needs to be met from the very beginning.

Primal Perceptions

In the preceding chapter, we saw that the senses of the little one come on line remarkably early. Perception may begin even before conception! Babies seem capable of perceiving before their organs of sensation develop. Physiology also cannot explain the compassion, empathy, telepathy, and astute observational abilities often present in early memories (Chamberlain 1990, 1999d, 1999e; Cheek 1992; Wade 1996). Reports from young children may include, for example, accurate details about parents' emotions during conception, discovery of the pregnancy, or birth (Wade 1996; Cheek 1992; Chamberlain 1990). Furthermore, the primitive state of visual processing neurologically at birth is contradicted by reports of detailed visual memories. Some prenatal memories include accurate descriptions of clothing or surroundings the prenate could have no neurological way of perceiving (Cheek 1991; Wade 1990). Reports often include a vantage point from outside the body of the mother, as well as one from inside the uterus (Wade 1996; Cheek 1986). They may include accurate medical details, which the reporter had no way to know, such as relative head-to-shoulders size, correct for the indicated fetal age (Wade 1996). This also applies to memories acquired while out of the body during surgery or near-death experience (Grosso 1982; Chamberlain 1990).

Little ones are present, perceptive, and responsive long before birth. With medical advances making it possible for very premature babies to survive, we now can peek into how prenates of the same age behave. Ultrasound has also enhanced our views into the previously hidden world of the unborn. A fascinating and informative study by child psychiatrist Alessandra Piontelli involved observing babies in the womb via ultrasound and following them up with regular observations at home up to age four. Her descriptions of how prenatal behavior matched behavior after birth is strong evidence for prenatal memory presented through enactment. For example, one pair of twins loved playing through a curtain, much as she had seen them interacting through the membranes in the womb (Piontelli 1992). Other observations of twins in utero have revealed other interactive movements, ranging from punching to kissing (Chamberlain 1999i). Apparently, such behaviors begin in the womb, and are remembered and reenacted later in life.

Prenatal studies in recent decades have shown that unborn children are capable of learning, are responsive to prenatal "lessons," and show signs of remembering what they have learned (Chamberlain 1998; Verny and Kelly 1981; Verny 1987; Van de Carr and Lehrer 1997). Observing babies' behavior after birth gives us further hints as to their abilities in the womb. Babies apparently remember stories, music, and languages they have been exposed to prenatally (Babic 1993; Parncutt 1993; Gellrich 1993; Blum 1993; Van de Carr and Lehrer 1997; Chamberlain 1992, 1998, 1999b). When given an opportunity to choose a story by changing the rhythm of their sucking, they demonstrate preferences for stories their mothers have read to them before birth, as well as for their mother's voice (De Casper and Fife 1980). Newborns have also been shown to recognize and respond to specific words (Chamberlain 1998).

It has been suggested that children's amazing ability to learn language depends on their prenatal exposure to it (Kovacevic 1993; Childs 1998). This notion is supported by the unusual cries and language of deaf children or children of deaf mothers (Chamberlain 1992). Hearing children of deaf mothers do not react muscularly to the sound of phonemes for the first two or three months after birth. They apparently need this time to catch up with babies of hearing mothers, who are exposed to these phoneme sounds in utero, and demonstrate muscular reaction to them starting in the seventh month (Pearce 1991). Furthermore, an aborted five-month-old fetus was found to have a cry matching its mother's voice characteristics, suggesting it had already started learning her language (Chamberlain 1999c). Children have also been noted to comprehend or speak their first words in a language they could only have heard in utero (Babic 1993).

Understanding of neonatal perception and awareness has grown as researchers have learned more about nonverbal learning and memory and how to assess infant responses (Bauer 2006; Courage and Howe 2004). For example, researchers record changes in babies' sucking in response to images shown to them, or the direction of their gaze. The remarkable intelligence of babies can no longer be denied in the face of amassing evidence. Regressive therapies provide further information. Birth memories have been validated by comparison to medical records and memories of those present at the birth (Emerson 1998). In some cases, adults in regression accurately recall obstetrical procedures, which they have no previous knowledge of or are explicitly told were not used, only to have their memories later confirmed (Emerson 1996, 1998). Films of birth regressions have been observed and evaluated by obstetricians and neurologists, who have agreed that the movements, reflexes, facial expressions, breathing patterns, and sounds made by the regressees were all authentic for newborns, though such behaviors could not be produced voluntarily (Janov 1983; Chamberlain 1999a). This kind of somatic memory may emerge in session work as areas holding trauma surface for healing purposes.

Perhaps, one of the most inarguable sources of evidence of prenatal and birth memory comes from toddlers, who spontaneously tell accurate stories about their birth or events that occurred before they were born, including medical details they would have no other way of knowing (Chamberlain 1998; Chamberlain and Arms 1999; Chamberlain 1999f; Emerson 1998; Bowman 1997). While these children could be telepathically "reading" their mothers' memories, they often have no other access to these events, except through direct experience and memory. They may even remember correctly details that their mothers were unaware of (Chamberlain 1998). Particularly revealing are accurate reports from young adopted children, whose adoptive parents had no prior access to these children's birth histories, and, therefore, could not have been the source of this information (Emerson 1998).

The Prenatal and Perinatal Holding Field

Little ones perceive, learn, and develop in a relational field. In object relations and attachment theories, a child's developing sense of self depends on reflection and protection from an attuned, empathetic, and responsive holding environment. Frank Lake, Donald Winnicott, Ronald Fairbairn, and others emphasize the ground laid by this early relational experience, which Lake saw as beginning prenatally, even before conception (Sills 2008). Sheltered by the field from impingements, the baby can simply rest and be. The developing self-system organizes around a cohesive sense of being, and the little one learns to recognize and trust attunement. A receptive, responsive relational field in biodynamic sessions serves a similar purpose for the client, and may provide a safe container in which early wounding in this area may emerge and be resolved.

The immediate holding field of the little one is the mother, but the field that holds the child, from conception on, is much larger. The state of the mother is affected by the field around her, including the nature of her support, her relationship with her partner, her family, friends, work environment, neighbors, and neighborhood, as well as the time and circumstances of the pregnancy and the larger field of the culture and the planet. None of us exists in a vacuum. In Buddhist terms, we *interbe*. Babies live and grow in the milieu of all beings around them, including ancestors and the historical context of their family.

The nature of the holding field varies according to circumstances. The relational field generated by mother and primary caregivers shifts with their moods and experiences. Ideally, the infant is held in what Winnicott termed a "good enough" fashion, where mother contains and manages the baby's inner states through empathy and attunement to baby's feelings, needs, and impulses (Sills 2008). Mother generates a protective holding field by the way she holds, carries, feeds, moves, speaks to, gazes at, and responds to her infant. In this field, baby is protected from the impingements and extremes of daily life until developing adequate resources to not be overwhelmed by them.

Just as important as the maternal surround is the mother's partner, who has the essential role of protecting the mother-baby relationship from outer impingement. This enables the mother to rest in her own being-state, naturally sensing and resonating with her infant's being. This being-to-being field becomes the context for the developing self-system. In some cultures, maternal support is provided by other women or family more than by the partner, but an outer support system continues to be important.

When the holding environment is not attuned, the infant attempts to protect herself by entering defensive, reactive states. The developing self-system then involves coping and complying with the needs of others, without reference to inner needs. In the extreme, with repeated impingements or mis-attunements, the little one may experience relational shock, and is thrown into a traumatized state of emptiness, nonbeing, and annihilation.

I recently watched a YouTube video of a craniosacral practitioner working with a newborn baby. The baby and I both cringed simultaneously as the practitioner spun the baby into the position the practitioner desired. I was horrified by the complete lack of acknowledgment by the practitioner that she was picking up and holding a small human being with feelings. The baby was obviously terrified and screamed accordingly. The helpless mother tried desperately to soothe her baby. As the practitioner worked on a clearly biomechanical level, she happily noted changes in structure. Based on my own experience with clients who have spent years attempting to recover from just such handling, I found it hard to imagine anything was resolved for this little one on a deeper level. Perhaps the temporal bone was less compressed, at least temporarily, but where did the compression and the stress of the interaction with the practitioner go?

Prenatal and birth therapist Ray Castellino teaches what he calls "first touch." Here, the therapist gently, respectfully makes her hand available to the baby, offering the little one the opportunity to initiate contact (Castellino 1996). In my experience, babies always appreciate this gesture and enjoy initiating contact when they are ready, as they sense a trustworthy relational holding field. This is important to consider when working not only with infants, but also with adults who may regress to an infantile state on the treatment table. This relates to Winnicott's concept of object presenting (Sills 2008). For the infant, this refers to how the mother and other primary caregivers present themselves and objects to the baby. In a therapy session, practitioners offer their hands, objects the baby needs time to explore and consider. Allowing the baby to make a choice about contact is empowering, as with any object offered. For infants, this supports learning that they are separate yet connected to mother and others. It also empowers them to explore and learn about their world. The same is true for adults who have regressed into a less differentiated state or have trouble feeling safe or discerning between safety and threat. Where babies have developed in a less-than-good-enough holding field, where mother or primary caregivers were not attuned to the little ones' needs and pacing, children develop a sense of insecurity, yielding a disempowered self-system oriented to meeting the needs of others while denying its own.

Castellino points out that babies need extra time to process events around them. Their nervous system is immature and pathways not yet well established. They can be startled by fast or unexpected transitions, as when an anxious, detached, depressed, or self-absorbed caregiver lifts the baby before it is ready or thrusts a breast or bottle into its mouth without warning. Transitions also tend to activate unresolved birth trauma, as birth is a major early transition setting strong imprints for how transition occurs. If caregivers behave in insensitive ways with a baby who was handled with similar disregard at birth, they unknowingly touch on the baby's early trauma. This reinforcement of birth trauma is even more serious when the way the baby was met at birth was reminiscent of even earlier experiences, like discovery, implantation, or conception. Life for the little one can unfortunately become one experience of rejection or mis-attunement after another.

Prenatal Attunement

Babies are sentient and relational beings from the very beginning, and mothers can be attuned to them long before birth. Mother and baby are involved in a dance together from at least conception on. In her intriguing book *Soul Trek: Meeting Our Children on the Way to Birth*, Elisabeth Hallett includes numerous reports from surprised parents who saw, felt, or heard their child before conception occurred. These children presented themselves to their parents, often looking like the toddler they would become in two or three years. Some pleaded or persuaded their parents to have them! Others apparently responded to their parents' prayers or meditations inviting them to come into the family. In either case, parents and child seemed to be meeting before there was a physical child to meet! After conception, pregnant women frequently report dreams about their unborn child, which often enhance their sense of their little one (Hallett 1995).

If beings coming in can indeed visit their new parents even before conception, then parenting, bonding, and attachment may begin much earlier than is commonly believed. The holding field for little ones begins long before birth. As highly responsive beings, how could prenates not be affected by the field they grow in? There is ample evidence that little ones whose mothers experience love, nurturing, supportive relationships, and resources during pregnancy tend to develop into happier, more resilient individuals than those growing in a field of violence, abuse, war, chronic stress, discord, or fear (Karr-Morse and Wiley 1997).

On a physiological level, we can understand that the embryo grows in relation to the medium it floats in. For example, if mother uses alcohol, tobacco, or certain drugs, it will affect baby's development, and cause the newborn to go through withdrawal. On a psychological level, the mother's experiences also directly affect her unborn baby. The prenate's relational field includes mom's mood and stress levels. Children are commonly affected if mom is upset, angry, or happy. This connection is even stronger for babies in the womb. They bathe in the biochemicals of the mother, as well as her bioelectric field. If mom is exposed to ongoing or repeated prenatal stress, for example, her baby is affected. High levels of maternal cortisol, an important stress hormone, affect prenatal and infant cognitive development and attachment processes (Bergman et al. 2010). Prenatal depression, involving elevated maternal cortisol, affects fetal activity and growth, increasing risk of prematurity and low birth weight, with newborns showing a biochemical and physiological profile similar to their mothers' (Field et al. 2006).

The Raine Study, an extensive longitudinal research study in Australia, has followed 2,900 babies from in utero through their teens (Robinson et al. 2011). It has shown that the number of stressful events mothers experience in pregnancy directly relates to the risk of behavioral problems in their children. Events include things like marital or financial issues, death of a relative, or job loss. Behavior problems occur regardless of stress levels after the birth, indicating their prenatal origins. Ongoing prenatal stress affects the child's neurodevelopment and stress response later in life, as well as being linked to behavioral, emotional, and cognitive problems (Doughty 2007; Glover 2011). Prenatal stress can contribute to prematurity, involving placental production of cortisol in response to increased maternal cortisol production (Wadhwa 2005). Prematurity often involves developmental issues affecting learning, cognition, and behavior, as well as physical health (Maroney 2003), and can interfere with bonding and attachment.

Premature babies usually spend their first few weeks or months in an incubator, where, as the British name, *isolette*, implies, they are isolated. Their experience of touch is often traumatic due to their immature nervous system, as well as being poked and prodded by strangers for frightening and sometimes painful medical procedures. The noise and stimulation level of the Neonatal Intensive Care Unit (NICU) can be extremely overwhelming for these tiny ones. They tend to withdraw in shock and overwhelm, where they are less available for loving connections with mom and family. Fortunately, the practice of isolating these little ones is shifting in response to growing evidence that preemies do much better with skin-to-skin or *kangaroo care*, where they are held in close contact, usually with mom or another family member (Ludington-Hoe and Swinth 1996). Not surprisingly, kangaroo care also supports attachment (Johnson 2010; Feldman et al. 2003). When a baby is born prematurely, the birth and period of postnatal hospitalization are usually stressful for family as well as baby. It can be remarkably soothing for both mom and baby when mom is able to hold and be with her baby. Babies in kangaroo care are often discharged home sooner, potentially reducing stress further.

In *The Continuum Concept*, Jean Liedloff described beautifully the natural blueprint for a continuum of holding and connection beginning prenatally and continuing through the birth and months following. Both baby and mother long for what they know within themselves is natural and needed.

> The violent tearing apart of the mother-child continuum, so strongly established during the phases that took place in the womb, may understandably result in depression for the mother, as well as agony for the infant. Every

nerve ending under his newly exposed skin craves the expected embrace, all his being, the character of all he is, leads to his being held in arms. For millions of years newborn babies have been held close to their mothers from the moment of birth. Some babies of the last few hundred generations may have been deprived of this all-important experience but that has not lessened each new baby's expectation that he will be in his rightful place.
    (Liedloff 1977, p. 36)

Babies already know their mother well by the time they are born, even if they are premature. They have been in close proximity and communication with their mother for months. They need and expect this to continue. If their holding field is impinged on at birth, they suffer. On an emotional level, unborn babies and their mother are naturally highly attuned. Their special bond includes two-way biochemical communication, with the mediating placenta being an important aspect of the prenatal holding field. Babies not only respond to maternal emotional and stress states; they also contribute their own important biochemical messages to mom. Frances McCulloch Doughty points out that the maternal rise in cortisol in response to that of the prenate can be considered a prenatal equivalent to a caregiver reflecting back a child's happy behavior. This is an aspect of attuned holding (Doughty 2007) and is reminiscent of Lake's "womb of spirit," a bidirectional interactive field between the baby and mother, from conception through the first nine months after birth. It includes both what is transmitted back and forth via the umbilical cord and the more energetic, instinctual, intuitive, and spiritual connections that are present between mother and prenate as a field experience.

On the physiological and behavioral level, several researchers have underlined the importance of early maternal-infant attunement (Condon and Sander 1974; Hatch and Maietta 1991; Kang 1978; Karen 1994; Karr-Morse and Wiley 1997; Kestenberg 1987; Klaus, Klaus, and Kennell 1995; Pearce 1992; Stern 1985; Schore 2001a; Verny and Kelly 1981). The remarkable synchrony observed between mother and infant just after birth, and the precocious abilities of newborns and premature babies to imitate adult facial expressions and gestures, suggests that this interactive dance begins prenatally, before they can see each other (Chamberlain 1994; Hatch and Maietta 1991; Verny 1981).

Joseph Chilton Pearce suggests that the sound sensitivity attributed to the first embryonic cells may serve the purpose of picking up the "stimulus of the mother's heartbeat, needed to generate production of the embryo's own heart" (Pearce 1992,

p. 110). This could be an early example of infant following mother's movement (i.e., the movement of her heart). Recent research has shown that the fetal heartbeat synchronizes with the mother's heartbeat if her breathing is regular (BBC News 2010). As mother and baby "follow each other's movement on a continuous basis, the motion of one becomes the feedback upon which the other bases his or her motion. They become highly dependent on each other's motion input in order to control their own movement at every biological and social level" (Hatch and Marietta 1991, p. 259). A relationship has even been found between fetal movement, as recorded by pregnant women, and the quality of movement in the women's dreams (Kestenberg 1987). Not surprisingly, women often begin deepening their connection with the baby when the movement they have been unconsciously interacting with enters their awareness through ultrasound, quickening, or perceiving the baby's heartbeat (Klaus, Klaus, and Kennell 1995; Freud 1987). Their enhanced responsiveness to their baby serves to strengthen the holding field.

The subtle dance that mothers and babies engage in is apparently influenced by prenatal rhythms, including maternal sleep-wake cycles and hormonal fluctuations, her heartbeat, and the rhythmic uterine contractions of labor. Newborns have been found to subtly synchronize their movement with adult speech, as detected by microanalysis of films (Condon and Sander 1974). This ability suggests that the baby has been practicing in the womb. Based on this finding, Stanley Keleman concluded: "Motor behavior is the basis of human mothering and communication. Patterns of muscular-emotional behavior are the substrata of bonding of the mother and child." He saw this somatic patterning as "expand[ing] from basic intrauterine pulsations," beginning with how the egg connects with the uterus (Keleman 1974, p. 6). Frank Hatch and Lenny Maietta (1991) described the synchrony of movement as beginning as early as ovulation, fertilization, and cell division. As David Chamberlain writes: "In the womb environment life is interactive and relationships are everything. Never isolated from each other, fetus and mother eat, sleep, exercise, smoke, take medicine, and have accidents *together*, resulting in a build-up of intense rapport" (Chamberlain 1994, p. 17).

Little ones of any age need to feel met. They require a sense of mom/other as present and contactful with enough space in which to be. Because unborn babies are in direct contact with maternal emotions, it is important for both brain development and bonding that the mother do what she can to provide a supportive neurohormonal environment. In that mom's ability to take care of herself often depends on others around her, especially her partner, family, close friends, cultural milieu, and birth support team, the prenatal holding field must be considered to include this social support system, and the culture that enables it.

If the mother's surround does not support her in having her baby, bonding can be interrupted. Women expecting to have their baby taken away are likely to hold their unborn baby with at least some degree of fear, grief, or shame, whether this is due to the mother's young age, rejection by her partner, potential mental or physical disability, or cultural gender preference (as in China and India where little girls are abandoned or killed). While babies and mothers bond prenatally even if they are separated at birth, stress hormones can counter the biochemicals that support attachment. On the other hand, the opioids released when mom holds her baby are supportive of bonding.

Attachment and Bonding

Our ability and motivation to bond with another are affected by our earliest experiences. Knowledge gained from regressive therapy sessions suggests that relational imprints may be established as early as conception or even pre-conception. For example, a sense of expectancy, disappointment, or betrayal, or feeling invited, received, smothered, or rejected can all occur at conception, and be reinforced at implantation and again at discovery and birth. Relationships and intimacy may then be challenged by unconscious reenactments of the early experience. Intimacy that is so longed for may become terrifying and threatening, triggering an urge to withdraw and run away, or to lash out angrily in self-protection. Where safety and love are actually available, they may not be perceived and received due to these early imprints. Relationships may be characterized by painful ambivalence and confusion.

Without a safe relational field, infants lack a secure base. The resulting separation anxiety is demonstrated as protest, until babies give up on having what they need. Little ones seek proximity for safety, but they are also inherently loving beings. Fairbairn maintains that infants are naturally loving beings and that the greatest wounding occurs when this love is not recognized and received (Sills 2008). When infants are not held and received, defensive strategies develop, perpetuating the search, driven by deep needs for recognition, acknowledgment, acceptance, and love, as identified by Frank Lake (Sills 2008). Children seek to be with their attachment figures even if they are abusive or indifferent. Unable to tolerate the perception of a bad parent, children tend to see their parents as good, even if they must, in Fairbairn's terms, internalize the bad object in the process (Sills 2008).

Attachment theorists have identified four styles of attachment, relating to the style of early parenting available to them. These are derived from an experimental method called the Strange Situation, where 12–18-month-olds are observed while briefly separated and reunited with their mothers. Securely attached children are usually distressed by the separation, may protest, and on reunion actively greet their caregiver, allow themselves to be comforted if needed, and return to their play or activity. Their mothers demonstrate attuned, responsive attention, providing a good-enough relational holding field, a sense of safety with adequate, but not excessive, stimulation. The child successfully uses a social nervous system to get needs met, generally not having to default to a sympathetic state. On occasion when sympathetic protest is needed, the caregiver quickly responds to meet the child's needs.

Insecure attachment is divided into three categories. *Insecure avoidant* children show little distress upon separation and ignore their caregiver on reunion. They are watchful of the caregiver and inhibited in their play. This withdrawal pattern relates to the active-alert phase and flight reaction of the stress response, expressed in infants and young children as withdrawal and avoidance. Not having their needs met through a social nervous system, they default to a sympathetic nervous system response. Similarly, *insecure ambivalent* children are run by sympathetic reactions. They are highly distressed by the separation and not easily comforted upon reunion. They may seek contact, but also resist by kicking, hitting, or turning away, often alternating between clinging and anger. This oppositional pattern is tied to the active-alert phase and fight reaction of the stress response. The behaviors of *insecure disorganized* children include freezing, immobilization, extreme fear, or dissociation, relating to the shock-dissociation phase of the stress response.

These categories correspond to the stress response described by Stephen Porges. If the initial response with a social nervous system doesn't work, sympathetic fight-flight is attempted. Little ones are generally not sufficiently strong or mobile for successful fighting or fleeing. They tend to resort to a parasympathetic dissociation, lacking other options (Porges 2007). In insecure attachment, the social nervous system has failed, contact is perceived as threatening, and the stress response is always engaged. In the absence of a safe holding environment, the child is in a double bind, both dependent on contact and needing to defend against the danger associated with it. Children may have different attachment patterns with each parent or caregiver, but by eighteen months old, attachment patterns are relatively stable, with maternal patterns predominating.

Early attachment patterns continue to present in adult relationships, including in therapy. Attachment issues commonly arise in sessions as the gentle, respectful, and negotiated approach to contact in biodynamics may activate old patterns before the client is able to begin resting in the safe relational field provided. Specific styles present particular challenges:

- Avoidant attachment clients may be remote and defensive, associating intimacy with pain and expecting rejection or disapproval from the practitioner. Trauma work geared to complete the flight response and mobilize frozen energies can be helpful.

- Ambivalent clients may be resistant, projective, and suspicious. They may struggle with sensing the safety the relational field offers but not trusting the practitioner or the situation. Trauma work using mobilization exercises geared to complete the fight response can help.

- Disorganized-dissociative clients may be very fearful of intimacy, easily overwhelmed by arising processes. Building resources and learning to differentiate self-other and past-present helps in processing cycling autonomic energies coupled with the disorganized behavior.

In all insecure attachment forms, exercises geared to resolve active-alert states, down-regulate the orienting response if hyper-aroused, and re-establish the primacy of the social nervous system are essential.

For each style, holding the client with an understanding of possible early origins of behavior can enhance a sense of safety and being met. While attachment theory developed through observation of babies after birth, more recent research into earlier prenatal and perinatal origins of attachment behavior has enhanced therapeutic practices. Lake, based on his experience with regressive therapy, outlined in detail how personality styles develop in relation to prenatal and birth experience. He described wounding at the level of being beginning with pre-conception and conception. Depending on how the little one is met and responds, Lake described a transmarginal hierarchy, including four levels of response: *ideal, coping, oppositional,* and *transmarginal* (Lake 1979; Sills 2008). The generation of personality systems relates to the level of the stress hierarchy engaged in each of these levels as the infant experiences impingements. At the most extreme, or transmarginal, level, the experience is shocking and overwhelming beyond the margins of the little one's ability to cope or oppose the incoming sense of badness. Both oppositional and transmarginal states can lead to insecure attachment and overly defended personalities.

Umbilical Affect and Toxicity

> It could be said that the whole process of attachment and implantation is oriented to these islands of stillness on the inside of the chorion and what are called lagoons of stillness on the outside of the chorion. This is the deepest metabolic connection that the embryo has with the mother—the blood and its stillness.... Two people—via the mother's blood and an embryo's blood—are growing toward one another via multiple points of stillness around the entire circumference of the embryo.
>
> (Shea 2010, p. 81)

Umbilical affect is a term first used by Lake to describe the effects on the unborn and newly born of maternal sustenance and feelings flowing in through the placenta and umbilical cord (Lake 1979). This connection actually starts very early as mother and embryo begin to interact via blood islands that will develop into the placenta and cord. Lake described umbilical affect as positive, negative, and strongly negative, extending for nine months postnatally. During this time, the little one continues to experience a connection with mom as if the umbilical cord were still present. Lake believed this early umbilical experience sets the ground for secure or insecure self-systems.

How the baby is affected by maternal affect relates to the nature of the holding field. A good-enough field provides a context of trust and continuity within which negative affect can be absorbed. A less attuned holding field and/or more negative affect, especially a strongly negative affect, increases the likelihood of little ones entering defended states too early, developing a defended personality with insecure attachment. In biodynamics, the practitioner similarly creates a negotiated holding field with an intention to generate a sense of safety and trust. The holistic shift has difficult occurring without this.

Lake pointed out that little ones lack ego defenses adults depend on. Their defenses are somatic and visceral in nature. He described three basic prenatal and infant responses to intrusive or overwhelming input—withdrawal, displacement, and dissociation. Exposed to uncomfortable input, such as loud noise, quarreling, or rough handling, infants withdraw by turning away, disengaging their attention, or in the extreme by dissociating. Little ones also displace incoming bad umbilical feelings into other areas of their body. It is common to encounter these displaced strong feelings or defensive reactions to them when meeting a client's liver, intestines, or other organs. The heart, as discussed earlier, often holds very early wounding, particularly pertaining to discovery and rejection. It is essential that the practitioner is aware of, and can hold the emergence of, these early defensive processes. They commonly emerge in adult session work, presenting a depth of inertia, nervous system activation, and strong emotional states. We must learn to hold the little one who is suffering here, along with the adult who is presenting these conditions.

Babies from conception through the first two years are directly attuned to maternal feelings. Fairbairn saw infants as being in a state of immature dependency, unable to differentiate their feelings and needs from those of mother or other primary caregivers (Sills 2008). In session work, it is not uncommon for clients to revert to an early state where they again need support in differentiating. They may try to sense what the practitioner needs or feels, in order to know whether they are safe.

As little ones, we are dependent on the field we grow in for survival and growth. On a physiological level, we take in nutrition and let go of wastes via the umbilical cord. We also receive via the cord the biochemical expressions of our mother's emotional state. This includes her feelings about the pregnancy and our existence, as well as her life and how she is treated. If mom experiences threat, baby is affected. If maternal perception of threat is ongoing or extreme, the little one prepares to enter a threatening world. If mother experiences being nurtured, supported, and loved, the little one relaxes into being, preparing for a loving world (Lipton 1998).

Threat may relate to any aspect of the holding field. The mother may be in an abusive relationship, or under chronic stress at her job. She may be pregnant during a war or drought without enough food. She may be grieving the loss of her partner or a close relative. We cannot blame the mother for her experience and what is passed on to the baby, as the baby cannot differentiate its experience from hers. The holding field for the baby includes not only the mother but also all who are holding the mother. On the other hand, we can support mothers and others in differentiating for the baby. For example, mother might say to her baby: "This is my sadness. It's not about you. You don't need to worry about it or take it on." Babies of any age respond to this kind of reassurance.

The exquisite sensitivity of little ones must be considered in prenatal medical tests and interventions. Amniocentesis, widely used for early detection of abnormalities, provides valuable information for parents and doctor, but the baby's experience of the event is rarely taken into account. Thomas Verny reports that babies may withdraw from or push away the amniocentesis needle, and take the danger as originating with their mother. This may result in later avoidance or fear of mother (Verny 1986). Unfortunately, such well-intended action on the part of parents and doctors may negatively affect bonding and attachment. If amniocentesis is deemed necessary, it would be easy to reduce potential trauma for the baby simply by explaining to the little one what is happening. A baby could cooperatively move out of the way if told why the needle was there. This could provide an imprint for future cooperative relationship rather than angry rebellion or frozen withdrawal.

While technology, both prenatally and at birth, can interfere with bonding and attachment, at least one form seems to support it. Ultrasound, although not necessarily as safe as commonly believed, gives parents an early visual of their baby. This fosters awareness and parental bonding long before the baby's kicks are felt or the pregnancy is visible to others (Verny 1986; Goldberg 2007). This can be particularly helpful where the mother or parents are ambivalent or worried about the health of the baby. Asking the mother about her sense of her baby, and acknowledging the prenate in session work, can also support maternal awareness of the little one within.

An important aspect of umbilical affect is the feeling of being wanted or welcomed, or not. Like any child, prenates want to be acknowledged. In that prenates are dependent on the maternal holding field for both physical health and development of a stable self-system, maternal rejection can be shocking. The unwanted child is bombarded by extremely negative, toxic affect. The most severe situation a baby can survive is an abortion attempt. Babies have been described by mothers and physicians as thrashing about and kicking violently in response to saline injections, chemicals, forceps, or knife during abortions (Ankerberg and Weldon 1989). These babies are clearly aware of the attack on their lives. They react with distress and apparent attempts to ward off the threatening instruments. Babies subjected to unsuccessful abortion attempts or thoughts of abortion are equally aware and disturbed. Adult abortion survivors often present as hypervigilant and sensitive. In session work, they may need especially careful negotiation around contact, with an immense amount of energetic space, and be easily activated by any unexpected sound or movement. Gradually, they learn to perceive and settle into the safety of the therapeutic field.

Being unwanted is a powerful imprint. Babies unwanted during pregnancy are more likely to die during the first month of life, while babies whose conception was planned (and presumably wanted) have shown higher levels of cognitive processing and greater attachment to their mothers at three months compared to unplanned babies (Bustan and Coker, cited in Chamberlain 1995). Studies on children whose mothers had requested and been refused abortions demonstrate that such unwanted children are more likely to have psychosocial problems, do poorly in school, demonstrate delinquent or criminal behavior, and have more difficulty coping with stress and frustration (David et al. 1988). Rejecting or negative attitudes in mothers have been associated with deviant behaviors in newborns, such as excessive crying, sleep problems, irritability, digestive and feeding difficulties, as well as prematurity (Freud 1987). It is important to be aware of these dynamics when working with clients who have been adopted, or encountered other forms of early loss or rejection.

Haunted by the Past

Babies in the womb grow not only in mom's body and emotional field, but also in a historical field. The baby may have been conceived after another baby was lost due to miscarriage, abortion, or adoption. In this case, the little one often encounters a "haunted womb," with resonances of the unresolved loss still lingering (Emerson 1995). When the parents have not worked through their grief and other feelings, the little one marinates in these in the womb. Feelings of the previous inhabitant may also be present, including terror, shock, and rage. Because babies do not differentiate between the emotions of others and their own, they experience these leftover feelings as their own, without an understandable context. Post-traumatic stress disorder (PTSD) is common in pregnant women who have had complications in previous pregnancies, which can be an additional source of stress for both mother and baby (Forray et al. 2009).

A woman who has lost a child to miscarriage often fears a recurrence. Some women admit being afraid to bond with their baby until they know it will survive. They have already experienced the severe emotional pain of losing a child and defend against feeling it again. Some women may claim to be thrilled to be pregnant but cannot allow themselves to truly celebrate their new little one because they are too afraid of another loss. Other women react to the loss by clinging so tightly that the little one feels smothered. As adults, these individuals may have difficulty trusting or avoid getting too close to others. They may be slow to trust the relational field in session work, and need extra energetic space. Consciously negotiating contact can be profoundly healing, as well as activating.

Life in the womb may also be haunted by the baby's own memories or experience of loss. Little ones coming in may not come alone. Over half of human conceptions are multiple, while most births aren't. This means many of us have had a twin in the womb who did not make it to birth. Sometimes, the mother is aware of the twin and consciously grieves the loss. A second baby may have been seen in an ultrasound, or a second heartbeat heard. Then it disappears. Some twins simply vanish. Their bodies are reabsorbed into the mother, or leave with some first-trimester bleeding. Some are absorbed into the surviving twin's body.

Later in pregnancy, the loss of a twin is apparent as a miscarriage, with significant bleeding. A tiny embryo dying, however, is less obvious. Often it is washed away with an expected menstrual period. The mother may not even be aware of being pregnant, let alone of having twins. Only the surviving baby knows. The grief and loss of this experience haunts many of us throughout our lives, without having conscious understanding of what we are missing or longing for. We may seek our twin in love relationships, being repeatedly disappointed when our mate does not live up to expectations. The kind of intimacy one experiences with a twin is hard to match. We may also learn to act in ways that protect us from having a similar fate to our twin, holding ourselves small in life, and avoiding danger. Or we may take the opposite route, as if trying to live two lives to make up for the one our twin didn't get to live, or being counterphobic as part of a survival mechanism of denial.

While we may learn about intimacy from a twin experience, twinning is not always an appropriate way to relate. It tends to lack boundaries needed in adult relationships, and comes with expectations that our partner will behave like our twin, for example, by understanding and being like us, or by dying or abandoning us. This may also affect boundaries, trust, and safety in the intimate context of session work.

A special case of twin loss occurs with in vitro fertilization when several embryos emerge ready to be implanted. It is not unusual for the "extras" to be killed. I have seen little children conceived this way acting out their loss. Twin toddlers, for example, would always drop three teddy bears, or balls, or whatever they were carrying. They always chose five and dropped three. Then they wanted to go back to get the dropped ones, but something seemed to stop them. They became agitated, clearly expressing their feelings about the three that had dropped. Their emotional reaction was far out of proportion to the dropping of teddy bears. They were expressing their grief about having lost three siblings.

This kind of grief is seldom acknowledged in families where there was such a strong longing for a baby as to warrant IVF. The tendency is to celebrate the successful fertilization. The loss remains in shadow. The surviving twin or twins then have no reflection of their painful feelings of loss, and cannot fully process or integrate them. On the other hand, when this topic is raised in the family, as in the play above, with supportive, knowledgeable practitioners as part of the holding field, the parents as well as the surviving twins can more fully integrate their experience of loss.

A similar dynamic occurs with adoption. Adopted babies usually come into a family that has been longing for a child. The parents often have little or no awareness that their new baby is in shock and intensely grieving the loss of the mother with whom the baby spent nine months in intimate contact. Even if the mother was a drug addict who would be abusive to her child (and already was by exposing her unborn child to her drug of choice), the baby still experiences loss. When adoptive families do not discuss the child's family of origin, the child remains haunted, longing for something unidentifiable. The child's personality and relationships organize around this extreme shock and loss, with ongoing seeking for contact or withdrawing from repeated disappointment.

Fetal Development: Emerging into a Sense of Self and Other

As personality develops in the prenate, a little body is also forming. The two are intimately connected. The embryonic body starts as an undifferentiated mass of cells, gradually specializing into different types of tissue. The sense of self also clarifies over time. The little one begins in an undifferentiated primordial state of spaciousness and oneness. These early roots of emotional life often emerge in session work as the body begins to release its hold on history. Those regressing to conception or early in the first trimester may experience being close to spirit or the creative forces of life, floating in vast space, outside the realms of time, with a sense of boundarilessness, completeness, and wholeness. Trauma at this time can affect one's ability to embody and fully enter into life, arising in session work with enhanced body awareness.

Implantation and discovery, both occurring in the first month, can both have profound impact on the little one's personality. Early shocking experiences of smothering or rejection influence how the individual later seeks and perceives contact and intimacy, contributing to insecure styles of attachment, again easily activated in the relational field of a session.

As the first trimester progresses, prenatal senses are maturing, enabling the prenate to receive sensory information as well as being umbilically affected by maternal emotions. The maternal-fetal relational field is established, affecting early conclusions about intimacy, contact, safety, and receptivity. By the end of the first trimester, the little one already has a sense of self and other. The baby's relationship with mom and the holding field deepens in the second trimester, setting the ground for future relationships. By the third trimester, the fetus has increasing awareness of the outside world, being able to hear, see, smell, taste, and feel. Preferences are established as the little one orients to dad's voice if available, prefers sweet tastes in the amniotic fluid, settles with soft music, and withdraws from loud sounds. The stress response and implicit memory system are also established.

Experiences of goodness or badness at this time can influence personality and behavior throughout life. In session work, clients may spontaneously regress to a prenatal state as their body becomes more fluidic. There may be a sense of holding a vulnerable and aware little one, along with the fears, shocks, or joys of that time. It is important to realize that, as you hold the therapeutic space for clients, they may project this experience onto you, perceiving the goodness or badness as directly coming from you. It is essential to recognize this, to acknowledge the presence of their little one and how it might have been "back then," and to help clients explore the arising feelings in present time, and to further support them in orienting to present experience.

As the pregnancy progresses and birth is near, the prenate experiences the womb becoming increasingly constrictive. Depending on earlier experiences in the womb, as well as the mother's attitude and external events, the prenate may have a sense of curiosity, anticipation, excitement, or fear and anxiety.

The Dance of Birth

The birth process is explored in great detail in the next three chapters, where clinical issues and practitioner skills are emphasized. Here, however, I would like to introduce an overview of birth and birthing with an emphasis more on the baby and mother's experience, as it will create a wider ground and introduction to explorations in the next three chapters.

For nine months babies and mothers are in close contact with each other. As contractions begin and the baby senses pressure and movement through the birth canal, the journey can be experienced as a continuation of an attuned, resonant dance together. Baby initiates labor when ready, mom's uterine wall responds to baby's push, and the forces and constriction function like a strong, deep massage, igniting the baby's system and enhancing health. The baby emerges wide-eyed and curious, with mom and baby happy to see each other and rest together after the energetic ordeal. The sympathetic charge needed to push through birth can then relax as parasympathetic relaxation takes over. A newborn placed on mom's belly will instinctively crawl to mom's breast and self-attach for a first feeding when ready. Some little ones prefer to gaze into mom's eyes before latching on. Throughout this process, the pleasurable sensations of oxytocin, known as the love hormone, supports bonding.

This lovely scene is natural but not as common as we might wish. The ease and satisfaction of birth for both mom and baby are affected by many factors. While modern medical procedures can save lives and enhance health, medical anthropologist Robbie Davis-Floyd has written in *Birth as an American Rite of Passage* a revealing account of how common obstetrical interventions are not only generally unnecessary, but also lead to a sense of failure or dissatisfaction for new mothers (Davis-Floyd 1992). This topic has been thoroughly examined in the field of pre- and perinatal psychology, including traumatic birth from the baby's perspective (Emerson 1998; Verny 1981; Chamberlain 1998). Medical interventions and birth issues become even more significant when the prenatal journey has been problematic.

The nature of the prenatal holding field and maternal-infant attachment and communication lay the ground for birth. As mentioned earlier, prenatal stress increases the risk of prematurity, which leads to other complications interfering with attachment. In a safe field with ongoing reassurance and explanations to the baby, birth difficulties can be less traumatic and overwhelming. The birthing mother depends on the holding field as much as the baby does. Research has shown fewer complications in births attended by doulas, who are there to support and be present with mom. A strong, supportive presence from the father, midwives, doulas, and/or other birth team members facilitate the birthing mother being able to rest into her instinctive knowing of how to birth her baby. As midwife Ina May Gaskin, puts it: "… the presence of even one person who is not exquisitely attuned to the mother's feelings can stop some women's labors.… Many labors stopped or slowed down when someone entered the birth room who was not intimate with the laboring mother's feelings" (Gaskin 2003, p. 138).

When mom is moved to the unfamiliar environment of hospital, particularly where the doctor has highest authority, she easily loses touch with her inner process and her baby. Contractions commonly slow down or stop during this process, which may in itself lead to medical interventions. The natural timing of birth is often overridden by the needs and perceptions of hospital personnel, while the experience of the baby is completely ignored or denied. Mothers and babies are designed for birth, which can enhance their bond.

> The bonding process gains momentum with delivery because the events surrounding birth provide a good atmosphere for attachment. The hard work of labor, crowning, pushing, the mother's heightened excitement, her baby's cry, and the extreme alertness of the infant contribute to the strength of the bonding between mother and infant.
>
> (Kang 1978, p. 71)

In a small percentage of births, interventions are required due to potential life-threatening conditions, such as placenta previa, cord wrapped around the neck, and so on. Where the natural course of birth is interrupted, however, a complex process designed over millions of years is affected on multiple levels. Babies often have their natural timing interfered with and experience shocking interventions and rough handling, accompanied by the panic or at least high activation level of birth attendants. Speed, change, and high levels of stimulation can easily overwhelm them, activating shock and withdrawal reactions. This is common as babies emerge from their relatively sheltered, fluid home of nine months into a hospital delivery or operating room.

Birthing women are also in an altered, highly sensitive state that can be interrupted by changes in nurses, examinations, or even talking. These distractions can separate a woman from her instinctive knowing, contributing to anxiety and stress, which are passed on to her baby. Losing her inner focus can also interfere with a birthing mom being able to sense and stay present with the baby. She may touch on her own birth history, becoming overwhelmed and withdrawing into her own dissociative state. She may also be less conscious due to drugs administered to calm her or reduce the pain.

In a speedy, impersonal, unfamiliar, and busy medical environment, women and their babies often experience fear and anxiety, stimulating a stress response. This slows or stops the process of labor, and disturbs the mother-baby relationship. Oxytocin is less available or effective under stress. Intimacy, whether it be with a lover or one's baby, becomes more difficult. A mother worrying about what the doctor is saying or what the fetal heart monitor is showing is less aware of the sensation of her baby within. Her uterine wall may be less responsive with stress, as circulation is shunted from the uterus and other organs to the large muscles needed for fight or flight (Verny 1986). The baby in this case is then less met, and less responded to. Emerson notes a change occurring here from mother-infant cooperative pushing—where baby pushes with its legs as mom's contractions are sensed—to an uncoordinated and confused process where baby and mother's pushing is unsynchronized (Emerson 1996, 1998).

In regression work, people often sense this lack of being met and have a sense of futile pushing, where one is pushing against resistance, rather than being supported by cooperative uterine contractions. Likewise, people accessing their birth process may feel themselves pushing against a uterine wall that is unresponsive—either being overly hard and resistant or too soft and flaccid. The latter occurs when anesthesia has been administered to the mother. Such drugs are designed to reduce sensation. While this may be a helpful resource for the birthing mother, it also renders her less able to feel her baby. The muscle tone of the uterine wall also decreases, leaving the baby with nothing to push against and less able to make progress. This is one reason such drugs often lead to cesarean section, forceps delivery, or vacuum extraction.

I have encountered this territory in many sessions, where adult clients experience a lack of space and a need to push with their legs. This must be held in present-time resources and negotiated slowly, so the client feels physically prepared to push and then slowly pushes out with the legs, perhaps with some resistance via a large cushion. The practitioner then monitors both the expression of the fluid tide and the action of potency in resolving inertial birthing forces in the system. Potency may orient to almost any area of inertia—commonly shifting to specific vertebral areas, occipito-atlanteal joint, occipital and cranial bases issues, and so on.

When labor stops, slows, or is later than predicted, birth may be induced by synthetic oxytocin, a drug called pitocin. Unlike natural oxytocin, this drug does not support bonding. It tends to disrupt the maternal-infant connection, interrupting natural rhythms that provide resourcing pauses, and instead causing unbearably painful, strong contractions that can be overwhelming for both mom and baby. In each case, the dance of birth has been interrupted, or at least its style has been changed.

Birthing babies may experience terror, abandonment, shock, confusion, and disorientation. They may feel anger at the doctor or deep grief on being separated from mom. Feeling-tones from earlier experiences, particularly conception and implantation may be restimulated during the birth process, especially the early stages when pressures build and a perception of endless entrapment or engulfment can permeate the experience. Strong relational imprints may be established as the baby is pulled out with cold instruments, met with masked faces, and whisked away from mom by strangers. These can affect how we expect to be treated, attitudes toward authority figures, and receptivity to intimacy and contact. All of these territories may arise in the context of session work and must be heartfully acknowledged, received, and inquired into on a felt-level.

Birth occurs in the context of the prenatal holding field. Where it has been supportive, babies and mothers have more resilience to endure whatever challenges birth presents. Where there have been earlier issues, as with implantation and discovery, birth may reinforce prenatal lack of trust, safety, and welcome. These may permeate later relational and personality styles as well as patterns of reacting to stress, establishing imprints of dissociation, addictive tendencies where there has been anesthesia, expecting to be rescued with emergency cesarean section, and so on. These may be expressed in session work where the practitioner can be perceived as being like the doctor or mom. Clients may tend to dissociate during sessions, have difficulty initiating or carrying through and completing with a series of sessions, or arriving on time. They may never feel complete upon ending a session, always feeling they need more time. It can be helpful to acknowledge what may have occurred in the past and support the client in accessing the little one within who is still organized around the wounding and to orient to present time, direct felt-experience, and resource.

And Beyond Birth: Postnatal Bonding and Attachment Issues

Babies are social nervous system beings. Upon emerging from the birth canal, healthy undrugged babies immediately seek mom's face and contact. Babies are also right-brain beings. The right cortex, oriented to holistic awareness, mediates sensory information, without separating the different senses out, or differentiating one's experience from that of others. Babies perceive holistically, with all sensations and emotions present at once and outer world not differentiated from inner. While the right brain is also involved in affect regulation, this takes two to three years to develop. The baby's emotional world is therefore immediate, with no ability to regulate responses or feelings, or to contextualize and differentiate experience or understand whose feeling is whose. Babies, like adults who have reverted to an infantile state in sessions, need others to differentiate and regulate their feelings for them.

Babies arriving via a medicalized birth often emerge sluggish due to a combination of drugs and shock. Infant development has been viewed through the lenses of a hundred years of hospital birth. Babies were not expected to be able to focus their eyes, lift their heavy heads, or initiate contact. Drugs at birth can interfere with the newborn's natural urge to crawl to mom's breast. Undrugged newborns also enjoy gazing into their mother's eyes, and their eyes focus well at 8–10 inches, the distance from mom's breast to her face. They easily recognize and prefer their mother's face and voice, as well as stories and songs they have heard in the womb (DeCasper 1980; Chamberlain 1998; Klaus, Klaus, and Kennel 1995).

These newborn abilities facilitate bonding and attachment. When interfered with by drugs, shock, maternal issues, or separation from mother at birth, both mother and baby suffer. For babies, separation from mom at birth can be terrifying and shocking. All that has been familiar to them for nine months is suddenly gone.

They have no reference point. Likewise, new mothers who are separated from their babies also experience disorientation and discontent. Their bodies are designed to be with their babies as much as babies are meant to be with their mothers. Oxytocin produced when baby breastfeeds both supports bonding and facilitates birth of the placenta. When baby is not available, mother may hemorrhage due to placenta retention, and her body reacts as if her baby has died. Biochemicals supportive of bonding and attachment diminish. When the baby is returned later, bonding may be difficult due to the lack of biochemical support.

Further challenges of medicalized birth not only affect the baby's ability to orient to and relate to mom, but also involve the possible undermining of mom's sense of power and authority, affecting her confidence as a mother. In the medical model of the hospital, the doctor is in charge and the patient is sick. Sickness is not to be trusted. Women in this context lose trust in their innate knowing of how to give birth, an important ground to their knowing how to mother.

Another important process occurs just after birth. When the umbilical cord stops pulsing, there is a synchronous ignition of potency in the baby's fluid system that allows the baby to be an independent, energized, physiological being. Not only is this essential ignition process often muted by drugs, overwhelm, and specific medical interventions, but mother's ignition of motherhood is also affected. The two may have difficulty meeting after birth. Some women become depressed and less able to reflect or meet the needs of their babies, interfering with bonding and attachment. (See Foundations Volume One, Chapter 20 for a discussion of ignition processes.)

Due to the work of Marshall Klaus and John Kennell, hospitals have made efforts to provide bonding time as soon after birth as possible (Klaus and Kennell 1976). Although critics have objected that there is no proof of a "sensitive period" for human bonding, it appears that being together immediately after birth facilitates bonding. For example, one study found that mothers whose infants touched their nipples in the first hour chose to keep their babies in their own room longer (Klaus, Klaus, and Kennell 1995). Rooming-in has been associated with mothers being more confident, feeling more competent in taking care of their infant, being more sensitive to their infant's cries, and being less likely to abandon their infant (Klaus, Klaus, and Kennell 1995; Klaus and Kennell 1976). Without this early contact, bonding is possible, but may be more difficult.

From the baby's perspective, birth anesthesia dulls the baby's responsiveness for some time after birth, interfering with bonding. In the quiet, alert state usual for undrugged babies immediately after birth, newborns actively seek contact with their parents and are "capable of intimate engagement, self-assertion, and, to the limit of [their] strength, even companionship and entertainment" (Chamberlain 1998, p. 62).

In session work with individuals born with anesthesia, drug affect may arise, along with dissociative tendencies. You may, as practitioner, sense a depth of inertia and stasis and have the experience that "there's no one home," as thinness and diffusion are sensed in and around the client's system. An understanding of dissociation and appropriate verbal skills may be helpful here, encouraging the client to explore the immediacy of the experience via feeling-tone, sensation, and imagery. Orienting to inhalation stillpoints in dissociative states can also help the client's dissociated psyche re-embody. As potency builds in the client's system, the drug affect tends to clear and the client can be more present. Coupled with this, feelings associated with being unable to properly bond with mom often arise in the relational field of biodynamics.

When working with babies and adults, birth trauma often emerges. Babies express their pain somatically through crying, fussing, being extremely quiet, sleeping, "spacing out" (dissociating), extreme startle responses, arching or stiffening when held, severe colic, and other behavior (Castellino 2000, 1995; Solter 1984). Common issues that may bring babies for sessions—including feeding and sleeping difficulties and colic—can relate to birth trauma, separation at birth, and prenatal stress or anxiety (Lifton 1992, p. 18; Verrier 1993).

Again, the relational holding field for baby and mother can have profound impact. Both babies and mothers who have experienced birth trauma can resolve it more readily in a loving, nurturing field of support. In view of potentially devastating developmental complications ensuing prenatal and birth stress and trauma, it seems imperative that young families, from before conception on, be held in a supportive field. If society cannot find its way to make this a number one priority, at least practitioners can offer understanding and support in the relational field we provide. Birth trauma commonly emerges in biodynamic session work and the practitioner must be well versed in this area, in order to support the processing of unresolved birthing forces. The birth process and practitioner skills in this area are discussed in detail in the next three chapters.

CHAPTER 4

Infants, the Birth Process, and Trauma

As introduced earlier, birth is one of our most formative experiences, a universal rite of passage that can have significant lifelong physical and emotional consequences. The birth process has a central role in psycho-emotional, physiological, and structural development and patterning—strongly influencing attachment processes and ego development. Craniosacral biodynamics offers profoundly effective support for resolving issues generated by the birth experience. Working with babies, children, and adults who are resolving birthing forces and their repercussions is one of the most significant and gratifying experiences available to practitioners. The following sections are meant to orient us to the physical and developmental aspects of birth and to the formative psycho-emotional processes it underpins.

Introduction

As we enter this area, it is important to again acknowledge that babies are conscious and aware little beings. Conventional medicine's historical view that babies have little awareness or intelligence is a gross misconception leading to enormous damage, even today. Hospital personnel and parents may routinely handle babies insensitively and administer medical procedures as if the child has no awareness and is not affected. However, as we have seen in Chapter 3, the research evidence is overwhelming that babies are extremely aware, even as prenates in the womb. They perceive threats, register pain, and even comprehend verbal and nonverbal messages with astonishing sensitivity, in some cases even greater than an adult's (Verny 1981; Chamberlain 1998).

Similarly, current medical beliefs can underestimate prenates and babies' emotional and physiological needs for a safe holding environment—one that encourages bonding, secure attachment, the avoidance of major threats and pain, and a growing trust in the caregiver relational field. Yet even today, medical interventions are often delivered as if the baby's basic attachment needs are not a priority, and nurseries may lack essential arrangements for his or her human contact and bonding needs. The medical community's historical resistance to well-researched facts in this area is still one of the mysteries of our times. Suffice it to say, if you are a pregnant mom or know any pregnant moms, and you encounter a health professional who says that (or behaves as if) babies have no feelings, don't experience or remember pain, don't really need full and immediate skin-contact bonding, and/or do not comprehend the psycho-emotional content of their surroundings, find a provider with a different belief-system.

The damage done to babies—and the hidden societal costs of all this—are enormous. I suspect that a good percentage of infant, child, and adult health issues may be traced to natural and unnatural events surrounding pre- and perinatal experience. These effects live on long after the circumstances of the womb experience and birth are forgotten, and may manifest in defended personality forms and tendencies, in psycho-emotional dysfunction, in nervous system sensitivity and activation, as well as structural issues, later in life. There is good news as well. In my experience, craniosacral biodynamic treatment of infants is clearly effective in resolving prenatal and birth-related issues, and treatment at any time of life can be immensely supportive.

Working with the impacts of the birth process often invokes issues for the practitioner. This is true for many other therapeutic situations, but it is especially relevant when treating babies, or when an adult client's birth process comes to the forefront. The problem is that our own unresolved birth issues may arise. I always recommend that practitioners work with their own birth issues in order to understand the birth process more clearly, and to be more able to hold a neutral ground for clients in treatment sessions. This means a commitment to taking on our own unresolved prenatal and birth issues and the related forces and psycho-emotional structures still at work in our systems. This can be done with cranial sessions, psychotherapy, or other therapeutic methods. I have done personal work around my own prenatal and birth trauma over the years and have even sensed and worked with my earliest felt-sense experience of conception and implantation. This exploration has been critical in understanding and opening up my personality structure and is an ongoing process. It has also greatly enhanced my ability to empathize with infants and adults, and to hold a steady neutral ground with their sometimes very intense processes.

Life Takes Shape

It is the nature of life to take shape. We are conscious, sentient, living beings. As we meet our world and have experience, we tend to take shape in response or reaction to what is experienced. These responses are developmental, psycho-emotional, physiological, and structural. So, as we have experiences, we make decisions about them, and shape ourselves in response to them.

Neonates and birthing infants are conscious, sentient beings who make decisions about their experience and take shape accordingly. Over the last thirty years much evidence has accumulated to show that neonates and infants are aware of their environment and register and respond to their sensory experiences. In this vein, I would like to quote Raymond Castellino DC, from his paper, Somatotropic Facilitation of Prenatal and Birth Trauma:

> Evidence is mounting that prenates are sentient, conscious, feeling beings who have much to express to those who receive them into their arms at birth. David Chamberlain PhD, has amply pointed out to us that, at seven weeks, prenates [the baby in the womb] have been observed to be sensitive to touch and at fourteen weeks prenates have been observed to move away from light sources even though their eyelids are still closed. At fourteen weeks prenates have clearly responded to sound. Thomas Verny cites cases which more than suggest that language development begins in the womb.... David Chamberlain cites other video ultrasound studies where prenates appear to be expressing affection and emotions such as joy, gladness, fear, anger and sadness. Prenatal twins have been observed gently caressing each other in the womb. In another case a prenate has been observed making a fist and actually hitting the shaft of an amniocentesis needle invading his womb space.
>
> (Castellino 1998)

A wealth of empirical evidence over the last four decades from the field of prenatal and birth psychology points to the sentience of prenates and newborns. As introduced in earlier chapters, William Emerson PhD, a dear friend and foremost pioneer in the field, has gathered voluminous evidence over a forty-year career in his egression work with clients, and with direct work with infants, that points to this conclusion. I have had the privilege to work and collaborate with Emerson and Castellino, and I can confirm their observations, in both my personal and clinical experience. In my own work with infants, it is clear to me that they respond directly to the quality of presence of the practitioner, understand what is said and communicated to them, and will express their needs to you, if you are open to their communications. Emerson writes about the prenate in a similar manner:

> The prenate (i.e., the unborn baby) is vulnerable in a number of ways that are generally unrecognized and unarticulated. Most people think or assume that prenates are unaware, and seldom attribute to them the status of being human. I recall a recent train trip, where an expectant mother sat in a smoking car filled with boisterous and noisy people. I asked her whether she had any concern for her unborn baby, and whether she thought the smoke or the noise would be bothersome to her unborn child. Her reply was, "Well of course not, my dear. They are not very intelligent or awake yet." Nothing could be further from the truth.... Theory and research from the last twenty years indicates that prenatal experiences can be remembered, and have lifelong impact.
>
> (Emerson 1998)

There is no longer any doubt that newborns must be related to as sentient, aware beings who deserve the best of our attention, respect, and understanding. In a baby's presence, it is important to slow oneself down—a baby's inner pacing is much slower than an adult's—and to enter a state of attunement and resonance to the baby's presence and needs. It is also important to communicate to babies as if they understand your words, because—in my experience—they are able to derive your intended meaning and are certainly able to attune to your presence and intentions. Similarly, communicate in a style appropriate for a small person, using a soft, gentle, slow voice that respects their extraordinary sensitivity and slow pacing. Avoid the practice of talking about babies in their presence as if they are not there and cannot understand your words—respecting how we would naturally feel uncomfortable if someone did this to us. I always model this with parents who bring their baby in to see me. I include the baby in all conversations with caregivers, and also ask the baby questions about its own birth experience—"Gee, as mom shares that, how is that for you?"

Experiencing babies as sentient, aware beings—even in the prenatal period—is a great paradigm shift with the capacity to revolutionize our pregnancy, birthing, and childcare practices. This is the foundation of craniosacral biodynamics with babies—babies are intelligent, sentient beings who understand your intentions and will express their needs. Please make this understanding the foundation of your work.

Empathy and Negotiation of Boundaries

The baby's acceptance of a practitioner is of critical importance, so special attention must be given to the negotiation of the relational field, contact, and touch. The infant has not come to the session of its own accord, but rather its parents or primary caregivers have brought it. We thus have to gain the baby's permission for the session work. Again, include baby in all conversations with caregivers, remembering that he or she will be able, at some level, to understand your words. Introduce yourself to the baby. Explain what is happening and describe your intentions, as the infant will understand all this, in its own way. In addition to verbal communication, your quality of presence is paramount; the slowness of approach and a gentle touch and clarity of intention help develop the baby's trust and participation. The infant must sense our integrity, full attention, and communication skills. Sincere enjoyment of being with babies is also an essential support in creating a trusting relationship.

Negotiation of boundaries with an infant is quite different from creating a relationship with an adult. As we have introduced in Chapter 3, the world of prenates and infants is totally unified. They perceive and sense everything all at once in present time. All input has equal weight and intense input—like a contact made too quickly, or your loud voice—can be overwhelming. It is important to respect this when approaching infants. Furthermore, their world is undifferentiated from their mom's world. They are truly a unified field of consciousness. Their physical and psycho-emotional world is not separate from mom's or primary caregiver's presence. So approaching the baby means approaching mom, dad, and any caregivers present, and vice versa. If trust is well established in the whole family field, the baby will gradually recognize the practitioner as part of the whole system.

Babies' Neurology: Present-Time Social Beings

It is important to understand the infant's basic neurology as we orient to its world of relationship and experience, directly pointing to the infant's ability to be present, process information on a felt-level, and respond to arising conditions. The infant's cortex is not yet fully developed. His or her left cortex will eventually encompass rational thinking and the ability to contextualize experience. This ability takes two to three years after birth to develop. Thus a baby cannot think logically, cannot contextualize its experience, and cannot differentiate what it is feeling from what others around are feeling.

Babies are, however, very much right-brain beings. The right cortex is oriented to holistic awareness—the ability to perceive everything all at once. Sensory information—both from its outer and inner worlds—are mediated by the right brain, again without the ability to separate the different senses out, or to differentiate one's experience from that of others. The infant's world is thus a holistic experience, where every sense is present all at once—seeing, hearing, smelling, tasting, touching, feelings, and emotions—and where the outer world cannot be differentiated from the inner world of feeling and emotion. Furthermore, the right brain is also involved in affect regulation, but this also takes two to three years to develop. Thus the emotional world of the infant is immediate, without ability to regulate responses or feelings, and without ability to contextualize and differentiate its experience or to understand whose feeling is whose. What is sensed "out there" is experienced as "in me."

Babies are also *social nervous system* beings. We discuss the social nervous system in Chapter 20, which explores what is known as the polyvagal theory in some detail. Researcher Stephan Porges has reclassified the autonomic nervous system usually discussed in terms of the sympathetic and parasympathetic system into three aspects—the social, sympathetic, and parasympathetic systems (Porges 2011). This makes much more sense of the actual nuclei and nerves involved, and is pivotal in understanding a baby's response to its relational world.

The social nervous system is mediated by nuclei in the brain stem, which provides nerve innervation to neck muscles, to the baby's ears, eyes, mouth, and to the heart and lungs. It allows baby to orient and respond to a caretaker's presence and to make its needs known via facial expression and vocalization—via social communication and the communication of feelings and inner states. If needs are not met at this level, if the baby feels unseen, abandoned, or unreceived, its nervous system may shift to a sympathetic response with shouting, crying, and anger. Its last defensive response, if needs are still not met or overridden, will be to default to the parasympathetic state of withdrawal, dissociation, and freeze. These early experiences and inner states set the tone for personality tendencies and defensive processes later in life (Figure 4.1).

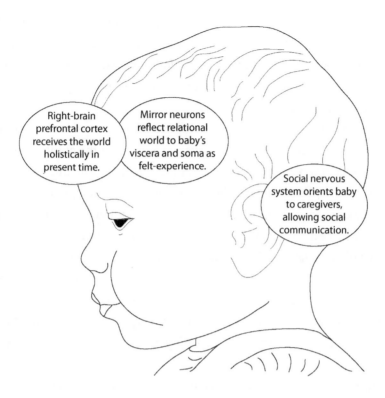

Figure 4.1. Baby's basic neurology.

Babies' Ability to Attune and Respond to Caregivers

Babies directly attune to the caregiver's presence, their relational world, and outer environment as direct felt-experience. It is thus important to explore this process of attunement and response as we orient to the prenate and infant's relational world. Researchers are still working out the basic neurological processes involved in felt-experience and felt-knowing of both our inner states and the states of others. I am offering the best synthesis here that I can at this time, and would like to thank Dr. Daniel Siegel for his writings in these areas (Siegel 2007, 2010). He also teaches a sophisticated integration of mindfulness practice and psychoneurology.

The basic idea is that, as babies sense the actions and intentions of others around them, specialized neurons called *mirror neurons* come into play. These are the starting point for a complex matrix of interrelated neurological responses, which I would like to describe and directly relate to babies' experience. Researchers discovered and named mirror neurons in the 1980s and 1990s. In neurological research with monkeys, Giacomo Rizzolatti and his team of researchers discovered that, as the monkeys perceived significant actions of those in their environment, particular cortical neurons fired in their brain. The neurons seemed to be mirroring the actions of others and preparing the monkey to perform similar actions—they acted as a bridge between what is perceived and a mirroring motor response to significant experience (Rizzolatti 1996, 2004, 2008).

Later researchers related these findings to human experience and extended this territory to include early attachment processes and the ability to attune and emphasize with others (Iacoboni 2008). Beyond mirroring and imitating the behavior of others, mirror neurons also help us sense, feel, reflect, predict, and respond to the intentional actions and states of others. They initiate an inner felt-sense and feeling-knowledge of interpersonal experience, and help us organize both internally and externally in relationship to this felt-experience of others. Babies' relational world is very much organized around this process—its perception of caregivers and significant events in their world is directly sensed as inner felt-experience. This is the ground for their response to relational process and caregiver intentions and actions. This is clearly also the felt starting point for both self/ego formation and attachment processes.

In human beings, mirror neurons fire in response to our perception or experience of the intentional actions and states of other people, especially significant others. This is obviously a critical ground for babies' relational experience. This information goes to various areas of the baby's cortex and, most tellingly, is directed downward into the body. The perceptual input of others—especially mother's and caregivers' intentions and actions—then becomes a felt-bodily experience, which helps the baby sense and know the actions, states, and intentions of others very directly. These feeling states are relayed back upward to the prefrontal cortex, which mediates present-time awareness, and then becomes "felt-knowing"—both of the baby's internal states and the actions and states of others. These then become the ground for the babies' internal organization and responses to their external relational world. Let's tease out some of the basic neurological dynamics of this process in terms of everyday experience.

As we perceive relationally relevant experience, our mirror neurons fire and interact with the superior temporal cortex. The temporal lobe in general, especially the temporal cortex and hippocampus, gives a historical context to present experience. It helps us predict and appropriately respond to the outcomes of relational experience. One of the prime functions of our brain is to predict and prepare us for the outcomes of experience. Thus our current experience can be contextualized relative to our history. This may unfortunately also set us up to experience current relational process through the filters of our past, and lead us to misinterpret the relational intentions of others. We will come back to this important territory later.

The perceptual information is then sent to both the motor areas of the frontal cortex, which primes us for motor responses to perceptual experience, and to the anterior insula, which is involved in awareness of our inner states (interoception) and the contextualization and processing of our emotional experience. From here the information continues to descend through the limbic system and brain stem into the body. Our perceptions of other's intentions, actions, and inner states are now present as sensation, feeling-tone, and emotional qualities in our viscera and soma. This is called *internal simulation*—our body resonates with our external experience and inner feeling states result.

Next, these sensations and feeling-tones are relayed back up to the insula and prefrontal cortex via nerves called *interoceptors*. This gives us a felt-perception of our inner states. Internal felt-information from muscles, viscera, nociceptors (also called pain receptors), and facial expressions goes through the spinal cord to the brain stem, hypothalamus, the parietal cortex, insula, anterior cingulate cortex, and prefrontal cortex. A complex of responses then occurs.

The hypothalamus—the master regulator of our interior world—responds to these interior feeling states via changes in hormones and hormone regulation. The parietal area is believed to be involved in self-awareness and self-identity—hence, as felt-information states ascends to the parietal area, our self-view and identity also become a felt-experience! This is very pivotal in the baby's developing sense of selfhood and the unfolding of attachment processes.

The anterior cingulate cortex and insula are involved in our awareness of these inner states and the processing of sensory information into an emotionally relevant context, which is pivotal in affect regulation. The totality of all of this is sent to the right prefrontal cortex—the mediator of present-time awareness—and a direct felt-knowing of our relational world is experienced. Thus when we perceive and attune to another, we are actually attuning to our own inner states and feeling-tones. This is very important to understand in terms of a baby's direct experience of its outer and inner world. All interoceptors in the body go to the *right* prefrontal cortex—remember that babies are right-brain beings and thus have the ability to directly sense their inner felt-world via their right-brain orientation holistically, which is not sensed as separate from their outer experience of caregivers or significant events (Figure 4.2).

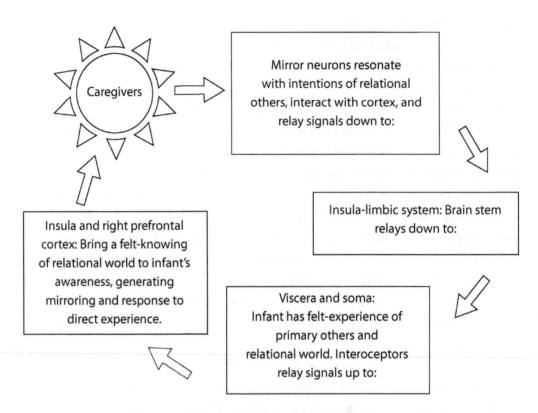

Figure 4.2. Baby's relational experience and interoception.

When felt-experience is perceived via the right prefrontal cortex, another important process is initiated. The prefrontal cortex, along with the anterior cingulate cortex, relates current experience to our historical map of relationship mediated by the temporal lobe. We then have a holistic picture of our present relational experience held in the context of history and time. Babies thus build an inner felt-experience of their world, which they can gradually relate to their current relational experiences. This is both the ground for early ego formation and attachment process—and for our experience of relationship throughout life. The baby thus builds an inner picture of its world based on direct felt-experience, which is pretty much in place by two to three years of age. This process then sets the stage for how we experience others, attribute states to them, and predict possible outcomes of relational interchange. It also helps both baby and adult read the inner states of others, empathize with their emotions and life experiences, sense their intentions, and predict the outcomes of experience.

All of this is critical in our lives on many levels. Very early in life, it sets the stage for our later response to intimate others, to caregiving, to friends and family—indeed to all those we meet in our relational world. As we mentioned above, there is, however, a caveat to be very aware of. From our earliest experience of caregiving, mediated largely through the neurology discussed above, we get a felt-experience of our inner and outer world and begin to form a self-system with its attachment processes. This early conditioning will color our later relational experience and we may make the felt-mistake of attributing past relational pain to current relational experience. We may see-sense danger when none exists, read other's intentions and inner states through the filters of these past experiences and act inappropriately toward others. In the extreme, if an overly defended, insecurely attached ego system evolved out of early relational pain and/or confusion, then current relational processes may be misread and defensive ego processes engage when there is no real relational danger present.

Therapeutic Intentions

Working with newborns and infants requires particular practitioner listening skills and intentions. In this, we seek an openness and receptivity through all of our sensory doors, simultaneously. We listen and communicate through all of our senses—in resonance with baby's holistic sensory state—compensating for differences in infant and adult communication. Put yourself in the baby's place and imagine how sensory input is a totally integrated experience, relatively undifferentiated, and not yet biased in favor of words and interpretations. We use the same basic skills in all craniosacral biodynamics, but they are used with particular delicacy and insight when working with newborns and infants. How we work communicates how we attune to and receive the infant, and how we respond to what is received. Castellino writes:

> The practitioner perceives visually, aurally, and kinesthetically. The practitioner sees, listens, and feels. The way the practitioner uses his or her attention during treatment sessions has profound effects on the course of treatment. It is the practitioner's responsibility to pay attention to and learn how the application of their attention affects the course of treatment.
> (Castellino 1998)

The first therapeutic intention is to settle into stillness and to be empathetically present with clear intention in a wide perceptual field. As we settle into an attuned, receptive relational state with infants, they will begin to show us their prenatal and birth history in macro- and micro-movement patterns. They will communicate via sound, feelings, facial expression, and body motion. Initially, simply appreciate the unfolding story—attuned to the baby's three bodies—oriented to mid-tide and Long Tide. The action of potency—the related fluid fluctuations and membranous-connective tissue patterns—will clarify and further convey their stories. Let the sessions unfold with pacing and therapeutic orientation that is noninvasive and appropriate to the infant's emerging process.

As mentioned above, practitioner pacing is of critical importance. In working with babies, we discover their great sensitivity. In their intrauterine watery life sounds were muffled and environmental changes were largely buffered and slowed. In the outside world a more intense pacing prevails. Sounds are louder and environmental changes arise much more quickly. Babies therefore appreciate a slow pacing consistent with world-as-womb. Practitioners can establish such pacing through truly slowing down their inner state, generating a still and receptive perceptual field—and through soft, low voice tones, slow movements, and gradual, negotiated slow-motion actions. Again, most important is the practitioner's inner state of receptivity and attunement—and his or her appropriate response to baby's arising process and needs. All of this is invaluable in work with infants, and is also essential with adults when early history is encountered.

The sensorial basis of the infant's reality leads us to another territory. The baby's ego/self-form and psychological defenses are not formed until later in early childhood. As discussed earlier, infants experience everything on a bodily felt-level via affect, feeling-tone, and sensation. There is no clear differentiation between self and other. Emerson, in his prenatal and birth psychology, calls the nature of the prenate and newborn ego system a *body ego*. The baby's experience is mediated entirely through its body senses. Therefore the craniosacral biodynamic skills of listening and sensing through actual contact can be extremely valuable, meeting babies in their own natural medium of felt, sensory awareness.

Infant Resources

It is important to appreciate the resources of the baby—including the nature of its home environment and family field—as session work must be carried out in the resources available to the infant. A safe holding environment is by far the top priority, the preeminent resource for babies. Practitioner skills of presence, contact, and negotiation can establish safety in sessions for the infant. Over time, the infant may begin to experience your presence and touch as a resource. Young infants have recently experienced a dramatic change of environment from inside to outside, and the journey is usually strenuous at best. In the birth process, their survival system—mediated largely by the limbic and autonomic nervous systems—has been at the least engaged, and more commonly fully taxed. Even mom—the heart of a baby's instinctual survival orientation—may have been exhausted and anesthetized during birth, even feeling endangered or threatened, with intense emotions generated. These combinations of factors can leave a deep impression in baby's mind-body system, which may affect subsequent bonding and attachment processes. The practitioner can provide a much-needed counterbalancing field of presence and safety, attunement, and resonance for the baby and its family.

Session work without a firm basis in relational safety can be retraumatizing. Infants can re-experience their unresolved prenatal and birth issues as if the events are happening all over again. Remember that a baby's consciousness is totally present-time oriented. What arises from the past feels like it is happening in the present. They do not yet have the left-brain ability to contextualize or differentiate their experience. Because of this, as the practitioner begins to work with unresolved prenatal or birth forces, the baby may start to become overwhelmed. The signals of overwhelm are generally quite visible, giving the practitioner plenty of opportunity to guide the unfolding process to a favorable completion. These signs are outlined below. The practitioner sees the signs of activation and helps the infant stay resourced in present time. This can be done as long as the relationship is secure and positive; if the baby experiences the practitioner as invasive or disrespectful, the whole process is jeopardized.

In addition to the primary resources of contact with mom and dad—assuming bonding and safety have been established—and quality of attention and relationship with the practitioner, babies may have other resources that can be cultivated in the session environment. The baby may prefer to lie on one side more than the other, like to move in a certain direction, or enjoy contact in a certain location. These kinds of preferences are commonly part of the *birth schema,* a term coined by Emerson and referring to the internalization of the birth experience by the infant. This may include such things as the nature of resource or traumatization held in the baby's system, related motion patterning, tissue patterns, and psycho-emotional effects. Likewise, there may be a certain way of being held or approached that resources the baby, including certain sounds, songs, textures of cloth, soft toys, or other factors.

The intention is to follow babies' processes, to support their healing, and to respond appropriately to their individual trauma patterns and birth schema.

Trauma Impacts

Parts of the birth process can be perceived to be traumatic by the infant, even in the best circumstances. The forces of birthing can be intense, and the nature of the experience can be overwhelming. Therefore, working with babies often means working with trauma and states of limbic and autonomic activation. Babies may express strong feelings and emotions, autonomic activation and sensitization, and, in the extreme, dissociative states. Babies have not yet organized ego defenses—their most primary response to overwhelming experience is to withdraw, disconnect, and dissociate. In dissociation, the little one literally splits off from its current overwhelming experience. The nervous system expresses parasympathetic shock and freezing states, as stress-related hormones flood their system. We explore these kinds of states in our last chapters on trauma and trauma resolution.

If stress-related, traumatized states arise in infant session work, the practitioner must maintain the receptive state of attunement and help baby return to present-time awareness and resources. Sometimes this can be accomplished through Long Tide awareness and stillness, through one's soft voice, with reassurance and renegotiation of contact and the relational field. Sometimes the baby is so overwhelmed that it has to be gently removed from the session environment—reconnected with mom and family field—and regrounded in a new sense of safety. All of this can be truly challenging for the practitioner and family alike and needs sensitive negotiation.

Working with babies at this level is a tremendous service to the baby and the family, as these states, if not resolved, may have significant long-term consequences. Practitioners will need all the skills we have discussed and competences in trauma resolution strategies to really meet a baby's arising healing needs. After a difficult birth, a baby's limbic and autonomic systems can reset in the ambiance of mother's loving presence and a safe, resourceful home environment. Unfortunately, conditions are not always ideal, and additional assistance can have tremendous benefits.

Stress Response Basics

The autonomic nervous system can become strongly engaged and sensitized in a baby's birth experience. Practitioners need to be able to recognize the various signs of activation and respond appropriately. The large topic of autonomic function is covered in later chapters, but a brief overview here will set the stage for understanding aspects of craniosacral biodynamic treatment methods.

The autonomic nervous system is part of our repertoire of survival mechanisms, constantly operating beneath our conscious awareness. Autonomic functions are deeply imbedded in our neurophysiology. If we feel threatened, the intelligence of our system immediately invokes a series of responses to address the situation, initiating a cascade of neuroendocrine-immune changes that we experience as physical and emotional shifts. Normally the system shifts back to a baseline state after the danger is passed, but if the threat is overwhelming, the system can become fixated at a particular phase of the autonomic cycle, constantly attempting to fulfill its natural sequence. These autonomic issues can be at the root of many health problems.

The autonomic nervous system evolved over the entire history of life forms, and three distinct aspects have been identified. Conventional anatomy and physiology recognizes only two of these—the sympathetic and parasympathetic nervous systems—but relatively recent research by Stephen Porges PhD (Porges 2011) has explored a third aspect, the *social engagement system*. This newer orientation is extremely important in understanding human stress responses and defensive tendencies. We discuss this concept in much more detail in Chapter 20.

The social engagement system is evolutionarily the newest and most sophisticated autonomic function—manifesting in babies via instinctual maternal bonding strategies. Babies know how to recognize mom both visually and aurally, how to find mom's breast, and elicit her attention and affection (via oxytocin and endorphin inducement). The social engagement system coordinates babies' orienting response when they seek mom's attention—neck muscles, eye movement, inner ear muscles, vocalization, and facial expression are all coordinated by the nuclei of the social engagement system.

If the social engagement strategies do not work, babies will turn to their older autonomic layer, the sympathetic nervous system, best known as the locus of fight-or-flight capabilities. It is common to hear angry cries coupled with physical motions when a baby's needs are not being met. Babies can express anger and fear, but their real effective usage of this layer is minimal, since they are physically incapable of either fight or flight. However, the neurochemistry of fight-flight—cortisol, adrenaline, norepinephrine, and related neurotransmitters—is still activated even if physical action is not possible, and a protective contraction of the muscles and connective tissues inevitably arises.

Assuming failure of the sympathetic nervous system to solve the problem, the system has one card left to play, the parasympathetic response. This is the evolutionary oldest layer of the system, present in simple, relatively immobile organisms. The parasympathetic response is to "play possum"—to engage freezing and immobilizing strategies—in hopes that the danger will pass on its own. In infants, dissociation, freezing responses, and withdrawal are primary examples of this response. Traumatized babies may thus sleep a lot, or be very quiet and slow in orientation. They may, however, be sensed to make poor contact, have bonding or attachment issues, or to be very distant or listless.

The autonomic system is designed to deal with ordinary novelties and threats, and generally functions quite well to keep us alive and operational. However, extreme circumstances can overwhelm the capacity of the autonomic system. *Overwhelm* is the distinctive point at which novelty and stress become trauma. When the system is overwhelmed and has inadequate resources to cope with the event, stress nuclei may become sensitized and stuck in the protective response. They continue to cycle the need to protect, but cannot complete the intention. This is the ground for the emergence of a whole spectrum of post-traumatic stress symptoms and is the key factor in traumatization.

Generally, babies' autonomic nervous system experience is underestimated or unrecognized in modern health care. I am convinced that simple awareness of autonomic effects of various birthing and infant-care events would have a huge benefit for our society and world.

Autonomic Strategies for Babies

Let's go through these stages in relationship to baby's experience in more detail. The social engagement system is baby's first orientation in getting its needs met. It will seek caregivers' attention and express its needs via voice, motion, and facial expressions. Unfortunately, this level is frequently overridden by routine birthing procedures, and much more so by events arising from major medical interventions. Babies need and expect protection from pain and nurturance from their mothers. But if mom is in pain and anesthetized, her capacity for meeting baby is at least compromised, and baby's capacity for meeting mom can be equally reduced because the anesthesia is fed to the baby through the umbilical cord.

If baby is immediately removed from the mom for cleaning and examination, the needed bonding contact with mom may be interrupted. If painful pressures, suctions, surgeries, or shots are given without sensitivity, the need for protection and safety is at least undermined. All of these may be experienced as a betrayal of the bonding and attachment process at the time of birth. It may even be experienced as a devastating abandonment by caregivers. When this occurs, the social nervous system and its orientation to safety, contact, and nurturance may be overwhelmed. Once non-protection and non-connection are experienced at a social autonomic level, the baby may respond to current novelty and stress by bypassing the social engagement system, engaging sympathetic nervous system activation. This is a survival ploy based on the experience of overridden needs and lack of security I suspect that this is a root source of childhood attention deficit and hyperactivity issues.

The sympathetic system in babies lacks muscular coordination and strength to implement survival intentions. The neurochemistry is present, but there is little chance for actual fulfillment. In session work, sympathetic nervous system issues in babies commonly present as hypertonic or tense tissues, sleeplessness, extended inconsolable crying, and similar excited states. The infant's cries may seem anxious and angry.

Limbic emotions commonly co-arise with the sympathetic response. The amygdala—the baby's limbic sentry for sensory and environmental danger and novelty—will couple sympathetic activation with feelings of fear and anger—all oriented to survival. Fight-flight responses thus have direct resonance with anger and fear and—in the extreme—rage and terror. These states—sensed as tensions, with autonomic and emotional activation—are clearly sensed as they arise in baby sessions. As they arise, the practitioner must have patience, presence, and empathy for the little one's arising process.

The parasympathetic state is the default strategy of last resort for the baby. Unable to make contact, unable to move, the baby deals with perceived threat—absence of mom, physical pain, and so on—by entering a dissociative and immobilized state. In sessions this can present as non-contact—a sense of withdrawal and distance—inability to orient, hypotonic tissues, excessive sleeping, inability to move the head, and similar placid states. Ironically, these babies may be identified as "good" babies, and indeed the neurochemistry of parasympathetic response (serotonin, dopamine, endorphins) is generally pleasurable in the short term. If the baby is stuck in a parasympathetic protective response, its ability to orient to mom and to get needs met via the social nervous system are severely challenged. In the extreme, a fixated parasympathetic state is dangerous because metabolic function slows down to the point where the heart-lung supply of oxygen-rich blood to the brain is too low. I wonder if parasympathetic shock may be a factor in sudden infant death syndrome?

Parasympathetic-overwhelmed children are commonly not recognized as having problems until later in life. They may appear as quiet babies who sleep a lot and give no trouble, and if they do not like your contact they are likely to just turn away instead of crying. But later they may have learning difficulties, and in adult life may have issues such as chronic fatigue, endogenous depression (atypical depression), and states of low energy and low motivation. This may also be a factor in the development of autistic states. Adults stuck in cycling a parasympathetic protective response tend to collapse under stress and can sleep for weeks on end in response to stressful or threatening life experiences.

The remarkable endurance of pre- and perinatal stress has been well established by Emerson, Castellino, Chamberlain, and others. A *trauma schema*—when the person responds in the present as though their trauma is still happening—may become a habitual way of responding to threat and may strongly shape the person's experience of everyday life. Under stress, the child or adult begins to live in *trauma time*—again living as though the threat is still present—and the ability to respond to current stress is greatly diminished. Researchers have proposed that an autonomic set point or adapted default strategy can be instilled semi-permanently so that the individual habitually goes to sympathetic or parasympathetic strategies instead of having the full autonomic repertoire available. Studies have shown that early trauma can be the root of later childhood dissociative and attention deficit disorders (Perry and Pollard 1998). My experience is that the inherent potential for a full spectrum of autonomic responses, including a full return to social engagement system strategies, is never lost. Healing modalities—such as craniosacral biodynamics, mindfulness-based therapies, and trauma resolution work—have great potential for healing the resonances and fixity of traumatic cycling and its repercussions in our mind-body system.

Physical Trauma

The birth process is a very physical experience. Strong forces are present, even in the most ideal natural scenario. In a vaginal birth, strong forces are encountered as the baby moves though the birth canal. In obstetric procedures, these can be greatly compounded. Contractions of the uterus are intense and forces will be introduced into the baby's body as it meets the inner surfaces of the womb. Mom's sacrum and pubic bone are powerful contact points. All of these forces are intensified if the baby becomes temporarily stuck in the birth canal, or held in one position over a length of time. Even in optimum conditions, passage is likely to involve uncomfortable, straining pressures and positions. Upon exit, drastic changes of environment are encountered, including different air pressure and temperature. The baby ideally resolves these forces naturally via mom's welcoming contact, bonding, and nurturance.

The more common experience involves a host of other physical challenges. Labor may be induced, disrupting the natural neurochemical prerequisites for natural self-regulation. Anesthesia may be used, generating dissociative experiences at the very time when authentic contact is most needed. Physical means of extraction such as forceps may be used, painfully squeezing the cranium. If vacuum extraction is used, the fluids and contents of the brain are literally sucked cephalad. Cesarean births pose a whole cluster of different issues, which vary depending on whether the infant was engaged in the birth canal. The list of physically stressful or painful possibilities goes on and on, including the customary examination, air passage suction, inoculations, and, just a bit later, circumcision for the boys. All of these physical experiences may generate protective tissue contractions and psycho-emotional tendencies that can endure for a lifetime, especially if bonding and attachment are sub-optimum.

From a biodynamic viewpoint, as the birth process proceeds, the field of potency coalesces and becomes inertial in order to center the various forces and disturbances in the system. The forces of the birthing experience are centered and contained in ways that are appropriate to the resources of the infant. As potency condenses to center and accommodates the shock in the system, protective energetic and tissue patterns are generated as the trauma becomes bound in the system. As the biodynamic practitioner meets a baby's system, his or her main orientation is to these forces at work in the system, to deepening states of equilibrium and stillness, to the expression of the fluid tide and its potency, to Long Tide phenomena and to the resolution of the birthing forces maintaining the patterning and autonomic activation in the baby's system.

Recognizing Traumatization and Shock Affects

Recognition of trauma's telltale signs in babies is an essential skill for effective treatment. *Shock affect* means any physical, physiological, emotional, or psychological aftereffect of limbic-autonomic nervous system overwhelm. These affects are often clearly observable. The following description of important shock affect characteristics in infants is gleaned from the work of Emerson and Castellino, with additions and clarification from my own experience. Sadly, we have become so used to seeing traumatized babies that many of the following affects are thought to be normal.

Motion Affects

Discontinuous patterns of motion are an early indicator of a traumatized infant. The traumatized infant's motion patterns may seem jerky and have clear breaks in body motion continuity. The infant may tend to move more easily toward one side as opposed to the other. She may lose orientation when moving toward the midline. For example, the infant may tend to stay on her left side. As mom moves to the right, she may express jerky motions or trembling as she approaches the midline. She may express jerking and/or shaking motions of the extremities and be unable to physically orient herself. Traumatized infants will thus not be able to coordinate their physical responses to the environment or to a caretaker's movements. At the other end of the spectrum, in parasympathetic shock, infants are overly quiet and placid. Their muscle tone may be hypotonic, and they may be developmentally slow in motor skills.

Traumatized infants also have difficulty holding their heads up. This shock affect is also so common that it is thought to be normal. An untraumatized infant can partially hold its head up and can turn its head from side to side to orient itself to its environment at will, without breaks in motion continuity. I have seen untraumatized infants lift and turn their head to orient to my voice, mom's presence, and other sound.

These kinds of shock affects are so common that it has become assumed that it is normal for an infant to express discontinuity of physical movement and jerky, disoriented motions. However, untraumatized infants will not express such discontinuous motion dynamics. I have had the pleasure to attend to a good number of infants who had relatively untraumatized births. In all cases their motions were smooth, they could make eye contact, they could orient to their environment, and they did not express startle reflexes inappropriately.

Motion affects often have coupled tissue affects, such as compression on the birth lie side, vertebral and pelvic distortions, and various cranial molding issues. As the child grows older, if the forces present remain unresolved, these can become formalized as intraosseous distortions, spinal issues, unsymmetrical structures, or other tissue patterns.

Reading these breaks in continuity and ease of movement has great clinical importance. Become sensitive to them and be able to see and feel babies' birth schema as you watch their motions and notice breaks in the continuity of their movement patterns. These motions and patterns are communications. They tell the story of the birth and its unresolved issues and are a call for attention and help.

Hyper- and Hypotonicity and Skin Color and Tone

Infants with shock affects may exhibit hypertonicity or hypotonicity, or a blend of the two. For instance, there may be a general hypertonicity present with specific areas of hypotonicity. Alternatively, hyper- or hypotonicity of tissues may be localized to areas that met the forces of birth. Hypertonicity is an expression of the sympathetic nervous system's protective tissue tension held in relationship to the forces and pressures of the birth process, while hypotonicity is an expression of the collapse into parasympathetic protection.

In hypo-states, tissues lose their tone and resiliency. There may also be a lack of skin color, paleness, or a mottled look to the infant's skin. Coloration can also be mixed—red for sympathetic, pale for parasympathetic—and occasionally the coloration can seem to flash back and forth.

Hyper- or hypotoned tissue in the occipito-atlanteal junction and occipital triad generally is a common manifestation of this affect (Schneier and Burns 1991). The occipito-atlanteal junction is under extreme compressive force during the birth process. Potencies will condense in the occipito-atlanteal (O/A) area and occipital triad in response to the birthing forces. The tissues of the O/A junction respond to the birthing forces by contracting to protect the infant from traumatic compressive forces. If the birth process is excessively prolonged, a hypertonic defensive contraction can become locked into the O/A junction and the occipital triad as a compressive strain pattern. This is often coupled with intraosseous occipital distortions. If the system went into shock, the tissues may alternatively collapse under the continual compressive forces and a hypotonic, hypermobile-floppy state may result. I have personally noticed this hypotonic affect in many infants. Castellino cites the study of Schneier and Burns as a basis for suggesting that hypotonicity at the O/A junction is implicated in sudden infant death syndrome (Castellino 1998).

When you meet an infant's system, you are basically in relationship to a fluid-tissue-potency field. The intention is always to re-establish the relationship of the fluid-tissue field to potency and the bioelectric matrix. In hypertonic states, it may be beneficial to work with exhalation stillpoints, deepening states of equilibrium, and augmentation of space. In hypotonic states, inhalation stillpoints and augmentation of fluid drive may be very helpful. The intention is to re-establish the relationship of hypotonic tissues to the fluid tide and its potency. Of course, the ability to be still and listen to the deeper forces at work is the foundation of treatment. I basically work with infants through heartfelt presence, attunement, stillness, and the offering of space.

Sensory and Attention Affects

Traumatized infants' eyes may seem glossy and dissociated, as though they are not fully present. Untraumatized infants' eyes are clear and fully present. The eyes of infants who have experienced shock trauma may not converge normally, but may cross or split as they move their head. This is both an expression of dissociation and of physical birth trauma involving the sphenoid bone, the frontal bone, the superior orbital fissure, the cavernous sinus, and the cranial base generally. Similarly, the infant may not be able to orient to its environment. There may be total or partial inability to orient to visual, auditory, and tactile stimuli. This is again an expression of traumatization, overwhelm, and dissociative states.

Attention affects are another trauma indicator. An infant may seem unable to be fully alert during waking states, unable to hold an object in her attention for even the briefest moment, or may shy away from any eye contact at all. Infants may have difficulty holding an object in their visual field, or maintaining contact with an object. Infants may also have difficulty in voluntarily holding or shifting their attention from person to person. They may have difficulty in negotiating a shift of attention from their inner world to the outside world, or vice versa. They may seem disoriented and spaced-out much of the time. Difficulties in areas of alertness and attention are signs of dissociative processes, and are all signs of traumatization and of the presence of either hyper- or hypoarousal states.

Sensitivity to Contact and Touch

Traumatized infants are highly sensitive to boundary issues and may be retraumatized by touch or contact. Babies relate to the world much more directly through the body than adults do. Their world is literally mediated through their felt-sensory experience, not through their mind and thought processes. They may be very sensitive to near or direct touch, especially if contact is made inadvertently on trauma sites and force vector pathways. Unconscious contact with these sites can be experienced as overwhelming by the infant and can touch off a stress response.

Castellino notes another important touch or contact affect. He writes that traumatized infants may have "total or partial inability to match gentle pressure from direct touch with extremities, head, or trunk of the body" (Castellino 1998). In other words, traumatized infants cannot appropriately respond to your touch. They may recoil, become agitated, or express discontinuous motions when touched. Touch may invoke their trauma schema, and they may then become lost in their shock response.

I sometimes find that I have to first make contact with traumatized infants via their local energetic field. It is sometimes easier for the infant to initially negotiate contact with an off-body touch. Emerson calls this *far touch.* Far touch can be surprisingly effective in revealing the nature of the force vectors present, areas of traumatic impact, and even cranial patterns. Some infants will begin to process their shock affects even more with this kind of touch than with physical contact. For these babies, actual physical tissue contact may become appropriate gradually, over a period of sessions.

Crying Affects

Many times parents will bring their baby in to see me because of issues around the infant's crying. The baby may cry almost constantly, or cry all night, or seem to become lost in the crying. These affects are commonly due to traumatization. Untraumatized infants cry according to their needs, and their crying varies according to what is being communicated. Traumatized infants may cry inappropriately. Their crying seems to be not about present time or present needs, but about the cycling of past trauma. Their bodies may hurt—their birth trauma may cloud their experience of the present—and it may even feel like the trauma is still happening, or that it may again happen at any moment. It is important to remember that in all of this, the baby is trying to communicate how it is, and it is important to learn to listen to this communication. They may express high-pitched, piercing crying, crying that is alternately weak or shallow, and crying that is frequent, perhaps almost constant and without apparent reason. In a cranial context, inertial fulcrums and their effects can actually hurt. These may be felt anywhere in the cranium, occipital triad, spine, pelvis, soma, and viscera—indeed, anywhere in the body! But please remember that we are not just treating physical patterns and symptoms. Babies are fully conscious beings, and their cries are attempts to communicate their suffering.

Thus traumatized infants may cry inconsolably and may get lost in their emotions. In this state they cannot make visual, auditory, or tactile contact and cannot orient to their present environment. They are not in present time, but are in trauma time. It is common in sessions with infants to have periods when these crying processes occur. If the infant gets lost in the trauma schema, it is important to bring him or her back to present time and to resource the infant in mom's presence, and in your present and conscious contact. One simple way of doing this, which can be successful in the short term, is to lift the infant and to consciously, slowly, physically and verbally bring him or her back into physical contact with mom.

Other Autonomic and Reflexive Affects

An infant expressing shock traumatization may display seemingly bizarre autonomic affects during sessions when birth trauma is re-experienced. The infant may have rapid involuntary changes in autonomic responses, such as rapid variations in pulse rate, respiratory rate, skin color, and pupil size. These are all autonomic functions still cycling from the stress response.

Inappropriate expression of the Moro reflex (the startle response) can also indicate trauma. Some traumatized babies may easily express this reflex when stimulated. Alternatively, they may also express the reflex while sleeping. This is so common that it is also often considered to be normal, but untraumatized infants only express this reflex when it is appropriate.

An infant may react to your presence with dissociative fear responses—going quiet and freezing. This is very common, and is not the sign of an accommodating and resourced infant. The intentions of the practitioner can be too overwhelming for infants' systems. They can experience the practitioner's presence as a new invasion or new stress upon their system. It seems to happen more when the practitioner gets into a "doing" mode without really listening and negotiating relationship and contact. The infant becomes overwhelmed by the practitioner's presence, goes into parasympathetic affect states, dissociates, and becomes seemingly accommodating. The practitioner may interpret this passive state as positive and apply more techniques. The structural issues may be helped, but the trauma is driven deeper and the child may even be driven into deeper hypo-states. These infants may sleep better after sessions, but this is the sleep of parasympathetic affect, not of resolved trauma, and they may be actually set up for future problems. Do not confuse the hypo-state with a quiet, resourced, and present baby.

Sleeping, digestive, and eliminative problems may also be present in traumatized babies. Respiratory affects are another common sign of trauma. These may include difficulty breathing, fitful breathing, mouth breathing, and other expressions of respiratory dysfunction. These affects may be due to the cycling of sympathetic energies in the brain stem and its effects on the autonomic nuclei of the central nervous system. They may also be generated by various cranial issues. Compressive fulcrums in the cranium may generate pressures that impinge on major cranial nerves. For instance, compression of the occipital base, intraosseous distortions of the occiput, temporal, or sphenoid bones, medial compression of the temporal bones, occipito-atlanteal compression, and almost any other kind of cranial base pattern can induce compression into the jugular foramen and vagus nerve, leading to digestive, respiratory, and sleeping problems. Issues involving the glossopharyngeal nerve can precede difficulties with the sucking reflex and feeding, while spinal accessory nerve problems can affect the orienting response. These are very common affects left over from birth process, even relatively nontraumatic births. I have treated many babies whose parents brought their baby in because of these kinds of issues, all having their origins in compressive fulcrums affecting cranial nerve function.

Clinical Highlight

I have treated many infants who expressed hypertonic spasticity throughout their bodies and especially in their limbs. This is a sign of frozen fight-or-flight stress responses. In a natural birthing process, babies will push with their legs in conjunction with mother's contractions. This engages and empowers them in their own birth process. This self-empowering process is strongly challenged by traumatic impacts, anesthesia, and autonomic overwhelm. The following clinical highlight describes one such baby and her healing process.

A good number of years ago, I worked with a newborn infant who expressed the startle response with any contact and had continual spasticity in her upper and lower limbs. She could not orient and inappropriately expressed fear responses and displayed almost continual shaking or trembling. Orthodox medical investigation did not uncover neurological damage or pathology. This seemed to be a situation in which her system was continually trying to resolve its shock, but did not have the resources to complete the process. She was caught in a hyperarousal stress response. The trauma-bound energy in her central nervous system could not successfully be processed, and this affected the cerebellum and midbrain structures that relate to muscular coordination and tissue tonicity. This was all coupled with a limbic and autonomic fear response. Her fluid tide was almost nonexistent, with much potency bound up in centering the activation present.

It took a number of months of slow and careful work for her to resolve a large part of her trauma and to orient to her world appropriately. What seemed most important was the slowness of my approach to her, my receptive and attuned state, the establishment of a resourced space with infant, mom, and myself, and the very gradual negotiation of physical contact. The negotiation of contact was most critical so that the cycling energies in her system were not driven deeper by a fear response to my presence. She needed to be empowered to say yes or no in her own way.

Long Tide orientation, stillpoint process, and stillness generally were all useful starting points. Over a good number of sessions, the baby began to orient to present time and settle into contact much more easily. She also began to complete her need to push and kick—which was overwhelmed in the birth process—by slowly pushing against my hands while in eye contact with both mom and myself. We worked on various inertial fulcrums, birth movement patterns, and cranial issues, and over a period of six months her fluid tide expressed itself with much more potency and she was more able to express her needs via the social engagement system. She resolved a great deal of her sympathetic cycling, her spasticity softened, and her development sped up. She was able to bond with her mother, sleep better, and orient more easily to her environment.

The Birth Schema

The concept of the *birth schema,* as developed by Emerson in his work with babies, covers a huge territory. It encompasses the whole matrix of interwoven effects of birth—the totality of all physical, physiological, and psycho-emotional effects left over from birth process. Physical components may involve physical pain, inertial patterns, restrictions, fixations, and specific motions. Each person's birth schema is unique and personal and relates directly to responses and reactions during the birth process.

To appreciate the full scope of a birth schema, we need to expand our horizons beyond the actual birth event. Subtle factors from the earliest stages of incarnation—including conception, implantation, and the womb experience itself—may color and even shape the baby's experience of birth. The parents' relationship may be a factor, as may mom's experiences during pregnancy such as a physical injury, stress, illness, or major family or societal events. The baby is an energetic-emotional-physical composite expression of all these factors.

I have worked with a good number of adults in Britain, who were in their mother's womb during the Second World War and the bombing of British cities. This clearly affected their early experience, attachment issues, and ego formation. It also generated real limbic and autonomic stress issues that were still cycling in their systems, with a real need for resolution. The following is a summary of some important aspects of the birth schema.

Birth Schema Components

- Psychological correlates and trauma memory

- Shock traumatization

- Force vector patterns and related inertial fulcrums

- Ignition issues

- Patterns of energy, fluids, and potency

- Birth lie position

- Conjunct sites (sites of impact)

- Conjunct pathways

- Inertial patterns and micro-movement patterns

- Macro (gross) movement patterns and body position, tissue tone, and patterns of tension, contraction, and flaccidity

Psychological Correlates

Psychological correlates are the attitudes and expectations that we hold, derived from family, culture, and other sources. These can set the stage for a person's sense of self, attachment processes, and how we perceive our world. The experience of the prenatal and birth period sets a tonal quality for our perception of ourselves, our world, and other people. Life statements such as "the world is good" or "the world is bad" or "I always get what I need" or "life is a struggle" can derive from our earliest experiences. Some psychological correlate categories are summarized below.

Mistaken Assumptions

These are beliefs about self or the world based on the limited perspective of the infant in the womb and in the birthing process. These may be things such as "I never get what I need" or "the world is a bad place and I want to escape it." These assumptions can infuse into our sense of self and of the world we live in, and into all our relationships.

Life Statements

These are deeply held beliefs about the world and our sense of self in the world based on our experience and reactions to experience in the prenatal and birth period. Life statements like "I always get hurt in intimate relationships" or "the closer I get to someone, the more threatened I get" or "the closer I get to someone, the more space I need" can obstruct true intimacy. Such statements may be derived from the pain of the birth process, relating to the very intimate relationship with mom.

Character Formation and Psychological Strategies

The first period of life can color our early childhood experience as the foundations of attachment processes, character formation, and psychological defense systems are developing. These affect how we later negotiate our way through life. Psychodynamic strategies are based upon the foundation of our earliest experience. Prenatal and birthing experience must not be neglected when doing work in a psychological or psychotherapeutic context.

Emotional Patterns

The emotional effects of prenatal and birthing experience can be the foundation of our later emotional life and can underpin our childhood and adult feelings about our world and ourselves. How we negotiated the birth experience may set the stage for how we later negotiate our way through life and express or repress emotions. Indeed, we may live our life through the sensations and feeling-tones of birth—reacting as though the current situation is similarly threatening—expressing inappropriate states of anxiety, fear, and anger. Alternatively, these strong emotions may be perceived to be overwhelming and life threatening, and some people will organize their personality system, and their life choices, in ways that protect against experiencing them, and may even develop dissociative personalities. All of these processes may have had their roots in the prenatal and birth experience.

Boundary Issues

The birth process is the first real physical experience that brings us clearly into relationship with physical boundaries and potentially traumatic experience. How we negotiate this experience as an infant may set the stage for our later perceptions of personal boundaries and an integrated sense of selfhood. The birth process is commonly coupled with issues around how we negotiate interpersonal contact, how we come into new relationships, how we experience moving toward others or the things and processes in our lives, how we experience being approached by others, and how we sense the presence of another in our space—these are all aspects of boundary issues.

Orienting Issues

Loss of boundary—and the cycling of shock trauma in the system—can lead to difficulties in orienting. One level of autonomic processing is called the *orienting response*—the ability to scan our environment and respond to conditions. Babies use this response to orient to mom and caregivers and to environmental input. The orienting response is also part of our autonomic response to novel or potentially dangerous situations. It allows us to scan our surroundings and identify threat. People may lose the ability to orient to those around them, to stressful situations or processes, or even to life itself. People with orientation issues may set up their lives so that they live in a narrow band of experience that is easier or safer to manage. Unique or novel situations may be continuously experienced as threatening.

Alternatively, orientation issues may arise mainly when under stress. People may lose the ability to respond to situations that are stressful or novel and may even develop personality systems that avoid conflict or the need to assert themselves. They may have great difficulty in asserting their needs.

Intimacy Issues

The prenatal and birthing experience is one of the most intimate experiences of our lives. The intense intimacy of bonding with mom is perceived as critical to survival. How this is experienced sets the stage for later issues around intimacy. How do we enter relationship? Do we expect to have our needs met? Is there trust? Do we protect ourselves from intimacy? How do we do this? Do we find close and intimate contact painful or joyful? When a relationship gets "too close," do we withdraw and run away? These questions and related issues all can arise out of our earliest experience. For many people the most painful emotional and psychological life issues revolve around the safety and trustworthiness of intimate relationships.

Life Goals and Tendencies

Our sense of self in the world and our life goals and direction can be supported or impeded by our response and reactions to prenatal and birth experience. I have met many people who, whenever they attempted a new direction in life, were stopped by feelings of impending doom or suffocation. Likewise, they may feel suffocated in personal relationships, or stressful situations and tend to withdraw from intimacy.

Alternatively, I have met people who could not stick with the intensity or struggle of reaching their goals. All of these kinds of issues can reflect our birthing experience.

Trauma and Emotional Memory

The psychological correlates discussed above are commonly coupled with emotional memories of traumatic origin. *Trauma memory* refers to emotionally charged implicit memories derived from traumatic experience. These are often coupled with autonomic cycling and tissue patterns. It is important to understand that an infant's defensive and emotional responses to stress are fully operational during the birthing process. If the infant is overwhelmed, these unresolved memories and stress responses can continue to cycle in the infant's systems if not resolved during or soon after the experience.

Implicit emotional memories are generated by processing in the amygdala, which accesses the importance of an experience and gives it emotional tone, and the hippocampus, which relates the present experience to the past, leading to short-term associative processes. This eventually leads to long-term indexing and storage of the experience elsewhere in the cortex. Implicit, emotional memory processing is fully functional in the infant, even in the womb. In the presence of trauma, the homeostasis of this processing system can be disturbed. If the amygdala assesses an experience as an overwhelming threat, neurochemical changes occur that may continue to cycle in the system. Memory becomes less reliable, the system may become hypersensitive to sensory input, and responses may no longer relate to present-time life experience. Traumatized babies and children may then experience anxiety, hyperactivity, depression, hyper- or hyposensitivity, and/or dissociation, all unrelated to apparent current events. It is not uncommon during sessions for babies and adults to re-experience these early trauma memories as the forces are activated and resolved.

Conjunct Sites and Pathways

Emerson, in his years of work with infants and adults, developed a unique understanding of birth process, which found its way into many forms of work. He coined terms such as *conjunct site*, and *conjunct pathway*, in order to clarify the nature of birth process. During the birth process, the infant makes firm physical contact with mom's pelvis. The conjunct site is the site, or part of the infant's cranium or body, that makes contact with the maternal pelvis. High levels of force can be applied at these sites. Some babies show significant bruises at these sites when they first appear. The conjunct site patterns in the baby's body may show these points of impact, sometimes in great detail. The position of the baby in the womb and in the birth canal, the shape of the mother's pelvis, and the nature of the delivery—such as a mobile versus a restrained mom, a bed/dry birth versus a water birth, and so on—all contribute to the conjunct site content.

There are obviously many conjunct sites during the birth process. Various parts of the baby's body will contact specific parts of mom's pelvis. Some contacts are of particular significance in cranial molding and distortion patterns. Mom's sacrum and pubic bones are especially potent sources for conjunct sites and the introduction of strong forces into the baby's system.

Conjunct pathways are the pathways of conjunct sites, or parts of the baby's body that are in contact with mother's pelvic structures as the infant passes through the birth canal. There are typical conjunct pathways for the different stages of birth and for different maternal pelvic shapes.

If the infant experienced trauma at a specific conjunct site, it then is also a trauma site. Force vectors will become associated with it, and, if the infant is later touched at or near the site, a trauma response may arise. This may include a startle response or an expression of shock affect such as autonomic activation, dissociation, or strong emotion. If the infant was stuck at that site—and was overwhelmed by the experience—then hypersensitivity and autonomic activation are more likely. The site itself may be hypersensitive and become associated with trauma.

Force Vectors and Vector Patterns

The forces encountered as babies meet conjunct sites in the birth canal will introduce vector patterns into their system. These are sometimes called *force vectors*. A force vector is simply the pattern that a traumatic force takes as it enters one's body space. The force itself will be centered by potency in some way and generate an inertial fulcrum, or fulcrums, which is the heart of treatment process. Generally, when an inertial fulcrum resolves in a state of balance and deepening equilibrium, the vector pattern it took also resolves. Commonly as the traumatic force resolves, it will leave the body either via a general expansion and release of heat, or via the original vector pattern it took.

Force vectors can be important aspects of the total birth schema, as specific physical events during birth are registered in the tissues. In the birth process inertial forces—and the vector patterns they take—are generated as the baby meets the physical structure of mom's pelvis—so in the birth context we expect to find the origins in the baby's being pushed against mom's sacrum or pelvic bone, being pulled out with forceps or vacuum extraction, or experiencing similar external forces. Castellino writes about force vectors:

> If the baby's ability to integrate the experience psychically, emotionally, or physically is compromised, these vector patterns are especially amplified in the baby's memory systems. The vector forces actually transmit the trauma through the baby's structures. In the cranium the vector patterns will cause cranial lesion patterns which are birth-stage specific.
>
> (Castellino 1998)

Thus the forces introduced in the birth process literally transmit the traumatic experience throughout the body structures via the vector patterns they take. These vector patterns are amplified in the baby's memory systems. These memories are mainly emotional and physical in nature. The inertial fulcrums associated with force vectors also generate tissue contractions and patterns around the related inertial fulcrums, which get coupled with the implicit emotional memories of the original experience.

Remember that the infant experiences the world through its body and its felt-sensations. There will thus be psychological and emotional processes of traumatic origin coupled to the forces introduced by birth, and to the fulcrums and inertial patterns they generate. The whole of this is sometimes called a *force vector pattern*. A force vector pattern may seem to have a particular directionality to its expression, reflecting the actual lines of force and echoes of the original impact.

Force vector patterns are reflections of unresolved traumatic forces and the inertial fulcrums and tissue patterns they generate. They are also consistent with the trauma sites and movement pathways of the birth process as the infant passes through the birth canal. Babies will exhibit movement patterns that relate to the unresolved birthing forces and related vectors patterns held in their system. Thus, fragmented and discontinuous motion patterns are a direct expression of the birthing process and of the forces and vector patterns still held in an infant's body. These unresolved forces and vector patterns will commonly become coupled with fight-or-flight emotions such as fear and anger, and/or with parasympathetic freezing and dissociative states.

Connective Tissue Patterning

Connective tissue responds to the forces of birth—and the fulcrums they generate—by contracting. This is part of the overall protective response to overwhelming experience. If these forces remain unresolved, the resulting contracted tissue state may be held as a defensive tendency throughout life.

Connective tissue patterns are often coupled with emotional memory. The original stress elicits a sympathetic nervous system and emotional reaction—fight and flight being coupled with anger and fear—which are responses both to the overwhelming experience and to the unresolved forces introduced into the system.

For example, an infant may have experienced strong compressive forces during birth that were accompanied by fear and tissue contraction in the system. As an adult, the same person may respond to stress at work or in a close relationship in the same way that he or she responded to birth. Thus, under stress, the person may re-experience the shock trauma, may contract, may react emotionally and psychologically inappropriately, and may express physical symptoms such as headaches or digestive problems. This is because the forces of the original experience are still held in the neuroendocrine, fluid, and tissue systems, and they are physically expressed in protective connective tissue contractions and compressive issues in the body. These patterns will become set tendencies in the tissues of the body and will tend to become expressed as tension and strain in its defensive processes. Under stress, the system will tend to defend itself by contracting in the same historical, protective ways it already knows, which reinforces the existing trauma schema and physical tensions already present.

Fluid Shock

A traumatic birth process introduces systemic forces throughout the baby's system, which can generate what is known as *fluid shock*. Fluid shock occurs when overwhelming forces enter the system, generating systemwide shock. Potency in the fluid body then acts systemically to center the shock affects present and the fluid system locks down in protective response. This strongly affects the vitality of the fluid tide—further affecting the vitality of the whole system—and lowers available resources for life's activities.

In the birth process systemic shock is commonly centered in the cerebrospinal fluid. The infant's fluid core may seem to be inertial and the fluid tide may be difficult to perceive. This may be due to the fact that the axial forces of the birth process especially impinge upon the cranium and vertebral axis—the core of cerebrospinal fluctuation. I have held newborns' craniums that were dense and deeply inertial with a loss of resiliency and motility due to the presence of fluid shock.

Some babies I have seen have had such extreme fluid shock and related tissue compression that their heads felt like small cannon balls. This is especially the case in cesarean births, as the rapid change in pressure experienced induces a shock response in the core of the fluid system. It is sad and sobering to see this in such young infants.

Furthermore, venous sinus drainage may be compromised due to the strain placed on the reciprocal tension membrane system by the birthing forces and related inertial fulcrums generated. This can also lead to inertial cerebrospinal fluid, resultant fluid stasis and lowered vitality, and to lethargic and hypotonic babies. Coupled with shock trauma, fluid congestion can be a significant source of devitalization. The system may be unable to constitutionally resource itself, and thus potency cannot be fully expressed.

I have also noted traumatically induced fluid congestion and shock affects due to vacuum extraction (ventouse). The vacuum force placed upon the cranium is an abnormal force that the system is not naturally designed to meet. The Aqueduct of Sylvius (the great cerebral aqueduct) is sucked cephalad during the vacuum extraction procedure. Due to the induced shock affects, unresolved traumatic forces, and related membranous tensions and cranial molding patterns, the aqueduct may not fully return to its natural anatomical position. This can generate important repercussions, especially in later life as the expression of potency and fluid drive are compromised. The person may have backpressure against the normal circulation of CSF to the fourth ventricle, as well as compromised fluid fluctuation in the third ventricle. The result is lowered potency and vitality. Augmentation of potency and fluid drive through the aqueduct from above may be a useful starting point when you meet this condition in an infant or adult and is very effective in infant session work when appropriate.

Ignition Issues

Sutherland coined the term *ignition* to denote the lighting up or ignition of the forces of life in the cerebrospinal fluid. As described in some detail in Volume One, ignition is a primal process whereby the intentions of the Breath of Life manifest in form. There is an ignition process at conception in which the blueprint of the human system is laid down as an organizing field in and around the conceptus. It occurs as the Long Tide manifests its ordering winds, and a stable ordering matrix is laid down. A bioelectric ordering field is generated and organizing fulcrums and midlines are expressed. In this process, the Long Tide ignites an ordering force in the fluids of the embryo. Sutherland called this process of ignition of potency in the fluid system *transmutation*. Ignition processes, as described in Volume One, can be sensed throughout life. The bioelectric field and transmutation processes are continually maintained throughout life, from the moment of conception until the day we die. As introduced earlier, some wonderful new research at Tufts University has shown frog embryos being formed in the action of bioelectric fields not mediated by genes, but by a deeper ordering principle (Jonathan 2011).

A further important ignition occurs at birth. When the umbilical cord stops pulsing and the first breath is taken, a powerful ignition of potency occurs at the umbilical center along the midline of the newborn, allowing the infant to be a separate, fully functioning physiological entity. Birth ignition is an expression of our most fundamental empowerment to incarnate as a human being (Figure 4.3). If there is traumatization during the birth process, this ignition process may not be fully expressed. Negative umbilical affect, anesthesia, birth trauma, and too-early cutting of the cord will affect this ignition process. Lowered potency and vitality result. Birth ignition issues are very common. I have found many adults with chronic fatigue and exhaustion whose etiology traces back to ignition issues, birth trauma, negative umbilical affect, anesthesia, medical interventions during birth, and bonding-attachment issues.

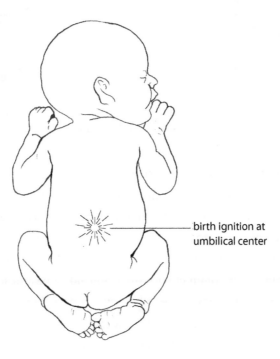

birth ignition at umbilical center

Figure 4.3. Ignition of potency after birth

Birth Lie Position

In the description of the birthing process, below, we use terminology that differs from that used in orthodox obstetrics. In orthodox obstetric terminology, the *lie position* relates to the general position of the infant in the womb. The traditional lies are *longitudinal*, in which the long axis of the infant is parallel to the long axis of the mother, and *transverse*, in which the long axis of the infant is perpendicular to the long axis of the mother (Figure 4.4).

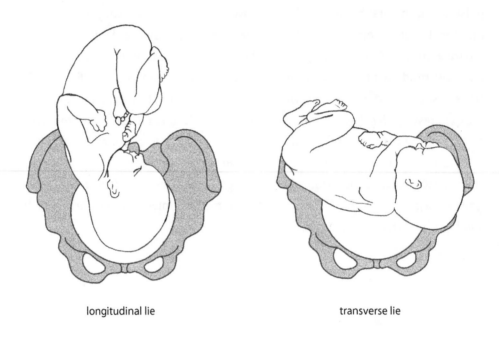

longitudinal lie   transverse lie

Figure 4.4. The longitudinal and transverse birth positions according to conventional obstetrics.

Our use of the term *birth lie* derives from the work of Emerson. In his paradigm, the birth lie of the infant relates to the aspect of the infant that is conjunct, or in relationship, with the mother's spine and sacrum. Hence, a *left birth lie* means that the left side of the infant's cranium is in contact with the mother's spine and lumbosacral promontory (see Figure 5.1). Alternatively, a *right birth lie* means that the infant's right side is conjunct with the maternal spine and sacrum. When I discuss specific birth dynamics in the following chapters, I use the term *non-birth lie side* to denote the side opposite the birth lie side. The non-birth lie side commonly conjuncts with the anterior aspects of the mother's pelvic structures, especially the pubic symphysis and the pubic arch.

The birth lie position is the starting point for the baby's journey through the birth canal. Determining the birth lie side helps us visualize, attune to, and empathize with the baby's birth process. Knowing the birth lie side gives a clear reference point for perceiving the rest of the baby's birth patterns and motions, and helps us orient to the whole birth process with greater clarity.

The True Pelvis and the Pelvic Inlet and Outlet

In classic terminology, the pelvis is divided into two basic areas—the false pelvis and the true pelvis. The false pelvis lies above the pelvic brim. The true pelvis lies below the pelvic brim and is the bony canal through which the infant must pass. The true pelvis is composed of the pelvic inlet, the pelvic cavity (mid-pelvis), and the pelvic outlet. The pelvic inlet is bounded anteriorly by the pubic symphysis and arch, laterally by the iliopectineal lines on the innominate bones, and posteriorly by the sacral ala and promontory. It is basically a plane between the sacral promontory and the pubic symphysis. The pelvic outlet is bounded anteriorly by the arcuate pubic ligament and the inferior aspect of the pubic arch, laterally by the ischial tuberosities and sacrotuberous ligaments and posteriorly by the tip of the coccyx. It is basically the plane between the most inferior coccyx bone and the inferior aspect of the pubic arch. The mid-pelvis is the space between these two (Figure 4.5).

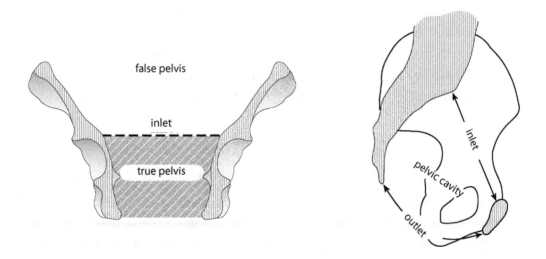

Figure 4.5. True pelvis and pelvic inlet and outlet.

Pelvic Shapes

Each birthing mother has her own unique pelvic shape and structure, and these are also part of the birth schema. Different pelvic shapes can have strong influences upon the birthing process. The pelvic shape categories were determined and named in the 1930s by medical researchers Caldwell, Moloy, and D'Esopo. They x-rayed and studied the pelvic shapes of more than 500 women in the era before x-rays were considered to be dangerous. They discovered four basic pelvic shapes that they called gynecoid, android, anthropoid, and platypelloid.

The *gynecoid pelvis* is apple or oval shaped. Its transverse diameter is a little longer than its anterior-posterior diameter. Its widest transverse dimension is located approximately one-third of the distance from the sacrum. It is the most common type. According to Harry Oxorn, it is present in fifty percent of Caucasian women (Oxorn 1986). Some other authorities cite fifty-five percent.

The *android pelvic* shape is sometimes called *heart-shaped*. It is triangular in shape, has a narrow pubic arch, and its transverse dimension is slightly wider than its anterior-posterior dimension. Its widest transverse dimension is closer to the sacrum than in the gynecoid pelvis.

The *anthropoid pelvis* is oval or olive shaped. Its anterior-posterior dimension is longer than its transverse dimension. Its widest transverse dimension is almost halfway between the sacrum and the pubic arch. It is the most common type in African and Asian women.

Finally, the *platypelloid pelvis* is plate-like, very flat transversely—a long transverse oval. It is long in its transverse dimension and short in its anterior-posterior dimension. It is the least common pelvic shape and is the most difficult for birthing. Each pelvic shape will be outlined in greater detail when we explore the various types of typical birth patterns in our next two chapters (Figure 4.6).

Synclitic and Asynclitic Positions

Just before labor begins, the infant's cranium and body may be in a number of positions relative to the mother's pelvic inlet. These positions relate to the angle in which, in a head-first birth, the infant's cranium enters the inlet of the pelvis. This is called the *angle of descent.* The angle of descent is defined by a flat transverse plane through the infant's head at the level of the sphenoid bone and the relationship of that plane to the mother's pelvic inlet. This transverse plane is called the *occipito-frontal plane.* The transverse diameter across the infant's cranium is called

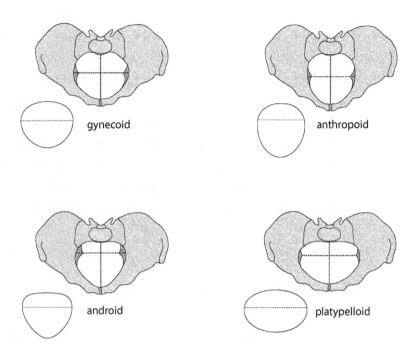

Figure 4.6. Pelvic shapes.

the *biparietal diameter* (Figure 4.7). The positions are named according to the angle this plane makes with the mother's pelvic inlet. These angles of descent have clear repercussions for the types of inertial patterns seen in infant and adult craniums. We will explore these in our next two chapters.

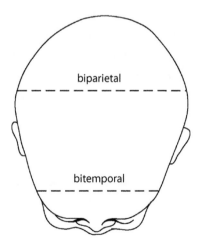

Figure 4.7. The biparietal and bitemporal diameters.

If the infant's occipito-frontal plane descends parallel to the plane of the maternal pelvic inlet, the entry is called *synclitic*. Synclitic births generally occur when the pelvis is spacious and there is plenty of room to descend. In synclitic births, the mother's uterus is basically perpendicular to her pelvic inlet, the infant's occipito-frontal plane is parallel with the mother's pelvic inlet, and its sagittal suture lies midway between the sacral promontory and the pubic symphysis.

If the infant's cranium descends into the inlet at an angle, it is called *asynclitic*. There are two types of asynclitic births, anterior and posterior. In most women, the pregnant uterus is held in a relatively upright position by the abdominal wall, parallel to the mother's spine, and it is in a posterior position relative to the plane of the pelvic inlet. This generally prevents the uterus from lying in a plane perpendicular to the inlet. As the infant descends in this position, the posterior parietal bone is lower than the anterior parietal bone, and the sagittal suture is closer to the pubic symphysis than it is to the sacral promontory. Thus, the posterior parietal bone descends first. The occipito-frontal plane is at an oblique angle to the pelvic inlet. This position is called *posterior asynclitic*. This is the most common position of descent.

In synclitic positions, the infant's parietal eminences enter the pelvic inlet at the same time. In asynclitic presentations, the parietal eminences enter one at a time, making the diameter smaller and less subject to pressure. There is thus a mechanical advantage in posterior asynclitic entries, with a narrower diameter presented to the pelvic inlet than that found with a synclitic position.

If the mother's abdominal muscles are lax—as is common in overweight women—the uterus and baby may fall anteriorly and the bulk of the baby's body is then held more anteriorly in the abdomen. In this position, the angle of descent is different from that of a synclitic or posterior asynclitic descent. The angle of descent is again oblique, but, unlike in posterior asynclitism, the anterior parietal bone descends first and is lower than the posterior parietal bone. The anterior parietal bone is conjunct with the pubic symphysis, and the sagittal suture lies closer to the sacral promontory than to the pubic symphysis. The descent is then called *anterior asynclitic* (Figure 4.8).

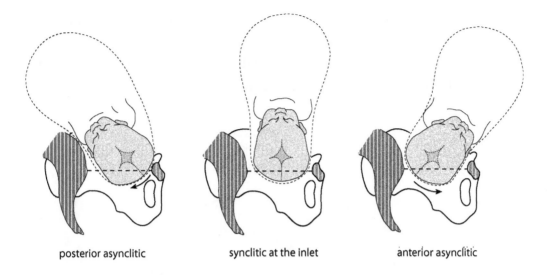

posterior asynclitic   synclitic at the inlet   anterior asynclitic

Figure 4.8. Asynclitic and synclitic positions.

Traditional Terminology for Position

In traditional obstetrical terminology, position is the relationship of a particular part of the baby, called the *denominator,* to the mother's pelvis. The terminology is used to describe the presenting position of the baby. The most common denominator is the occiput. Others are the *frontum* (forehead) for brow presentations and the *mentum* (chin) for face presentations. There are three sets of abbreviations used to describe the position of the baby as it presents to the obstetrician or midwife:

- *The denominator:* O = occiput, M = chin, Fr = forehead (frontal bone)

- *Contact or conjunct site with the mother's pelvis:* The side of the mother's pelvis that the denominator is in contact with. L (left) indicates the left side of the mother's pelvis, R (right) indicates the right side of the mother's pelvis, and no letter indicates that the dominator is directly anterior or posterior.

- *The position of the denominator relative to the mother's pelvis:* A (anterior) indicates that the denominator is in an anterior position in the pelvis, P (posterior) indicates that the denominator is in a posterior position in the pelvis, and T (transverse) indicates that the denominator is in relationship to the side of the mother's pelvis and the cranium is thus transversely oriented in the pelvis.

Thus, LOA indicates that the occiput is conjunct with the left anterior side of the mother's pelvis. In other words, the baby's occiput is pointing to the left anterior side of mother's pelvis. OA would indicate that the baby's occiput is directly pointing anterior and is conjunct with the pubic arch (Figure 4.9).

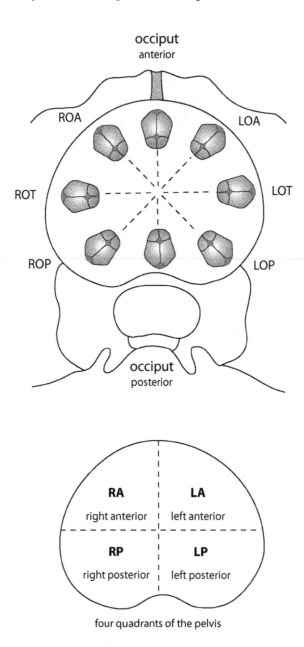

Figure 4.9. Classic positions of the occiput.

Station

The word *station* denotes the relationship of the presenting part of the infant to an imaginary line drawn between the ischial tuberosities of the mother's pelvis. This line is a reference point that helps obstetricians and midwives to talk about the depth of descent that the infant has accomplished at any time. The imaginary line across the ischial tuberosities is called *station zero,* or 0. Above the spines the next station is minus 1 (one centimeter above 0), and this continues to minus 5, which is an imaginary line across the pelvic inlet. Below the spines, the station is plus 1, 2, 3, and so on, until at plus 5 the infant is crowning at the pelvic outlet (Figure 4.10).

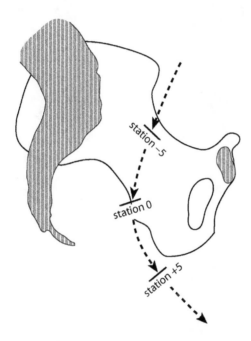

Figure 4.10. The "station" of the presenting part of the baby.

Inlet Attitudes

Inlet attitudes refer to the attitude or entry position of the infant's head at the beginning of labor. It indicates the position of the head as the infant enters the maternal pelvic inlet. The attitude of the infant as it enters the pelvic inlet can obviously have major implications for its experience of Stage One and the subsequent stages of birth (Figure 4.11). The basic attitudes are:

- The *military attitude,* or *median presentation:* The infant's head is aligned with its spinal axis. It is neither in flexion nor extension. The vertex of its cranium is centered in the inlet.

- *Bregma presentation:* The infant's bregma presents to the maternal inlet.

- *Brow presentation:* The infant's brow presents to the maternal inlet.

- *Face presentation:* The infant's face presents to the maternal inlet.

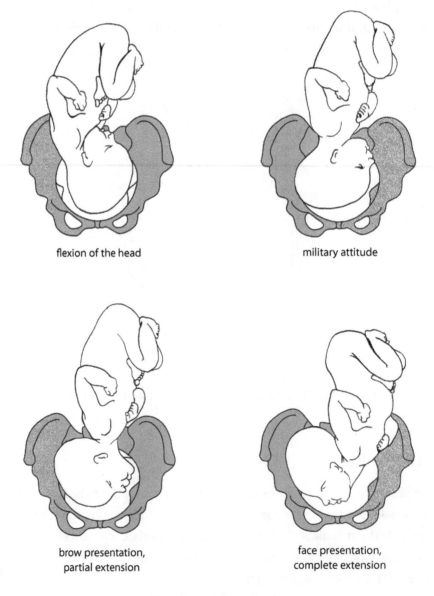

flexion of the head

military attitude

brow presentation,
partial extension

face presentation,
complete extension

Figure 4.11. Inlet attitudes.

Stages of the Birth Process

Different birthing dynamics occur in each region of the pelvis, as described by the *stages of birth*. Mainstream obstetrics uses a three-stage birth process description; however, I prefer the four-stage categorization developed by Sills and Emerson in the mid-1980s and further clarified by Castellino. It relates much more directly to the actual motions in the birth process and to the experience of the infant. Emerson has also outlined typical psychological correlates relating to each birth stage and to each pelvic type.

In the common obstetrical view, there are three stages of labor. The first stage begins at the onset of labor and ends at the complete dilation of the cervix. The second stage begins at the complete dilation of the cervix and continues to the birth

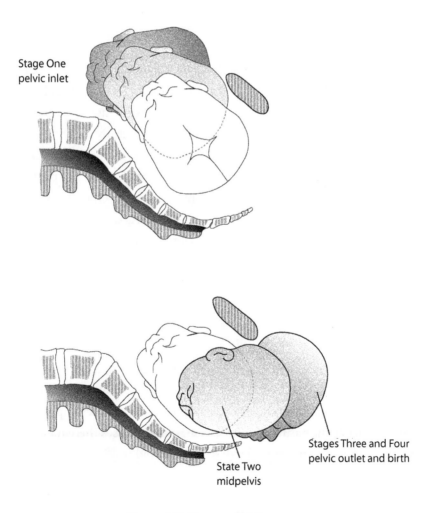

Figure 4.12. Stages of birth.

of the baby. Finally, the third stage begins at the birth of the baby and continues to the delivery of the placenta. Both Emerson and I have concluded that these stages do not give a clear description of the baby's journey and do not reflect the baby's own experience and the tasks that must be negotiated for successful birth and bonding. Having four stages seems to enable a more accurate description.

In the four-stage system, Stage One relates to the dynamics of the pelvic inlet, Stage Two relates to experiences of the mid-pelvis, Stage Three relates to the dynamics of motion around and through the pelvic outlet, and Stage Four relates to actual birth of the head and body, to umbilical issues, and to the entire process of bonding and attachment. These stages are summarized below and described in much more detail in the next chapter. Having an accurate understanding of these relationships helps in attuning to, and empathizing with, the infant's journey though them (Figure 4.12).

Stage One—Inlet Dynamics

Following the beginning of contractions, the infant descends into the pelvic inlet. This stage is therefore also called Stage One, inlet dynamics. The baby's head experiences the first of a series of compressive forces as the uterus pushes against the resisting pelvic tissues. In a gynecoid pelvis, it is generally a transverse or oblique descent, and this position will vary with each different pelvic shape. Stage One has two basic phases. Phase one is the descent into the pelvic inlet, and phase two occurs when the infant moves over the sacral promontory. Stage One ends when the cervix is fully dilated and the infant enters the mid-pelvis. As this occurs, the infant's head commonly begins to rotate toward the maternal sacrum. In Stage One the lie side cranium is in strong contact with the maternal lumbosacral promontory. If the infant gets stuck here, the conjunct site can become a strong source for generating inertial fulcrums, cranial patterns, and overwhelming experiences.

Stage Two—Mid-Pelvis Dynamics

Stage Two occurs mainly in the mid-pelvis. In Stage Two, the cervix is fully dilated and the infant's cranium commonly rotates toward the maternal sacrum. Stage Two ends when the infant is facing the sacrum. Different pelvic shapes and sizes will greatly influence the nature of this descent. In some cases there may be little or no rotation, such as in a posterior birth or platypelloid pelvis.

Stage Three—Outlet Dynamics

Here the infant must negotiate its way through the pelvic outlet. In this phase, the infant's cranium is typically oriented in an anterior-posterior position relative to the mother's pelvis. This stage also has two phases. In phase one, in a typical birth, the infant's cranium is in lateral flexion, and its nose is toward its shoulder. As the infant descends, its cranium must first go into a flexion position to negotiate its movement around the pubic arch. In the second phase the baby's head moves into an extension position in order to continue its descent through the arch. This stage can take the longest to negotiate, with infants frequently becoming stuck here for periods of time. Medical interventions such as forceps delivery commonly occur here.

Stage Four—Restitution, Head and Body Birth

This is the last birth stage and includes a number of processes. Restitution occurs when the baby's head is born and realigns with its shoulder position. The body is then born. Once the baby is born, its umbilicus must stop pulsating, the placenta must be born, and self-attachment and bonding to the mother occurs. Self-attachment denotes the baby's own intention to connect with mom and attach to her breast. The untraumatized baby will actually push itself up its mother's body to reach the breast and will naturally attach itself to her breast. This takes time and nurturing both for baby and mom and does not usually occur in hurried modern hospital births, a great loss for us all. Some authorities consider this process important in the bonding and attachment processes and in the empowerment of the infant to get what it needs. Medical interventions commonly occur here, interrupting the natural process of bonding in favor of examining and cleaning the baby.

Stage Four also includes the early months of life outside of the womb, a period in which loving contact and secure attachment can naturally heal much of the shock or trauma experienced during the birth process. In our next chapter, we will look at these stages in some detail in relationship to different maternal pelvic shapes.

CHAPTER 5

Basic Birth Dynamics

Using our overview of the birthing process from Chapter 4, this chapter presents the specific forces at work in each birth stage. A thorough knowledge of the birth process gives practitioners a deeper capacity for empathy and more accurate comprehension of factors affecting their clients, leading to more efficient clinical results.

This chapter's exploration makes use of terms from Chapter 11, where we discuss classic cranial base patterning in some detail. These include inhalation-exhalation patterns, side-bending, torsion, lateral or vertical shear, and compression. In clinical sessions, you will find that the most intransigent inertial fulcrums and related cranial base patterns are commonly generated from unresolved birthing forces. Because of this, in our foundation training, we discuss the process of birth before we present cranial base patterns.

In this chapter we describe how the forces introduced in the various stages of birth can generate these patterns. The inertial fulcrums that the birthing process introduces into the system also generate patterns of compression, traction, torsion, and shear throughout the body. As we describe all of this, please remember that cranial base patterns are not separate from connective tissue and membranous tensions and other fulcrums and inertial issues throughout the body.

To help understand the birthing process, I highly recommend a good textbook on birth and labor, such as *Human Labor and Birth* by Harry Oxorn (Oxorn 1986). Our chapters on birthing are not meant to be a full course on working with infants, but rather serve as an introduction to the subject. To work with infants, the best approach is to apprentice with an experienced practitioner and/or to take postgraduate courses in the subject.

Typical Birth Process

As introduced in the last chapter, we will begin our exploration of a typical birth process in terms of four stages. Again, these are not the traditional obstetrical stages, but are derived from an appreciation of the baby's physical and emotional experience during the birthing process. In this exploration we define the stages of birth in terms of the tasks the infant must complete in order to be born. During the birth process the infant experiences positional and movement changes as well as great variations in sensations of pressure, compression, torsion, and shear. All of these factors are expressed in every level of the system. The inertial forces generated by the experience affect potency, fluids, and tissues as a unified field. The whole tissue field—including bone, membrane, structural integrity and balance, CNS motility and function, and so on—is affected by and will express these birthing forces. The total response is not just structural or physical, but includes a full spectrum—from tissue and fluid effects, to emotional processes, to autonomic stress states, including both sympathetic and parasympathetic responses.

The infant begins the birth process in a variety of positions when true labor starts—when maternal contractions are regular and about twenty to thirty minutes apart. Many babies start in a posterior position and then rotate to one side or the other. The most common pelvic type in caucasians is the gynecoid pelvis, and the most common beginning position is baby lying with her left side conjunct to mother's spine. The left side of the baby's head and body contacts the mother's lumbosacral promontory and spine. Some variation of this starting position is seen in 50–55 percent of births (Oxorn 1986). We call this the *left birth lie* position (Figure 5.1).

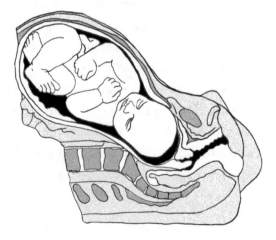

Figure 5.1. Left birth lie position: baby's left side is conjunct with mother's spine.

The common positions of entry into the pelvic inlet include *left occiput anterior, left occiput posterior,* and *left occiput transverse.* The following explanation is based on a common starting position, the left occiput transverse engagement (LOT). In this position, the infant's cranium is in a transverse relationship to the maternal pelvis; the sagittal suture of the infant is in the transverse diameter of the pelvis. Oblique starting positions are also common, as are posterior positions. Other common left birth lie positions include left occiput anterior (LOA) and left occiput posterior (LOP), each yielding an oblique orientation (Figure 5.2).

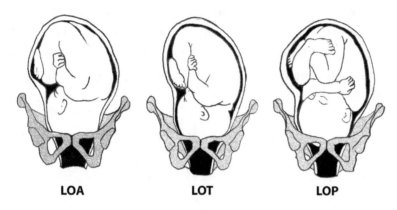

Figure 5.2. Typical left conjunct lie positions.

In the following sections, we will describe the dynamics of a birth through a *gynecoid pelvic inlet.* As described in our last chapter, the gynecoid pelvic inlet is an oval-round shape. Its transverse diameter is a little longer than its anterior-posterior diameter. It is sometimes called an apple-shaped pelvis. Its inlet shape is oval to round, and its widest transverse dimension is located approximately one-third of the distance from the sacrum (Figure 5.3). Many variations in positions and forms of movement are possible. The following sections describe typical birthing motions and emphasize the potential introduction of strong birthing forces, the vector patterns they take, and the inertial fulcrums they generate.

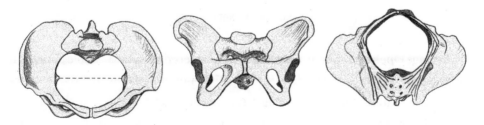

Figure 5.3. Gynecoid pelvic shape.

Stage One: Pelvic Inlet Dynamics

Stage One begins when contractions begin. In the LOT position, the infant's left side is lying against mother's spine with the left side of the head conjunct (in contact) with the maternal lumbosacral prominence. The infant's first task is to negotiate its way past the pubic arch so that it can enter the pelvic inlet. The posterior asynclitic entry position is the most common, with the baby's left parietal bone lower than the right and leading the way into the pelvis (see Figure 4.6). The infant generally starts the birthing process with her head partially flexed toward her body. The infant's occipito-frontal diameter is the common presenting diameter. As the pressures of descent build, the head is forced into increased flexion, the neck is more fully flexed, and the suboccipito-bregma diameter becomes the presenting diameter (Figures 5.4 and 5.1).

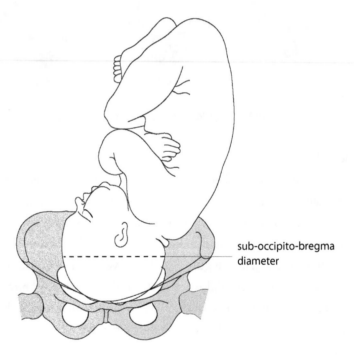

sub-occipito-bregma diameter

Figure 5.4. Outset of labor.

In Stage One's early phase, the infant's head meets the mother's pubic bone with the posterior parietal bone leading the way. The pubic arch is the first tissue structure met, which may generate strong resistance to movement. Either the sagittal area of the cranium, or the superior aspect of the right parietal bone, may contact the pubic symphysis (Figure 5.5).

If the sagittal suture is conjunct with the maternal pubic symphysis, birthing forces may be introduced into the baby's cranium in a caudal (footward) direction. The non-birth lie parietal bone (right parietal bone) may be subjected to strong pressures in both caudal and oblique directions via its contact with the pubic arch. Caudal vector patterns may affect the cranial base generally and generate compressive cranial base fulcrums; oblique vectors may affect the opposite (birth lie) occipito-mastoid and occipito-atlanteal areas. Compressive fulcrums may be introduced into these areas. This may give rise to cranial base and SBJ compressions and general compressive vectors through the longitudinal axis of the body. If the right parietal bone initially is conjunct with the maternal pubic bone, then oblique force vectors may be introduced into the cranium (Figure 5.5).

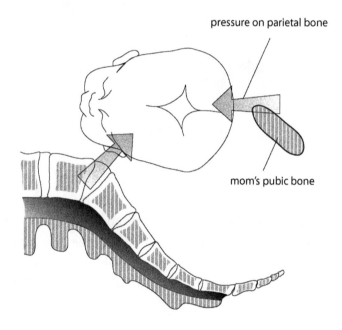

Figure 5.5. Early Stage One.

In the later phase of Stage One, the infant must change direction to pass under the pubic bone, rotating over the maternal sacral promontory (Figure 5.6). Both sacrum and pubis exert a dragging effect on the cranium as the baby passes. The baby's body rotates anteriorly, along with the mother's uterus. As this occurs, the infant's left parietal bone is conjunct with the maternal sacral promontory and may experience strong transverse forces. As the baby's cranium rotates over the sacral promontory, this transverse pressure moves caudal and creates pressure against the left temporal bone. Thus, a conjunct pathway is generated from the superior aspect of the left parietal bone caudal to the left temporal bone, forcing them into an exhalation pattern (internally rotated) with corresponding membranous tensions. The baby may be in this phase for some time; the longer a pressured contact is held, the more likely that the system will gather potency at the site to contain and manage the disturbance, leading to the generation of inertial fulcrums, vector patterns, and other effects. Commonly, as pressures are introduced into the left side of the cranium as it conjuncts with the maternal sacral promontory, a *right side-bending* pattern (a convexity bulge) may be generated on the opposite, non-birth lie side.

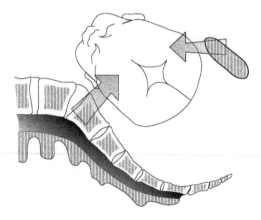

Figure 5.6. Middle Stage One.

At the end of Stage One, the infant is in a synclitic position and is fully engaged in the birth canal. If the infant is in this position for some time, strong transverse forces can be fed into the cranium, leading to medial compressive issues, temporal bone intraosseous compression, and exhalation patterns (Figure 5.7).

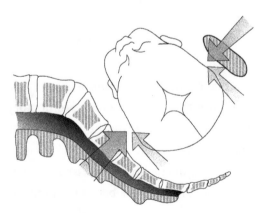

Figure 5.7. Late Stage One dragging and compressive forces.

Cranial Base Patterns in Stage One

In Stage One, compressive and dragging forces may be placed on the cranium and greater wing of the sphenoid on the birth lie side. As these forces are fed in via the conjunct site at the sacral promontory, a *right lateral shear* pattern may result, as may a *right side-bending* pattern. As the infant experiences dragging forces along this conjunct pathway, the left greater wing of the sphenoid may be dragged inferiorly on the birth lie side, generating a *right torsion pattern* (a superior greater wing on the non-birth lie side). The medially compressive forces introduced via the sacral promontory may also give rise to medial compression of the cranial base on the birth lie side. A medially compressed left temporal bone may be generated (Figure 5.7).

Stage One General Inertial Issues

- Exhalation patterns may be introduced into the dynamics of the cranium.
- Axial compressive issues are introduced into the body, especially on the birth lie side.
- Various cranial base patterns may be generated, usually on the non-birth lie side.
- Medial compressive issues may be generated, especially on the birth lie side.

Intraosseous Distortions of the Sphenoid in Stage One

Each stage of birth can introduce forces directly into the young bones of the baby's cranium. These can generate intraosseous patterns in particular bones, affecting the cranium as a whole. The term *intraosseous* denotes inertial fulcrums and related patterns located in the tissue of a bone itself. In this chapter, as we explore each stage of birth, we describe the common intraosseous issues that may be generated in that stage.

In Stage One, intraosseous compressions in the temporal and sphenoid bones are commonly created. At birth, the sphenoid bone is in three separate parts, the body and its lesser wing, and the two greater wing and pterygoid sections (Figure 5.8). During Stage One, compressive forces may affect these parts, and generate compression and shearing patterns in the dynamics of the sphenoid bone itself. Torsioning of the parts of the sphenoid, may occur in Stage One, but is more commonly generated in Stage Two during the rotation of the baby's head through the birth canal. These three parts then become distorted or displaced in relation to each other.

Vertical Shearing of the Parts of the Sphenoid

In one instance, as Stage one proceeds, the baby's greater wings can become held in medial compression while its cranium as a whole is experiencing downward forces. This can generate a shearing of the greater wings of the sphenoid relative to its body or cause the body to shear inferiorly relative to the greater wings. This will be sensed as a strong shearing force in the infant's cranium and will also persist in adults. Vertical shearing of the parts of the sphenoid can be found on just one side, if one greater wing is dragged inferiorly while the other is held fixed against the maternal sacrum or pubic arch. In the adult, as you sense a vertical shear pattern in the cranium as a whole, you may notice that its fulcrum is located in the sphenoid bone.

body and lesser wing section

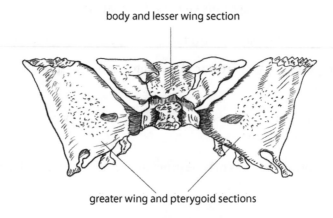

greater wing and pterygoid sections

Figure 5.8. The sphenoid bone is in three sections at birth.

Vertical shear in the sphenoid can produce dramatic effects in the facial area. The sphenoid wings pull the maxillae up via the pterygoid processes, while the sphenoid body pushes the vomer down. This situation can affect the vomer—leading to compression or an S-shape distortion—and cause restricted glide and range of motion between the pterygoid processes and the palatines. Facial effects of shearing can also be one-sided, corresponding the unilateral vertical shear of one greater wing only.

It is also possible to have a vertical shear of the wing sections relative to the body in the opposite direction, with the body pushed up and both or one of the wings pulled down. This occurs when the inferior dragging forces on the greater wings are stronger than the inferior compressive forces transferred to the body of the sphenoid. The greater wing sections are dragged inferiorly and the body is left in a superior position, creating a strong tension in the hard palate (Figure 5.9).

Medial Compression of the Parts of the Sphenoid

During Stage One, the greater wing sections of the baby's sphenoid may become medially compressed into its body. Negotiating the motion around the sacral promontory can place great pressure on the birth lie side—in this case the left side—generating intraosseous compression in the parts of the sphenoid bone. This can be a factor in intransigent side-bending and torsion patterns, generating great sensitivity to touch contact at the greater wings. Some people cannot initially be contacted at the greater wings due to these strong intraosseous forces and to the implicit memories that may be coupled with them. The vault hold may bring up a sensation of intense crowding and pressure. Contact needs to be carefully negotiated by the practitioner. We describe how to energetically relate to this in Chapter 6. In late Stage One, bilateral compression of the wing sections into the body of the sphenoid can also be generated (Figure 5.9).

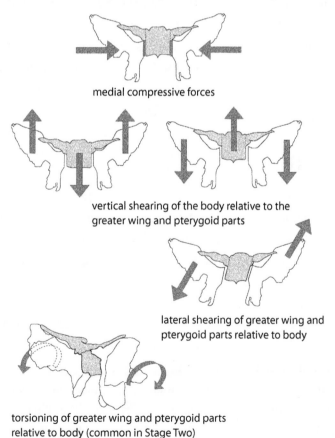

medial compressive forces

vertical shearing of the body relative to the
greater wing and pterygoid parts

lateral shearing of greater wing and
pterygoid parts relative to body

torsioning of greater wing and pterygoid parts
relative to body (common in Stage Two)

Figure 5.9. Common intraosseous distortions of the sphenoid bone.

Common Stage One Intraosseous Distortions of the Sphenoid

- Shearing patterns between the greater wings and the body of the sphenoid (various forms of lateral and vertical shearing).

- Compression between the parts of the sphenoid.

- Torsion patterns between the greater wings and the body of the sphenoid (more common in Stage Two).

Intraosseous Distortions of the Temporal Bone in Stage One

The temporal bone is originally composed of three parts, the petrous and squamous parts, and the tympanic ring. During Stage One, medial compressive forces may impact a temporal bone, inertial fulcrums may be generated, and its parts may become compressed together. Later, these temporal bone intraosseous issues may be the origin of persistent medial cranial base compression—with the organizing fulcrum located in the temporal bone itself. No matter how much attention is given to the cranial base as a whole, the pattern will not resolve until the intraosseous forces in the temporal bone itself are resolved.

Other Effects of Stage One Pressure

The TMJ may also be affected by Stage One dragging and compressive forces. The TMJ and its ligaments on the birth lie side may experience compressive forces, which generate local inertial fulcrums, and become compressed and hypertonic. The TMJ and its ligaments on the opposite side may then become tractioned and hypotonic in compensation.

In the late phase of Stage One, the infant's head is now in a synclitic position, with its head parallel to the pelvic inlet. If the infant becomes stuck here, strong medial forces arise from both the sacrum and pubic arch, which may generate bilateral medial compression of the cranial base. This can also generate an inhalation pattern—with the cranium held in an inhalation position with transverse narrowing of the cranium (Figure 5.7). Intraosseous distortions of the sphenoid and temporal bones may also be generated and either or both parietal bones may be flattened, puckered, or forced to overlap at the sagittal suture.

During Stage One, while this is occurring, the mother's pelvis must widen to receive the infant's head. This motion is called *counternutation.* The pelvis widens at the pelvic inlet and narrows at the ischial tuberosities. The sacrum moves into flexion and the ilea rotate externally (Figure 5.10). The infant has now descended into the pelvic inlet and is in a synclitic position (parietal bones level with each other). The infant will now begin its rotational descent in the mother's mid-pelvis, the beginning of Stage Two.

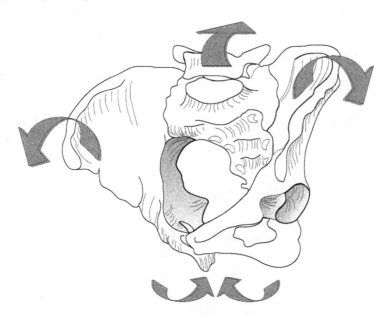

Figure 5.10. Inlet dynamics: counternutation of mother's pelvis.

Body Relationships

Spinal and Structural Repercussions

Infants experience strong compressive forces along their longitudinal axis throughout the birth process, leading to possible vertebral issues. Axial compression through the vertebral column is a common clinical finding in both children and adults, and birthing forces are a common origin. Specific vertebral fixations result, but commonly the axial force must be addressed as a whole for full resolution to occur. See Chapter 8 for clinical approaches to these issues.

These forces are especially felt on the birth lie side (Figure 5.11). As these axial forces are experienced, the infant may react to protect itself by contracting muscles and connective tissues on that side, setting up formative inertial patterns, and structural tendencies that can continue throughout life. In a left birth lie, this would manifest as left-sided body contraction, chronic tissue tension, and compensatory structural patterns. These forms of birth-generated contraction and tension become habitual modes of protection, which intensify in reaction to stress.

Axial compressive forces introduced on the birth lie side may later generate patterns of scoliosis and compressive issues affecting the spine and tissue system as a whole. These commonly manifest as compression and side-bending in vertebral relationships, especially on the birth lie side, with a possible narrowing of intervertebral discs on that side. A low shoulder, a generally contracted left side, and posteriorly rotated hip bone on the birth lie side will give the appearance of a "C" curve on that side of the body. If the sacrum is also posterior and inferior on the birth lie side as described below, then an "S" curve may be generated. A general pattern of contraction on the left side of the body may also commonly be seen (Figure 5.12).

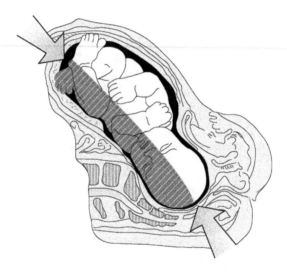

Figure 5.11. Stage One axial compression especially affects the birth lie side.

Compressive forces often generate inertial fulcrums in places of transition, such as areas of change in the spinal curve. Inertial forces commonly also lodge in specific areas of transition such as the occipito-atlanteal junction, the cervical-thoracic junction, and the lumbosacral junction. Compressive forces impinging on the occipito-atlanteal-axial area may generate compressive patterns in the occipital triad area, coupled with intraosseous fulcrums in the occiput.

As the birth process continues, axial forces are intensified by the ongoing nature of birth contractions. After birth, the leg on the infant's birth lie side is commonly

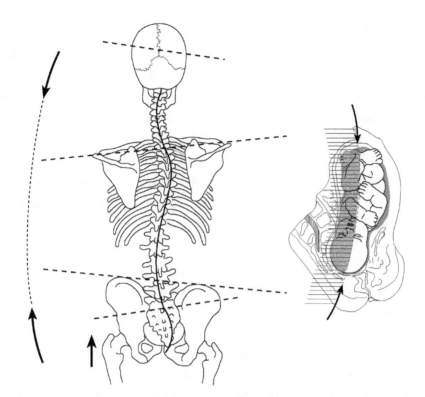

Figure 5.12. Adult structural distortion based on Stage One
experiences, left birth lie.

pulled up in a contracted manner. Babies who are born from a posterior presentation, and who remained posterior during the whole birth process, tend to pull both legs up and tend to suddenly pull their head posteriorly if they are startled.

In the infant these structural patterns are commonly sensed in session work as tendencies, not as full-blown structural issues. It may take years of growth and habitual maintenance of these forces before they are expressed as clear structural forms. I have treated many infants who retained these birthing forces in their spinal relationships. The sacroiliac pain or migraine headache of the thirty-year-old may have had its beginnings in the experience of birth.

Dural Repercussions

Compressive forces generated by the birth process can also affect the dural membranes. The dural tube may seem denser along its entire length due to the presence of these forces. Commonly, birthing forces come to rest in specific areas of the vertebral axis, generating local inertial fulcrums that generate dural tube contraction and local vertebral issues.

Central Nervous System

The central nervous system also experiences extreme compressive forces during the birth process. If these forces become entrapped in neural tissue, potency will condense to center the forces involved and the motility of the central nervous system will be affected. The ventricle system also has to organize around the unresolved compressive forces introduced. In a left birth lie, the infant experiences more intense forces on its left side. In this case, the left ventricle may be slightly contracted when compared to the right. A right side-bending pattern in the cranial base may be coupled with the narrowed ventricle. This will have ongoing repercussions for both infant and adult.

Pelvic Repercussions

Stage One forces especially affect the pelvis on the birth lie side, particularly at the hip and sacroiliac joints. In a left birth lie, compressive pressures build on the left side of the body and, as forces are introduced into the hip area, the left innominate bone may be forced to rotate posteriorly. This will also drag the sacrum on that side in a posterior and inferior direction. The patterns that are generated may include a posteriorly rotated innominate bone on the birth lie side and a torsioned sacrum. The sacrum tends to be held inferior and posterior on the birth lie side—the left side in the example here.

Both innominate bone and sacrum may express inertial patterns organized around left-sided inertial fulcrums, commonly located in the hip joint-acetabulum

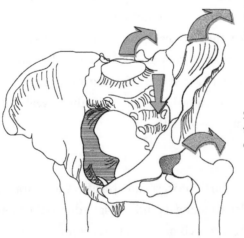

Left-side compressive forces force innominate bone to rotate posterior.

Sacral base on birth side is forced to rotate posterior and inferior, creating sacral torsion.

Figure 5.13. Pelvic repercussions.

area and sacroiliac joints. Posterior rotations of the hip bone and a posterior-inferior sacrum on the left side of the body are reported to be most common by osteopaths and chiropractors, probably because a majority of people start the birth process in a left birth lie position (Figure 5.13).

Psychological Considerations

As birth contractions build, the infant begins to descend toward a cervix that is not yet dilated. This is sometimes called the "no exit" phase of the birth process, as the infant meets strong resistance from the undilated cervix, and may feel stuck with no sense of completion or a clear way out. This can bring up feelings of confusion, loss, and even abandonment as the infant enters and moves through the birth canal. Some infants seem to have a clear sense that they are going to an outside world, but for others it can be a confusing and even terrifying experience as if they are entering a dark tunnel with no apparent end in sight (Grof 1993).

The infant may experience loss of contact with mom and this alone may be disorienting and scary. As we have seen, infants live in present time and cannot contextualize their experience. Strong forces and overwhelming pressures at any time in the birth process may have the sense of being endless. Furthermore, when these experiences are activated in clinical sessions, it may seem to the infant that the trauma is occurring again. It is extremely important to resource the infant in mom's presence and for the practitioner to gradually become a resourcing presence for them. The various stages of the birth process can also restimulate earlier prenatal trauma or stress. Stage One can restimulate conception issues as the infant is again in transition from one world to another.

SUMMARY OF STAGE ONE PELVIC INLET DYNAMICS

Summary of Motion (Figure 5.14)	Cranial and Tissue Impacts
Early Stage One Infant descends in posterior asynclitism, pressures against the left parietal-temporal and sagittal areas (Figure 5.5).	• Diagonal and oblique force vectors on cranium. • Occipito-atlanteal compression on birth lie side. • Occipito-mastoid compression of birth lie side. • Ongoing caudal compression yielding compressive patterns in the cranium and spine.

SUMMARY OF STAGE ONE PELVIC INLET DYNAMICS (continued)

Summary of Motion (Figure 5.14)	Cranial and Tissue Impacts
Middle Stage One Infant's cranium meets pubic arch, cranium rotates around lumbosacral promontory in lateral flexion (Figure 5.6).	• Medial compression of the left temporal bone and cranial base. • Intraosseous distortions of the sphenoid and temporal bones. • Right side-bending. • Right lateral shear. • Right torsion. • TMJ compression on birth lie side. • Intraosseous distortions of sphenoid and temporal bones.
Late Stage One Infant is in synclitic position and has descended into the pelvic inlet in a transverse position (Figure 5.7).	• Exhalation patterns. • Medial compression of the cranial base. • In all stages: possible over-riding of sutural relationships—sagittal suture is especially vulnerable—flattening or puckering of parietal bones.
Body Patterns (Figures 5.11, 5.12, 5.13)	• Compressions in the body on birth lie side. • Dural and spinal compressions. • Posterior innominate bone and inferior sacrum on birth lie side. • Short leg on birth lie side.

In early Stage One mom's pelvis expressed counternutation and the pelvic inlet opened. During the later stages of birth, the pelvic floor and outlet must begin to open, and nutation, which is the opposite of counternutation, occurs. In nutation, mom's ischial tuberosities spread apart, the sacrum moves into extension, and the two ilea move into internal rotation. The result is that, as the infant continues its descent in the birth canal, the pelvic floor opens to allow the infant easier passage (see Figure 5.24).

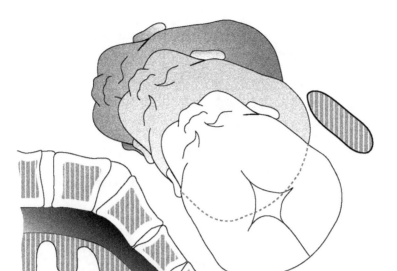

Figure 5.14. Summary of motions in Stage One descent.

Stage Two: Mid-Pelvis Dynamics

Stage Two begins the transition from an inside world of the womb to the out-side world. It begins when the infant moves through the pelvic inlet and begins to negotiate passage through the mid-pelvis. The pelvic inlet in the gynecoid pelvis is basically an apple-shaped oval with a transverse dimension slightly longer than its anterior-posterior dimension (Figure 5.3). The pelvic outlet, however, is an oval that is wider in the opposite anterior-posterior dimension (Figure 5.15). In order to more easily enter the pelvic outlet, the infant's head must turn in the birth canal so that its longitudinal dimension enters the outlet anterior-posterior. To do this, the infant will generally rotate its head posteriorly toward the maternal sacrum as it continues its descent through the birth canal. Rotation is mainly of the head, not the body, with strong cranial contact on the mother's sacrum and pubic arch. The whole process is facilitated by the shape of the birth canal and the downward force of uterine contractions working together to generate a firm corkscrew-like motion. Because of the rotation that commonly occurs in this stage, it sometimes is called *rotational descent.* By the end of Stage Two, the infant's head is facing the maternal sacrum (Figures 5.16 and 5.22).

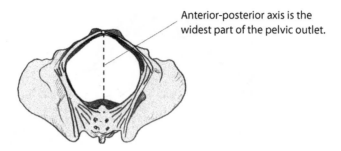

Anterior-posterior axis is the
widest part of the pelvic outlet.

Figure 5.15. Pelvic outlet in a gynecoid-shaped pelvis.

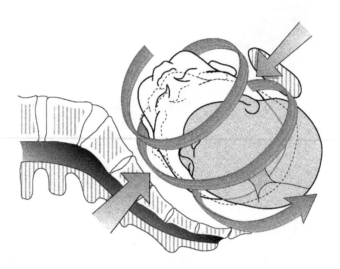

Figure 5.16. The corkscrew-like motion through the mid-pelvis.

Forces and Patterns Generated in Stage Two

Torsion

During Stage Two, rotational forces generate torsion in the infant's tissues, especially
in the reciprocal tension membrane, the cervical spine, and related connective tissues, and through the vertebral axis and dural tube generally.

Dragging Pressure

Dragging forces are generated by the contact with the sacrum and pubic bone on
the infant's cranium. Mom's sacrum becomes a moving fulcrum for conjunct sites,
intense forces, and force vector patterns. Pressure commonly begins at the baby's

parietal-temporal area on the birth lie side and moves inferiorly along the greater wing of the sphenoid, zygoma, and maxilla, and then the TMJ area. This generates a rotational and torsioning force against all of these structures. Meanwhile, a similar pressure can be exerted by the contact with the pubic bone on the posterior of the baby's head, at the parietal and occipital bones on the side opposite the birth lie. The dragging forces here move inferiorly and toward the occiput (Figure 5.17).

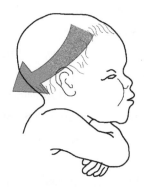
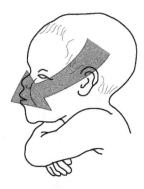

conjunct pathway with pubic bone
(left side lie)

conjunct pathway with sacrum
(left side lie)

Figure 5.17. Dragging forces in Stage Two.

Force Vectors

If the infant becomes stuck in any position during mid-pelvis descent, any area contacting the sacrum or pubic arch at that point may generate strong pressures, which may introduce intense inertial forces into the cranium. These compressive and rotational forces—and the vector patterns they take—may generate a variety of inertial fulcrums in the baby's system, producing compressive and torsional patterns throughout its tissues.

Sphenoid Patterns

As the baby moves over mom's sacral promontory, the left greater wing of the sphenoid may be dragged inferiorly on the birth lie side, giving rise to a torsion pattern on the opposite side. In a left birth lie, a *right torsion pattern* will result as the left greater wing is dragged inferiorly. The left side of the head will also experience strong lateral forces that may yield a right side-bending pattern, or reinforce an existing one generated during Stage One. These forces may also reinforce an existing lateral shear pattern, or may induce one. In this case, since the forces are directed from left to right across the infant's cranium, a *right lateral shear* will result. Intra-osseous distortions of the sphenoid bone may also be reinforced or generated here (see Figure 5.9).

Sphenoid-Maxillary Patterns

Another pattern that can be generated in Stage Two is sphenoid-maxillary torsion. As the infant's head corkscrews past the sacrum, the fulcrum of contact shifts from the left side of the head to the left side of the face. As this occurs, the head is also descending, and dragging forces are introduced from the greater wing of the sphenoid inferior across the zygoma and maxilla on the left. This can be visualized as a moving fulcrum of contact from the greater wing anteriorly and inferiorly across the left side of the face. If the forces are great enough, the maxillary complex may be forced into a torsioned relationship with the sphenoid bone. This is a true torsion pattern where the sphenoid-maxillary complex is forced to rotate around an anterior-posterior axis (Figure 5.18). This can also generate compression in the TMJ on the high maxilla side. It is thus common to see maxillary torsion in relationship

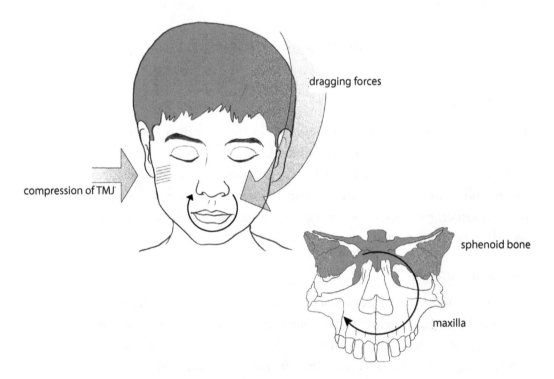

Figure 5.18. Sphenoid-maxillary torsion.

to TMJ compression. This is common in both infant and adult and can have important clinical repercussions. By the end of Stages One and Two, such intense forces may have been fed into the cranium that a "C" curve concavity is generated on the birth lie side of the infant's head.

Possible Stage Two Inertial Issues

- Rotational patterns throughout the cranium and body; rotational issues in the membranous-osseous system.

- Generation or reinforcement of cranial base patterns expressed on the non-birth lie side.

- Torsional issues that involve the sphenoid-maxillary complex leading to a true torsion of the maxilla and vomer relative to the sphenoid bone.

- Compressive issues in TMJ dynamics.

Intraosseous Distortions in Stage Two

Inertial fulcrums located in the tissue of the sphenoid, temporal, or occipital bones will generate distortions in the tissue of that bone and commonly underlie cranial base patterns. Almost any pattern, inhalation-exhalation, torsion, side-bending, shearings, and compressions can be organized around an intraosseous issue in either the occiput, sphenoid, or temporal bones, which are not yet fused into single bones at birth. The following sections review the creation of these intraosseous issues during birth process.

Intraosseous Distortions of the Occiput

The baby's occiput is in four distinct parts: the two condylar parts, the basilar part, and the squamous part (Figure 5.19). In Stage Two, the occiput's contact with mom's pubic arch can generate strong pressures across the back of baby's head. These forces can generate intraosseous inertial fulcrums in the occiput and its four parts, and affect its later coalescence into a single bone. In rotational descent, the squamous portion commonly encounters rotational forces as it conjuncts with mom's pelvic bones, while the downward pressures of birth contractions relatively fix the other occipital parts.

In a left birth lie—as these forces are encountered—the occipital squama may be rotated clockwise (when viewing it from the rear) as its right side is forced inferiorly into compression with the right condylar part. Meanwhile the left side of the occipital squama is forced away from the left condylar part. The infant would end up with compression between the right side of the squama and the right condylar part and a spreading, or wedging apart, of the left side of the squama and left condylar part (Figure 5.20). The spread side may generate more pain later in life than the compressed side. The forces of the birth process are literally introduced into the tissues of the occiput. These inertial forces, if not resolved, will maintain compressive and torsioned tissue patterns in the inner relationships of the occiput. These intraosseous issues may, in turn, generate various cranial base patterns, compressive issues in the occipital triad area, autonomic activation, and cranial nerve sensitization.

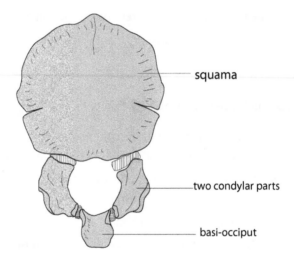

squama

two condylar parts

basi-occiput

Figure 5.19. The occiput is in four parts at birth.

Stage Two Intraosseous Distortions of the Occiput

- Rotation of the occipital squama relative to the condylar parts.
- Compression between the squama and condylar part on the non-birth lie side.
- Wedging apart of the squama and the condylar part on the birth lie side.
- Torsioning of the squama, condylar parts, and basi-occiput around the foramen magnum.

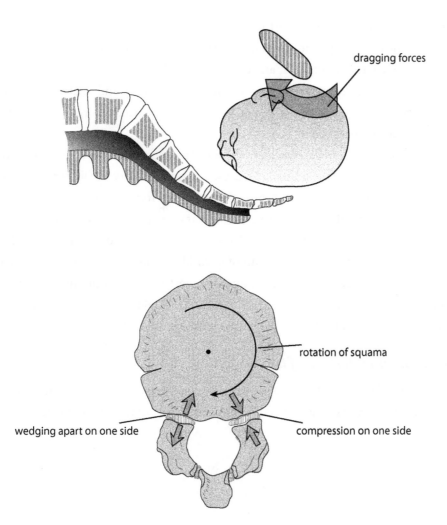

Figure 5.20. Stage Two rotational forces on occiput.

Intraosseous Distortions of the Sphenoid

In Stage Two the infant may also experience forces that generate tensions between the three parts of the sphenoid. The baby may have to pause or may become stuck at any part of its corkscrew-like descent, and the forces encountered may press the wings of the sphenoid in opposite directions, generating torsion between the wings and the body. This may also create torsion patterns in the dura, the cranial base, and the central nervous system.

If the infant's head is stuck in a position that generates medial pressures and force vectors from one side of the cranium toward the body of the sphenoid, then the greater wing can become medially compressed into its body. Almost any variation of intraosseous distortion can occur between the greater wing sections and the body of the sphenoid, creating torsion, vertical or lateral shear, or wedging of the structures in almost any direction (see Figure 5.9). These intraosseous fulcrums commonly organize wider cranial base patterns and related tensions in the membrane system and, in session work, can be sensed as organizing factors throughout the tissue field.

Intraosseous issues have both physiological and structural repercussions. Intraosseous distortions of the occiput can cause discomfort and contribute to compression of the vagus nerve at its exit through the jugular foramen. These pressures can also affect the spinal accessory and glossopharyngeal nerves. Symptoms of these effects in babies include digestive problems, colic, respiratory difficulty, and sucking problems. These can persist and manifest in children and adults as a potentially long list of problems, such as respiratory and/or digestive issues, migraine headaches, autonomic dysfunction, learning disorders, and even depressive states. I have seen such wide-ranging effects clinically in both infants and adults.

Intraosseous Distortions of the Temporal Bone

The temporal bone is subject to the same pressures as its neighbors and can also acquire intraosseous distortions in Stage Two. These may be new at this stage, or

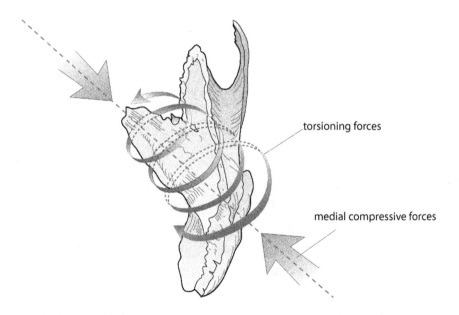

torsioning forces

medial compressive forces

Figure 5.21. Compressive and torsioning forces on the temporal bone.

they may be a continuation of the medial pressures described in Stage One. But Stage Two places special rotational pressure on the inner relationships of the petrous portion. The intraosseous forces present, and the resulting compression-torsion pattern in the temporal bone can generate symptoms for a long time. Intraosseous distortions of the temporal bone can manifest later as "glue ear," ear infections, tinnitus, and learning disorders (Figure 5.21).

Stage Two Intraosseous Distortions of the Temporal Bone

- Medial compression in the petrous portion of the temporal bone.

- Compression and torsion issues in the petrous portion.

- Inertial patterns between the petrous portion and the squama of the temporal bone.

Body Patterns in Stage Two

Birthing forces introduced in Stage Two dynamics may also affect the whole body, similar to the patterns described in Stage One. Strong downward pressures continue to compress the vertebral axis, particularly the cervical area. Meanwhile the rotational component—commonly found in Stage Two birth descent—adds to the picture. The baby's head turns while its body is relatively fixed, yielding torsion patterns in general—and torsion of the spine, dural tube, and pelvis in particular. Rotational patterns found throughout the vertebral axis are not uncommon, and are a clear consequence of the unresolved rotational forces met in Stage Two. Dural tension and torsion may also be generated and become coupled with vertebral torsion, pelvic compensations, cranial base patterns, and rotational patterns throughout the body. Stage Two torsion can also contribute to adhesions of the dural tube to the inner walls of the spinal column and to a torsioning of the denticulate ligaments in the dural canal. The respiratory diaphragm may also reflect the torsion pattern by tensing, leading to a host of secondary symptoms including shallow breath, tight chest, general inflexibility, and nerve sensitization. I have seen this as a common finding when working with infants and adults alike (Figure 5.22).

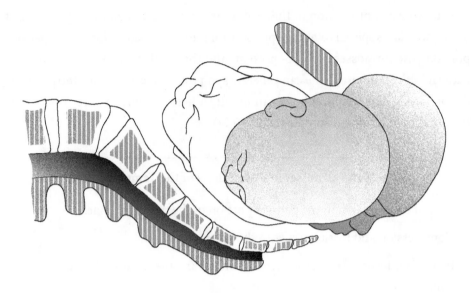

Figure 5.22. Stage Two motions.

SUMMARY OF STAGE TWO MID-PELVIC DYNAMICS

Summary of Motion (Figure 5.16, 5.22)	Cranial and Tissue Impacts
Cranial Patterns Infant's head is engaged in the pelvic inlet and must rotate toward the sacrum to enter the anterior-posterior diameter of the pelvic outlet (Figures 5.16, 5.17, 5.18, 5.20).	• Cranial torsion patterns on the side opposite the birth lie side. • Right side-bending. • Right torsion. • Right lateral shear. • Intraosseous distortions of the temporal bone, occiput, and sphenoid. • Torsion patterns across the foramen magnum and condylar parts, sphenoid-maxillary torsion, and TMJ compression.
Body Patterns Torsional and rotational forces are placed on the infant's body.	• Dural rotations. • Cervical compressions, rotations, and side-bending. • Pelvic torsions and shear. • Vertebral rotations. • Respiratory diaphragm torsions. • Whole-body torsions.

Stage Three: Pelvic Outlet Dynamics

At the end of Stage Two, in a left birth lie, the infant's head has rotated toward its left shoulder and her face is pressed against mom's sacrum, chin pushed toward the neck. The cervical area is compressed and torsioned though the body does not generally rotate very much. The baby is now in a position to descend through the pelvic outlet. Infants must negotiate their way around a ninety-degree angle at the pubic symphysis while their face is being dragged across the maternal sacrum and coccyx. Stage Three has two basic phases. In early Stage Three, the infant's head is in anatomical flexion. In late Stage Three, the infant's head moves into extension as it descends around the pubic arch (Figure 5.23).

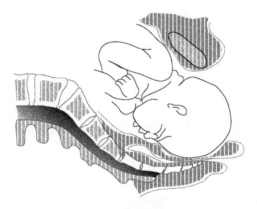

In early Stage Three infant's head is in
inhalation toward the sacrum.

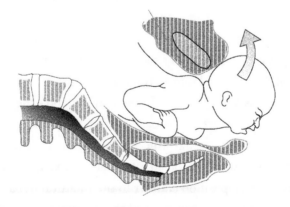

In late Stage Three infant's head descends into
exhalation to move around the pubic arch.

Figure 5.23. Basic movements in Stage Three.

Meanwhile, the mother's pelvis is shifting into nutation at this time with the iliac crests moving closer together and the ischial tuberosities moving wider apart. This helps the infant in its Stage Three descent as the pelvic outlet widens and opens to its motions (Figure 5.24).

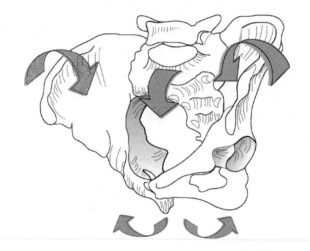

Figure 5.24. Nutation of the maternal pelvis.

Flexion Phase in Early Stage Three

In early Stage Three, the infant's head is in anatomical lateral flexion. Her head is oriented in an anterior-posterior position in mom's pelvis, with her frontal bone conjunct with mother's sacrum and occiput conjunct with mother's pubic bone. The compressive forces and pressures are mainly anterior-posterior in orientation. The conjunct pressures of mother's sacrum on the frontal area tend to drag the greater wings of the sphenoid into an inhalation position—forward, widened, and inferior—while its basilar aspect is high, and may also force the frontal area to bulge out. Meanwhile, the pressure on the occiput from the pubic arch tends to hold the occiput in exhalation—its basilar aspect is low while its squama is superior and narrowed. The sphenoid will be forced into relative inhalation, while the occiput is in relative exhalation, a position counter to their natural dynamics (Figure 5.25). This is the source of the superior vertical shear pattern described in Chapter 11. This will occur if the infant is stuck in this position for a period of time and if the forces involved could not be processed at the time or immediately thereafter. In this case the baby may have a distinctive bulge at the frontal area.

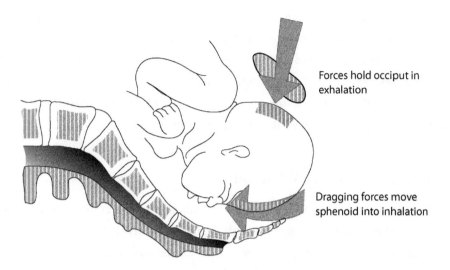

Forces hold occiput in exhalation

Dragging forces move sphenoid into inhalation

Figure 5.25. The generation of superior vertical shear.

During the whole of Stage Three, anterior-posterior forces can also generate compressive fulcrums in the sphenobasilar junction and occipital base. Thus, cranial base compressions can arise here. The falx can also go into a protective contraction, while the SBJ tends to be held in a relative raised, inhalation position.

As early Stage Three continues, the conjunct point against the occiput moves toward the foramen magnum and creates a moving conjunct point from the upper occipital squama toward the foramen magnum. The occipital base can become

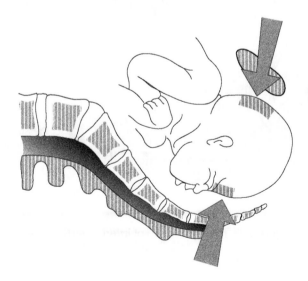

Figure 5.26. Strong anterior-posterior forces in Stage Three.

extremely compressed because of the forces introduced as this occurs. If the infant becomes stuck at any point, the moving conjunct point of the pubic symphysis on the occiput can fixed, introducing forces and related vector patterns affecting the occipital base, the cervical area generally, the O/A junction, and the occiput-C1-C2 (O/C1/C2) relationship. The forces involved can also affect the dynamics of C7 and T1 and the upper thoracic vertebrae (Figure 5.26).

Extension Phase in Late Stage Three

As the infant's head moves around mom's pubic bone, the conjunct site becomes the occiput and foramen magnum. This signals the arrival of late Stage Three and anatomical extension. This position generates a reversal of the forces experienced in early Stage Three, as the sphenoid bone is now held in relative exhalation (its wings narrow and superior and its basilar aspect low), while the occiput is held in relative inhalation (its squama wide and inferior and its basilar aspect high) because of the pressure against the pubic bone. This can give rise to an inferior vertical shear pattern. This situation is indicated by a distinctive ski-slope look at the frontal area at birth (Figure 5.27).

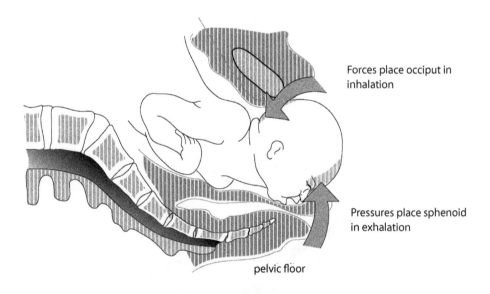

Forces place occiput in inhalation

Pressures place sphenoid in exhalation

pelvic floor

Figure 5.27. The generation of inferior vertical shear.

Meanwhile, as the baby continues its descent through the pelvis outlet, the anterior-posterior pressures also continue, with the baby's frontal bone flattened against mother's sacrum and coccyx. Compressive forces are experienced at the two parts of the frontal bone, but impact the sphenobasilar junction and the occipital base. The infant's vomer may be pressed into the body of the sphenoid. This is a relatively common inertial issue—baby's thumb-sucking can be a natural self-corrective attempt to alleviate the discomfort of sphenoid-vomer compression. These forces can also generate contraction and compression in the falx and tentorium, the ethmoid bone, and the ethmoid notch of the frontal bone.

The mandible, sphenoid-maxillary relationships, and TMJ are also affected by the birthing forces of Stage Three. The pressure of the face against the sacrum and pelvic floor can travel through the mandible into the TMJ, affecting one or both sides. The same pressure on the face can push the maxillae firmly into the palatines and the pterygoid processes of the sphenoid bone.

Body Patterns

During Stage Three compressive forces are introduced commonly into the O/A junction, occipital triad, cervical area generally, upper thoracic area, and lumbosacral junction. The C/D junction (C7 and T1), and T2–T3 are particularly vulnerable to compressive forces at this time. These forces can later generate vertebral compression and fixation and become the basis for possible sensitization of spinal nerves and CNS nuclei.

The downward pressures described for Stages One and Two continue in both early and late phases here, so the earlier discussion of cervical and occipital issues—impingement of cranial nerves at the jugular foramina—is equally true in Stage Three. Similarly, vertebral and dural tube issues described in the prior stages are equally possible here. Inertial fulcrums generated along the vertebral axis will affect both vertebral and dural dynamics. Also, the respiratory diaphragm may be tensed in response to these compressive and torsioning forces.

In any birth stage, compressive forces may be transferred to the infant's sacrum, sacroiliac joints, and lumbosacral junction. Intraosseous distortions of the sacrum are not uncommon. If the sacrum is fixed in its articulations or holds intraosseous forces, the motility of the central nervous system can become compromised. The sacrum will not be able to express its natural rising in the inhalation phase of primary respiration, and a dragging force may be generated and transferred to the spinal cord via the lamina terminalis.

Intraosseous Distortions in Stage Three

As in previous stages, the compressive forces introduced in Stage Three can generate intraosseous distortions in cranial bones, especially in the occiput and sphenoid. We explore these possibilities below.

Intraosseous Distortions of the Occiput

Stage Three birthing forces can deeply affect the occiput due to a phenomenon known as *telescoping* in which the occipital squama is so firmly pushed against the condylar parts that they become wedged together and forced anterior. They in turn press against the basilar part and the body of the sphenoid, and all of these structures telescope together in compression. Thus telescoping is another type of intraosseous distortion of the occiput, where its primal parts are all wedged together in compression. The birthing forces involved will also wedge the atlas into the condylar parts of the occiput and generate occipito-atlanteal compression. The axis can also become involved due to the ligamentous continuity between the occiput, C1, and C2.

Telescoping may produce a range of symptoms—discomfort, headaches and even migraines, cranial nerve entrapment, and limbic and autonomic activation. Resultant issues in infants may include sucking problems, respiratory problems, digestive problems, and even later learning disorders.

The infant may also experience a shelving of the occipital squama relative to the condylar parts. Here the squama, which is separate from the condylar parts at birth, is flattened due to the pressures encountered as the infant moves around its mother's pubic arch. A part of the squama becomes flattened and an angular indented shape is created instead of the normal smooth curve. At the level of inion and the transverse sinuses, as the squama is stabilized by these structures, a literal folding of the squama at inion may result. I have treated a good number of infants with this pattern. Strain patterns will then be introduced in the dural membrane and this can even affect the central nervous system There are inevitably emotional and autonomic issues coupled with these intraosseous distortion patterns (Figure 5.28).

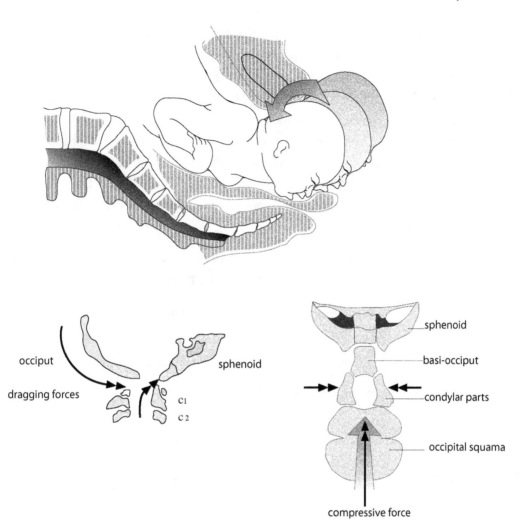

Figure 5.28. Intraosseous telescoping of occipital base structures.

Intraosseous Distortions of the Sphenoid

In early Stage Three, a *superior vertical shear* pattern may be generated in the sphenoid bone itself. If compression is present between the body of the sphenoid and the occiput, the sphenoid's body will follow the occiput. In this case, while the greater wings of the sphenoid may be forced into an inhalation position by the pressures from the frontal bone, the body can be forced into a relative exhalation position by the occiput. This is more likely to happen if there is a telescoping of structures as described above. The infant may then be left with a superior vertical shear pattern whose fulcrum is in the sphenoid itself.

Likewise, in late Stage Three an *inferior vertical shear* pattern in the sphenoid bone may be generated. In this case, while the greater wing portions are forced into an exhalation position by the pressures from the frontal bone, the body of the sphenoid is forced into an inhalation position by the occiput. An inferior vertical shear pattern is generated with its fulcrum in the sphenoid itself.

Alternatively, almost any kind of intraosseous pattern in the sphenoid bone may be generated. The most common kinds are shearing patterns between the sphenoid's greater wing sections and its body. The greater wing sections may shear superiorly or inferiorly relative to its body, dependent on the inertial forces present (see Figure 5.9).

Stage Three Intraosseous Distortions

- Telescoping and wedging together of the axis, atlas, occipital squama, occipital condyles, basi-occiput, SBJ, and body of the sphenoid bone

- Formation of an internal shelf on the occipital squama.

- Various intraosseous sphenoid issues.

SUMMARY OF STAGE THREE PELVIC OUTLET DYNAMICS

Summary of Motion (Figure 5.23)	Cranial and whole-body impacts
Cranial Patterns, Early Flexion Phase A-P descent in the flexion position; face is conjunct with the sacrum; occiput is conjunct with the pubic symphysis (Figures 5.23, 5.25, 5.26).	• Superior vertical shear, flexion patterns. • Compression at the SBJ. • Compression at the occipital base and through the falx. • A-P compression in cranium. • Ethmoid compression in ethmoid notch of the frontal and in glabella area. • Vomer-sphenoid compression. • Vomer-maxillary compression.
Cranial Patterns, Late Extension Phase A-P descent in extension, cranium rotates around the pubic arch (Figure 5.27).	• Inferior vertical shear. • Flexion or extension patterns. • Compression at cranial and occipital base.

SUMMARY OF STAGE THREE PELVIC OUTLET DYNAMICS

Summary of Motion (Figure 5.23)	Cranial and whole-body impacts
	• A-P compression through falx.
	• Intraosseous distortion of occiput that telescopes the squama, condylar parts, basilar part, body of sphenoid, and C1 and cervical structures.
	• O/A and O/C1/C2 compressions.
	• TMJ compression.
	• Flattening of frontal bone.
	• Shelving of frontal bone.
	• Shelving of occipital squama.
	• Compression of ethmoid into the ethmoid notch and sphenoid.
	• Compression of the vomer into the body of the sphenoid.
Body Patterns, Both Phases	• Continued compression through the body yields occipito-atlas and axis compression, and cervical and upper thoracic (C7, T1, T2, T3) compression.
	• Sacroiliac and lumbosacral compression and torsion of the sacrum in the ilea.
	• Compression in respiratory diaphragm, dural tube, and ribs.

Stage Four: Head Birth, Restitution, Body Birth, and Bonding

The baby's head is born at the end of Stage Three, signaling the beginning of Stage Four. Relieved of pressure, the infant's cranium springs open in an expansive inner breath. Ideally, any birthing forces present are resolved as this occurs, and the infant's cranial structures remold and orient to the midline and natural fulcrums. However, during head birth intracranial pressures are dramatically lessened, and the sudden change may elicit a systemwide defensive response in the baby's fluids, as potency condenses to protect against the sudden pressure change. The state of *fluid shock*, described in Chapter 4, then results. This protective response may also generate compressions in cranial bones, dural tension, and CNS activation. This can further affect the motility of the central nervous system and the fluid drive of primary respiration, and can strongly affect birth ignition. Fluid shock is also very common in cesarean births.

Restitution occurs next. In restitution, the infant's head rotates and realigns with the rest of the body. If the midwife or doctor forces restitution, a strain can be fed into the cervical area or can reinforce compression and strain patterns already held in the cervical vertebra. Dural torsion can also be exacerbated (Figure 5.29).

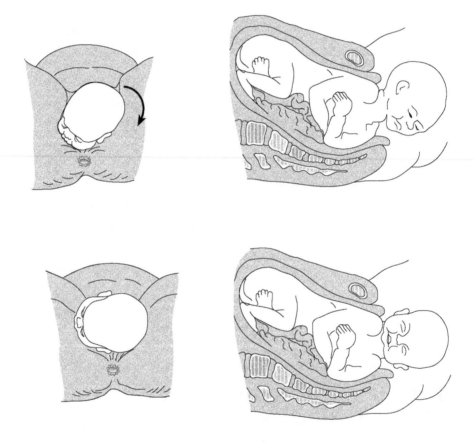

Figure 5.29. Restitution: the head rotates to the natural position relative to the shoulder.

Birthing the body involves several events. First, the baby's anterior shoulder must be born. In our current left birth lie description, the baby's right shoulder is anterior and conjunct with mother's pubic symphysis. The infant's shoulder may become stuck at the pubis, and the forces involved can generate a low shoulder on the side opposite to the birth lie side. Midwives and doctors often try to help here by pulling the baby's head posteriorly, to help the infant's shoulder clear the pubis. The forces applied can yield shoulder strains, sprains, and even cervical damage, usually on the side opposite the birth lie side. Clavicle fractures can also occur. Other interventions here can also be problematic. Strong contact attempting to help the movement may generate forces leading to an internal rotation of the shoulder. Lifting via the armpit can generate rotator cuff strain. Other strain patterns that can arise due to intervention at this point include rib head strains and shoulder muscle damage. In discussions with Castellino, he has described an adult condition, which he terms *pseudo cervical disc syndrome.* The symptoms mimic cervical disc syndrome, but on investigation the discs are not pathological. When these individuals resolve the original traumatic forces generated during birth, marked improvements in symptoms are gained.

Next, the other shoulder is birthed. The posterior shoulder has been conjunct with the maternal coccyx and perineal floor; now it must move anterior (in relation to mother). Patterns may arise that are similar to those described above, but here they are usually less intense, and they are located on the birth lie side.

Finally, the infant's body comes out. If the baby is pulled out with excessive force, a protective contraction can occur throughout the body, and further compression, rotation, and torsion patterns may be fed into the infant's system. A compressive pattern yielding a "C" curve on the side opposite to the birth lie side is also sometimes induced.

Umbilical Issues

Now the baby is born, still attached to mom via the umbilical cord. If the umbilical cord is cut before it stops pulsing, it may be experienced as very shocking. The connection with mother is suddenly ended, and the pulsing of her blood in the cord is suddenly stopped and not allowed to gently cease. Most important, when the cord is suddenly cut, the baby's system is not given an opportunity to adjust to its new relationship with its mother.

When the umbilical cord stops pulsing, and the first breath is taken, there is a natural ignition of potency at the umbilical center along the baby's midline. This is called umbilical or birth ignition. This generates a strong intensification and expression of potency in the fluid midline, cerebrospinal fluid, and fluids in general. The fluids of the baby become infused with potency, as the newborn is empowered to be an independent physiological being in its new relational world. If birth ignition is only partial, low vitality and lethargy may result in later life. Vitality issues may even arise in early childhood. Issues of low ignition are commonly generated by birth trauma and fluid shock. Anesthesia in the infant's system is also a common origin of partial ignition, evidenced by a dampened fluid tide with sub-optimum drive.

Respiratory issues such as breathing difficulties and asthma have been noted by practitioners in relation to this type of trauma, as have digestive and eliminative issues. I have treated a number of adult colitis cases that had their origin in umbilical shock. Once the shock resolved, the system was relieved of the colitis. Likewise, I have noted cases of depression in adults, which had their origin in birth trauma and low birth ignition. See Volume One for a more detailed clinical discussion of ignition issues.

If the cord was wrapped around the infant's neck, specific issues may result. I have experienced this kind of trauma in adult clients who experience feelings of suffocation, umbilical tension, and solar plexus activation as these forces are accessed. They may even be the source of a general sense of compression in life—and relational issues around safety in intimacy may also be generated—as intimacy may be experienced as suffocating. Clinically, it is important to help resource the client, to slow activation down, and to make a sensitive relationship to the umbilicus and the forces and shock affects present.

Umbilical shock can lead to various umbilical affects—including low vitality, sensitivity, tissue contraction, poor sense of personal empowerment, low esteem, and lumbar vertebral issues, to name but a few. Sensory nerves may become sensitized, as may sympathetic nerves, and the solar plexus and diaphragm may contract in a protective response.

As mentioned above, low potentization of the fluid system—with resultant low fluid drive and vitality—is another possible outcome. This has two major origins. One relates to interference with the ignition process as previously discussed. Another has to do with the nature of umbilical energy. Randolph Stone noted a spiral-like pulsation that naturally surges from the umbilicus as birth ignition occurs (Stone 1999). This is easily sensed in the space above the umbilicus throughout life. When the cord is cut too soon, it as though the infant has had to draw this umbilical energy inward in order to survive. This sense of umbilical *implosion* can be very palpable in session work. Later in life a sense of low energy, low motivation, and lowered vitality—coupled with low self-esteem and a sense of disempowerment—may result.

If umbilical shock arises during a session, you may see the infant or adult spasm around the umbilicus and solar plexus area. Autonomic and emotional responses such as hyperarousal and fear may also emerge. Again, it is important to slow things down, reassure the infant or adult with your voice and contact, help in resourcing generally, and help resolve the forces and CNS activation present. The obvious preference is to avoid these issues in the first place by allowing the infant's umbilicus to stop pulsating naturally as the baby is brought into contact with the mother. The only medical justification for the immediate cutting of the cord is real danger to the infant or mother's life, yet the practice of early cord cutting is still common in general obstetrical practice.

Bonding

Bonding is also part of Stage Four dynamics. Mother and baby need time and space to establish their new relationship. This entails a shift from womb-as-world, where mom and prenate are in direct umbilical connection, to an outer being-to-being, interpersonal relationship. Successful bonding is essential for secure attachment processes and nervous system fluidity and development, and interrupted bonding may be perceived by the baby as a direct threat to survival, with potentially devastating consequences. Changing birthing practices to actively encourage bonding may be one of the most significant reforms available in support of large-scale public wellness. Letting baby and mom rest together undisturbed, in skin-to-skin contact for a lengthy time after delivery, gives the natural bonding impulses a chance for fulfillment.

Self-attachment is a relatively new concept relating to infant-mother bonding. Research has shown that when a newborn baby is placed on mom's belly, with a gentle supportive contact from mom, it will naturally move to the breast on its own, and doing this successfully seems to have repercussions for later life (Righard and Franz 1995). Infants who can successfully self-attach have fewer medical complications and seem more able to mobilize themselves to get what they need in later life. In contrast, babies who experienced anesthesia or shock lie passively on mom's stomach with little sense of orientation and no capacity for self-propulsion to the breast, and these babies show lower motivation, with more difficulties in getting their needs met later in life.

Bonding continues to mature for at least the first two to three years after birth. This period is called the *attachment period,* where the infant hopefully develops an inner sense of security and safety—called secure attachment—in the good-enough safe holding field of mom and early caregivers. It is an important period of neural maturation and the development of a secure and fluid self-system. This essential territory was discussed in some detail in Chapter 3

STAGE FOUR HEAD BIRTH, RESTITUTION, AND BODY BIRTH

Summary of Motion (Figure 5.29)	Cranial and whole-body impacts
Head Birth Cranium is born through the pelvic outlet.	Cranial expansion—possible shock affects expressed in dura and fluids.
Restitution Head realigns with the body	Cervical sprains and strains; dural torsion.
Body Birth Body is born, anterior shoulder first..	Shoulder strain, sprain. Clavicle damage. Pseudo cervical disc syndrome. Umbilical trauma, umbilical affects generated, bonding issues.

Pelvic Shapes and Alternative Birthing Motions

In our birth process descriptions, we have oriented to the most common birth, a left birth lie through a gynecoid-shaped pelvis. However, different maternal pelvic shapes have a marked influence on the baby's birth process. We introduce some of the basics of birth through the different pelvic shapes below.

The Anthropoid Pelvic Shape

The birthing dynamics in an anthropoid pelvis can be subtly different from those in a gynecoid pelvis. As you may remember, the anthropoid pelvis is oval shaped. Anthropoid pelvises are more common in Asian women. Due to its relatively wide anterior-posterior inlet dimensions, it is not uncommon for a baby to enter an anthropoid-shaped pelvis in a posterior position. She may remain in that position throughout the birth. Births may be slow, yet paced to the baby's needs. Cranial base patterns tend to orient to exhalation patterns, cranial base compression, medial compressive issues, and intraosseous forces introduced into the dynamics of the occiput, temporal bones, and sphenoid bone. The most common intraosseous occipital distortion is the telescoping of structures. These relate to the anterior-posterior forces introduced throughout much of the posterior birthing process.

If the mother's pelvis is ample in size relative to baby's head, then a number of other dynamics may arise. Here, the infant may start out posterior, and begin a long slow rotation right though the end of Stage Two and with even some rotation in Stage Three. The rotation may begin in Stage One and can continue for much of the birth. Here, there may be a long rotational descent right from the very beginning.

Other dynamics are also common. Again, if the mother's pelvis is ample, the baby may engage in almost any position. Posterior positions are most common, but the infant may engage in an oblique position and begin a long slow rotation to the occiput anterior (OA) position at the beginning of Stage Three. Again there may even be rotation in Stage Three. The baby's head may even continue to rotate in the pelvic outlet in such a way that its head passes the midline in rotation.

Let's briefly describe some typical cranial repercussions for a baby who has negotiated its way through an anthropoid pelvis. A long, slow birth with much rotation is common. Rotational forces are introduced relatively high up on the baby's cranium and descend in an arc from the parietal bone to the mandible. The rotational forces can be strong and can last longer than those of a gynecoid pelvis birth. These forces can lead to strong rotation and torsioning in the cranium and dural membrane, and the tissue system in general, in both baby and adult. Torsional issues in the cranial base, temporal bones, sphenoid bone, maxillae, and TMJs are common, as are those in the vertebral axis and pelvis (Figure 5.30).

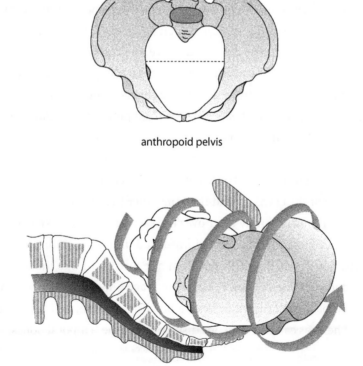

anthropoid pelvis

Figure 5.30. There is commonly much rotation through an anthropoid pelvis.

The Android Pelvic Shape

The android pelvic shape can introduce very intense birthing forces into the baby's system. As seen in Chapter 4, the android pelvis is triangular in shape and the pelvic yoke is very narrow. This leads to both a tight pelvic inlet *and* outlet within which intense forces may be generated. In Stage One, the infant may find it difficult to find an entry point into the inlet. The triangular shape can be very tight here. She may actually take a long time finding a way in. In this period, the infant's head may rotate back and forth against the pelvic inlet until engagement occurs. This can lead to rotational forces introduced high in the baby's cranium. Unlike the anthropoid pelvis, where the infant may descend in rotation right from the beginning, here the infant is not descending. Her head rotates back and forth, and a high, circular-like force is generated in the membrane. I have treated adults who had a feeling they were wearing a very tight skullcap located relatively high up on their heads. There were strong rotational forces in their membrane system and a sense of torsioning and twisting throughout the cranium. The origin of this pattern was found in Stage One of the birth process as they tried to enter their mother's android-shaped pelvis. Here, unlike Stage One of a gynecoid pelvis, there may be rotation right at the beginning of Stage One and it is located high up on the head in a circular pattern.

After the rotation process described above, once a way into the pelvic inlet is found, the baby commonly enters the pelvis in an oblique or transverse position. Due to the triangular pelvic shape, an oblique engagement is the most common. As the baby enters the pelvic inlet, since the android pelvis is triangular and narrow, triangular force vectors are commonly introduced into the cranium. This is because the baby's head meets three points of contact: both pelvic bones and the sacrum. The practitioner may perceive sometimes confusing force vectors that seem to bounce off first one side of the cranium and then the other in a triangular manner. As the baby descends, it must literally lever over the sacrum to enter a synclitic position, and this can lead to very strong forces introduced into the cranium. One colleague of mine calls this a "can opener" effect. I'm not sure that I like the image, but the forces introduced by the conjunct sacrum in Stage One can be extremely intense. Strong cranial base patterns, such as side-bending, torsion, and lateral shear, can be generated here, as can intraosseous distortions of the temporal bones, sphenoid, and occiput.

In an android pelvic shape, there is commonly not very much rotation in Stage Two. This is different from that of the gynecoid or anthropoid pelvis, in which there is rotational descent in Stage Two. Here, due to the tightness of the android pelvis, the baby's head may not rotate very much, and strong medial compressive forces may be fed into the cranium. Exhalation patterns are commonly introduced both here and in Stage One. The baby may remain in an oblique position all the way to the pelvic floor and outlet. Its head may then very quickly rotate so that it faces the sacrum, or may remain oblique throughout Stage Three. The pelvic yoke is very narrow, and strong forces are commonly introduced in Stage Three as the infant negotiates its way under a narrow pelvic arch. A tight android pelvis is a

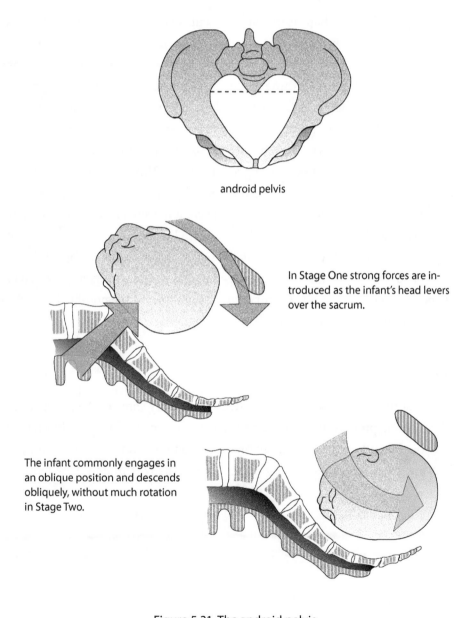

android pelvis

In Stage One strong forces are introduced as the infant's head levers over the sacrum.

The infant commonly engages in an oblique position and descends obliquely, without much rotation in Stage Two.

Figure 5.31. The android pelvis.

very difficult pelvis to be born through. This can lead to variable forces entering the cranium, depending on the position and the length of time in that position. If the infant rotates its face to the sacrum, strong vertical shear patterns are commonly generated. Intraosseous distortions of both the occiput and sphenoid bone are also commonly introduced here. Cesarean births, either planned or elected, are not uncommon due to this tight pelvic shape (Figure 5.31).

The Platypelloid Pelvic Shape

The platypelloid pelvic shape is the most difficult shape to be born through. Platypelloid means *plate-like*. This pelvic shape is wide transversely, and very narrow and tight. This is the kind of pelvic type in which, in earlier days, mother and baby may have died during the birthing process. Elected cesareans are the norm here. Fortunately, a pure platypelloid pelvis is relatively rare. Something like 5 percent of the female population has this kind of pelvic shape. If the baby births through the tightly transverse pelvis, she will enter the pelvic inlet in a transverse position and will remain in that position throughout the birth. This leads to extraordinarily strong medial forces being introduced into the baby's head. Exhalation patterns are the norm. The sacrum becomes a very strong conjunct site and side-bending, torsion, and lateral shear patterns, all to the non-birth lie side, are all coupled together. Medial compressive issues in the cranial base and intraosseous distortions of the temporal bone are also common here. The adult may have a strong, narrow, exhalation look to their face, with a "C" curve that bulges toward the non-birth lie side. I have heard this ignobly called a banana face (Figure 5.32).

Conclusion

I hope that this chapter served to introduce and clarify some of the issues related to the birthing process. Please have patience. It may need a few read-throughs, as it may be difficult to visualize these motions. You may want to buy a soft pelvic model and properly scaled baby model to take the "baby" through these motions.

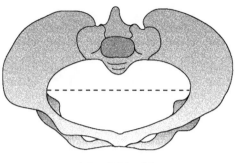

platypelloid pelvis

The infant descends and births in a transverse position with little or no roation.

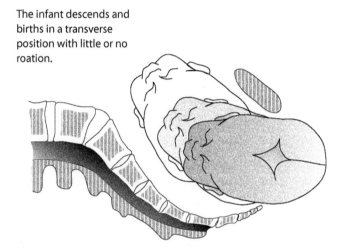

Figure 5.32. The platypelloid pelvis.

CHAPTER 6

Treating Infants and Intraosseous Issues in Adults

In this chapter I would like to introduce clinical orientations to infant and adult birth issues. We start by forming and negotiating a conscious relationship with infants—which recognizes their sentience and presence—and will then turn our attention to session work, including various intraosseous issues. As stated earlier, I always advise new practitioners, if they are interested in working with infants, to be supervised by a senior practitioner who has experience in this area. Supervised clinics are another avenue, as are post-graduate courses. I find that infants place me on the cutting edge of my knowledge and personal process, and a gradual approach to working with them builds confidence and allows the sessions to be a resource for all concerned, including the practitioner.

General Guidelines for Treating Infants

As introduced in earlier chapters, the foundation of care for infants is the recognition that they are feeling, sentient beings. Babies recognize the presence of the practitioner and contact must be negotiated sensitively. The best approach is to wait until baby acknowledges our presence and invites us to make contact. In some hospital births, babies may have experienced being handled as unfeeling objects, with little recognition of their awareness or choice. So if practitioners behave in a similar manner, they may activate baby's traumatic implicit memories, including fear and anger.

Working with babies requires a slower pacing than normal. A soft, slow-motion presence and very gentle contact is essential. Among other factors, the birthing process is often quite a hectic scene—especially in the hospital setting—with midwives, obstetricians, and other staff acting quickly and efficiently. A slow, deliberate contact can serve as a counterbalance for the baby's impressions of this kind of birth experience.

This is especially true for traumatized infants. In initial sessions we may not be able to touch their cranium or body at all. Instead, we may have to use Emerson's *far touch* by slowly meeting their local field energetically with our touch and presence. Until it is clear that a baby is receptive to our touch, we might work off the body using intention and proximity. As the baby begins to experience far touch as noninvasive, she may become more receptive to the practitioner's presence and actual physical touch. Negotiated far touch may also lead the practitioner to areas of the baby's body where touch is experienced as noninvasive and nontraumatizing.

In working with infants, respect their relationship with mom, who is ideally their major resource. Babies' use of their mother as a resource is usually quite evident. They will turn their heads to watch mom, follow her voice, and continually monitor her presence. Include both in all communications and include mom in your contact—including touch—with infants. Always work in relationship to baby and mom as a holistic unit.

The baby commonly resources itself by seeking the most comfortable position and most secure relationship. For most babies this means turning to their lie side (see the next section) and being in close visual, auditory, and physical contact with mom. In working with babies, we try to observe how the baby resources—and then resonate with those behaviors. Practitioners ideally work in the range and nature of the baby's resources and find that a baby will begin to sense the practitioner and the sessions as another resource over time.

As discussed earlier, babies are conscious, sentient beings who seem to know exactly what I am saying. They are responsive to my voice in clear ways. I know that babies' nervous system is immature at these early stages of life, yet I also know that they largely understand my communications. Because of this, I always talk directly to babies and also let them know my intentions, which they clearly seem to understand. It is likewise also important to not talk over them as though they are not there. They recognize this and may become disturbed and distrustful. Instead, include them in conversations with mom and dad and other caregivers. Over a number of sessions, they will gradually come to recognize you as a person who respects their presence and listens to their communications. The only time this is not evident is if the infant presents dissociation and parasympathetic shock affects due to the overwhelming nature of their experience. They then cannot orient to me, my intentions, or my words. Gentle stillpoints via the sacrum and appropriate birth ignition intentions may be very helpful here.

Babies will describe their history and clinical issues through movement, sound, and orienting actions. They may direct us to sites of discomfort or focus, or reenact portions of their birth process. I have had many babies take my hand and place it over the place "where it hurts," or take my hand away if they are not ready for contact where I am touching, or if the contact is too intense or overwhelming. Work in the resources of infants and respect their "no" statements. If a baby does not want you to touch in a certain place or manner, respect that. If they say "no" by pushing your hand away, or by a traumatic activation, please back off. The baby may need to deal with other things first, may not be resourced enough in your presence, or may simply need more time and space to settle, resource, and tell his story.

Babies will show motions relative to their traumatization and related inertial fulcrums. They may express disjointed motion and loss of orientation when they meet the edges of their motion dynamics. Notice these often subtle expressions and respect them as valid communications, as we would naturally do if they were coming from an adult. Hear their sounds, movements, crying, gestures, and facial expressions as communications that are definitely not arbitrary. Listen for how the infant needs to resolve its trauma. Remember that trauma is not just physical. It resonates with every aspect of a baby's being. They may need to express their fear or anger, and/or they may need to resolve some sympathetic or parasympathetic shock affect.

Inhalation oriented stillpoints are helpful in parasympathetic dissociative shock states—where baby seems far away, disoriented, and not fully present. Exhalation oriented stillpoints can generally help resource and slow down sympathetic arousal—where a baby is expressing strong emotions, with crying and disjointed movements. When babies settle out of a dissociative state, they will commonly let you or mom know how painful their experience was. Again, they may describe this in their movements, emotional states, in crying, and facial expressions. Please stay present, use a soft and calm voice, resource baby in mom's presence, and let babies know that they are in control. The more baby can come into oriented, present-time awareness, and directly express its experience, the sooner related nervous system cycling can resolve and clear.

In session work, infants' systems will most clearly orient to mid-tide and Long Tide phenomenon. The Long Tide is very evident in their local field. As baby's system deepens, it is thus important to orient to Long Tide as a tidal body that is supporting the baby. Babies will naturally orient to this most fundamental level of primary respiration, if given the opportunity. Maintain your wide perceptual field, sense the space around and in the baby's system, and simply be present.

Babies are also fluid-tide/fluid-body beings. Their sutures are not yet formed, the fontanels are large, and the cranium is basically a fluidic-membranous system, as is their whole body. It is thus important to orient to their bodies as a fluidic field suspended in the tidal body, where an appropriately light touch is used—hands floating on tissues, suspended in fluid. In this ambiance, we patiently offer our presence and stillness.

In sessions with babies, the action of potency in the fluids is very evident. As specific inertial fulcrums, vector patterns, and related compressive issues clarify in session work, fluctuations of potency and fluid will commonly lead you to these inertial sites. Work will orient to deepening states of balance and equilibrium and the appropriate augmentation of space and fluid drive if needed. Remembering that the baby really is a holistic fluid body, sometimes augmenting the drive of potency and fluid from the sacrum superiorly at the height of inhalation—while also holding baby's occiput—may help resolve compressive forces in the cranium. Subtly augmenting space and the action of potency in and around specific compressed areas can also be helpful.

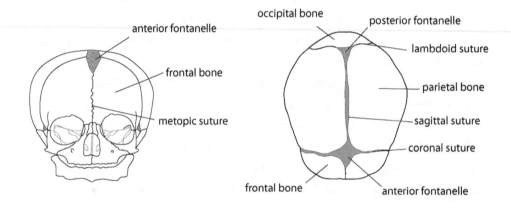

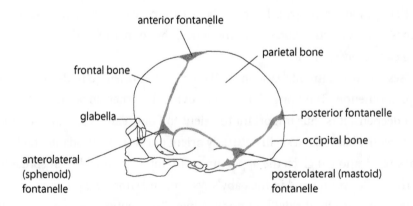

Figure 6.1. The fetal skull.

Don't try to do too much in a session. It is also important that you like infants and that you like to play. The infant learns that the session is resourcing and that you are fun. Then, when difficult edges arise, they will look to you as a resource, not as the cause of their pain (Figure 6.1).

The Field of Orientation

I have repeatedly observed that infants have a *field of orientation* arising from unresolved traumatic experience. One direction of motion and orientation will be comforting, while another is difficult. For instance, babies commonly orient more easily to their surroundings from their birth lie side. This is because the forces of birth tend to generate compressive tensions through baby's body, which creates a "C" curve, with the concavity on the birth lie side (see Figure 5.11). It is easier for the baby to orient from that side, being naturally pulled toward it due to the presence of compressive forces. If mom is positioned on the birth lie side, baby may orient to her as a resource more easily. As mom moves to the opposite side—and baby's head rotates toward its midline as it follows mom's movement—baby may begin to become disoriented and express disjointed motions and distress. This is perhaps why many babies prefer feeding on one breast more than the other. By noticing the field of orientation and locating ourselves in that area, practitioners can more easily cultivate a trusting relationship. We are making it easier for babies to relate to us by letting them use their visual, auditory, and kinesthetic senses from their most resourced space.

Similarly, babies may have a *position of orientation*. For example, if they were born in a posterior position, (i.e., occiput posterior throughout the birth process) they may feel most oriented and prefer to lie in this position.

Look for the baby's more oriented side and/or position, or their field of orientation (Figure 6.2), and initially work from that side or position. In early sessions I always work with the baby being held by the mother. In later sessions the baby could be placed on a mat or pillow, with the mother located nearby in the field of orientation. Gradually, the positioning of the mother becomes less significant as the baby begins to recognize the practitioner as a resource. For example, if the baby orients most easily to the left side, work from that side and have mom in baby's visual field on that side. Also ask mom to talk to her baby from there so that the baby can orient to her voice as a resource. Hearing mom's voice can elicit a primal orienting response and evoke feelings of being nurtured.

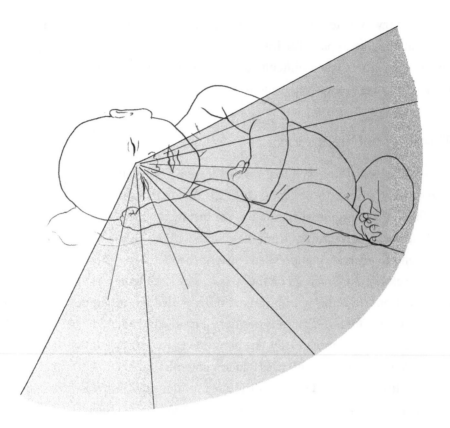

Figure 6.2. The infant has a field of orientation.

Common Inertial Fulcrums and Issues in Infants

A large variety of inertial fulcrums and patterns may be observed in babies. These generally relate to the shape of the mother's pelvis, the nature and progression of the birth process, and medical interventions that were used during birth. The following are common cranial issues that practitioners may sense or observe in newborns and infants.

Cranial Overriding and Molding Patterns

Overriding refers to the slippage of one cranial bone over the other, instead of their normal abutment positioning. Almost any kind of cranial overriding or molding pattern can result from the forces experienced in birth. Common examples include overriding of parietal bones and of the two parts of the frontal bone. Overriding is not just a matter of bony relationships; the membranes are also involved. Bones are perceived as denser places in the membranous whole and the combination of bone and membrane is a holistic form. Treatment of overriding is relatively straightforward, involving placement of two fingers of the same hand on either side of the relationship involved. For example, if the two parietal bones have overridden at the sagittal suture, place a finger on each bone. At the height of inhalation, orient to the augmentation of space across the relationship while augmenting fluid drive fluid to the site with the other hand at the occiput. It is really a matter of orienting to the drive of potency and fluids in the system.

Cranial *molding* issues generally relate to forces lodged in a particular bone and in the membranous-osseous system as a whole. For instance, a raised aspect in a bone such as a parietal bone may seem to be puckered-up. This is not just a structural or tissue form; it is an energetic expression of the presence of potency and inertial forces in an inertial fulcrum. Treatment of molding involves placing your fingers in a circular ring around the puckered area, or to either side of it. Potency processes the inertial forces in the bone, and helps the membranous-osseous system reorient to natural midline phenomena.

A similar cranial molding pattern has to do with flattened areas. It is not uncommon to observe a flattened occiput, parietal, or frontal bone resulting from the birthing forces placed against the membranous-osseous system. Again, we approach these with recognition that bones, membranes, and fluids are one continuous whole. For treatment of a flattened area, place your fingers in a circle around the area, or to either side of it, and augment fluid drive toward the flattened site as you also allow your fingers in contact with the area to resonate with the natural motility of the bone, augmenting space in its tissues at the height of inhalation. Your fingers, suspended in fluid—in resonance with the action of potency and tissue motility—are subtly spread apart by the action of the fluid tide and its potency, augmenting the expression of potency in the site. This is very delicate work. The potency does the work, not your finger pressure or intention.

Compressive Issues

All sorts of compressive issues may arise from the unresolved forces of the birthing process. The following is a simple pointer to some of the more common issues, not a comprehensive list of all possibilities.

Sphenoid-Vomer Compression

It is common to find compressive issues between the vomer and the sphenoid bone. In a gynecoid pelvis shape, the forces generating this kind of compression are generally introduced in Stage Three when the baby's face is conjunct with the mother's sacrum. An inertial force between the body of the sphenoid and the vomer may be sensed in any number of ways—an inertial pattern and motion organized around the area, backpressure, density, and barrier below the sphenoid bone, or lateral fluctuations of fluid and potency around the area. Treatment involves placing an index finger in the infant's mouth. This must be negotiated with extra care, as babies use the mouth as a primary medium for interacting with the environment. I do not like to use finger cots with babies because they generally do not like the taste. There are several ways to work around this problem. We can wash our hands really well with antibacterial soap and then carefully rinse the soap off well, or we can wash the finger cot once it is in place. The cotted finger can also be dipped in mother's milk or a familiar-tasting formula.

An infant often accepts the finger as a sucking reflex and even as a knowing attempt to get relief from the sensation of vomer compression. Relief of vomer compression can be a factor in the impulse for thumb-sucking. Even if your finger is easily accepted, settle, orient, and wait before doing anything. Negotiate your intention here; listen and wait for a sense of negotiated contact. When the relationship seems well established, very gently contact the baby's upper palate with that finger.

With your other hand at the top of the infant's head, subtly augment the action of fluid drive and potency toward the sphenoid-vomer interface. At the height of inhalation, sense the presence of potency as a bioelectric-biomagnetic force in the

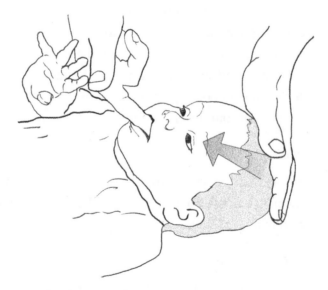

Figure 6.3. Augmenting fluid drive toward the sphenoid-vomer area.

fluids—allow your hand on top of baby's head to augment this drive toward the inertial spheno-vomer area by a simple orientation to it in the tissues of your hand or fingers. Simultaneously, allow your finger under the baby's palate to resonate with the action of potency at the height of inhalation and to breathe deeper in the natural inhalation motility of the vomer—inferior-anterior. Remember that, in inhalation, the rear of the vomer naturally rotates inferior at the back of the palate, while its anterior aspect rotates anterior-superior (see Chapter 14). Again, your finger is suspended in fluid, being breathed by the tide and moves like kelp in the sea in the inhalation direction of tide and motility. Use no force whatsoever, but rather let the fluids and potency do the work. Using force may simply enlist the baby's defensive processes and can even deepen the compression (Figure 6.3).

Occipital Base Compression and Intraosseous Distortions of the Occiput

Occipital base compression and intraosseous distortions of the occiput are common issues in infants, with wide-ranging implications as described above. Patterns include rotation of occipital squama, telescoping, wedging of condylar parts, occipito-atlanteal compression, and a general axial compression throughout the relationships of the occiput and sphenoid.

Occipital base compression affects nearby cranial nerves and can generate many issues including digestive—sucking and feeding, colic, and diarrhea—and respiratory breathing difficulties. It may also be coupled with poor sleep and autonomic activation in the baby's brain stem area. The occipital area can be very sensitive to the newborn and young infant, so all our considerations about careful negotiation and slow pacing apply.

One approach to occipital intraosseous fulcrums is to negotiate contact with the baby's occiput and orient to the augmentation of space in its tissues. For infants, place the index and middle fingers of one hand at the occipital base's two condylar parts so that the foramen magnum is between them. Place the other hand on the baby's frontal bone with the intention of augmenting fluid drive toward the occipital area. Remember that the occiput is in four parts here. See if you can sense those parts and their interrelationships as part of the whole membranous-osseous-fluid system of the cranium.

At the height of inhalation, allow your two fingers to be moved by the tide and take a deeper breath at its height. As this occurs, your fingers will be subtly spread apart in resonance both with the tidal surge and with the natural widening and space generated in the parts of the occiput at the height of inhalation. If no tide is present, allow your fingers to be suspended in fluid and to take a deeper breath as though the tide is moving them and they are breathing deeper in its inhalation direction.

Simultaneously, you can also augment fluid drive toward the occipital area via your contact on the baby's frontal bone. Again, this is accomplished via resonance with the action of potency in the fluid tide, and your hand/finger's orientation to the occipital area.

As this occurs, the potency centering inertial forces in the occiput will begin to process them and a spreading of the condylar parts, a de-telescoping of the occipital parts, basi-occiput, and body of the sphenoid bone will naturally occur. Again, let the potency do the work! The practitioner's role is to simply and intelligently augment naturally occurring processes (Figure 6.4).

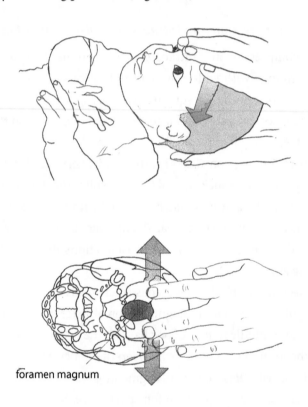

foramen magnum

Figure 64. Augmentation of space and fluid drive in occipital area.

Temporal-Occipital Issues

The temporal-occipital interface is another common area for inertial issues in babies. This junction will become the occipito-mastoid suture as the baby matures. The approach is similar to the one described above, with the index and middle fingers of one hand now on either side of the temporal-occipital interface. The middle finger is placed on the occipital squama while the index finger is placed on the temporal bone. The other hand is placed on the diagonally opposite frontal bone. After negotiating contact, we again orient to the height of inhalation and augment space between the temporal bone and occiput, simultaneously augmenting fluid drive toward the temporal-occipital area with our other hand. Again, this is a matter of resonance with the action of potency as it is expressed in the tide, and the natural space generated in the tissue field at the height of inhalation. Wait for the action of potency to manifest locally, and for the tissues to naturally spread apart as the inertial force is resolved.

Medial Compression and Intraosseous Temporal Bone Distortion

Intraosseous distortions of the temporal bone are common, as is medial compression of the cranial base. These often arise in the early stages of the birth process, especially in Stages One and Two when the baby experiences medial and rotational forces in the descent past the mother's sacrum. This can affect one side only or both sides. Again, there are a number of traditional approaches to these issues. Classically you can orient to both temporal bones, or to one at a time.

In the first approach, hold the baby's ears in your normal temporal bone ear hold. Allow your hands to resonate with the expression of tide and to augment the expression of potency and motility at the height of inhalation. Again, allow your hands to float on the baby's tissues, suspended in fluid—your hands take a deeper breath in the direction of inhalation tide and motility, which augments the action of potency locally and resonates with the natural expression of space in the tissue field. If no tide is present, allow your fingers, suspended in fluid, to take a deeper breath as though the tide is moving them and they are breathing deeper in its inhalation direction.

Alternatively, you can hold baby's temporal bones in a temporal bone ear hold—gently holding both lobes of each temporal bone. At the height of inhalation you allow your hands to resonate with the natural space generated in the temporal bones' relationship to the other bones in the cranial base. As the tide surges, your hands augment space as they are moved by the tide and resonate with the natural widening across the cranium along the 45-degree angle that each temporal bone makes with the occiput and sphenoid bones.

Another approach is to orient to one temporal bone at a time, especially useful if only one bone is inertial. Lightly hold the temporal bone involved by gently holding the ear lobe of that bone. Your other hand is diagonally located on the opposite frontal bone side. At the height of inhalation, the fingers of the hand at the baby's ear lobe are subtly moved by the inhalation surge and augment space as above—as inhalation is sensed, your fingers are moved by the tide and take a deeper breath as the cranium widens along the 45-degree angle that the temporal bone sits in. You can simultaneously augment fluid drive to the area with your hand on the frontal bone—again, allow the fingers of that hand to resonate with the action of potency in the fluids as they orient to the temporal bone on the opposite side of the head (Figure 6.5).

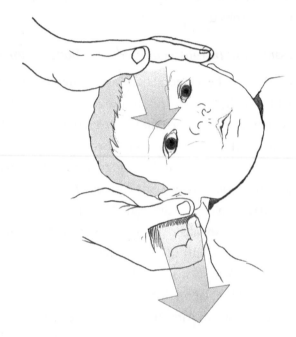

Figure 6.5. Augmentation of space and fluid drive toward one temporal bone.

Cranial Base Patterns

Any and all of the classic cranial base patterns may present in the infant due to prenatal and/or birthing process. I find that the most important thing for the practitioner to do is to orient to the pattern and to offer space. The most useful approach in infant work is to simply augment space in the cranial base as a whole. You can use either Sutherland's hold or Becker's vault hold. I find Becker's hold easiest with babies, as their heads are small compared to my hands.

In a gentle Becker's hold—hands floating on tissue suspended in fluid—allow all of your fingers to resonate with the tidal expression of inhalation. They are both moved by the fluid tide and its potency and take a deeper breath at the height of inhalation. All of your fingers suspended in fluid breathe deeply here—your thumbs at the baby's greater wings tend to spread anterior and slightly inferior as the tide takes them (Figure 6.6). This must be done with ultimate sensitivity. As your fingers resonate with the natural expression of potency and space at the height of inhalation, the action of potency is augmented and inertial forces begin to be processed and resolved.

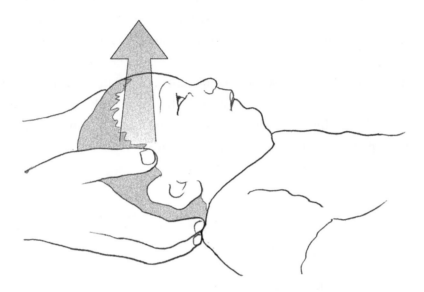

Figure 6.6. Augmentation of space and action of potency in vault hold.

Sacrum and Occiput

A simple *bipolar sacrum-occiput hold* can be a great starting point in orienting to a baby's system. Holding and orienting to the two poles of the primary respiratory system orients you to the core of baby's system and the primal midline, and can be very healing for the baby. Gently hold the baby's sacrum and occiput at the same time—allow your hands to be soft and suspended in fluid (Figure 6.7). It may be enough to simply hold the two poles and deepen into stillness and equilibrium. Alternatively, it may be helpful to subtly augment space between the two poles. Orient to the fluid body and fluid tide. As you sense the height of inhalation, allow your hands to be moved and to take a deeper breath. As you allow this, your two hands will seem to spread apart—your hand at the occiput being moved by the surge through the midline and natural rising of the tide. Alternatively, if no tide is clearly present, allow your fingers to take a deeper breath as though the tide is moving them and they are breathing deeper in its inhalation direction.

As this occurs the natural expression of potency and space through the midline is augmented, which will also augment the expression of potency through the midline and help resolve any compressive axial forces present in the baby's vertebral axis. If an axial compression is present in the vertebral midline, a general lengthening and expansion through the midline may be perceived. Midline axial birthing forces are common in both infants and adults. An alternative approach that sometimes works is to augment the action of potency cephalad from a sacral hold. At the height of inhalation, allow your hand at the sacrum to be moved by, and to follow, the rising of potency in the fluids. Again the felt sense of this is that your hand takes a deeper breath in that direction. This will augment the natural expression of potency in the inhalation surge. This commonly augments the fluid drive along the midline and helps resolve the axial forces present, and may even resolve compressive fulcrums in the cranium above.

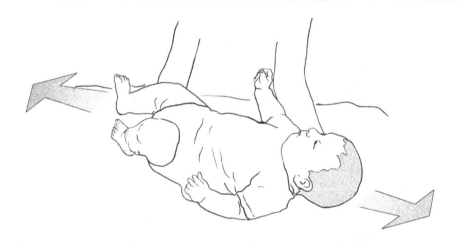

Figure 6.7. Augmenting space while holding the sacrum and occiput.

Other Clinical Issues

Forceps

The use of forceps to aid delivery has a long and complex history. Forceps are commonly used in urgent situations and are not always ideally applied to the infant's cranium. Many times, too much force is used to pull the infant out, and sometimes the obstetrician simply gets the direction and motion of the infant wrong and places extra forces upon her system, against the existing direction of natural movement.

I have seen diverse baby and adult outcomes relating to the use of forceps, both positive and negative. In some cases the use of forceps undeniably helped alleviate the suffering and pain of both mother and baby. I have even seen cases where the sensitive and gentle use of forceps helped the infant and left no cranial issues whatsoever. However, these seem to be the exception rather than the rule. Common issues that derive from the use of forceps include intraosseous distortions of various bones, tissue abrasions, and the introduction of compressive forces, which leave marks on the baby and generate various inertial issues in the cranium, cranial bone overriding, and the introduction of compressive force vectors into the infant's cranium. While working with adults, I have even seen forceps marks come out on their face as the forces involved were processed.

Cesarean Births

Cesarean births are becoming more and more common. If you see babies in your practice, you will certainly see many infants who have undergone this birthing process. There are two kinds of cesarean births: *elective* (in which the baby was not engaged in the birth canal), and *emergency* (in which the infant was engaged and may even have been far into its birthing process). Each kind of cesarean birth may generate different issues in the baby's system.

For both kinds of cesarean, the general anesthetic given the mother is also experienced by the baby. Anesthetic shock affects may arise. Anesthesia may generate a parasympathetic response in the baby, inducing a hypoarousal state. This is basically a state of parasympathetic shock. The baby may seem listless or sleep a lot, and she may not be able to orient to her mother, or to her essential needs such as feeding. Difficulties in feeding, dissociation, fluid shock, and poor ignition are possible affects.

I have held many cesarean babies whose heads felt solid, almost like a cannon ball. When I first encountered this, I was surprised. What happened to the baby as a fluid-sac pulsating with potency? Babies' heads are not supposed to feel like cannon balls! I really had to reorient to a new process here. This stasis and solidity is a direct repercussion of the fluid shock held in the core of the system. I found that I really had to orient to the Long Tide, to field phenomena, and to deeper resources. Inhalation stillpoints via the sacrum and gentle augmentation of space throughout the system—perhaps via the bipolar sacrum-occiput hold described above—may help free up some of the inertial potency and process some of the effects of the experience. Ignition is a real issue here, but some resolution of shock states must be accessed first.

In the elective cesarean, the baby is generally removed from the mother's uterus before it has entered the pelvic inlet and birth canal. When the surgeon opens up the mother's abdomen and uterus, a very rapid pressure change may be experienced by the baby. This can generate fluid shock. The potency in the fluid will become suddenly inertial in order to center the forces induced by the rapid pressure change. This may have strong repercussions for that infant, as fluid stasis results. The fluids lock up as the potency becomes suddenly inertial. This will strongly affect the ignition process at birth. The fluids may not fully ignite in the midline and the third ventricle when the umbilicus stops pulsing and the first breath is taken.

Another inevitable disadvantage of elective cesarean relates to timing. The baby has a key role to play in the birthing process. Both baby and mother mutually employ the naturally arising biochemical stimuli that initiate the birth process. Elective cesareans are commonly done for the convenience of the mother and the doctor, overriding the baby's role. The whole situation is a reflection of the belief system that babies have little intelligence or feelings, and can be treated as medical objects. It is a convenient blind spot by which the practice is perpetuated, without informed consent by the parents since the topic was never discussed. Unprepared for the birth and literally not biochemically ready, these babies often show autonomic distress and activation, not uncommonly manifesting parasympathetic shock.

In the non-elective, or engaged, cesarean section, usually in an emergency situation, the baby has entered the birth canal. Perhaps the birth has been going on too long, or the obstetrician felt that the birth process might be dangerous to the mother and/or baby if continued much longer. In this case the baby has encountered the forces and timing of a natural birth. The doctor may need to use great force to pull the baby back out of the birth canal.

The practitioner needs to appreciate the nature of the trauma here. The baby has been through an extremely difficult experience. There has been sudden disengagement from the mother and the womb experience. This is true in both kinds of cesarean section. In the case of an engaged cesarean, the disengagement process may have been experienced as a violent wrenching away from the mother and her pelvic canal. Unusual cranial patterns will be generated by the forces of the pull. These are not forces that the system is naturally designed to meet. Natural birthing forces generally drag caudal; they do not pull violently cephalad. This will most likely be shocking to the infant. Shock affects and dissociative processes are common here, compounded by the anesthesia used. The baby may be left with a poor sense of boundaries as its boundaries were violated in the process. When born, the infant may not be able to orient to the space around it or to mother, perhaps for some time after birth. Because of the emergency surgical setting, the baby may have no contact with mom at all for an extended recovery period in separate areas of the hospital. This may generate bonding and feeding issues. Either hyperarousal or hypoarousal states are common.

In emergency cesareans, the sympathetic nervous system is commonly engaged during the birthing process. But the parasympathetic nervous system may also suddenly surge to protect the infant. A coexisting parasympathetic shock response then overlays and masks the initial sympathetic response. After birth, the baby may seem dissociated and listless, yet under that, anger and fight-flight energies are still cycling. In session work, as the parasympathetic shock resolves, the underlying sympathetic cycling may come to the surface. What seemed to be a listless and dissociated baby is suddenly able to express its anger. The baby may also express pushing intentions during sessions, as these could not be completed naturally due to anesthesia and the cesarean section. Angry, pushing babies are thus more common in emergency cesareans, where the birth process was engaged but then interrupted. I always explain these possibilities to parents as they may blame me as practitioner, or the sessions, for their baby's anger. After all, they may have come with a placid baby who is now very angry. They need to be able to hear the anger of their infant, respond with reassurance and contact, and not take it personally.

In elected cesareans, pure parasympathetic shock is more common, as the baby's system was rapidly overwhelmed by the experience, setting the stage for later bouts of low motivation, low energy, and chronic fatigue. As described earlier, these children are commonly not identified as needing help because they sleep a lot and are perceived as good, quiet babies. They may later have learning difficulties and poor attention spans due to the parasympathetic shock affects and dissociative processes still cycling in their system. In these cases, I try to gently orient the infant to the possibility of movement and pushing in order to mobilize a more sympathetic nervous system response. I do this via gentle contact and upward pressure on the bottoms of their feet and the use of a reassuring and encouraging voice.

Vacuum Extraction

Vacuum extraction, or ventouse, is becoming more and more common. In this process a suction cup is placed upon the infant's head to enable a grip for pulling the baby out. The common thinking is that suction has less potential for damage than forceps. Unfortunately, I have found this to be incorrect. If forceps are carefully and sensitively applied, repercussions can be minimized. But I have never seen minimal repercussions with ventouse. The suction applied can have highly traumatizing consequences. There is commonly a local hematoma at the site of the application of the suction, but repercussions are deeper than this. The baby's system was not designed to meet these kinds of suction forces during the birthing process. Rather than dragging forces in the cranium and body, a strong suction is introduced into the baby's fluid system. This is experienced as a shock, and potency becomes inertial in the cerebrospinal fluid. Fluid shock and stasis result. This will strongly affect the ignition of fluids with potency at birth. Ignition will be dampened down due to systemic fluid shock.

The central nervous system is also affected by vacuum extraction births. After all, the cranial vault is made of soft bones, with large spaces between them. It is just a sheet of membrane, so the suction forces go deeply into the system and actually impact the brain. I have found in many cases that the Aqueduct of Sylvius is literally pulled up cephalad in this process and can remain in this position if not treated. If the inertial forces suctioning the aqueduct are not resolved, they will continue to generate a pulling force after birth. This pattern may stay with a person indefinitely, producing fluid backpressure and lowered fluid drive in the system.

The easiest way to relate to the Aqueduct of Sylvius is to place a finger, or fingertips, at the top of the baby's head. Place your other hand at the base of the occiput. In this position, form a general relationship to her fluid system. Let the fluids come to you; do not crowd or invade the infant's system. Once you have done this, see if you can sense the third and fourth ventricles. An initial visualization of these structures may help, but you must learn to actually sense the ventricles through direct perception. With the fingers at the top of the baby's head, augment a drive of potency and fluid downward toward and through the Aqueduct of Sylvius. After a while you may sense events such as expressions of potency, fluid fluctuations, a processing of the inertial forces present—perhaps as a streaming of energy and/or heat, a shift or settling in the aqueduct, and a settling of the nervous system as a whole. There may be a general sense of downward streaming in the body as the backpressure releases.

I have also seen cases in which the ventouse process has generated parasympathetic shock states. My sense is that the shock of the process elicits a more primitive response than fight-or-flight, or that the fight-or-flight response becomes overwhelmed very quickly and the infant enters a dissociative and withdrawn state. Sympathetic arousal may also be running under this, and after some of these issues are resolved, you may find yourself treating a very angry little person. This process can give rise to listless, dissociated babies, or to very angry, hyperaroused babies who do not sleep well.

Clinical Highlight

A good number of years ago, I helped set up a free clinic for infants and newborns. We called our clinic the Whole Family Clinic, because we recognized the powerful fulcrum the baby becomes for the whole family, not just for mothers. We always had at least two practitioners present so that the mother's process could be attended to if her own birth issues arose during the session work with her baby. We also tried to have fathers attend the sessions and we worked with the family dynamics cycling around the baby. The intention of the clinic was especially to cater to young parents and young single mothers who could not afford sessions. The team included myself, a cranially trained obstetrician (Dr. Martin Hunt), and another experienced cranial practitioner (Maria Harris). We each donated one morning a week to this clinic over a three-year period.

A nineteen-year-old single mother came into our clinic with her two-month-old baby daughter. The father had left her and she was on her own with the infant. She was a strong and bright young woman, but had no current source of income and was on welfare benefits. All of her energies were taken up by her new role as a mom. The baby's delivery had been an emergency cesarean section. The baby was pulled out after many hours of labor. It had been an exhausting and painful experience for both mother and baby. She brought the baby in because the infant was not sleeping and had a very strong case of colic. The mother also expressed her difficulty in bonding with the baby and in feeling the baby's bonding with her. This is not unusual in cesarean births. We began to see the two of them weekly.

Much was accomplished over the first two months. The colic was greatly reduced and the infant's sleeping began to enter more set patterns so that her mother had more space and more sleep for herself. Work initially revolved around a gentle negotiation of contact with the baby, as she was very traumatized by her experience. Initially it was hard to touch the infant without eliciting a fight-or-flight response. Her typical response was to turn her head away, cry, and go into dissociation. Babies cry for all sorts of reasons. Mostly it is to communicate something to us. I don't mind babies crying in sessions—it is part of the process—but not if they dissociate. Working while babies are dissociated can drive their trauma deeper. So initially it was a slow process of negotiating contact and short periods of hands-on clinical work. It was important for us to become a clearly felt resource for both mom and baby. This occurred over time. The infant became easy in our presence and accepted gentle contact for longer periods. It is patient work. Mom, in turn, was able to talk about her predicament. The sessions became a resource for her also. As time went on, some of the traumatic forces and fulcrums in the infant's system, and their related tissue affects, were resolved. There were also sessions devoted to the processing of her shock affects that were expressed as fear, crying, and dissociation. We had to help her slowly process all of this. Yet there was still something between mom and baby. The bonding had never really happened, and mom was acutely aware of this.

In one magical session, when the baby was about five months old, an extraordinary process ensued. We were attending to an intraosseous distortion of the occiput. It was a very deep pattern coupled to shock affects and fear. We were very aware of its dynamics and had worked with it in previous sessions. Mom was holding her baby upright against her body. I felt a streaming of energy out of the area and then baby focused her eyes on mom. This was something in itself, as the baby would very rarely look at her mother. Then she expressed incredible anger; rage is the best name for it. She began to beat mom with her tiny hands held in fists. She screamed in anger, and her mother was shocked. There was a deep fight-or-flight anger still cycling in the infant, generated at the time of the birth process. I held the baby while my co-worker supported the mother and I simply said to her, "You know mommy didn't mean to hurt you; it hurt her too." Then the mother, with tears in her eyes said, "Yes I would never hurt you; it hurt me so much too." A marvelous thing happened: the baby stopped hitting her mother and looked deeply into her eyes as the mother was looking at her with tears in her eyes, and literally melted into her arms. Her whole body softened for the first time in all these months. It was like the baby finally landed in her mother's presence and could feel her mother's heart and could finally feel safe. We all cried a bit together. After that, their relationship was completely transformed. I saw them a few years later and both were doing very well.

Intraosseous Occipital Distortions and the Occipital Base Spread

In Chapter 5 we discussed the possible introduction of intraosseous forces into the cranium, including the many significant repercussions and the wide range of symptoms that can result from related intraosseous issues. Now that we have an understanding of the clinical considerations in working with babies, let's explore treatment concepts for working with intraosseous issues in the adult. This section depends on

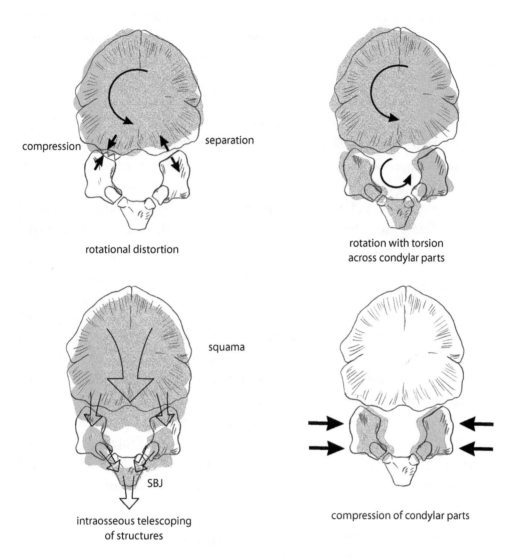

Figure 6.8. Common intraosseous distortions of the occiput.

knowing the specific anatomy of the newborn cranium as well as the specific forces at work during the process, as presented in Chapter 5. Following are summaries of the major possibilities for intraosseous occipital distortions (Figure 6.8).

Rotational Distortions of the Occiput

During birth process, the occipital squama may be forced to rotate clockwise or counterclockwise relative to the other parts of the occiput, with the inertial fulcrum generating the rotation located in the occiput itself. This can lead to compression between the squamous portion and the condylar part it is rotating toward, and a spreading pattern on the other side. Intraosseous rotation of the occipital squama commonly generates cranial base torsion. In this case the fulcrum of the torsion lies not in the SBJ relationships, but in the occiput itself.

Compression Across the Condylar Parts of the Occiput

Due to the rotational distortion described above, or other medially compressive forces introduced during birth process, the condylar parts of the occiput can become medially compressed and/or torsioned in relationship to each other. Telescoping of structure as described below is a common origin of compression of the condylar parts. Compression and/or torsion across the foramen magnum will result. This will literally wedge and compress the articular surfaces of the atlas into the condylar parts of the occiput.

Telescoping of the Occiput

As intense anterior birthing forces are introduced into the occiput—commonly in Stage Three—the squama, condylar parts, and basi-occiput may all be forced to compress together toward the SBJ. Compression across the foramen magnum may also result. This will commonly wedge the atlas between the condyles and compromise its free motion. It is very common for an intransigent SBJ compression to have its primary inertial fulcrum located in an intraosseous telescoping of occipital structure. It is no use working with the SBJ as the fulcrum of a cranial base compression if the forces at work are actually located in the occiput. The SBJ compression may be secondary to the intraosseous occipital distortion.

Working with Intraosseous Issues in Adults

Let's now turn our intention to addressing birth issues in the adult. If the forces generated by the birthing process have not been resolved, they will continue to be organizing patterns and tendencies in the person's system. Intraosseous distortions are manifestations of traumatic forces and related fulcrums that have lodged in bony tissue. Intraosseous fulcrums in the occiput, sphenoid, and temporal bones are commonly at the heart of cranial base patterns and tension patterns throughout the body. They are always of traumatic origin, often arising from pre- and perinatal birth events or early childhood. They can also be generated by later trauma, such as an accident or fall, and may even be a response to severe emotional shock.

In the adult, the traumatic forces that were introduced during their birth experience are still present, maintaining tissue compression and patterning in their system. It is important to remember that the origin of the pattern—unresolved birthing forces—is still held in the present. A biodynamic orientation to cranial work is not about the past—or what is left over from the past—but is about present forces still at work in the client's system. This reminder is especially relevant when we are encountering birth patterns in adults. The history may be compelling, drawing us out of present-time awareness, but the work depends on our being able to maintain orientation to the forces currently at work rather than with the story of how they got there. In the clinical exploration below, we present approaches to intraosseous issues in adult clinical practice.

Many times, as you hold the adult cranium, it may feel like you are holding an infant's head in your hands. It is important to receive this and to also hold the adult's infant in your heart-space. Deepening on the relationship I have with clients, I sometimes acknowledge that it feels like I am holding their infant in my hands, and may even help clients make a present-time relationship to the felt-sense of that little one in their own heart center.

Exploration:
Birth-Related Patterns in the Occiput_____

In this exploration, we are assuming that an inertial pattern organized around an intraosseous fulcrum located in the occiput has clarified as the inherent treatment plan unfolds.

After starting as usual, orient to the three bodies and holistic shift via contact with the client's feet. Let's assume that an inertial pattern clarifies with its organizing fulcrum located in the occiput. Move to the head of the table and place your hands in the occipital cradle hold previously learned. In this hold, the patient's head is resting on your hands as you simply cradle the occiput with your fingers pointing inferiorly. Be sure that the heels of your hands do not place any pressure on the occiput. Let your hands be soft, suspended in fluid and fluid body. Orient to the fluid tide and the motility of the tissue field and occiput in particular. Do not narrow your perceptual field or project your attention to the occiput. Let its dynamic come to you. Settle into your listening and orient to any inertial pattern that clarifies.

As a pattern clarifies, imagine-sense that the occiput is still in its four parts of infancy: squama, condyles, and basilar portion. How do these parts relate to each other? Do you sense the squama in rotation in relationship to the condyles? Do you sense a compressive or torsional force across the foramen magnum? Do you sense a telescoping of structure anteriorly toward the SBJ? As you listen, simply let the story unfold.

As inertial issues in the occiput clarify, notice the dynamics that arise. The squama may rotate inferiorly in one direction, the condyles may torsion, or they may be sensed to be wedged together, and there may be an anterior drag in the squama as you sense a telescoping of occipital base parts as described above. These are all expressions of unresolved birthing forces.

Deepen into your still and receptive state and allow the system to settle into a state of balance—a dynamic equilibrium of the forces in the fulcrum generating the pattern. As this occurs, the inertial fulcrum uncouples from other fulcrums in the system and becomes suspended in its tissue field—which is now, in turn, suspended in the fluid body, which is likewise suspended in the tidal body of Long Tide—all fields entering a state of equilibrium. Allow the process to deepen and orient to any level of healing process that clarifies. Potency in fluid will be expressed, Long Tide phenomenon engage, and a deepening into Dynamic Stillness may occur. Listen for the processing of the inertial forces involved and for the stage of reorganization and realignment to midline.

_____

Exploration:
Augmentation of Space _____

Many times the inertial forces maintaining intraosseous distortions and their related tissue effects are deeply entrenched, as are the fulcrums they generate. The compressive forces may be so deep that the state of balance cannot be easily accessed or deepen. In this exploration, we will orient to an augmentation of space in the dynamics of the occiput itself. Here the intention is to help the inertial potencies in the fulcrum access space and enter a deeper state of balance and/or process the inertial forces involved.

An effective way to work with infants is to offer space and stillness. In this exploration, you will orient to the inertial fulcrum in the occiput, with the intention of augmenting the expression of potency and space in its tissues. We are assuming that you are holding the occipital cradle as above, are in relationship to an intraosseous fulcrum in the occiput, and that the system could not settle or deepen into a state of balance and equilibrium.

Holding an occipital cradle, again settle into a still and receptive state—with your hands and fingers suspended in fluid. Orient to the fluid tide and the motility of the occiput and cranium in general. As the inertial pattern clarifies, orient to the basic tissue organization around the inertial fulcrum/inertial area in the occiput. You may sense rotations in the squama, compressive issues in the condyles and a quality of telescoping of the parts of the occiput toward the SBJ—all indications of unresolved birthing forces.

At the height of inhalation, allow the fingers of your hand to be moved by the tide-like kelp beds in the ocean—as they take a deeper breath with the tide. As this occurs, your fingers widen apart and move posterior, mirroring and augmenting the action of potency and space in the tissue of the occiput. You don't have to follow the particular tissue patterns present as in a biomechanical approach—simply be moved by the tide and allow your fingers to resonate and respond. Again, if no tide is present, allow your fingers to take a deeper breath as though the tide is moving them.

Be open to any healing process that clarifies. The inertial forces in the occiput may be processed and resolved—you may sense heat, pulsation, shifts of potency in the inertial area and fluids in general, or the process may deepen into a state of equilibrium as different levels of the healing process are engaged. Orient to the resolution of inertial forces and the reorganization, realignment stage (Figure 6.9).

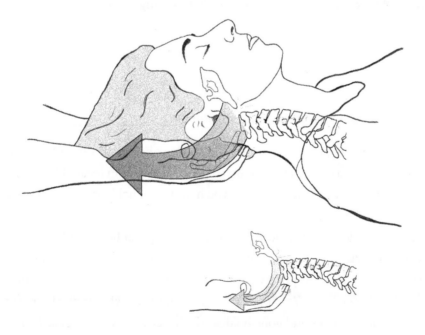

Figure 6.9. Augmentation of space in the occiput.

Exploration:
Intraosseous Fulcrums in the Temporal Bone _____

The temporal bone is next in our inquiry into intraosseous issues. The temporal bones are in three parts at birth: the squama, the tympanic ring, and the petrous portion. Intraosseous forces can be introduced into these tissue relationships during the birth process. Intraosseous temporal bone issues commonly arise due to medial compressive forces and rotational forces in Stages One and Two. As we have seen, during the first stage of birth strong medial forces can be placed on the baby's cranium. Rotational and compressive forces can also be experienced during the mid-pelvic descent as the baby rotates toward the pelvic floor (see Figure 5.21).

Intraosseous fulcrums and distortions of the temporal bones can have profound effects on the system. In infants, compressions at the jugular foramen and hypoglossal canal may generate entrapment neuropathy in the vagus, hypoglossal, glossopharyngeal, and spinal accessory nerves, leading to digestive problems such as colic, sucking problems, and respiratory symptoms. In adults, intraosseous temporal bone issues may generate chronic cranial base patterns with resultant symptomologies, migraine headaches, digestive disorders, respiratory issues, fluid congestion, tinnitus, or other hearing problems, chronic fatigue, and low potency.

Exploration:
Augmentation of Space in the Temporal Bones _____

In this exploration, we are assuming that you have been working with a client and an inertial pattern clarified, organized around a fulcrum located in a temporal bone. Sometimes this may clarify as you hold a vault hold, or the temporal bones in a temporal bone hold.

Let's assume you are holding the general temporal bone hold and an intraosseous fulcrum and its pattern clarify. As you hold the temporal bones, this may be sensed as a compressive force or medial pull and/or a rotation, or inner spiraling, in the bone. You may even sense a corkscrewing type of force in the tissue. From the temporal bone hold, as the intraosseous pattern clarifies, move to the specific temporal bone where the inertial fulcrum seems to be located.

Maintain your hold, with middle finger in the ear canal, at the temporal bone involved. Move your other hand to the opposite frontal eminence. The frontal contact enables an augmentation of potency and fluid drive toward the temporal bone in question.

Again orient to the fluid tide and tissue motility. At the height of inhalation, allow your hand at the temporal bone to resonate with the tide, and take a deeper breath at its height. Again, this has a very fluid feel to it—your hand is suspended in fluid, moved by the potency and tidal surge of inhalation. Your hand follows the inhalation motility of the temporal bone, and augments its expression as it resonates with tidal forces. Your other hand simultaneously orients to the drive of potency in the tide and augments its expression toward the temporal bone simply by orienting to its present.

This has a bioelectric-biomagnetic quality to it—as you orient to the temporal bone at the height of inhalation, you will sense a shift of potency in the fluids toward that area. As the forces in the inertial fulcrum respond, orient to whatever level of healing process clarifies. Commonly, you may sense inertial forces being processed, leaving the cranium in the vector pattern they originally entered. For instance, you many sense a spiral-like force literally shifting out of the temporal one, leaving the cranium (Figure 6.10).

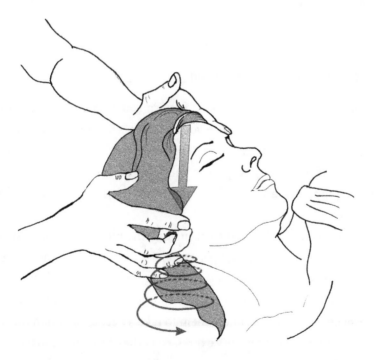

Figure 6.10. Augmentation of space in the temporal bone.

Intraosseous Distortions of the Sphenoid Bone

As we've described, intraosseous distortions of the sphenoid bone are very common and can affect all other parts of the system. The sphenoid bone is in three parts at birth: the body/lesser-wing section and the two pterygoid/greater-wing sections (see Figure 5.8). The sphenoid bone is subject to many forces during all phases of the birthing process. In the pelvic inlet it is commonly exposed to medially compressive and shearing forces. In the mid-pelvis, rotational and lateral shearing forces are often encountered. In the pelvic outlet, vertical shearing may arise (see Figure 5.9). The effects are numerous and wide-ranging. In fact, many cranial base patterns have intraosseous issues as their fulcrum. For instance, a torsion pattern in the cranial base may be an expression of torsion between the greater-wing sections of the sphenoid. The following exploration assumes that you are at the vault hold and perceive an inertial pattern clarifying, whose inertial fulcrum is located in the sphenoid bone itself. You may also notice a pattern in the sphenoid bone clarifying. For instance, you may sense, as you hold a Sutherland vault hold, that the greater wings between your index fingers express a torsioning or shearing pattern around a fulcrum in the sphenoid.

Exploration:
Intraosseous Fulcrums in the Sphenoid _____

Let's imagine that you have sensed a pattern clarifying in the cranium and are moving to a vault hold. Negotiate your contact with the greater wings—either with your thumbs or index finger depending on the vault hold you are using (Becker's or Sutherland's). Approach the greater wings of the sphenoid bone as you would approach an infant's, fingers suspended in fluid gently floating on the tissues.

Orient to the fluid tide and then include the motility of the tissues. As you sense an intraosseous sphenoid pattern clarifying, orient to the fulcrum in the bone that organizes it. At the height of inhalation, allow your fingers at the great wings to really be suspended in the tide and to be moved by the potency in it. As they resonate with the tide, allow them to take a deeper breath in the inhalation direction of tide and the motility expressed at the great wings, augmenting space locally in the tissue of the sphenoid bone. This will augment both the action of potency at the height of the tide, and the inner relationship to space in the tissue of the sphenoid bone.

As inertial forces are processed, listen for a reorganization of the tissues of the sphenoid and allow time for the whole of the cranium to reorganize and realign with natural fulcrums and the midline. This is very important. An intraosseous fulcrum in the sphenoid may be the focus for any number of cranial patterns. Be patient and allow the tissues, fluids, and potencies to reorganize their relationship to natural fulcrums and the primal midline.

Some people are very sensitive at the greater wings of the sphenoid. It may seem impossible to negotiate a comfortable contact via a vault hold or similar contact. These sensitivities are usually expressions of strong compressive forces in the tissue of the sphenoid, especially in the greater-wing sections. One or both greater-wing sections may be compressed into the body of the sphenoid during the birth process.

You can work bioelectrically-biomagnetically to orient to these situations. Potency is essentially bioelectric-biomagnetic in quality. As you sense the potency in the fluids surging at the height of inhalation, imagine that your thumbs are like magnets. Subtly intend the two greater wings laterally apart via an intention of lateral space at the height of inhalation. It is as if the potency in the sphenoid is like a pond and you are touching its surface tension. Subtly widen the surface tension sensed laterally. As you bring this biomagnetic intention to the fluids, potencies, and inertial tissues—while oriented to the inertial fulcrum in the sphenoid bone—you will sense the potency in the inertial fulcrum beginning to shift, resolving the inertial forces present. As this occurs, you may sense heat, pulsation, and inertial forces literally leaving the tissue of the sphenoid bone along the original birth vector pattern. Again settle into stillness and orient to any level of healing process that emerges.

CHAPTER 7

The Dural Tube

In preceding chapters we oriented you to the earliest experiences of life, the pre- and perinatal period, and birthing dynamics. As we have seen in these chapters, and in Foundations Volume One, Chapter 19, embryonic tissue development is organized around a crucial midline that we call the *primal midline*. The primal midline is the midline of the wider bioelectric ordering field that the Long Tide lays down at conception and can be sensed throughout life as a spiral-like, uprising force ascending from the coccyx, through the center of the vertebral bodies, bending at the occipital base, continuing to ascend through the center of the cranial base and ethmoid bone, and diffusing back into the wider bioelectric field around the body. The primal midline is the ordering midline within which the notochord is formed, and is the main organizing midline for tissue organization throughout life. The next few chapters explore the tissue forms directly organized around this midline and the notochord it generates. This includes the dural tube, the vertebral column, the pelvis, and cranial base. In each case we will also describe how these structures respond to the birthing process and the patterning that birthing forces may generate in the young system.

Perception of the primal midline as the ordering midline for the tissue field gives the practitioner a wealth of information. When an inertial force is processed, the tissue field does not have to organize around its presence anymore, and reorganizes relative to the primal midline and natural automatically shifting fulcrums. This shift in relationship to the primal midline is palpable, and gives the practitioner clear indications as to the new organization of the tissue field. Likewise, awareness of the primal midline also gives the practitioner clear indications of inertial issues in and around the midline. For instance, as we shall see, if there are inertial forces present in vertebral dynamics, the primal midline may become obscured to the practitioner's awareness, indicating where midline inertia and compressive forces are located. In the following explorations, the primal midline is a prime orientation for practitioner awareness. See Foundations Volume One, Chapter 19, for detailed descriptions and explorations of the midline.

The Core Link

This chapter orients to the dural tube, which is classically called the *core link*. The dural tube is a natural linking structure for the whole tissue field as all membrane, fascia, and connective tissues in the body are continuous with its tension dynamics. The dural tube is continuous with the inner layer of dura that surrounds the brain. It follows and surrounds the spinal cord as it leaves the cranium, extending all the way down into the sacral canal between the cranium and pelvis (Figure 7.1).

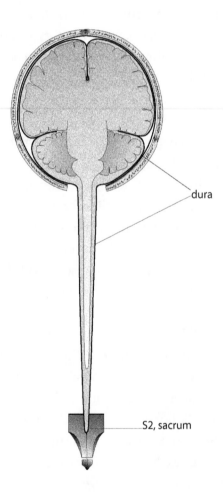

Figure 7.1. The dura and dural tube.

The dural tube expresses a natural reciprocal tension throughout its form and motility. It naturally rises and settles in the inhalation and exhalation phases of primary respiration (Figure 7.2). As it expresses its motility and mobility, it should be relatively free to glide in the vertebral canal. If there are inertial issues anywhere along its length, its natural reciprocal tension motion will be compromised and inertial fulcrums may be perceived in its dynamics. Likewise, the dynamic tension balance in the membranous-osseous system of dural membrane and bone will also be affected.

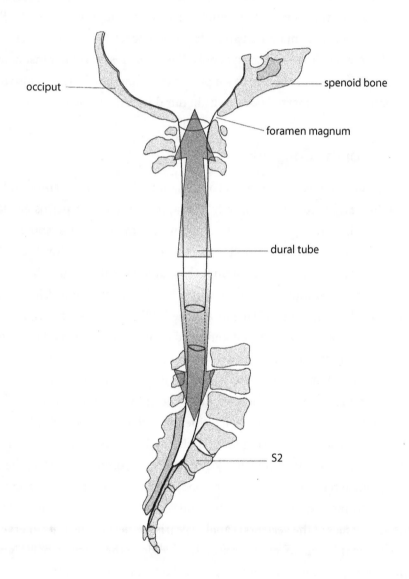

occiput — spenoid bone

foramen magnum

dural tube

S2

Figure 7.2. The dural tube as a reciprocal tension structure.

If the reciprocal tension dynamics in the core link become conditioned and strained, the whole tissue field will have to compensate in some way. Since the dural tube directly links the occiput to the sacrum, occipital patterns will be directly reflected in the sacrum, and vice versa. Furthermore, a most important activity also occurs as the dural sleeves follow nerve roots out of the vertebral canal—small quantities of cerebrospinal fluid follow the dural sleeves out of the vertebral canal via diffusion all along the length of the spine. This is an expression of the radiance and infusion of potency all along its length from core to periphery, and is a manifestation of the continuity of fluid dynamics throughout the body. Experienced practitioners maintain that an exchange—potency to fluid to nerves—occurs along all nerves and especially at synapses. It is an expression of a transmutation of potency from fluid to nerve, which supports nerve function. This may also become compromised due to inertial issues within dural tube dynamics.

Anatomy of the Core link

The dural tube can be considered a continuation of the inner meningeal layer of cranial dura and is composed of only one layer. The outer, or periosteal, layer of cranial dura is interrupted at the foramen magnum and, in the spinal column, the periosteum of the bone functions as this outer layer. The dural tube is thus continuous with the inner layer of dura that surrounds the brain. The dural tube extends from the foramen magnum, where it is firmly attached at its dural ring, into the sacral canal, where it is firmly attached at the second sacral segment. There are also attachments at the second and third cervical vertebrae and lower lumbar areas. Dural sleeves also follow nerve roots out of the spinal canal, and this provides continuity with all of the fascial relationships of the body (Figure 7.3).

There is a layer of loose fatty tissue in the epidural space between the dura mater and the connective tissues that line the inside of the vertebral canal. This fatty tissue acts as a lubricating layer, assisting in the ease of dural glide in the spinal canal. As you move your body and bend your spine, the dural tube should be able to glide relatively freely. As the body responds to experience and trauma, inertial fulcrums may be generated and adhesions between the dural tube and the connective tissues of the vertebral canal may arise, especially near its intervertebral foramen, and this will affect the ease of dural glide in the spinal canal (Figure 7.4). Connective tissue drag in other parts of the body may also be transferred into the dural tube via the continuity of dura and connective tissue. Vertebral fixations can also generate dural adhesions and restrictions to dural glide. Inertial fulcrums in

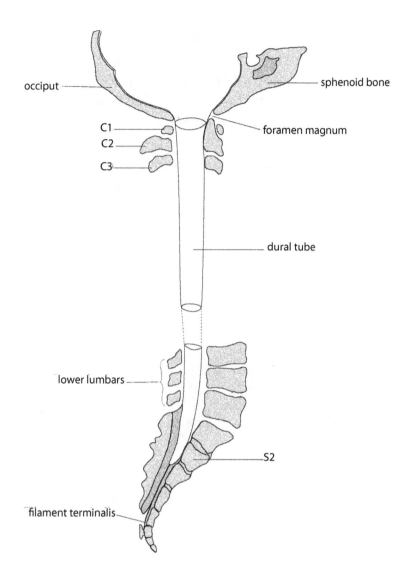

occiput

sphenoid bone

C1

foramen magnum

C2

C3

dural tube

lower lumbars

S2

filament terminalis

Figure 7.3. The attachments of the dural tube.

the dynamics of the dural tube will also affect the expression of the fluid tide and its longitudinal fluctuation. Potency may become inertial in the core of the body in order to center the forces involved. Obviously this may have profound implications for the biodynamics of the whole system.

Finally, there are fine ligaments called denticulate ligaments along the spinal cord, which arise from the pia mater around the cord. These anchor the spinal cord to the arachnoid and dural layers. Twenty-one pairs of these ligaments arise laterally between spinal nerve roots. Their function is to stabilize the spinal cord in the dural tube (Figure 7.4). I have seen dissections of the spinal canal in which these internal ligaments have been severely torsioned, generating adhesions between the meningeal layers. This was clearly because of torsioning of the dural tube as a whole. Rotational and compressive birthing forces commonly produce these patterns as the baby moves through the birth canal. Unresolved birthing forces can generate a torsioned relationship between the occiput and sacrum, and compression, torsion, and rotation between vertebrae. Adhesions in the meninges due to the denticulate ligaments being torsioned will have a profound effect on the dynamics of potencies, fluids, and tissues. The drive of the fluid tide may be affected as potency becomes inertial in order to center the forces at work in the core of the system.

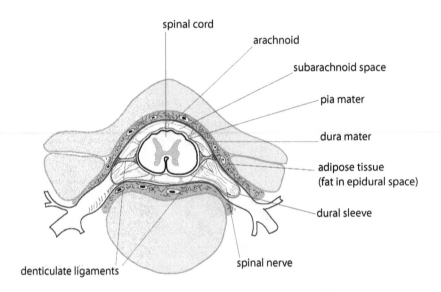

Figure 7.4. Dural sleeves and fatty tissue.

These kinds of issues will also directly influence the motility of the central nervous system. At the most caudal end of the dural sac, in the sacral canal, the pia mater pierces the dura to form the filum terminalis that anchors the end of the spinal cord to the coccyx. It is covered with a thin investment of dura as it forms the filum terminalis. Any tethering of the filum terminalis due to compressive forces in the sacroiliac joints or pelvis will have a strong effect on the central nervous system and on the fluid drive and biodynamics of the system generally (see Chapter 9 on pelvic dynamics).

Motility of the Dural Tube/Core Link

Like all connective tissues, the motility of the dural tube ideally has its natural point of reciprocal tension balance at the anterior aspect of the straight sinus—Sutherland's fulcrum. As we have seen, the leaves of the reciprocal tension membrane can be thought of as being suspended from the straight sinus and Sutherland's fulcrum. (For a review of Sutherland's fulcrum and the motion dynamics of the reciprocal tension membrane, see Foundations Volume One, Chapter 13). In the inhalation

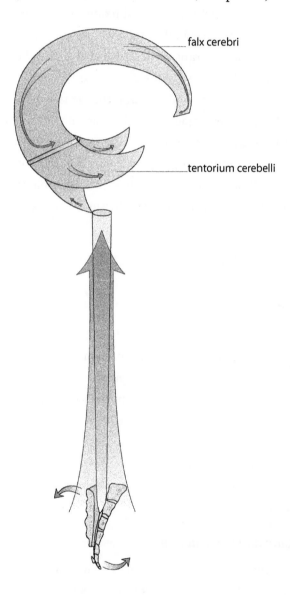

falx cerebri

tentorium cerebelli

Figure 7.5. The reciprocal tension membrane and dural tube in inhalation.

phase, the dural tube generally rises superiorly. Simultaneously, the spinal cord subtly shortens toward the lamina terminalis of the third ventricle, and the fluid tide ascends. None of these dynamics are separate. They are generated all at once by the action of potency in the fluids (Figure 7.5).

Common Inertial Issues Relating to the Dural Tube

There are common inertial issues that may affect the dural tube and its ease of motility and glide. These include vertebral fixations, adhesions in the meninges and connective tissues in the spinal canal, local toxicity, and edema and fascial-connective tissue resistances transferred to the area from other parts of the body. Please remember that all of these tissue changes are due to the presence of unre-solved inertial forces and the inertial fulcrums they generate. Traumatic forces, such as those encountered in car accidents or falls, may induce protective responses in dural tissues. This is most obvious in whiplash injuries, when the cervical fascia and dura are strongly impinged upon, generating protective contractions in their relationships. Acute illnesses, such as meningitis or encephalitis, may also generate changes in the quality of dural tissue and adhesions in dural relationships.

Common Inertial Issues Affecting Dural Motility and Glide

Vertebral Fixations

Fixation in vertebral dynamics can affect dural tube motility and ease of glide. Vertebral fixations and their related inertial patterns can be transferred to the dural tube via the dural sleeves that surround spinal nerves as they exit the vertebral canal. Thus, if vertebral dynamics are compromised, dural motility and mobility will also be compromised. Furthermore, vertebral fixations can directly affect the central nervous system. Their dynamics can be directly transferred to nerves as they leave the vertebral canal. Facilitation-hypersensitization of nerves can result, as we will discuss in our later chapters on vertebral dynamics and nociception (Chapters 8 and 20).

Fascial Adhesion and Contraction

The dynamics of the dural tube are continuous with all of the connective tissue relationships of the body. Any pattern of fascial strain and inertial tensions can be transferred to the dural tube. Similarly, any inertial pattern in the dural tube can be transferred into the general connective tissue relationships of the body.

Dural Sleeves

It is not uncommon to sense adhesions between the dural tube and the connective tissues that line the spinal column. This is most common at, or near, intervertebral foramina. As spinal nerves leave the spinal canal, they are invested with a sleeve of dura. These dural sleeves are continuous with the connective tissues that surround the spinal nerves and with paravertebral connective tissues. As the fatty tissue that separates the dura from the connective tissues lining the spinal canal thins out near the intervertebral foramina, the dural tube is most vulnerable as its sleeves follow nerve roots out through these foramina. Somatic dysfunction in vertebral or paravertebral relationships can be fed into the dural tube at these locations. Inertial fulcrums affecting vertebral dynamics and paravertebral connective tissues are commonly transferred to the dural tube. Dural adhesions may be generated, and the dural tube's ability to glide freely will become compromised.

Transverse Relationships

Along the dural tube are various transverse relationships that can directly affect its dynamics. Compressive fulcrums at either end of the dural tube will strongly influence its ease of glide. This includes the relationships of the occipital triad (occiput, atlas, and axis) at the superior pole, and the lumbosacral junction and sacroiliac joints at the inferior pole. These are very important areas to be aware of and to respond to clinically. Other transverse relationships include the thoracic inlet, the respiratory diaphragm, and the pelvic diaphragm (perineal floor). Contraction and adhesion found in any of these areas may compromise dural mobility and function. We will look more specifically at these dynamics in later chapters.

Sacrum and Occiput

The occiput, sacrum, and dural tube are totally integrated in their motility. Ease of motility in occipital and sacral dynamics, and ease of dural glide in the spinal canal, are essential for a balanced and integrated expression of motility. Any inertial issue in the dural tube will directly affect the sacrum and occiput, and vice versa. The sacrum, occiput, and dural tube should ideally express their motility in an integrated and synchronous way. Inertial patterns from either side of this relationship will cause asynchronous motion.

Denticulate Ligaments

As described above, resistances and adhesions between the layers of meninges in the spinal canal are commonly found in relationship to the denticulate ligaments. The denticulate ligaments arise from pia mater all along the spinal cord, pierce the arachnoid layer, and anchor to the dura mater. They stabilize the spinal cord in the spinal canal. Any pattern of tension, compression, or congestion in these relationships, and in vertebral or paravertebral tissues, will be transferred to the dural tube and it denticulate ligaments. These will also strongly influence the fluid dynamics in the subarachnoid space.

Tissue Changes

In all of these instances, the dural membrane may manifest local or global qualitative tissue changes. These may include loss of elasticity, a leathery feel to the tissues, densification of tissue, and even a sense of the dural tissues drying out and hardening. I have noted that extended usage of certain drugs—marijuana is one and heroin another—can generate an extreme sense of dryness and loss of elasticity in dural tissues. This will strongly affect the biodynamics of the system, and the person involved may experience lowered constitutional vitality. I have also noted that meningitis and even low-grade inflammation can generate densification in the dural membrane.

Facilitated Segments

Vertebral fixations, dural adhesions, and visceral issues all may generate, and be generated by, nerve facilitation-hypersensitization. In osteopathic terminology, the sensitization of a spinal nerve loop is called a *facilitated segment*. A facilitated segment is a segment of the spinal cord, including both sensory and motor nerves, that has become hypersensitive and has a lowered threshold of stimulation. Very small stimuli may cause the nerves involved to overreact and fire excessively. Vertebral fixations, dural adhesions, and visceral issues can all generate overstimulation of a spinal nerve segment. This, in turn, will overstimulate the organs or muscles that relate to that segment, and a vicious cycle can be set up. The spinal nerve becomes hypersensitive and highly excitable. The hyperactivity in the spinal segment causes hyperactivity in the organs or muscles involved. The overstimulated organ or muscle sends back sensory stimuli to the spinal segment that keep the cycle going (Figure 7.6). These can generate spinal fixation and dural adhesion. We will discuss this in great detail in Chapter 21.

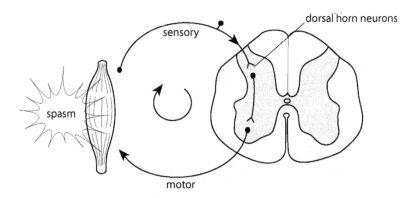

Figure 7.6. Sensitized nerve loop.

Birth Trauma

Birth trauma is another factor that influences dural tube motility and the dural membrane generally. The body of the birthing infant is truly a fluid-tissue-membranous unity. I have had the pleasure of assisting William Emerson PhD over the years in seminars dealing with prenatal and birth trauma. I was first amazed, and then deeply appreciative, of his ability to read the whole of a person's prenatal and birth history via the patterns held in the body, both energetically and via his perception of cranial, dural, vertebral, and pelvic dynamics. Dural membranes, both locally and as a whole, will directly express all of this in some way. After many years of observation, I have also seen how our earliest experiences are directly expressed in the fluids and tissues of the body, and how the dynamics of dural membranes are shaped by prenatal and birth experience.

During the birth process, the young system has to contend with extreme forces as it passes through the birth canal. Compressive forces during the birth process can introduce inertial forces into the system. These forces can generate compression, torsion, and shear in the baby's tissue systems. This is especially true if the birth was experienced as traumatic and there was some shock and traumatization involved. In relationship to the dural tube, these inertial forces may set up patterns that become habitual and restrict both dural motility and mobility in later life. It is not uncommon to find a dense and compressed dural tube whose etiology can be traced back to the compressive forces of birth. As practitioner, you may sense a shortened and dense dural tube whose compressive issues seem to be held in itself. The vertebral column may also hold axially compressive forces originating in the birth process. You may actually sense that potency has become inertial all through

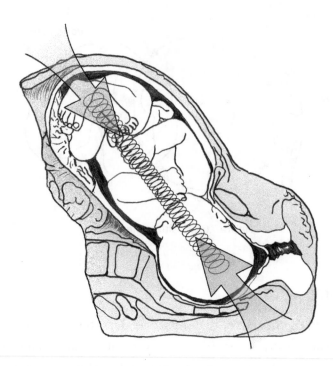

Figure 7.7. Axial birthing forces.

the core of the body in order to center unresolved axial compressive forces. These potency-fluid-tissues patterns will be coupled with the original birth trauma and related psycho-emotional states, and thus must be held empathically by the practitioner with a clear awareness of the potential depth of wounding present (Figure 7.7).

The inertial forces generated by the birth process are generally not solely located in isolated fulcrums. Rather, these forces are commonly spread throughout the core of the body along its longitudinal-vertebral axis. Whole areas of the spine may go into compression due to these unresolved axial forces. Although these forces will generate localized fulcrums in vertebral and dural dynamics, these axial forces must be related to holistically. Working with the augmentation of space through the whole vertebral axis can help in their resolution. We will describe this both in this chapter and in Chapter 8, on vertebral dynamics.

Torsion and side-bending patterns in the sacrum or occiput can originate in the birth process, and these can give rise to twists and torsions in the dural tube itself. This will affect the dynamics of the denticulate ligaments, and meningeal adhesions can result. Whole-body torsions that arise in the birth process can also be fed into the dural tube and affect the dynamics of the sacrum and occiput. As seen in our earlier chapters on the birth process, all of this depends on the length of time in labor, where and for how long the infant was stuck in any position, the relationship and connection between mother and baby, and whether any of this was experienced traumatically by the baby.

Thus there are many factors to consider when you are looking at the dynamics of the core link or dural tube. All and any of the above dynamics may generate inertial issues at the core of the system. Reduced motility and ease of glide of the dural tube in the vertebral canal is a common result and everything attached to and in the dural membrane system may become affected. This includes the relationships of the cranial bones, the motility of the central nervous system, and the motion of the sacrum between the ilea. Indeed, any inertial issue in any of these tissues will affect the motility of all the other structures. Dural tube inertia will strongly affect the relationship between the sacrum and the occiput and the ability of the sacrum to express its motility, generate stagnation in the lumbosacral waterbed, and strongly affect the expression of potency in the system as a whole. Inertia in the dynamics of the core link can thus become an important fulcrum for the whole system. Reduced fluid drive, lowered expression of potency, and a general devitalization of the system can occur. This is probably the most important repercussion of core link inertial issues.

Exploration:
Orienting to the Motility of the Dural Tube _____

In this exploration you will first tune into the expression of the primal midline and then orient to the dural tube as it expresses its motility around it. Do not narrow your perceptual field as you orient to the primal midline, as you may be sensed as an outside force and potency will coalesce around the midline in a protective response. This will have the effect of shutting things down and little motility will then be perceived. We expand upon the importance of the primal midline as an orienting principle in later chapters.

One way to begin to tune into dural tube motility is to place your hands on the sacrum and occiput of your client in the side-lying position.

After your client's system has settled into the holistic shift, move to the side-lying sacro-occipital hold. In this position, place your cephalad hand over the occiput with your fingers pointing superiorly and your caudal hand over the sacrum, fingers pointing inferiorly. Holding a wide perceptual field, orient to the fluid and physical bodies in the wider tidal body (Figure 7.8).

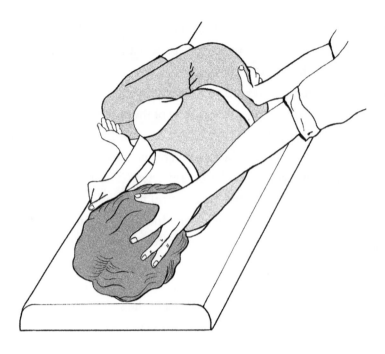

Figure 7.8. Sacrum and occiput hold, side-lying position.

First let your hands float on the tissues, suspended in fluid. As explored in Volume One, in your wide perceptual field, gently orient to the primal midline as an uprising force in the center of the vertebral bodies. This is the primary midline around which the dural tube expresses its motility.

Settle into this awareness and then, still maintaining your wide perceptual field, sense the motility of bone and membrane in the phases of the mid-tide/fluid tide. First orient to the fluid tide, and then generally include the tissues in your perceptual field. You are already used to sensing the motility of the sacrum and occiput. In the inhalation phase, the squama of the occiput and the sacral base may be sensed to widen and rotate posteriorly into your hands, as the sacrum subtly rises. This may feel like a filling and rising in your hands.

Once you sense this, then include the dural tube in your perceptual field. Sense the occiput, sacrum, and dural tube as a unified dynamic. In the inhalation phase, the dural tube will be sensed to rise, while the sacral base and occipital squama will be sensed to rotate into your hands. The distance between the sacrum and occiput may be sensed to shorten as the sacrum and dural tube subtly rise. The reverse will happen in the exhalation phase.

See if you can sense the motility of the dural tube rising and settling in inhalation and exhalation. Just let your hands float on the tissues you suspended in fluid, and orient to the space between them. Let yours hands be moved by this expression of primary respiration and orient to any healing processes that emerge.

Exploration:
The Augmentation of Space and Dural Tube Dynamics _____

In this exercise we are inquiring into the ease, or lack of ease, in the ability of the dural tube to express its motility and ease of glide in the vertebral canal. Dural sleeves are in intimate relationship with local paravertebral tissues and are continuous with the connective tissues that cover nerves as they leave the spinal canal. Thus, inertial fulcrums located anywhere in the body may affect the dural tube and its ease of motion.

The following exploration is a continuation of the one above where you oriented to dural tube motility in the side-lying sacro-occipital hold. As you orient to dural tube motility in this hold, you may sense inertial patterns organized around particular fulcrums. These inertial fulcrums may be present anywhere along the length of the spinal canal. They will affect dural tube motility and may generate adhesions of the denticulate ligaments and dural sleeves with the connective tissues that line the spinal column. This is most likely to occur at the spinal foramina where dural sleeves follow nerves out of the spinal canal, and the protective fatty tissue that lines the canal is thinnest. You may sense this as resistance in dural motility. For instance, as you orient to the phases of inhalation and exhalation, you may perceive that the dural tube cannot fully ascend in the inhalation phase. You may also sense resistance in dural motility as inertial tension patterns organized around inertial fulcrums in the vertebral axis and spinal canal.

If, in the side-lying sacro-occipital hold used above, you sense resistance to dural motility and ease of glide in the spinal canal, you can subtly augment space along its length. Again, sense that your hands are suspended in fluid and that you and your client are suspended in a wider tidal field. Holding a wide perceptual field, orient to the inhalation and exhalation phases of the fluid tide and the motility of the dural tube. At the height of inhalation, subtly augment space in dural dynamics by allowing your hand at the occiput to resonate with the inhalation surge and take a deeper breath in the cephalad direction. Your hand follows the ascending of the tide through the fluids and dural tissue and subtly breathes/deepens into that headward, ascending direction.

As space is augmented in dural dynamics, you may sense inertial forces being processed and dissipated back to the environment. This may be perceived as heat

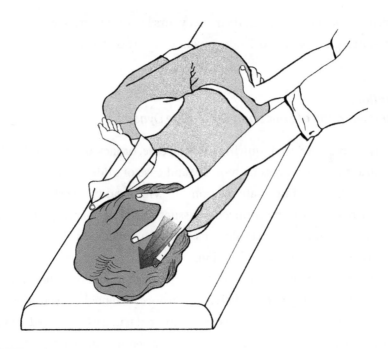

Figure 7.9. Augmentation of space in dural tube dynamics.

or force vector dissipation that is commonly sensed as a streaming of energy and/or heat out of the body. You may then sense a softening, expansion, and resolution of the inertial forces and tissue resistances in and along the spinal canal and vertebral axis. You may also sense a surge in the fluid tide, and the dural tube may then be sensed to soften, subtly expand, and glide more easily in its motility. When you sense the dural tissues reorganizing, can you sense a new relationship to the midline and to Sutherland's fulcrum? Has the quality of the fluid tide changed?

This approach can also be used more specifically by placing your cephalad hand under the vertebral level where dural resistance is sensed, rather than at the occiput. We explore this more specific approach in our next chapter where we expand this work as we orient to vertebrae and vertebral dynamics. The clinical explorations described in that chapter also relate to dural tube issues, as vertebral and dural dynamics cannot really be separated out from each other. When vertebral fixation and inertial fulcrums are perceived, they inevitably include dural issues (Figure 7.9).

CHAPTER 8

Vertebral Dynamics

In this chapter, you will continue to orient to the primal midline as a crucial ordering principle, and form a relationship to vertebral motility and inertial vertebral issues that may have coalesced around it. The initial intention in clinical work described below is to orient to the primal midline as an uprising force through the center of the vertebral bodies and to notice areas where its presence is not clear. Potency will become inertial in and around the areas of the midline where conditional forces have not been resolved, and the uprising force, although always present, may then become obscured to your awareness. As you tune into the primal midline, you may then sense areas where it seems absent or unclear, or sense gaps in its expression.

As seen in earlier chapters, birthing forces are a prime example of forces introduced into the midline of the system, whose unresolved presence may obscure the primal midline. These forces are very strong, commonly affecting the whole vertebral axis. Potency may become inertial along and in the vertebral axis to center these forces in some way. If unresolved, inertial fulcrums will be generated, manifesting as compression and inertial patterning. Areas of tissue density or dryness, structural fixation, and fluid congestion are expressions of these forces at work in and around the primal midline. Axial compressions along whole areas of the vertebral axis are also a very common finding in clinical practice.

Vertebral Discs and Suspended, Automatically Shifting Fulcrums

In the embryo, the vertebral bodies, and vertebral column as a whole, form around the primal midline and notochord. This embryological imperative continues to be the primary organizing axis for cells and tissues throughout life (Figure 8.1). As we have further seen, tissues also organize in relationship to automatic shifting fulcrums along the midline. Some classic automatic shifting fulcrums are Suther-land's fulcrum—located at the anterior aspect of the straight sinus—and fulcrums located at the sphenobasilar junction (SBJ) and the lamina terminalis.

However, there are many other natural fulcrums throughout the body. Stone noted that the disc between each vertebra acts as an orienting fulcrum for that local vertebral relationship. The intervertebral disc is literally a remnant of the notochord. The fulcrum in the disc can be thought of as a point of potency located in its center (Figure 8. 2). This is a suspended automatic shifting fulcrum that shifts in the phases of the tide. It rises cephalad in inhalation and settles in exhalation.

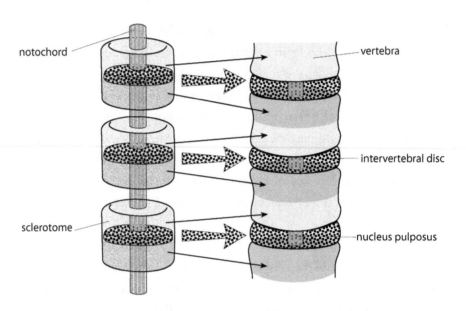

Figure 8.1. The vertebrae form in relationship to the notochord.

The vertebral column thus expresses its motility in relationship to the primal midline and to automatically shifting fulcrums. The SBJ is classically considered to be the most cephalad orienting fulcrum for vertebral dynamics. An awareness of the nature of these fulcrums can give the practitioner important information about the overall organization of the system. For instance, after an inertial fulcrum has resolved, you may sense the vertebral column shifting and reorganizing relative to the midline and automatically shifting fulcrums. After a dense inertial issue has resolved, you may also more clearly sense the cephalad rising of vertebrae in inhala-tion as the vertebral column as a whole subtly shortens toward the SBJ.

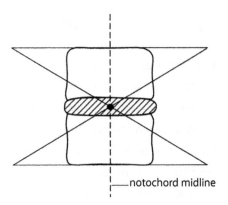

—notochord midline

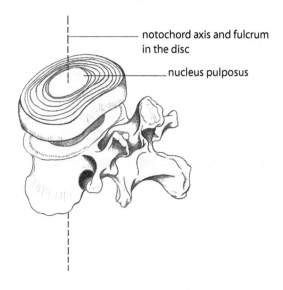

— notochord axis and fulcrum in the disc

— nucleus pulposus

Figure 8.2. The automatically shifting fulcrum in the disc.

Vertebral Fixation and Inertial Issues

Vertebral fixations are called lesions or somatic dysfunctions in classical osteopathy. These terms denote an area of clinically significant tissue and fluid change and may include connective tissue contraction, bony fixation, local edema, fluid congestion, tissue adhesion, and tissue changes such as thinning, dryness, and/or densification. As seen in Chapter 7, if vertebral dynamics are compromised, dural tube motility and mobility may also become compromised, leading to wider inertial issues. Furthermore, vertebral inertia can impinge upon nerves as they leave the vertebral canal, causing nerve sensitization and directly affecting the functioning of the central nervous system.

Vertebral fixation is an expression of tissue organization around inertial forces and related fulcrums introduced into the system via falls, accidents, toxins, or birth process. Postural issues and genetic overlays will also come into play. Some spinal issues will even have their origin in the prenatal experience. Individual vertebral fixations commonly relate to inertial forces affecting a wide area in the spine and midline. Traumatic forces introduced into the longitudinal axis—commonly called axial forces—can generate compressive issues in the vertebral column. Again, birthing forces are a common origin for the introduction of these kinds of axial forces into the system. In our first clinical exploration below, you will orient to the primal midline to gain information about inertial issues along the vertebral axis.

Structural Balance

All structural dynamics relate to how vertebrae, and tissue structures generally, orient to the primal midline, automatic shifting fulcrums, and unresolved inertial forces. If a system is totally free of inertia, an ideal balance of structure, function, and motion ensues. If no inertial issues are present in the body, the organization of structure around the midline is more likely to be symmetrical with an easy balance relative to the forces of gravity. Reciprocal tension motion would be completely

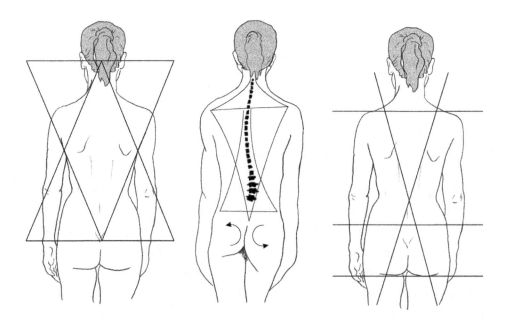

Figure 8.3. Images of structural balance.

oriented to the midline and to suspended automatically shifting fulcrums in an easy and balanced way (Figure 8.3). However, we incarnate into a life that is replete with conditions and contingencies. As we meet life's inevitable circumstances, and inertial fulcrums are generated, our mind-body system must shift to a compensated balance, and structural compensations inevitably arise.

This does not mean, however, that we become inherently unbalanced or fragmented. The Breath of Life and its potency always sustains a balance of structure and function, and wholeness is always maintained, albeit in a compensated manner. But there is a price to pay for the need to compensate for unresolved forces and the fulcrums they generate. Potency becomes bound in centering the conditions present, tissues change in quality, fluids become inertial, form distorts, and vitality is reduced. The stage is set for the arising of pathology and pain. But even in the most pathologically desperate and painful conditions, health is never really lost, the midline is ever-present, and a reorientation to the imperative of the Breath of Life is always possible (Figure 8.4).

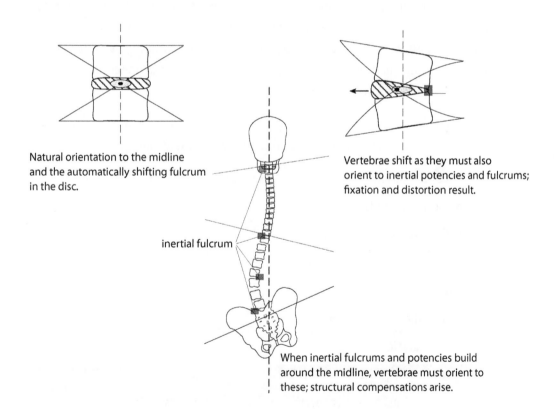

Natural orientation to the midline and the automatically shifting fulcrum in the disc.

Vertebrae shift as they must also orient to inertial potencies and fulcrums; fixation and distortion result.

inertial fulcrum

When inertial fulcrums and potencies build around the midline, vertebrae must orient to these; structural compensations arise.

Figure 8.4. Structural compensation.

The clinical issue is never about ideal structural balance, nor about vertebral sub-luxations, tissue and fluid changes, and pathology. A biodynamic approach orients to health and Intelligence in all conditions—the perception of primary respiration and stillness is our foundation. In the midst of a busy clinical practice, we must remember that the Breath of Life centers all of the conditions present—all at once—in the totality of our body-mind-spirit experience. The anatomical form of our body is an embodiment of the interchange between the ordering forces laid down by the Breath of Life and the impact of conditional forces. Structural balance is a direct manifestation of this dynamic and clearly expresses life experience. The ability to relate to structural patterns and structural balance is thus a necessary clinical skill.

Understanding structural relationships gives the practitioner an entry into the nature of that person's embodied experience and healing needs. Structurally oriented healing forms, such as osteopathy, chiropractic, and Rolfing have evolved due to the importance of structural balance and midline inertial issues in the overall function of the body-mind. Structural readings are an essential part of the diagnostic process in these systems. Structural awareness is also seen in many forms of indigenous bodywork, such as Thai massage and manipulation, Chinese massage and acupressure, Ayurvedic massage, and many others evolving over many centuries. A working knowledge of structural issues is also essential for clinical efficiency in the biodynamic craniosacral approach.

Common Origins of Vertebral Fixations

Vertebral fixation and inertia can arise from many factors, including:

- Unresolved birth trauma
- The forces of accidents and falls
- The forces of traumatic experiences
- Postural issues
- Shock and traumatization
- Fluid congestion
- Inflammatory processes and related tissue changes
- Compensations for other inertial fulcrums and processes in the body
- Pathogens and degenerative diseases
- The forces of genetics

Biomechanics, Biodynamics, and Specific Vertebral Dynamics

In order to have a clear clinical relationship to vertebrae, it is useful to have an awareness of their mobility dynamics. I would like to first differentiate between biomechanics and the voluntary motion of the vertebrae, and the biodynamics of motility as involuntary motion generated by primary respiration. Biomechanics is about how we orient to gravity, how we use leverage, and how we move through life. Joints have mobility and allowable motion. We can flex and extend our arms and legs and we can voluntarily move ourselves through the world.

In a purely biomechanical orientation, the human system might be conceived to be a mechanism with clock-like parts. This idea is derived from a vision of the universe that goes back to Déscartes. A human being is likened to a clock mechanism, and perfect health is likened to the perfect functioning of all its parts. In a classical biomechanical framework, the practitioner commonly orients to the allowable motion of joints and sutures and conceives of that motion in relationship to axes and direction of motion around those axes. Clinically, the practitioner may tend to orient to motion testing, resistance, and boundaries. The work then becomes based on releasing resistance and shifting lesions.

In a biodynamic context, the motions we listen for are those of primary respiration and the tide-like motility it generates. Rather than analysis and motion testing, we wait for the holistic shift to deepen and for the inherent treatment plan to unfold. Motility will become conditioned relative to the forces at work in the system and will express motion relative to these forces. Mobility restrictions and voluntary axial motion are expressions of this deeper dynamic.

In the following sections, we will introduce the basic biomechanics of vertebral relationships so that you can be clearer about the nature of vertebral fixations. This will support a more precise orientation to the inertial forces and the fulcrums and patterns they generate as they come into your awareness.

Vertebral Motility and Mobility Dynamics

As we have seen above, vertebrae express their motility relative to the primal midline and automatic shifting fulcrums. In inhalation, there is a subtle rising and shortening of the vertebral axis toward the SBJ. Each vertebra individually expresses a shortening top-to-bottom and a widening side-to-side. The shortening of the spinal axis is similar to the shortening of the neural axis in inhalation toward the lamina terminalis.

Each vertebra has four sets of articular surfaces called facets, two articulations with the vertebra above and two with the vertebra below, and a disc above and below also. Thus each vertebra typically has six joint relationships, although there is no disc between C1 and C2. In the inhalation phase, space is generated in these joint relationships.

The mobility and voluntary motion of the vertebrae are largely governed by the facets of the articulations between them. In the lumbar area these facets are largely oriented vertically in an anterior to posterior plane. This allows for little individual rotation. The lumbar spine will generally rotate as a whole. It also gives some protection in lateral bending and allows the lumbar spine to express a good forward and backward bending. The motion of the thoracic spine is largely governed by the more transverse orientation of its facets, and by its relationship to the rib cage. The thoracics allow for more rotation and lateral bending than the lumbars. This helps compensate for the stability and containment offered by the ribs. The cervical area has the most allowable motion. Its facets are oriented more or less transversely, and this permits much rotation and lateral bending. Much rotation is also allowed around the dens of the second cervical vertebra.

The ease of motion in the cervical area allows mammals to easily orient to their environment and to danger. In their orienting response, animals will momentarily freeze and then will calmly rotate the head via their cervical area to scan their surroundings. This high degree of cervical freedom has a cost. The cervical area is most vulnerable to whiplash injuries and to tension introduced via the stress response. Proprioceptive and motion information goes directly from the cervical area to the locus ceruleus, an important pair of nuclei in the stress response. As part of the orienting response, neck tension is read by these nuclei as potential danger in the environment. A feedback loop can be created in which neck tension stimulates the stress response, while the stress response maintains neck tension to ready the organism for possible danger. Thus tension held in the neck area is commonly related to unresolved stress and autonomic cycling and, if chronic, can even help perpetuate it. Due to all of these factors, it is important to resolve the forces that generate patterns of tension in the cervical area. The cervical area also bears the weight of the head and is thus vulnerable to postural stress.

Vertebrae move in relationship to each other in very specific ways. Vertebral relationships, like any other joint dynamic, will have a natural range of motion and mobility. These dynamics are dictated by the relationships of the articular facets to each other, by the intervertebral discs between vertebrae, by adjacent structures such as ribs, and by the connective tissue and muscular relationships between and around them. The basic mobility movements possible for the vertebrae are forward and backward bending (which occurs around a transverse axis), rotation or torsion (which occurs around a vertical axis), side-bending (which occurs around an anterior-posterior axis), anterior-posterior glide, and lateral glide. Finally, compression can occur between vertebrae, when one vertebra is compressed superiorly or posteriorly in relationship to another (Figure 8.5).

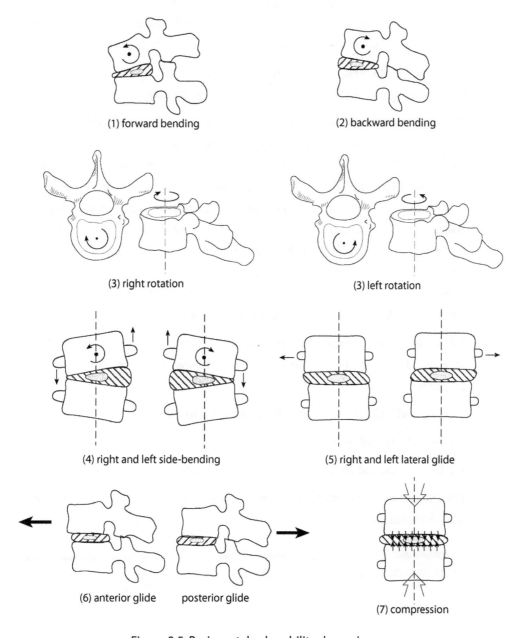

Figure 8.5. Basic vertebral mobility dynamics.

With the above introduction to the primal midline, vertebral dynamics and potential inertial issues, we will begin a clinical exploration fully oriented to primary respiration and the primal midline it generates.

Locating Vertebrae Via Spinal Landmarks

- Atlas: The atlas has no palpable spinous process. You can feel its transverse processes and articular masses slightly posterior to the mastoid process of the temporal bone (in the groove just posterior to the mastoid process).

- Axis: This is the first spinous process that you can palpate just below the foramen magnum. Lateral to this, you will be on its articular masses.

- C7: The next landmark is C7, the vertebra prominens. It is called this because it is usually the most prominent vertebra at the top of the shoulders, although sometimes T1 is actually more prominent. You can determine the vertebra prominens with the client in a sitting position. Place one fingertip on the most prominent spinous process and another one on the spinous process above it. Then have the client move his head forward and backward. When the head moves backward, if the upper vertebra is C6, it will move anterior and seem to disappear. If the upper vertebra disappears, it is C6 and the vertebra prominens is C7. If the upper vertebra does not "disappear" to your touch, it is C7, and in that case the vertebra prominens is T1.

- T7: In the prone position, T7 is commonly level with the bottom of the scapulae. In the sitting position, T8 is usually level with the bottom of the scapulae.

- T12: To find T12, follow the last floating rib up to the spine.

- L3: Usually located at the level of the waist.

- L4: Usually located level with the tops of the iliac crests.

- L5: The spinous process of L5 is often hard to feel. It is located in the hollow just above the sacrum.

Exploration:
Orienting to the Primal Midline and Vertebral Dynamics _____

In this exploration you will make a relationship to the primal midline, the vertebral axis, and any inertial vertebral issues that may clarify. As the primal midline comes into your awareness, it may be sensed as an uprising force in the centerline of the vertebral bodies. I have heard practitioners describe it as a spiraling wind in the midline, as a geyser, or—as Randolph Stone described it—the fountain spray of life. He also noted that what he called the *neuter essence* is found at the center of the midline (Stone 1986). This is an expression of Dynamic Stillness as a creative ordering principle constantly centering the primal midline in its bioelectric field.

The primal midline may be experienced as an airshaft in which air is always rising. As you step into this airshaft with your awareness, it is like hitching a ride in the air stream. As you orient to the primal midline, it seems to ascend from the coccyx and disappear into space at the ethmoid bone. The structural axis of the body forms in relationship to it, from the coccyx through the vertebrae and the cranial base. Review Foundations Volume One, Chapter 19, for an overview of both midline dynamics in general, and the primal midline in particular. Let's explore its relationship to the vertebral axis now.

While holding the client's feet in the supine position, allow the holistic shift to deepen and move to the sacral hold using your caudal hand. As you widen your perceptual field, orient to the client's three bodies—physical body suspended in fluid body, suspended in tidal body of Long Tide—with the client's midline in the center of your field of awareness.

Maintaining a wide perceptual field, orient more to the physical and fluid bodies—the client's biosphere—and the local bioelectric ordering field (Figure 8.6). As you settle into this awareness, orient to the midline from the coccyx through the center of the vertebral bodies and cranial base. Do not narrow your perceptual field as you do this. Simply orient to it in a wide field of awareness and let the felt-sense of the midline come to you. Have patience; don't immediately try to sense anything. This may take a number of minutes and/or a number of practice sessions.

Once you begin to sense the uprising force in the midline, notice how it is expressed. You may sense a smooth expression rising through the midline and vertebral bodies. You may also sense areas of backpressure or gaps in its expression. These indicate the presence of inertial forces and fulcrums along

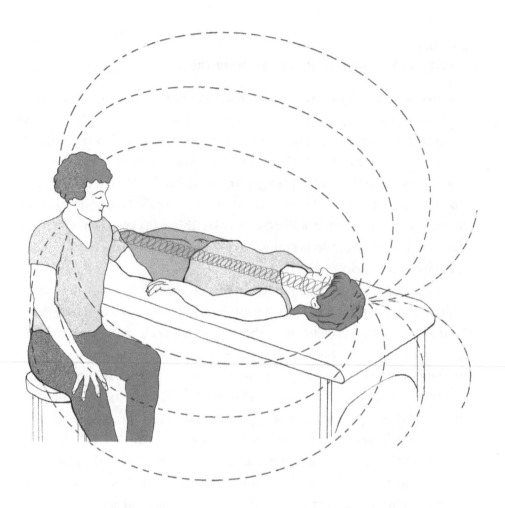

Figure 8.6. Sacral hold with orientation to the ordering matrix.

the vertebral axis. These commonly manifest in compressive fulcrums, vertebral fixations, and congestion. Inertial issues in different areas of the spine will mask the expression of the primal midline and make it difficult to perceive.

Wherever you sense a gap, absence, or backpressure, place your other hand under the spinous processes of that vertebral level and orient to its dynamics. Spread the palm and fingers of your cephalad hand under the vertebrae in this area. Really let your hand and fingers be suspended in fluid, even with the weight of the body on them. Settle into your wide perceptual field, and orient to the inertial dynamic at that vertebral level (Figure 8 .7). Again holding the three bodies in your awareness—physical body suspended in fluid body, suspended in tidal body—sense how the inertial fulcrum or fulcrums involved becomes suspended in this wider field as the forces in it enter equilibrium—the state of

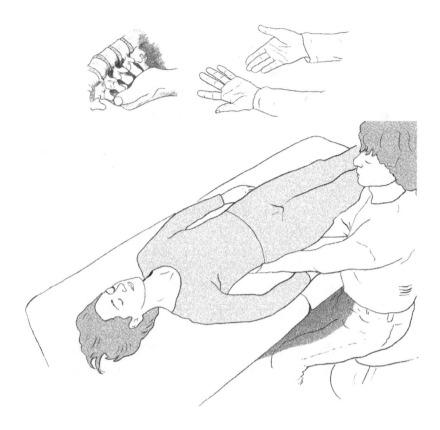

Figure 8.7. Sacral-vertebral hold.

balance. Deepen into your own midline and stillness and see how healing intentions clarify. While you do this, try to maintain awareness of the midline and of the larger whole.

Without losing your awareness of the wider field, and of the client's midline at the center of that field, orient to the fluid body and the potency expressed in it. Can you sense a deeper equilibrium emerging? Does the inertial potency in the inertial fulcrum begin to resolve the conditioned forces? How do you sense this? Does the potency in the inertial area seem to "come alive"? Perhaps you sense local pulsation, or heat being released? Do you notice a permeation of potency into that area? Does the Long Tide begin to express itself through the midline and shift through the area?

After a while this perceptual process becomes very organic and your perceptual field will naturally orient to the appropriate healing level and process emerging in and around the client's system, whether mid-tide or Long Tide, with a natural orientation to Dynamic Stillness.

As the inertial forces resolve in the fulcrum, notice how the midline manifests. Is there a clearer expression of the primal midline through the area? Does its uprising force clarify? Once the inertial issue is resolved, can you sense tissues reorganizing and realigning to the primal midline? Finish with your hand at the sacrum and note the expression and quality of the fluid tide as the session completes for the day.

It is not uncommon for vertebral dynamics to be deeply inertial and compressed. In the following sections you will learn to orient to entrenched compressive issues in the vertebral column.

Vertebral Compression

The vertebral column ideally functions as though each vertebra is hung from above. The joint relationship between each vertebra is then allowed space, and the disc and nucleus between vertebrae act as a hydraulic piston that spreads the compressive gravity force through the disc and maintains the joint space and flexibility (Figure 8.8). Adding to this fluidic sense is the fact that each vertebral articular joint is a synovial joint. In essence, vertebrae are ideally floating in their joint relationships.

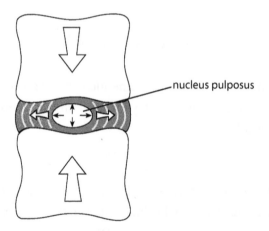

nucleus pulposus

Figure 8.8. The intervertebral disc and its nucleus as a hydraulic piston.

As we experience life, unresolved inertial forces commonly build up around the vertebral axis. This can begin with the womb experience and continue through the birth process and onward. In addition, the vertebral column is always under gravity pressure when we are in the upright position. As inertial forces are introduced into the vertebral axis, more and more potency becomes inertial in response and the joint spaces and hydraulic action of the discs become compromised. Vertebral relationships in the spinal column then become inertial and compressed and a loss of mobility is inevitable. This can lead to lowered vitality and lowered fluid drive and the fluid tide may be sensed as depressed and sluggish.

Augmentation of Space in Vertebral Dynamics

Working with Specific Vertebral Fulcrums (1)

In the sacral-vertebral hold used above, you may have sensed a vertebral area that was deeply inertial and compressed. Augmentation processes can be extremely helpful in these deeply inertial cases. In the following sections, we give examples of a number of augmentation approaches to entrenched inertial fulcrums in vertebral dynamics. The first approach follows on from the session work described above via the sacral hold

Let's say that you have been orienting to the primal midline via a sacral hold as in the above exploration, and noticed that the midline was not clear in the mid-thoracic area at T5–T6. Perhaps you also noticed backpressure or fluid fluctuation in the area and/or a pattern of tissue organization clarifying around an inertial fulcrum at T5–T6.

While still holding the sacrum, place your cephalad hand and fingers under the mid-thoracic area, T5–T6. You may also rest your palm under the vertebral area for a more general contact. Let your hand soften under the client's body, sensing it to be suspended in fluid. Settle into a wide perceptual field, orient to stillness and primary respiration, and see if the inertial forces enter equilibrium as above. If the inertial fulcrum is very dense and the forces cannot access a state of balance, then an augmentation of space at the height of inhalation may help initiate a healing process.

Orient to the inhalation phase of mid-tide and fluid tide. At the height of the inhalation phase, subtly augment space in the mid-thoracic area. Allow your hand and fingers to be moved by the inhalation tide like kelp beds in the ocean. At the height of inhalation, the vertebrae in the area will naturally rise and widen, with space accessed in their disc relationships. As you follow the quality of the fluid tide and the local vertebral motility, allow your hand and fingers to be breathed more deeply by the tide and to take a deeper breath with it. As you resonate with this, your hand and fingers will spread apart and subtly rise, augmenting the expression of potency and space in the local vertebral dynamic. This augments the natural rising and widening of the vertebral axis in inhalation, both in general and in its local dynamics. Allow your hand to relax and soften as the inhalation surge subsides.

Again, if no expression of fluid tide is clearly present, allow your fingers, suspended in fluid, to take a deeper breath as though the tide is present. Again, settle into your wide perceptual field, to the action of potency and to any level of healing process that emerges and deepens as space is accessed.

As the conditional forces within the fulcrum are attended to, you may sense pulsation, heat, and shifts in the expression of potency, tissues, and fluids. As these forces resolve, orient to the reorganization and realignment of the vertebral axis and note the expression of the primal midline. Is the primal midline clearer in the area? Is there less inertia or compression in local vertebral dynamics? Wait for the fluid tide to express itself and notice changes in its drive and quality.

Exploration:
Augmentation of Fluid Drive_____

Another approach via the sacral-vertebral hold used above, is the augmentation of fluid drive toward the inertial vertebral area. Let's again assume that you have one hand under the client's sacrum and the other under the mid-thoracic area. Allow your hands to be as soft as possible, suspended in fluid. Orient to the fluid tide and to the drive of biomagnetic potency in it, and to the motility of the sacrum and vertebral areas you are holding.

As the tide surges in inhalation at or near its height, allow your hand under the sacrum to resonate with the surge. As you allow this, your hand—suspended in fluid and moved by potency—will subtly rise cephalad as your fingers spread apart. This will augment the drive of potency in the fluids toward the inertial site, and stimulate the expression of inertial potencies within the inertial fulcrum, thus helping in the resolution of entrenched conditional forces.

You can simultaneously augment space at the vertebral area above by allowing your cephalad hand to synchronously be breathed by the tide and to subtly spread apart, as described above. Again, notice how potency responds in the local vertebral area and orient to any level of healing process that emerges.

Working with Specific Vertebral Fulcrums (2)

In the next exploration, you will orient more specifically to compressive forces affecting particular vertebrae and the relationship between two vertebrae. This approach is especially useful in the lumbar and thoracic areas. We will orient to the cervical area more specifically in a later section.

In this exploration it is important to remember to orient to the natural widening, shortening, and rising of vertebrae and the vertebral axis during the inhalation phase, and that, at the height of inhalation, space is naturally generated between vertebrae in the disc areas. Remember also that the SBJ is the natural, automatically shifting fulcrum for vertebral organization and motility. In the inhalation phase, you will notice that, as the SBJ rises, the whole vertebral column subtly rises toward it. The following exploration is especially useful when compressive fulcrums are sensed in the dynamics of two or more vertebrae.

Exploration:
Augmentation of Space between Two Vertebrae _____

After the holistic shift, move to the sacral hold and again orient to the three bodies—physical body suspended in fluid body, suspended in tidal body—and the primal midline and its uprising force. As you orient to the midline, see if an inertial vertebral relationship clarifies—you may sense a gap in the expression of the midline at a particular level of the spinal axis, or sense fluctuation of fluid around a vertebral area, or sense the tissue field organizing around a particular vertebral relationship. Notice where the midline is not obvious or where its expression is masked or obscured.

Ask the client to roll over to a prone position. Standing at the side of the table, using your caudal hand, place your index and middle finger over the inertial vertebral area. An alternative hold is to use your thumb and index finger. See which hold is most comfortable and clear for you. Place your fingers over the transverse processes of the vertebrae involved. This will be in the hollows on either side of the spinous process (Figure 8.9). The first stage is to simply deepen into your listening to the dynamics that emerge. See if the vertebral area enters equilibrium in the wider field and healing processes clarify at some level.

If the inertial fulcrum is very dense and the system cannot deepen into the state of balance, then augmenting space between the two involved vertebrae can be very helpful. Place the index and middle fingers of one hand over the transverse processes of the caudal vertebra, and then place the index and middle fingers of the other hand over the cephalad vertebra. Alternatively, you can use the thumb and index finger of each hand. Maintain a wide perceptual field and orient to the biosphere and mid-tide. Maintain an awareness of the physical and fluid bodies suspended in the wider tide (Figure 8.10).

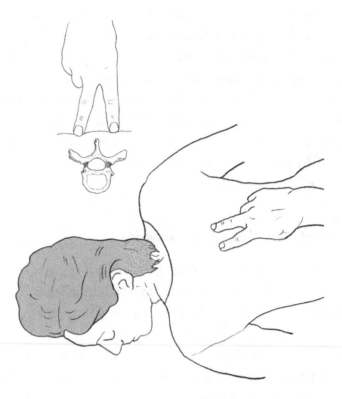

Figure 8.9. Thoracic and lumbar hand position.

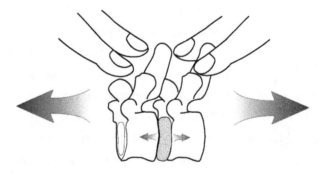

Figure 8.10. Augmentation of space in vertebral dynamics.

In the phases of primary respiration, sense the motility of the vertebrae you are holding. Can you sense the vertebrae breathing? Is there a quality of a subtle rising and widening during inhalation, and a sense that space is naturally generated between the two vertebrae in their disc area?

At the height of inhalation—oriented to the disc and space between the two vertebrae—let your two hands and fingers subtly breathe in opposite directions. This is as though your fingers are being moved/breathed by primary breath at the height of the inhalation surge and subtly widen apart. If no tide is present, allow your fingers, suspended in fluid, to take a deeper breath as though the tide is moving them. Your fingers are very fluidic and are resonating with the quality of space present.

When space is accessed, a number of processes may come into play. You may sense an expression of space clarifying in the disc area between the two vertebrae. You may also notice an intensification of potency in the inertial fulcrum being oriented to, and/or a permeation or drive of potency into the inertial area. The system may deepen into a state of balance, or inertial forces may be processed in the context of the shifting of potency in the fluids. When inertial issues have been processed, orient to the reorganization of the vertebrae and vertebral axis to the primal midline and for a clearer expression of motility and fluid tide.

Working with Cervical Patterns

The cervical area has a relatively free range of motion compared to the rest of the spine. Furthermore, the cervical area is a connecting link where the spinal cord, the throat, and many major nerves and vessels negotiate their way through a relatively narrow area. As described above, the neck and cervical area is an integral part of the stress response and its neural feedback loops, and can hold related tensions due to unresolved stress and trauma in a client's system. The cervical area is thus a very common place for stress to be expressed as physical tension, vertebral fixation, and connective tissue restriction. Indeed, in your explorations above, you may have sensed inertial fulcrums and related compressive issues and tissue patterning clarifying in the cervical area.

The intense and sometimes traumatic forces of the birth process can also leave an imprint in cervical dynamics. The cervical area often holds birth-related forces and the related affects they generate—such as compression, torsion, and neck tension and pain. Tension headaches commonly have origins in these cervical dynamics. Due to the continuity of connective tissue and membranous relationships, inertia in the cervical spine directly influences the dural tube and dural membrane in general, and also affects the cranial base—affecting the dynamics of the sphenoid, occiput, and temporal bones. This obviously has important repercussions for the

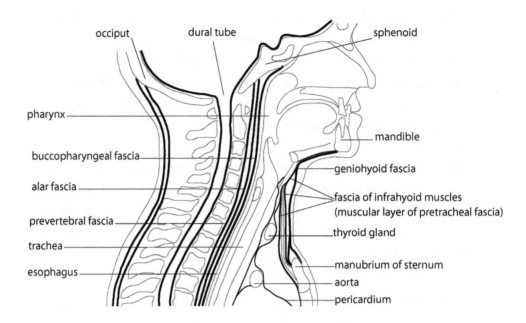

Figure 8.11. Continuity of fascial relationships.

whole system. The fascia of the cervical area is also continuous with the fascia of the cranium, neck, thoracic, and abdominal areas. There are continuous fascial relationships from the base of the skull, through the cervical fascia, to the thoracic inlet, pericardium of the heart, the thorax, the respiratory diaphragm, the abdomen, and pelvis (Figure 8.11).

Other considerations may also be important when relating to the cervical area. Tibetan Buddhists consider the neck to be the seat of ego. We "take it in the neck" when our ego processes are overwhelmed by our experience. The neck is also the traditional location of the throat chakra. This chakra is closely associated with issues revolving around space and boundaries. Thus issues that especially relate to space seem to affect the neck and its tissue relationships. When the feeling of space in life closes down, the cervical area closes down. The cervical area tenses and contracts in response to stress and overwhelm. We contract to protect. It is a manifestation of an attempt to "hold things together." All of these stresses and lifestyle issues are part of the therapeutic inquiry.

The cervical area will also mirror other issues held elsewhere in the body. For instance, pelvic issues and patterns will be directly reflected, as will issues relating to the lower lumbar spine. The vertebral column functions as a single unit oriented to the primal midline and inertia in any part will be reflected in the whole.

Explorations:
Cervical Holds _____

We orient to two cervical holds below: the first exploration is a hold for the cervical area as a whole, and the second allows orienting to specific vertebral issues and relationships. In each exploration, you will begin by orienting to primary respiration and the primal midline via the occipital cradle hold.

General Approach to the Cervical Column and the Augmentation of Space in Cervical Relationships

The cervical vertebral column can become inertial and tense as a whole. In these cases it is useful to have a way to orient to the cervical area as a whole. This is also useful as a general starting point when orienting to any cervical issue. Common origins of general cervical inertia, compressive fulcrums, and neck tension include whiplash and the birth process. For example, the birth process may place the baby under continuous compressive forces affecting whole areas of the spine. If these forces are not resolved at the time of the impingement, articular masses of the cervical column and their individual joint facets can become chronically compressed and fixed, losing independence and general flexibility.

This first exploration orients to inertial forces and tensions present in a wide area of the cervical column and will help you relate to wider issues of axial compression. You will first orient to any inertial fulcrums or patterns that clarify, and to the deepening equilibrium of the forces involved. If these forces cannot enter equilibrium, we also include an approach for the augmentation/exploration of space in the cervical column as a whole.

After the holistic shift, move to the occipital cradle hold and orient to the client's biosphere—the physical and fluid bodies—as suspended in the wider tidal body. Don't force your perceptual field to be wide—simply orient to the biosphere with a wider perspective. As you settle into this orientation, allow the primal midline to also enter your perceptual field. Can you perceive this midline rising through the cervical area? Do you sense an uprising force in the vertebral and cranial base midline? Are there gaps in its expression? See if a specific area of the cervical spine, with a specific vertebral relationship, comes to the forefront. You may also sense a more general quality of inertia through the cervical area, or more specific areas of restriction.

Move from the occipital cradle hold and place your fingertips longitudinally (vertically) along the articular masses of the cervical vertebral column. Your

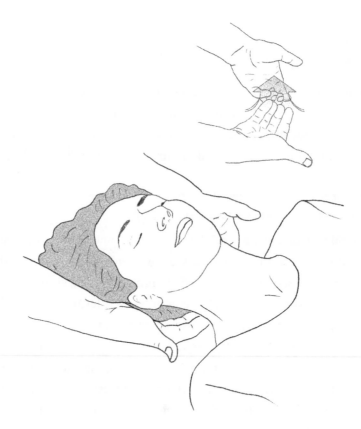

Figure 8.12. General cervical hold.

fingers should be gently spread pointing anterior (toward the ceiling) in relationship to the client's body (Figure 8.12). As you place your fingers in this position, subtly lift them anterior (toward the articular masses) to make a clear, but gentle contact.

Settle into your wide perceptual field, orient to the fluid tide, and include the tissues and their motility. You may sense the cervical spine rising and widening in the inhalation phase. Maintain your wide perceptual field and orient to any inertial patterns and fulcrums that clarify. Orient to the forces in the fulcrums that clarify, and the sense of the inertial fulcrum being suspended in the wider field as the forces in the fulcrum enter equilibrium. Allow this to deepen into stillness, and orient to any level of healing process that emerges.

If you sense that the inertial issues are very dense, expressed in multiple vertebral fulcrums and/or general axial compression, then you can explore the augmentation of space in these relationships. Maintain the same hand position, with your fingers gently spread under the articular masses. At the height of the inhalation phase allow your fingers—suspended in fluid and moved by the fluid tide—to take a deeper breath, while subtly spreading apart. This has the quality of resonance with the expression of inhalation and the space naturally generated between vertebrae at the height of inhalation. The cervical area ideally expresses its motility in inhalation by subtly rising and widening, with space generated between each vertebra.

Again settle into your perceptual field and orient to whatever level of healing process emerges. You may sense potency in inertial areas expressed as pulsation, inertial forces resolved, and heat generated, and/or a shifting of potency in the fluids into inertial areas. Likewise, the inertial forces in the cervical area may enter equilibrium and deepen, and healing processes may emerge from any level. You may sense the Long Tide entering the midline and shifting in a wind-like manner to resolve inertial forces, or deepen into stillness, which then becomes the fulcrum for the emergence of healing processes.

After the forces are resolved to the degree they can be in that session, orient to the reorganization of the cervical area, and vertebral axis in general, and for their realignment to the primal midline. How does the cervical area now express its motility? Does the fluid tide emerge with grater drive and clarity?

Specific Approach to Cervical Vertebral Inertia

As you orient to the cervical area from your occipital cradle hold, you might want to relate to a particular cervical vertebral issue and its dynamics. To do this, change your hand position from the occipital hold to that specific vertebral level. Place the index and middle fingers of both hands on either side of the spinous process of that particular vertebra, over its articular masses. If you are working with the atlas, place your fingertips in the hollows under the occiput just posterior to the mastoid processes. You can also relate to the atlas by placing all of your fingertips under the occipital base pointing anterior toward the atlas (Figure 8.13). As you do this, maintain your wide perceptual field and orientation to primal midline, fluids, and tissue motility.

Settle into a state of interior stillness and maintain a wide perceptual field. Orient to the physical and fluid bodies in the wider tidal body and to the primal midline at the core of the vertebral axis and cranial base. Allow the felt-quality of the inertial fulcrum, its tissue elements, and the energies that organize it, to come into your wider awareness. Notice if the forces, fluids, and tissues enter a state of equilibrium. Remember Becker's three stages of seeking, settling, and reorganization and realignment. See if a deeper sense of equilibrium and stillness begins

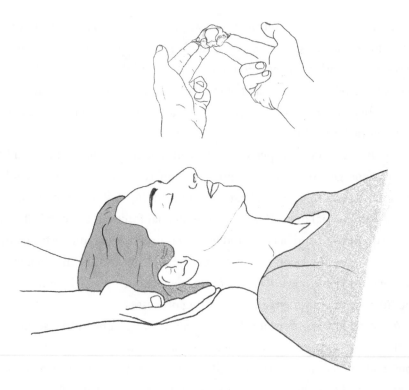

Figure 8.13. Specific cervical hold.

to emerge and deepen into this arising state. Note the expression of potency and be open to any level of healing process that emerges.

If the forces in the fulcrum are very inertial, and the state of balance cannot deepen, you can then orient to the augmentation of space as suggested above. Change your hand position to the general cervical hold and, at the height of inhalation, allow your fingers to breathe more deeply as they subtly widen apart. Notice how the potency, fluids, and tissues respond to this augmentation intention. Again, if no fluid tide is expressed, allow your fingers to resonate with the space present, and to take a deeper breath as though the tide is moving them.

Return to the original specific cervical hold, and again deepen into a still and present relationship to the inertial site. See if the forces can deepen into equilibrium, and if potency is more available in the initiation of healing processes. Again be open to any level of healing process that emerges.

Finish at the sacrum or sacral-occipital hold. Again, orient to reorganization, realignment, and the expression of the fluid tide—its quality and drive.

Augmenting Fluid Drive in the Cervical Area

In the descriptions above, you initially oriented to the cervical area via an occipital cradle hold. One clinical option is the augmentation of fluid drive toward an inertial cervical area. The most natural way to orient to this intention is in the exhalation phase. In exhalation, potency is returning to the midline and receding footward.

Let's say that you are holding a specific cervical vertebra, perhaps C4, as described above, with the palms of your hands still at the occiput and your fingertips either side of the midline at C4. In the exhalation phase, the palms of your hands follow the receding of potency through the cervical area while maintaining an orientation to the inertial issue at C4. This simple orientation, both to the receding of the fluid tide and its potency *and* to the inertial site, will augment the action of potency in inertial fulcrum being oriented to.

Axial Forces and the Augmentation of Space

It is not unusual to encounter unresolved longitudinal or axial forces affecting wide areas of the spine. These axial forces may, in turn, generate various kinds of inertial fulcrums and compressive issues along the vertebral axis. Axial compressive forces commonly originate from unresolved birth trauma or other traumatic or shocking experiences. Potency will act to protect the notochord/primal midline, and areas of condensation and compression result. This need to protect the integrity of the midline must be appreciated and respected. Our work is not about fixing anything; it is about the resolution of traumatic forces and unresolved experience.

One way to approach inertial issues in and around the midline is to orient to the axial forces present holistically. Thus the intention in the exploration below is the augmentation of space in the vertebral midline as a whole. The inertial forces present may generate specific inertial fulcrums in vertebral dynamics, but the forces involved must first be holistically oriented to for efficient clinical results.

Exploration:
Augmentation of Space in and around the Primal Midline _____

In this exploration we are assuming that you have sensed inertial issues in the vertebral midline. Perhaps you have sensed areas where the primal midline is not clearly perceived along the vertebral axis, or have perceived wide areas of vertebral inertia as you listened from a sacral, occipital, or sacral-occipital hold. Sensing this, in this exploration you will orient to the inhalation phase of the fluid tide/mid-tide and augment the natural expression of space in the vertebral midline.

After the holistic shift, place your hands in an occipital cradle hold. Establish elbow fulcrums and avoid backpressure in the fluid system via the heels of your hands. Let your hands float on the tissues, suspended in fluid, and orient your perceptual field to the biosphere (physical and fluid bodies).

Orient to the primal midline from your occipital hold. Notice how it manifests as an uprising force through the vertebral and cranial base axis, and areas where it is obscured to your perception.

From your occipital hold, orient to the inhalation phase of the fluid tide/mid-tide. At the height of inhalation allow your fingers and hands, which are under the occiput, to take a deeper breath in the cephalad direction as the midline reaches the peak of its inhalation rising. The intention is to orient to the rising of the fluid tide and the natural space generated in vertebral dynamics at the height of inhalation and let your hands and fingers breathe with the inhalation surge. Hold the whole of the vertebral axis in awareness as you allow this (Figure 8.14).

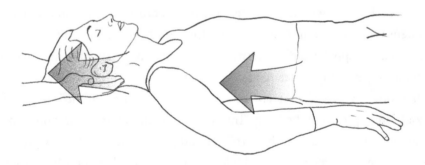

Figure 8.14. Augmentation of space in the vertebral midline
via the occipital cradle.

As space is accessed, you may sense a drive of potency in or through the vertebral axis and a natural resolution of inertial forces may occur. As this occurs, you may also sense a lengthening throughout the vertebral axis. This may herald the completion of the session, or you may sense the system further deepening into a state of balance and dynamic equilibrium and other expressions of healing processes may emerge from any level of action. Potency may shift in the fluids toward specific fulcrums, the Long Tide may express healing intentions through the wider field and midline, or the system may deepen into stillness as the Dynamic Stillness comes to the forefront. Allow your perceptual field to be open to any level of healing that emerges.

An alternative approach to axial compression is the same as that described in our last chapter, on the dural tube. With the client in the side-lying position, place your lower hand over the sacrum and upper hand over the occiput. At the height of inhalation, allow your upper hand to follow the inhalation surge, and augment space through the midline, by breathing deeper in the cephalad direction. Your hand followed the ascending of the tide through the fluids and dural tissue and subtly breathed/deepened into that headward, ascending direction. (See Figure 7.9.)

Our next chapter orients to the inferior pole of the primal midline, the pelvis, and pelvic dynamics.

CHAPTER 9

Pelvic Dynamics

The pelvis is located at the inferior pole of the primal midline, vertebral axis, and cerebrospinal fluid core. It is a foundation for midline structural dynamics and a common site of inertial issues. It commonly holds inertial forces related to the birth process, falls, and general tissue tension. Inertial issues here will directly affect the reciprocal tension membrane system via the firm attachment of the dural tube at S2. Compressive issues in pelvic dynamics will also affect the motility of the central nervous system via the connection of the filum terminalis to the coccyx, which can then tether the spinal cord and dampen down CNS motility. Sacral compression can also lead to hypersensitization of brain stem nuclei, and initiate a stress response in the system as a whole, due to constant drag on the central nervous system. We delve deeper into this possibility in Chapter 21 on nociception and the stress response.

Inertial forces held in the pelvis and sacrum will also strongly affect the expression of the fluid tide throughout the system. As we have seen, the fluid systems of the body convey the potency of the Breath of Life to all cells and tissues. The lumbosacral waterbed is a key site for the building of potency at the beginning of inhalation, generating a strong inhalation surge. Inertial potencies held in pelvic dynamics may thus affect the drive and vitality of the whole system.

Energetic Dynamics

In classic traditions such as the yogic system of India, the sacrum and lumbosacral waterbed are considered to be sites of powerful potential energies. This energetic quality is represented as a coiled serpent, the kundalini energy of the sacral area. The sacrum is also considered to be a site of crystallized energy and of life force held in reserve. The pelvic chakra (water chakra) is traditionally located at the base of the sacrum in the lumbosacral junction. The root chakra (earth chakra) is located between the apex of the sacrum and the coccyx. *Chakras* are organizing fulcrums along the midline that order specific orbs of structure and function. The pelvic chakra classically relates to grounding energies, nurturing feelings and intentions, sexuality, and self-view. The root chakra relates to foundation, support, and a sense of stability and centeredness in life. Inertial fulcrums in the pelvic area can thus be an expression of deeper issues relating to safety, foundation, self-view, support, and nurturance in life. Traditional cultures looked at the human system as a conscious energy system, and the pelvis was considered to be a root, or foundation, of that system. In a craniosacral biodynamic context, the water chakra between L5 and the sacrum is considered to be the primary fulcrum of the fluid tide. Inertial issues here will dampen down the expression of potency in the tide, affecting the whole system.

These dimensions may come into play when working with the pelvis, and the pelvis can reflect these in its patterns and shapes. I have had many clients, with issues relating to self-worth, past abuse, self-confidence, ability to nurture and be nurtured, and loss of ground and contact, who have benefited greatly from session work oriented to pelvic dynamics.

As in all of our work, the chakras can be sensed by orienting your perceptual field to these phenomena. One way to do this is to hold your hand a few inches above the client's spine. Let your awareness encompass the whole biosphere and wider bioelectric field. Starting from the coccyx, slowly move your hand superiorly. Do not narrow your field of awareness as you do this. Move from the coccyx to the occiput slowly a number of times. After a number of passes, you may begin to sense localized vortexes and/or pulsations along the midline. These will have different qualities expressing their distinct locations and functions. Randolph Stone clearly oriented to these vortexes in his polarity therapy.

Anatomical Relationships

As we have seen, the physical body is a unified field whose tissues manifest holistic organization and motility. Likewise, the entire pelvic bowl—including bones, joints, muscles, connective tissues, and viscera—manifests a unified dynamic. A strong ligamentous stocking of connective tissue unifies all of the structural components, supports the lumbar vertebrae, surrounds the sacrum, anchors the muscles, and stabilizes all the osseous relationships. The sacrum can be visualized as hanging from the lower lumbar area in this stocking (Figure 9.1). As it hangs, it ideally floats in the fluids of its joint relationships (Willard 1995). It is important to understand the ligamentous relationships of this stocking and to be able to sense its integrated dynamics. Ligaments that stabilize the relationship between the fifth

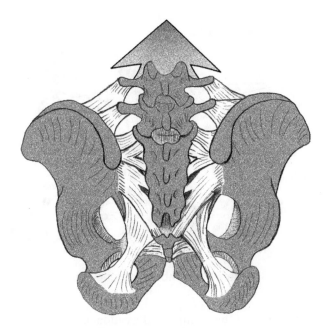

Figure 9.1. The sacrum hangs in the ligamentous stocking
from the lumbar vertebra.

lumbar vertebra and the pelvis and those stabilizing the relationships between the
bony structures of the pelvis are of particular interest.

Lumbosacral Junction

The primary joint between the pelvis and the lumbar vertebrae is the lumbosacral
junction, including all joint and connective tissue relationships between L5 and
the sacrum. The two articular facets and the intervertebral disc between L5 and
the sacrum are often found to be in compression. Conditional forces of trauma and
stress are commonly expressed as inertia in these pelvic tissues (Figure 9.2).

The ligamentous relationships of L5 and the pelvis include:

- Caudal continuations of the anterior and posterior longitudinal ligaments that
  connect the body of L5 to the first sacral segment

- The ligamentum flava that connects their laminae

- The inter- and supraspinous ligaments of the spinous processes

The iliolumbar ligament stabilizes the relationships of L5 to the pelvis. It radi-
ates laterally from the transverse processes of L5 via two main bands. The cephalad

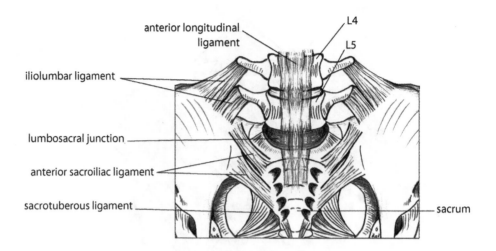

Figure 9.2. Lumbosacral junction.

band attaches to the crest of the ileum and the caudal band connects to the base of the sacrum where it blends with the anterior sacroiliac ligament.

The Sacroiliac Joint

The sacroiliac joints form another major joint relationship of the pelvis. Each S/I joint has L-shaped articular surfaces that allow for the variety of pelvic motions required for walking, running, sitting, and stretching. The joint allows both rotational and gliding motions. It commonly has a lower and upper compartment. These compartments are usually formed by concavities in the articular surfaces of the sacrum and convexities in the articular surfaces of the ileum. However, many variations in the internal topography of the joint surfaces are possible. For instance, some people have one large compartment rather than two. Some have a small third compartment at the level of S2, and some have one type of articular surface on one side of the pelvis and another on the other side. It is also possible to find that the sacral surface is convex rather than concave and that each S/I joint surface of the same sacrum is different (Figure 9.3).

The articular surface of each bone is covered with a cartilaginous plate. The cartilage covering the sacrum is thicker than that found on the ileum. The cartilaginous plates are in close association and are connected by softer fibrocartilage. At the anterior and posterior ends the joint surfaces are connected by fine interosseous fibers. Posteriorly, at the level of S2, these interosseous fibers thicken to form

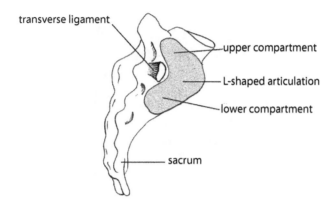

Figure 9.3. The sacrum, its articular surfaces, and the transverse ligament.

what is sometimes called the axial or transverse ligament of the sacroiliac joint. The transverse ligament helps to create the sacrum's transverse axis of rotation at S2.

The S/I joints are synovial joints. There are joint capsules (fluid-filled sacs) around each S/I joint. Fluidic potency and circulation are thus essential in their functioning. The synovial fluids enable ease of motion and the mobility necessary in the dynamics of the joint. These fluids carry the potency of the Breath of Life, and the quality of fluids is a major factor in the maintenance of joint mobility.

The sacrum and its S/I joint surfaces form a wedge-shaped, upside-down pyramid that is wedged into the innominate bones at the sacrum's articular surfaces and secured by its connective tissues. A series of coronal sections through the S/I joints shows this wedging mechanism. At the first section, at the level of S1, the distance between posterior S/I joint margins is slightly greater than the anterior margins. This is the start of the anterior-posterior wedge shape (Figure 9.4a). At this level the articular surfaces of the S/I joints also narrow closer together as they move inferiorly, so there is also an upside-down pyramidal wedging of the sacrum into the innominate bones.

In a second section through S2, the posterior width is distinctly greater than its anterior width and the two joint surfaces again narrow together medially (Figure 9.4b). So at the level of S2, there is a clear wedging of the joint surfaces. A third section, through S3, shows an interesting change. At this level, the anterior width is greater than the posterior (Figure 9.4c). There is generally also a wider dimension transversely across the two joint surfaces. This change in the wedging at S3 in the joint surfaces helps to stabilize the joint in its motion. The wedge shape of the sacrum's joint surfaces, and their interlocking concave-convex form, resist downward pressures of weight, and the second sacral segment (S2) thereby becomes the

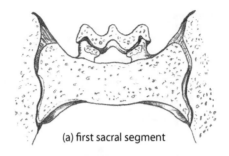

(a) first sacral segment

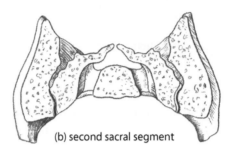

(b) second sacral segment

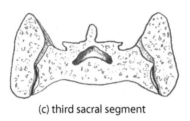

(c) third sacral segment

Figure 9.4. Coronal sections through the sacroiliac joints.

natural axis for the motion of the sacrum. This is reinforced by the interosseous transverse ligament at the level of S2.

Although this is a general description of typical joint surfaces, variations in joint structure are extremely common. The wedging can be opposite to that described above. In bony specimens, I have even seen different directions of wedging from one side of the same sacrum to the other. Variations of the topography of the articular surfaces have been mentioned above. The sacral surfaces are generally concave, commonly with two joint concavities, many times with one long L-shaped concavity and sometimes with three concavities. I have seen many variations of these surfaces and have seen specimens with convex rather than concave surfaces.

As introduced above, there are commonly two "legs" of the L-shaped sacroiliac joint: an upper, relatively horizontal leg, and a lower, relatively vertical leg. Each leg commonly has a compartment or depression corresponding to the shape of the iliac articular surface. The presence of inertial forces in these compartments will generate compressive issues in their dynamics.

The legs can hold compression independently of each other. Compressions of the upper leg of the L tend to be transferred to the upper aspects of the ligamentous stocking that maintains stability in the lumbosacral relationships. The iliolumbar and lumbar vertebral ligaments can become involved, and lower- to mid-lumbar pain, tissue and fluid congestion, and nerve facilitation may result.

Compression in the lower leg of the L will tend to be transferred to the sacroiliac ligaments such as the sacrospinous and sacrotuberous, and sciatic pain radiating in the buttocks and legs may result. Bilateral compression of both legs of the L is also common and can result in pain distribution in any direction. The interosseous ligaments around the joint may also become involved, with resulting restriction in mobility. Pain is often transferred to the opposite side of the pelvis, away from the compressed sacroiliac joint. The compression can also be transferred diagonally across the ligamentous stocking to the opposite side.

Ligaments Connecting the Sacrum to the Ilia

Understanding and accurately visualizing the relationships of the ligamentous stocking that connects the lower lumbar area, the sacrum, and the innominate bones together can inform clinical work. The ligamentous stocking helps to stabilize the pelvis and its joint dynamics. The transfer of the downward force of weight through the lumbar area to the pelvis is buffered and resisted by the connective tissue structure. This helps to stabilize the sacrum and its sacroiliac joints and allows them to float in synovial fluids. We are first going to look at the ligaments that connect the sacrum to the ilia around the S/I joints themselves. These are the anterior sacroiliac, posterior sacroiliac, and interosseous ligaments. Although we describe them individually, all these ligaments function as one ligamentous unit (Figure 9.5).

Anterior Sacroiliac Ligament

The anterior sacroiliac ligament consists of numerous bands that form a sheet-like ligament. It connects the anterior surface of the lateral aspect of the sacrum to the margin of the auricular surface of the ileum and its preauricular sulcus.

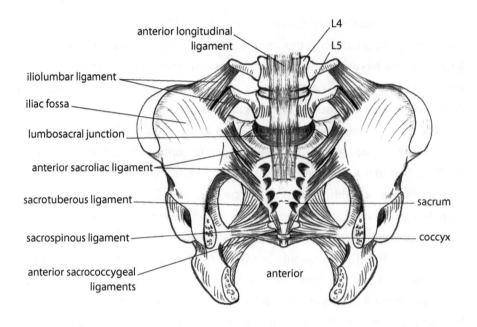

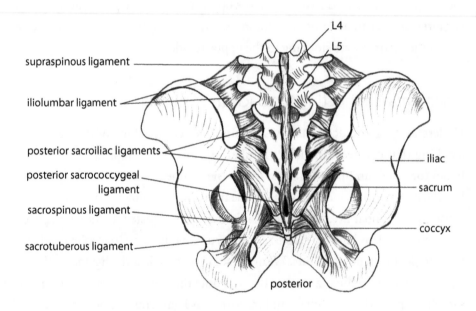

Figure 9.5. The major ligaments that stabilize the sacroiliac joints.

Posterior Sacroiliac Ligament

The posterior sacroiliac ligament consists of numerous fibers oriented in many directions. Its superior part is sometimes called the *short posterior sacroiliac ligament*. It is nearly horizontal in orientation and connects the first and second transverse tubercles of the posterior surface of the sacrum to the tuberosity of the ileum. Its inferior part is sometimes called the *long posterior sacroiliac ligament* and it is oblique in orientation. It connects the third transverse tubercle of the sacrum to the posterior superior spine of the ileum and merges with the superior part of the sacrotuberous ligament. It is a strong ligament, creating one of the chief bonds of the joint.

Interosseous Sacroiliac Ligament

This ligament consists of a series of short, strong fibers that connect the tuberosities of the sacrum and ileum. It lies deeper than the posterior ligament and connects the borders of the joint. It creates a strong band posterior to the articular surface at the level of S2 and defines the classic osteopathic axis of rotation for the motion of the sacrum.

Ligaments Connecting the Sacrum to the Ischium

The ligaments connecting the sacrum to the ischium help to stabilize the joint. They are an integral part of the ligamentous sock that holds and stabilizes the lumbosacral area. These include the sacrotuberous and sacrospinous ligaments.

Sacrotuberous Ligament

The sacrotuberous ligament is a broad fan-shaped complex of fibers that connects the posterior inferior spine of the ileum, the fourth and fifth transverse tubercles of the sacrum, and the caudal (footward) part of its lateral margin and the lateral margin of the coccyx, all to the inner margin of the tuberosity of the ischium. Its caudal border is continuous with the tendon of origin of the biceps femoris muscle and many of its proximal fibers are continuous with the posterior sacroiliac ligament and sacrospinous ligament. It is also continuous with the interosseous ligament and joint capsule.

Sacrospinous Ligament

The sacrospinous ligament is a triangular sheet that is attached at its base to the lateral margins of the sacrum and coccyx and at its apex to the spine of the ischium. Its fibers are continuous with the sacrotuberous ligament and also blend with the sacroiliac joint capsule.

These ligaments form a unified ligamentous stocking that holds and stabilizes the sacrum and lower lumbar vertebrae, and also affords attachment for various pelvic muscles. The ligamentous stocking is an important aspect of the self-bracing mechanisms of the pelvis and its integrity is essential for ease of lumbosacral and craniosacral functioning.

Neuroendocrine-Immune Implications

The sacrum ideally floats in its joint relationships. If it cannot, the dural tube and CNS can become tethered in their expression of motility and mobility. As described earlier, this can become a major inertial factor in the system, leading to hypersensitization in brain stem nuclei and the activation of the stress response.

Chronic lumbar muscle contraction will be transferred directly to the ligamentous stocking and can cause related contractions in ligamentous fibers. The contractions can then be transferred to the sacroiliac joints. Chronic tissue contraction can generate nerve sensitivity and inflammatory responses. These will cause chronic nociceptive input (pain input) to be sent to the dorsal horn cells of the spinal cord. These cells may then become sensitized, and chronic pain and a vicious cycle of facilitation may result. Similarly, vertebral fixations can generate nerve sensitization, hyper- or hypotonic nerve response, tissue contraction, and chronic inflammatory responses.

Frank Willard PhD points out that the ligamentous structures of the lumbosacral area contain many nociceptive nerve fibers (pain receptors) and efferent sympathetic fibers. These are capable of secreting proinflammatory neuropeptides that interact with immune cells in the surrounding tissues. Chronic stimulation through nerve facilitation and tissue contraction can result in chronic low-grade inflammatory responses that are thought to play a major role in chronic pain and degeneration in the lumbosacral area (Willard 1995).

Furthermore, chronic nociceptive input into the dorsal horn neurons of the spinal cord can generate wider effects in the system. Cycles of central nervous system facilitation can be set up and the hypothalamus-pituitary-adrenal axis can become sensitized. The neuroendocrine-immune system will become adversely affected, and the system may become overwhelmed. See Chapter 21 for a full discussion of these topics and clinical approaches.

The Motility of the Sacrum

The sacrum is a roof more than it is a back wall for the pelvis. It is situated in a relatively oblique position in the pelvis with its base (top) much more anterior than its apex (bottom). As a midline structure, the sacrum's motion is classically described in terms of flexion and extension. In mid-tide dynamics, its motility is sensed to be more holistic and cellular in nature, not separate from the whole tissue field, and is best described in terms of the inhalation and exhalation phases of the tide.

In inhalation, the sacrum subtly rises cephalad and expresses an intraosseous widening as its segments uncoil. In inhalation, the sacrum also expresses rotation around a transverse axis located at S2 (the second sacral segment). Its base rotates in a superior and posterior direction, while its apex rotates in an inferior and anterior direction around S2. In our description of the anatomy of the sacrum and its ligamentous relationships above, you may remember that its wedge-shaped articular surfaces, and the transverse ligament located at the level of S2, help to generate this axis of rotation.

More simply on a felt-level—while holding the sacrum—in inhalation, you may perceive a subtle quality of filling and rising, widening, and uncurling of the sacral segments. In the exhalation phase, the opposite may be sensed; you may sense a subtle quality of emptying as the sacrum settles, narrows, and curls up.

The cephalad rising of the sacrum in inhalation is an important motion. If the cephalad lift of the sacrum in the inhalation phase is restricted by inertial issues, such as sacroiliac compression, the motility of the central nervous system will be directly affected. The central nervous system is connected to the coccyx via a continuity of pia mater called the filum terminalis (Figure 9.6).

The motility of the sacrum is accompanied by movement in the surrounding tissues. As the sacrum expresses its motility, the innominate bones simultaneously widen in inhalation and narrow in exhalation (Figure 9.7). Likewise, as the fluid tide ascends in inhalation, the sacrum, dural tube, and central nervous system also ascend as they shorten and widen. This is all an expression of the holistic nature of motility and is ideally oriented to the primal midline.

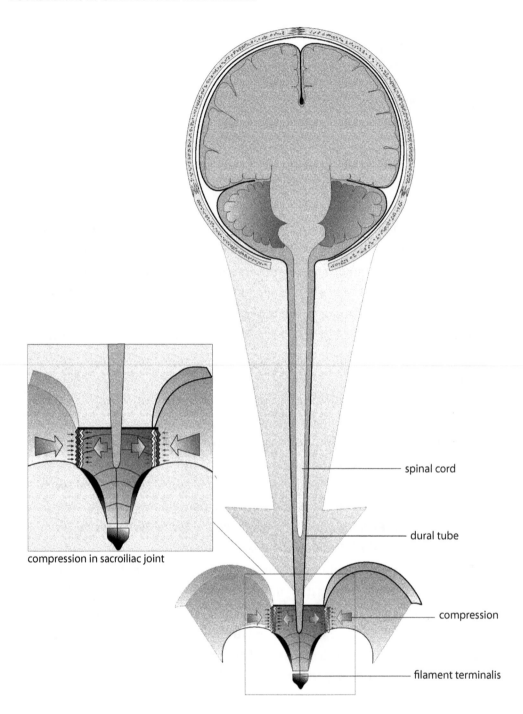

compression in sacroiliac joint

spinal cord

dural tube

compression

filament terminalis

Figure 9.6. Tethering of the central nervous system.

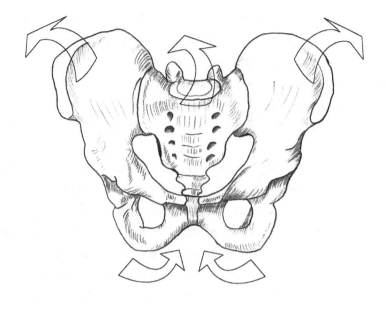

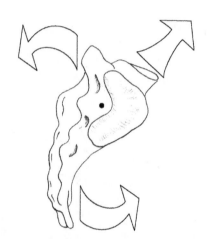

Figure 9.7. Inhalation of the sacrum in the innominate bones.

Motility of the Sacrum and Inertial Issues

It is very common to encounter clients whose sacrum cannot express motility clearly. Instead of sensing rising-widening-uncurling and settling-narrowing-curling in the phases of the tide, the sacrum's motility may seem inertial. Sometimes it may even be hard to sense motility at all.

This is commonly a consequence of birthing forces, or other traumatic forces of some kind that are present in the tissues and joint relationships of the sacrum. These inertial forces can generate many clinical issues in the client's system. Due to the presence of inertial potency and related fulcrums, inertial sacral issues will strongly affect the expression of potency in the fluid tide, commonly damping down its inhalation surge. A flat or thin quality of inhalation surge will then be sensed.

On a tissue level, spinal nerve roots leaving the sacral canal can also be affected by sacral inertia. This may manifest as nervous system hypersensitivity, sensorimotor nerve facilitation, local inflammation, sacroiliac and low back pain, sciatica, and various kinds of pelvic visceral symptoms. Sacral inertia can also be transferred superiorly and be expressed in the dynamics of the occiput, cranial base, and CNS. Furthermore, as discussed above, the inertial issue may contribute to a tethering of the central nervous system via the filum terminalis. Thus, the motility of the CNS may be compromised.

Sacral Mobility Dynamics

Before exploring the motility dynamics of the pelvis, it is also useful to have a general understanding of its basic mobility. As we have seen, the sacroiliac joint

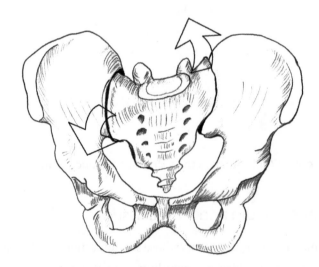

torsion composed of side-bending
and rotating components

Figure 9.8. Torsion in sacral dynamics.

is L-shaped and allows both gliding in its articular surfaces and rotation around its axis of rotation at S2. If you are sitting down and your ischial tuberosities (sitz bones) are fixed, as you bend forward and backward, the sacrum moves around the fixed ilia. The sacrum simply forward-bends and backward-bends on the ilia around S2. But as you walk, or move freely without fixing the ilia, the two bones move in relationship to each other with both rotation and gliding at their L-shaped joint surfaces. Due to the L-shaped joint structure, and to the combined rotation and gliding dynamic of the joint, the sacrum both rotates and side-bends at the same time as it expresses movement in relationship to the ilia. Fixations of the sacrum are thus commonly expressed as forward-bending or backward-bending fixations *combined* with torsion where there is both a side-bending and a rotation component (Figure 9.8).

Sensitivity in Explorations

The pelvis can be a sensitive and/or emotionally charged area for many people. When approaching the pelvis, the practitioner must keep this in mind. The pelvic area may hold issues relating to sexuality, self-worth, and nurturing. Negotiating safe contact is critically important here. The pelvis can hold a history of trauma that may involve birth trauma, physical and sexual abuse, falls, and accidents. It is important to explain your intention to your clients, and why you are contacting this area. It is also important to give them some power in the relationship by giving them easy ways to signal any discomfort, such as lifting a hand or simply saying "no." At every step, explain how and why you are about to engage in a particular contact, and negotiate that gently and gradually. Do not attempt to override protective patterns—you might overwhelm the client.

Clients may not verbally communicate feeling overwhelmed to you, but the system will. The goal is to access the health within, not to activate symptoms or emotional processes. If emotional processes arise, know what you are in relationship to. There is a huge difference between a true emotional completion and a traumatic recycling of emotional energies. In a true emotional completion it is clear that the client is grounded in the present. There is a sense of something moving through the system and completing as space is accessed. In a traumatic recycling of emotional energies, things may speed up dramatically and the client may seem to be caught up or lost in emotions with little space. It may seem as though the client is re-experiencing the trauma rather than processing it and letting it go. (See Chapters 18–21 on the stress response, neurophysiology, traumatic impacts, and activation states.)

Exploration:
Sensing the Motility and Motion of the Sacrum _____

The sacrum ideally hangs freely in its ligamentous stocking and floats with ease in its synovial joints. In this exploration, listen for this ease of floating as the sacrum expresses motility. If it cannot float freely, as is often the case, then the fluidic nature of the joint relationship is compromised. Also listen for a subtle rising of the sacrum at the beginning of the inhalation phase. If the sacrum cannot express this, the central nervous system may be tethered and its motility will be affected.

Starting at the feet, notice the quality of the suspensory field that emerges after the holistic shift has deepened—physical body suspended in fluid body, suspended in wider tidal body—one of the crucial starting points in session work. Move to the sacral hold after the holistic shift deepens. As described in Volume One, sit at the lower caudal (footward) corner of the treatment table with your chair pointing toward the diagonally opposite shoulder. Ask the client to lift the pelvis off the table so you can place your hand under the sacrum. Your fingertips should be pointing cephalad and the client's sacrum should be comfortably nestled in your hand. The heel of your hand should not be pressing against the sacrum or coccyx. Your elbow should be near or under the client's knee so that your wrist is not bent at a sharp angle. Your hand should be comfortable. After establishing your wide perceptual field, imagine that your hand is sinking under the table, suspended in fluids.

In your wide perceptual field, orient to the client's biosphere as a unified potency-fluid-tissue field and to the quality of the fluid tide. You may sense this as a subtle rising-filling in inhalation and receding-emptying in exhalation. Once you have a sense of the fluid tide, add the sacrum and its motility to your orientation. Notice how the sacrum expresses its motility in the cycles of the tide. Do you sense a subtle rising at the beginning of inhalation and a widening and uncurling of its segments, or the reverse in exhalation? Is motility oriented to the midline, or is it expressed in some patterned fashion—as is commonly the case?

As you settle into this awareness, does an inertial pattern of some kind clarify? You may notice that the sacrum manifests its motility and motion in an eccentric fashion and that, as the inherent treatment plan clarifies, the whole fluid-tissue field begins to organize around it. These patterns may include rotations, torsions, compressive issues, and related connective tissue pulls and strains. For instance, as you sense a torsion pattern in sacral dynamics, you may sense a related contraction or tension pattern in the ligamentous sack within which the sacrum is supported, and a wider tension pattern throughout the body.

As you sense a pattern clarifying, orient to the inertial fulcrum around which it is organized. This inertial fulcrum may be a local one, in the sacroiliac or hip joint for instance, or may be related to a more distant fulcrum elsewhere in the body.

As the system continues to deepen, you may sense a state of equilibrium emerging in and around the inertial fulcrum—the state of balance—as the forces in it access equilibrium. As this occurs, you may then sense the fulcrum to be suspended in its wider field—physical body suspended in fluid body, suspended in tidal body, suspended in Dynamic Stillness. As this suspensory system deepens, listen for the level of healing process that emerges from the deepening stillness.

Notice the action of potency in and around the inertial fulcrum and the resolution of inertial forces. This may be perceived as pulsation, permeation, fluid drive, fluctuation, heat, expansion, or other expressions.

As the inertial forces are resolved by the action of primary respiration, notice the reorganization and realignment of the tissue field to the midline and for greater ease in sacral motion. You may also notice a fuller sense of surge in the inhalation phase of the tide and a greater sense that the sacrum is floating in its joint relationships. Finish either at the sacrum, or at the sacral-occipital hold and feet.

Kundalini Forces

Sacrum literally means "sacred bone." It is the traditional seat of vitality in the human body. It is also the classic location of what is called *kundalini* energy in yogic philosophy. In biodynamic terms, kundalini energy is an expression of the storehouse of potency in the lumbosacral waterbed. Potency builds here at the beginning of the inhalation surge of the fluid tide. Randolph Stone described a process in which the practitioner holds both sacrum and occiput, and orients to the cisterna magna and lumbosacral waterbed until a dynamic equilibrium is accessed (Stone 1986). One way of doing this is to deepen into Dynamic Stillness as you hold this awareness. This helps resource the system by building potency in the fluids in a balanced and therapeutically significant way.

Mystical and tantric traditions have practices to rapidly open this storehouse of vitality. These practices are not to be taken lightly and must be learned under the guidance of a master of those traditions. Forces can be unloosed too quickly and disturbances can arise in the body-mind process. I have had a number of "kundalini refugees" whose systems became very disturbed with the use of extreme breathing practices geared to "raise the kundalini." They commonly presented extremely unintegrated, agitated, and dissociated systems. In the Zen tradition, this is called *Zen sickness*—a consequence of excessively forced meditation practice. Clinical work involved slowing down activation, working with felt-resources and stillpoint processes, and orienting to Long Tide and Dynamic Stillness as starting points in clinical work.

Innominate Bone Motility

The innominate bones have a number of important articulations: the two sacroiliac joints, the pubic symphysis, and the hip joints. The S/I joint was described above. The pubic symphysis is the articulation between the two pubic bones. It has a fibro-cartilaginous disc that connects the two bones and allows slight movement. The hip joint is a ball-and-socket joint. The acetabulum is a cup-shaped cavity on each innominate bone that receives the head of the femur. The acetabulum is anteriorly located on the innominate bone and is also located anterior-inferior to the axis of rotation of the innominate bone as a whole (Figure 9.9). In inhalation, the ilia of the innominate widen apart transversely; in exhalation, the innominate bones narrow transversely at the ilia (see Figure 9.7).

Innominate Bones and Inertial Issues

Possible inertial issues between the sacrum and the innominate bones at the sacroiliac joints include anterior and posterior rotation and gliding motions around the sacroiliac joints, lateral shifts or shears, and superior and inferior shifts or shears (vertical shifts). The relationship between the sacrum and innominate bones can become fixed in any of these directions. Vertical shifts always originate in external trauma, usually occurring due to falls or accidents (Figure 9.10). Any fixation in the S/I joints will be transferred to the pubic symphysis and the hip joints, and can generate compensatory fulcrums in these areas. Furthermore, these issues can generate compensatory patterns in cervical, occipital, and cranial base dynamics. Any of these patterns may be encountered in a general exploration of the motions of the pelvis.

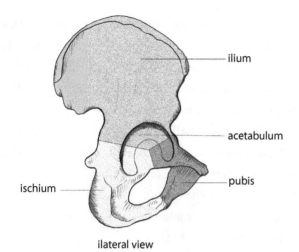

ilium

acetabulum

ischium

pubis

ilateral view

Figure 9.9. Anatomy of an innominate bone.

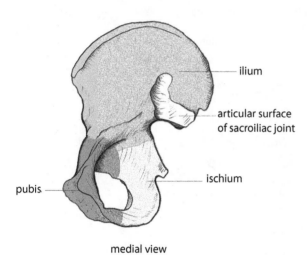

ilium

articular surface
of sacroiliac joint

pubis

ischium

medial view

Figure 9.10. Superior vertical shift of the
sacrum in the ilia.

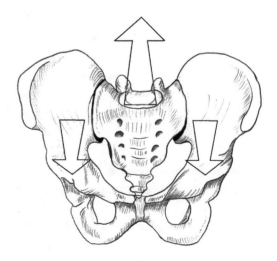

It is common for one innominate bone to prefer, or be fixed in, posterior rotation while the other prefers, or is fixed in, anterior rotation. This generates, or is part of, torsion across the relationships of the pelvis. It is also common for both innominate bones to prefer posterior rotation, with one more posterior than the other. This also generates torsional forces across the pelvis.

When torsion occurs, the sacral base is usually forced into a posterior and inferior position on the most posterior innominate bone side. This is because as the innominate bone rotates, its posterior superior iliac spine rotates posteriorly and inferiorly, and the sacroiliac joint follows. As the sacrum is forced inferiorly and posteriorly by the innominate bone, it must rotate and side-bend at the same time. It is then forced into a torsioned position (Figure 9.11).

Posterior rotation of innominate bone
forces the sacrum to rotate posteriorly
and inferiorly, creating sacral torsion.

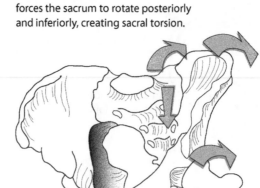

Figure 9.11. Mechanics of sacral torsion.

The leg on the side of the posteriorly rotated innominate bone is usually found to be physiologically short (as opposed to anatomically short). That is because the acetabulum follows the posterior rotation of the innominate superiorly, and the head of the femur is rotated relatively superior, generally yielding a short leg on that side.

Thus, a common structural picture on the side of a posteriorly rotated innominate bone is:

• A physiologically short leg on that side

• An inferior and posterior sacral base on that side

• A torsioned relationship between the sacrum and innominate bones

Exploration:
*Sensing Motility of the Innominate Bones*_____

This exploration focuses on the motility of the innominate bones at the ilia.

While holding the client's feet, after the holistic shift is accessed, you may start to perceive the motility of the pelvis as a widening in inhalation and narrowing in exhalation. Move to a pelvic hold by placing your hands over the anterior aspects of the pelvis at the anterior superior iliac spines (Figure 9.12). Again, let your hands float on tissues, suspended in fluid, with you and your client suspended in a wider tidal field. In your wide perceptual field, again orient to the biosphere and fluid tide. Once you have a general sense of the fluid tide, orient to the tissue field. Settle into this awareness, really let your hands be suspended in fluid, and see if you can sense the motility of the pelvis more directly. As the ilia transversely widen apart in inhalation and narrow together in exhalation, it may seem as though your hands are being gently moved in those directions like a boat suspended in water, moved by the tide. You may also become aware of various shapes and patterns of motion. For instance, you may sense that one ilium prefers inhalation and the other prefers exhalation. You may also sense torsioned, sheared, and compressed tissue patterns. Simply listen to the motility of the innominate bones in the phases of primary respiration.

Listen, remain oriented to the wider biosphere and the expression of inhalation and exhalation, and wait for an inertial pattern to clarify. Some of the issues

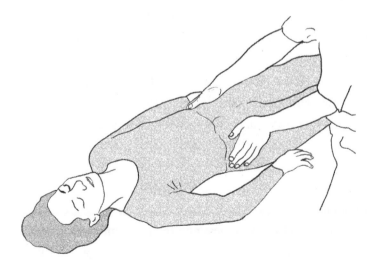

Figure 9.12. Hand position for the innominate bones.

described above may clarify. One ilium may be more posteriorly rotated than the other. The pelvis as a whole may be side-shifted either left or right, or one or both innominate bones may be vertically shunted. Notice all of this. See if you can sense the related organizing fulcrums.

As an inertial fulcrum clarifies and the system deepens into equilibrium and the state of balance, again remember Becker's three-phase awareness, while being open to any level of healing process that emerges. Finish the session at the feet and notice how motility is sensed from there. Do you note any changes in its expression?

___

Exploration:
The Pelvic Diaphragm and Sacro-Pelvic Patterns _____

In this exploration, we orient to both sacral motility and the related motility of the pelvis as a whole. You will be holding the transverse structures of the pelvic diaphragm and its related fascia as well as the bony structures of the pelvis. In this position, you will maintain a wide perceptual field—holding all three bodies in awareness—with an orientation to the fluid and physical bodies (Becker's biosphere). The intention is to orient to primary respiration and see what healing priorities emerge. As we orient to pelvic tissue dynamics, it may be helpful to review the anatomy of the fascial and connective tissue relationships in the male and female pelvis.

After the holistic shift has been accessed at the client's feet, move to the sacral hold. With one hand under the sacrum as in the sacral hold, place your other hand over the pubic symphysis (sacro-pelvic hold). Slowly move the heel of your hand caudal (footward) from the abdomen until the edge of the heel of your hand is over the pubic symphysis. Your fingers are generally pointing cephalad, away from the pelvis (Figure 9.13). In this position, allow your hands to float in fluids. Orient to the fluid tide and then notice how the pelvis expresses its motility in inhalation and exhalation. See if you can sense the potencies and fluid drive underlying the tissue motions. Notice how all of this is organized in relationship to the primal midline.

As you settle into this awareness and the inherent treatment plan emerges, what inertial patterns clarify? What inertial forces organize this? Patterns of inertia throughout the pelvis may clarify, including tensions and fulcrums in the pelvic diaphragm, connective tissues, and organs. The pelvis may express

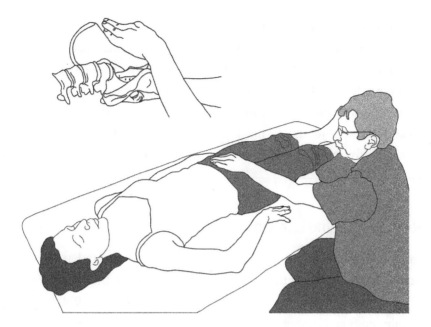

Figure 9.13. Sacro-pelvic hold.

almost any kind of motion, and this may be organized around an inertial fulcrum located almost anywhere. Very commonly, you may note compressive forces in the sacroiliac joints, hip joints, and lumbosacral junction.

As the system continues to settle, notice how the forces in the inertial fulcrum settle into equilibrium and orient to any level of healing process that emerges. The inertial potency in the fulcrum may begin to express itself, you may sense pulsation and heat being released, there may be an experience of potency shifting in the fluids toward the inertial area, and/or you may sense the system further settle into Long Tide and Dynamic Stillness. Finish at the sacral-occipital hold and/or feet.

As you continue to practice this work, you will discover that there is a huge potential for various kinds of inertial patterning in this area. You may perceive tissue compressions, tensions, and related inertial patterns involving not just the joints and connective tissues in the area, but also the viscera that are suspended in their midst. For instance, on a tissue level, you may perceive the sacrum pulling up into the lumbar area, or moving around the lumbosacral junction in some fashion. You may also sense the sacrum pulling into, or expressing motility around, one of its sacroiliac joints. It is not uncommon to perceive torsioning throughout a client's pelvic dynamics. For instance, in the female pelvis you may notice a torsioned sacrum and pelvis, continuous with torsioning through the broad ligament and female pelvic organs. Alternatively, you may sense a general lack of motility and motion of any kind. You may also notice these issues via fluid fluctuations, spiraling of fluid, and fluid rebound. These are common phenomena in the pelvis. In the following clinical explorations, we will orient to inertial issues, especially the presence of compressive forces, in the lumbosacral junction and sacroiliac joints, the major joints of the pelvis. We will learn some new pelvic holds for these areas and the augmentation of space in their relationships.

Relating to Specific Lumbosacral Issues

The lumbosacral junction is the transition point between the lumbar vertebrae and the sacrum. It is at this point that the weight carried through the bodies of the vertebrae above is transferred to the sacrum and pelvic arch (Kapanji 1974) (Figure 9.14).

Membranous and ligamentous strain patterns from other areas of the body are often transferred to the lumbosacral connective tissues. Postural issues and trauma of various sorts, including falls and accidents, can be reflected here. Birth trauma and birthing forces are another potential source of stress here. These various experiences introduce inertial forces into the tissue field that may affect the dynamics of the lumbosacral junction in many ways. Remember the discussion above about the ligamentous sock that surrounds the sacrum and lower lumbar area. Also remember that many nociceptive fibers are found in these connective tissues.

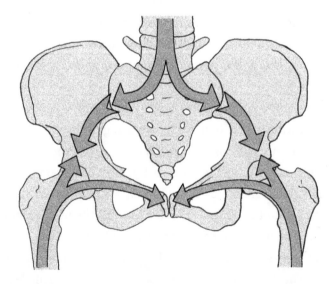

Figure 9.14. Weight transfer via the lumbosacral junction.

While orienting to sacral motility, you may have sensed a pull into the lumbo-sacral junction, or various kinds of tension patterns organized around it. These are almost always a consequence of unresolved compressive forces held in the junction. These commonly generate tissue compression, fluid congestion, and tension patterns in surrounding connective tissues. These can also be the origin of nerve sensitivity and lumbar pain.

In the following explorations, we are assuming that the client's system has deepened into the holistic shift and the healing process has begun to orient around the lumbosacral area. As session work unfolds, you may be drawn to the lumbosacral junction while holding the sacrum, or via an awareness of tissue patterns organizing around it, via shifts in potency and fluid fluctuations and/or via awareness that the primal midline is obscured as it rises through the area. In the explorations below, you will first orient to the lumbosacral junction from your sacral hold, and then learn a new lumbosacral hold in order to explore augmentation of space in its relationships.

Explorations:
Lumbosacral Motility and Augmentation of Space _____

Orienting to Lumbosacral Motility

From your sacral hold, orient to the motility expressed in the sacrum and lumbar spine. As the sacrum expresses its motility, you may also perceive a rising and widening through the lumbar area. As you settle into this awareness, you may sense that the sacrum expresses patterns organized around the lumbosacral junction. For instance, you may sense a cephalad pull toward the junction, or a pattern of motion organized around it. If the compressive forces are dense, you may not be able to sense much motion at all. The motility and mobility of the sacrum and pelvis may seem to be compromised.

As the inertial fulcrum in the lumbosacral junction clarifies, and the system enters equilibrium, be open to any level of healing process that emerges. Finish at the sacral-occipital hold and/or feet.

As the system settles into the state of balance, inertial potencies will commonly be expressed, and you may sense a welling up and permeation of potency in the joint relationship. As things deepen, this may include your awareness of the Long Tide and Dynamic Stillness. You may sense the inertial forces in the fulcrum being dissipated back to the environment. As the compressive forces resolve, the lumbosacral junction may be sensed to soften and expand.

It is not uncommon, however, to find that the compressive forces present are so dense, and the tissue and fluid effects so chronic, that an augmentation of space in the joint relationship may be very helpful. In the next part of the exploration you will augment space in the lumbosacral area. We are assuming that, in the sacral hold above, you sensed an intransigent compressive fulcrum in the lumbosacral area.

Augmentation of Space in Lumbosacral Dynamics

With one hand under the sacrum as above, place your other hand in a partial fist under the lower lumbar vertebrae. Your fingers should be against the spinous processes from L2–L5. If the lumbar curve is too flat to allow this, let the spinous processes fall in the indentation between your fingers and the heel of your hand, or just use your fingers to make contact with the client's lower lumbar spine. The inferior aspect of your upper hand should be just touching or very close to your lower hand at the sacrum (Figure 9.15).

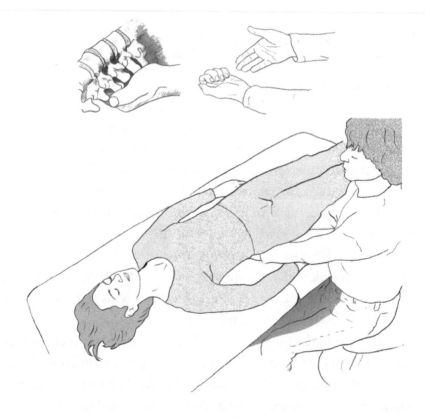

Figure 9.15. Lumbosacral hold.

Maintain your lumbosacral hold as above. Settle into an awareness of the inhalation and exhalation phases of the tide. At the height of inhalation, allow your two hands, suspended in fluid, to deepen into the expression of inhalation both at the sacrum and lower lumbar area. It is as though your two hands take a deeper breath, or are breathed more deeply, as the sacrum expresses the fullness of inhalation as it widens and uncurls, and the lumbar area rises with the tide cephalad. In resonance with the tide and its fluid drive, your hand at the sacrum widens and rotates posteriorly, while your other hand under the lumbar area subtly rises. Again, if no tide is clearly present, allow your hands, suspended in fluid, to take a deeper breath as though the tide is moving them. This really has a doing-not-doing quality to it, where your fingers are very fluidic and are resonating with the quality of space present.

As space is augmented, listen for expressions of health, the expression or permeation of potency in and around the area, and for a softening and expansion of the tissues. As space is accessed, the sacrum may be sensed to literally soften and float toward the feet and to express its motility with greater potency and drive. Again, finish at the sacral-occipital hold and/or feet.

Primary and Secondary Coupling of Compressive Issues

It is common for secondary fulcrums to be generated in compensation for a primary issue. Potency acts as a unified field to maintain order and the best possible balance. As the system holds local inertia, other areas will also become inertial in order to compensate for the forces present in the primary fulcrum. In this compensatory process, compressive forces will be transmitted through the tissue field to other tissue relationships.

Lumbosacral compression is thus often coupled or associated with other compressive issues in the body—such as occipito-atlanteal compression (compression between the occiput and atlas), intraosseous occipital issues, and compression at the SBJ. Likewise, compressive forces held anywhere in the midline of the system will be mirrored throughout the midline. If the lumbosacral compression is primary, the others tend to express a compensatory compression.

Lumbosacral compression may strongly affect dural function and ease of dural glide. Chronic low-grade inflammation and pain are also often associated with lumbosacral inertia. In the presence of unresolved compressive forces, local connective tissues go into protective contraction, muscles spasm, and joint compression results. Nerve facilitation and pelvic visceral issues may also arise, all generated by lumbosacral compression.

In yogic philosophy, the lumbosacral junction is commonly considered to be the site of the swadhisthana chakra, located between L5 and the sacral base. This is a classic site for the generation and maintenance of creative forces. As noted above, in a biodynamic context, the lumbosacral junction is an important fulcrum area for the fluid tide. If there is compression in the junction, the fluid tide is commonly compromised and its vitality or drive will be affected. Thus lumbosacral compression may have detrimental consequences for the expression of potency in the fluids and for the general vitality of the system.

Sacroiliac Joints, Compressive Forces, and the Augmentation of Space

Compressive issues in sacroiliac joints are common. In previous explorations, as you oriented to sacral motility, you may have noticed that the sacrum expressed some form of inertial pattern around a compressive fulcrum in an S/I joint. You may have likewise noticed connective tissue strains or pulls oriented to an S/I joint area. A sense of torsion in sacral dynamics may have been perceived, or perhaps a hinge-like motion between the ilia, around an S/I joint. You may even have sensed a compressive wedging of the sacrum between the ilia. Very little motility will then be perceived.

Compressive forces in S/I joints may be very dense and the tissues of the joint may undergo real qualitative changes, becoming chronically contracted, compressed, and inertial. The space in the joint may literally close down, and the fluids in and around the joint become static. Potency may become very inertial, centering the forces involved, and the state of balance may not easily deepen.

In the next exploration, you will orient more specifically to compressive forces found in S/I joints. You will learn a new innominate bone-sacral hold, called the sacroiliac hold, in order to explore the augmentation of space in S/I joint dynamics. In the exploration we assume that you have been orienting to sacral motility, a strong inertial fulcrum has been perceived in an S/I joint, and the state of balance cannot deepen.

Exploration:
*Sacroiliac Joints and the Augmentation of Space*_____

The sacroiliac hold is a new hand position for exploring S/I patterns. Maintain contact with the client's sacrum in the sacral hold—place the forearm (near the elbow) of your other arm on the lateral aspect of one iliac crest and the fingertips of the same arm on the lateral aspect of the other iliac crest. Your arm is arched over the pelvis and bridging the space between the two ilia. You now have a clear relationship with the two iliac crests as you maintain your original sacral hold (Figure 9.16).

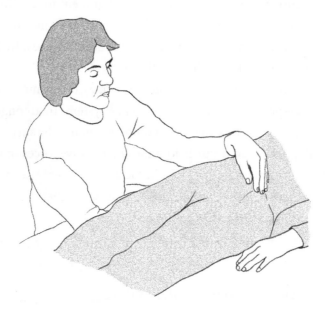

Figure 9.16. Sacroiliac hold.

Settle into this hold and orient to the motility of the sacrum and innominate bones in inhalation and exhalation. Your contacts at the ilia, simply by their presence, gently stabilize the client's innominate bones. At the height of inhalation, allow your hands and forearm to take a deeper breath with the inhalation motility and fluid drive sensed. Your hand under the sacrum augments the quality of sacral motility perceived, as you sense the widening and filling quality of potency, fluids, and tissues. I tend to take a deeper physical breath as my hand intends a deepening into inhalation. Again, here we are in relationship to the natural space generated in all tissue relationships at the height of inhalation. Likewise, if the fluid tide is not clearly expressing itself, allow your fingers to resonate with the space naturally present in the sacroiliac joints, and to take a deeper breath as though the tide is moving them.

Once space is accessed, orient to any level of healing process that emerges. You may sense expressions of potency, forces shifting, heat being released, fluid fluctuations, tissues reorganizing and realigning to midline, and so on. The system may also settle into Long Tide or Dynamic Stillness as a state of balance, a state of dynamic equilibrium in the whole system, deepens. As inertial forces resolve, you may sense a softening in tissue relationships and an expansion of the tissue field. You may also perceive that the sacrum begins to float more easily in its synovial joints, and hangs more freely in its ligamentous stocking.

After the reorganization of tissues and realignment to midline completes, what do you notice has changed in sacral dynamics? Is its motility expressed in a more balanced fashion? Has the inertial issue been fully resolved? Is potency more available? Is there better drive in the fluid tide?

Be patient—the resolution of inertial forces may take a number of sessions to complete. Respect the timing of the client's system. In an ongoing clinical practice, as the inherent treatment plan unfolds, you may be surprised to notice that something else must occur before the compressive forces in the S/I joints can resolve. This "something else" may be located anywhere else in the body. For instance, you may sense potency shifting to other areas that need attention first, before the sacroiliac issue can be addressed.

Exploration:
Sacroiliac Joints and Augmentation of Fluid Drive _____

Another classic approach to deeply inertial fulcrums in S/I joint dynamics is the augmentation of fluid drive toward the area. This augments the action of the potency in the inertial fulcrum, can assist in the resolution of the inertial forces involved, and can help the state of balance to deepen. In this clinical exploration, you will be orienting to the sense of potency and fluid drive relative to the inertial area.

Maintain your sacral hold and place your other hand on the front of the client's body with your palm over the inguinal ligament area anterior to the S/I joint being addressed. Settle into your awareness of the inhalation and exhalation phases of the fluid tide (Figure 9.17).

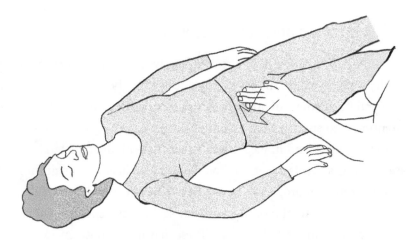

Figure 9.17. Augmentation of fluid drive toward a sacroiliac joint.

As you sense the fullness of the inhalation surge, and the drive of potency in it, subtly augment the expression of drive toward the sacroiliac area from your anterior hand. Your hand orients to the S/I area and resonates with the energetic drive of the potency in the fluids toward the inertial S/I joint. This occurs largely via your awareness of the electromagnetic quality of potency in the fluids in the inhalation surge and your orientation to the S/I area. Once you sense that potency is being expressed in the joint relationship, and that inertial forces are being processed in some way, remove your anterior hand and proceed as usual.

An alternative to the above process is to make a more direct relationship to the S/I joint. To do this, move your hand from the sacral hold. Place your cephalad hand under the S/I joint being addressed and create a "V"-shaped spread under the joint, using your index and middle fingers to span the joint with the posterior inferior iliac spine between these fingers. Place your caudal hand over the anterior inguinal area as above. The palm of that hand should be centered over the inguinal ligament. Your posterior hand is monitoring the expression of potency as the process unfolds. Then, with your anterior hand, augment fluid drive toward the inguinal area to the V-spread as above. Sense the response of potencies and fluids to this intention. Wait for a sense of expansion and welling up of potency in the V-spread area.

Lateral Fluctuation and Sacroiliac Issues

If, as you orient to sacral motility, the compressive forces are so dense that little or no motility is perceived, or the state of balance cannot be accessed, the augmentation of lateral fluctuations of potency in and around the joint area may be helpful. The intention is to augment the action of potency in the inertial fulcrum as the fluctuations build around it. Please remember that enhancing lateral fluctuations can be activating, and this intention should be avoided in acute or painful situations. This process is most appropriate for very inertial, cold, and dense areas.

As you orient to sacral motility, you may sense various forms of fluid/potency fluctuations around an inertial fulcrum. These may take almost any form. They may be pendulum-like, swinging back and forth, or they may be expressed as figure-eights or spirals. These fluctuations are the expression of potencies and fluids in direct relationship to the inertial fulcrum and inertial forces being addressed. As you hold the client's sacrum, you can augment the fluctuations sensed around the area by using the thumb and little finger of this hand. Again sense your hand to be immersed in fluid. Augment the lateral fluctuations sensed by subtly enhancing the felt quality of the flux of fluid and potency between your fingers, first in one direction, then the other—like the swings of a pendulum. This generally encourages a greater expression of potency in the area. Any time the fluid fluctuation becomes stronger in an area, more potency becomes available. This may encourage expression of potencies in the inertial fulcrum. At first, the uptake of your suggestion may be sluggish. Gently persevere. The fluids and potency in the area will begin to respond. As this occurs, you may have a sense of potency welling up in the area.

Clinical Highlight

I'd like to share a relatively early clinical experience, which relates to sacral dynamics and helped my early understanding of the inherent treatment plan to clarify. A long time ago, in 1983, while I was working in a London clinic, a thirty-five-year-old man was referred to me. He had been suffering from ongoing sacro-iliac pain over a two-year period and had seen many other health practitioners. He remembered a fall off a horse four years before and a past sense of tightening in the area. When his pain was most intense, it was disabling, and he was in a depressed state. He entered my office bent over with contraction and pain and, after discussing his circumstances, needed to be helped onto the treatment table.

He was literally crying with pain and despair. The current intense bout had been going on for almost a month.

My first tendency at this early point in my clinical practice would have been, after some stillpoint process, to try to resolve the sacroiliac and lumbar pain by local work of some kind. I realized, however, that he had seen some very experienced osteopathic practitioners before me, so I was somewhat humbled by the situation. I decided to go slowly into the work and see what evolved. I found that his system was literally shut down; there was no expression of fluid tide, potency was locked up, centering the process he was experiencing, and there was both local inflammation and tissue shock in the lumbosacral and sacroiliac areas. There was also a general sense of autonomic activation throughout his body and he was experiencing anxiety and poor sleep patterns.

Over the first few sessions I helped him access a relatively comfortable position, and we worked verbally with felt resources and basic trauma skills. I helped him slow his process down and worked with some basic mindfulness processes within which he slowly learned to hold his pain more spaciously with less activation. Cranially, I mainly oriented to stillpoints, Long Tide, and Dynamic Stillness in these sessions. This gradually helped down-regulate his activation and help him access a sense of space and stillness within himself. I also showed him a parasympathetic recovery position from the work of Randolph Stone. This involved him lying on his left side with a pillow between his knees, placing his left hand over the rear of his neck and his right hand over his buttocks with his fingers in the crease between his buttocks. He found this a very comforting position to use at home.

He found that the sessions gave him some additional resources, and his S/I pain gradually lessened. By the tenth session his autonomic activation had greatly reduced, and his system was better able to orient to primary respiration and the inherent treatment plan could start to be expressed. For the first time, I was able to perceive the wholeness of his system and its suspensory nature. There was a sense that his tissue field was suspended in fluid and the Long Tide was more accessible. Then a powerful sequence of events took place. His system finally settled into a holistic shift and his potency began to shift in fluids toward the mid-thoracic area. I supported this process as thoracic compression softened and his structural midline lengthened. Potency again shifted and the tissue field then distorted around the right occipito-atlanteal area, as an old compressive issue was attended to. Once this completed, the potency shifted to the occipital bone itself and an intraosseous compression. As the intraosseous forces resolved, his potency oriented to the central nervous system, and an inertial pattern clarified, organized around the brain stem, along with a related cranial base pattern. The occipital, cranial base, and CNS issues were all related to very early experience and birthing forces. As these resolved, another level of autonomic clearing occurred with electric-like releases down the sympathetic chain. This all resolved over a number of sessions.

It was only then that potency shifted to the pelvic area and session work more specifically oriented there. It thus took many sessions for his system to do what it needed to begin to relate more directly to the S/I issue and the pain that it generated. Over a number of subsequent sessions I was able to support work in the pelvic area. An intraosseous birth pattern in the sacrum also came to the forefront, which seemed very connected to the previous work his system had undertaken. As this occurred, he had an early childhood memory of a bicycle accident and fall. It appeared that a coupling of a series of birth and childhood experiences had become coupled with his later horse accident, and his sacroiliac pain was an expression of all of this history. When these forces uncoupled, a general reorientation of his tissue field around the midline occurred, along with a real lightening of his sense of pressure and fragility. When the inertial forces in and around the sacrum finally resolved, a major shift in the tissues of his pelvis occurred, and the motility of the whole pelvic area realigned to the midline. By the twentieth session, his pain had completely subsided and his depression had lifted. Basically, he felt hopeful and had relief from pain for the first time in years. Over the course of the later sessions, I also taught him some gentle chi kung exercises that empowered him to relate to his sacroiliac area with much less fear.

The main points here are that the processes described above are used in the context of the unfolding of the inherent treatment plan, and that it is also helpful to give clients methods that empower them to take their healing process into their own hands.

Intraosseous Sacral Issues

As we have seen in our birth chapters, birthing forces can generate inertial fulcrums and distortion patterns within a bone itself. Intraosseous distortions in the sacrum are not uncommon and are an important territory to consider. Intraosseous issues in the sacrum can occur due to the inertial forces placed on the young sacrum by the birth process. Issues may also be generated during the toddler period when infants learn to walk and have many falls on the bottom, or later in life by trauma.

Exploration:
Intraosseous Inertia in the Sacrum_____

If a sacrum is holding unresolved intraosseous forces, its segments may seem compressed together, and its motility may be dampened down. The sacrum may feel lifeless and dull, or dense and compressed, even if it is expressing some kind of outer motion. Likewise, the presence of intraosseous forces in sacral tissue will affect the motility of the pelvis as a whole, and dampen down the fluid tide. This exploration orients you to the augmentation of space in its inner dynamics.

While holding the sacrum, you may notice that the quality and ease of its widening and uncurling in inhalation is dampened down, dense and resistant. This may indicate the presence of unresolved intraosseous forces. At the height of inhalation, allow your hand and fingers to follow the motility of the sacrum in its inhalation expression and to breathe more deeply in that direction. Your hand is responding to the motility of the fluids and tissues at the fullness of inhalation by augmenting the felt quality of the filling, widening, and uncurling of the sacrum. This again has a doing-not-doing quality to it. Ideally, you are bringing this intention of augmentation to the tissues without introducing any outside forces into sacral dynamics. The intention is to access the potential space available in the tissues of the sacrum.

Orient to expressions of potency in sacral tissue and note whether the inertial forces in the sacrum are being resolved. You may notice pulsation, heat, fluid fluctuations, and tissue motions, as this occurs. As inertial forces are processed, the sacrum may be sensed to soften, spread, and open like flower petals. When the process seems complete, orient to the motility of the sacrum and see if there is greater ease in its dynamics.

Intraosseous inertia in the sacrum can have important consequences for the vitality of the system. Inertia in sacrum-coccyx relationships will strongly affect the expression of the fluid tide and of tissue motility throughout the body. If the sacrum is holding intraosseous inertia, the ability of the whole system to express primary respiration may also be compromised. A long time ago an osteopathic oldtimer said to me, "If the system doesn't respond to your work, look to the sacrum!"

CHAPTER 10

The Occipital Triad

In this chapter we will complete our exploration of vertebral dynamics, continuing our exploration of the structures that develop around the primal midline and orient to the superior pole of the spinal column. This is the *occipital triad*, comprising the occiput, atlas (C1), and axis (C2). As with the inferior pole—the sacrum, L5, and L4—the three structures of the occipital triad are intimately linked together due to the continuity of their ligamentous relationships. This continuity is derived from their integrated embryological origins. The occiput originates from sclerotomes and can be considered to be a modified vertebra. The occiput, atlas, and axis form a functioning embryological unit intimately bound together in its dynamics. Inertial issues in the occipital triad will be directly transferred to the cranial base and the dural membrane system, and, most interestingly, will also be mirrored in the pelvic triad of L4, L5, and the sacrum. Thus the occipital and pelvic triads will directly mirror each other's dynamics. The old maxim "as above, so below" certainly holds true for midline structures.

The junction between the cranium and cervical vertebrae is commonly called the occipito-atlanteal junction. This highlights the close relationship of the occiput and its condyles with the articular surfaces of the atlas. However, it is of utmost importance also to understand the continuity of their relationship with the axis. These three bones and their associated connective tissues form a clear local unit of function (Figure 10.1).

It is important to orient to the fluid nature of these relationships to accurately understand their functioning. As we will discuss in Chapter 16, connective tissues are basically fluidic in nature. Their fibers float in a semi-liquid field and their interrelationships form a unified liquid crystalline matrix. Bone, ligaments, and membrane are all connective tissues and share in this fluidic nature. Ideally, the atlas is free to float between the occiput and axis in the synovial fluids of its joints, as the axis hangs suspended from the occiput by ligaments attached to its dens.

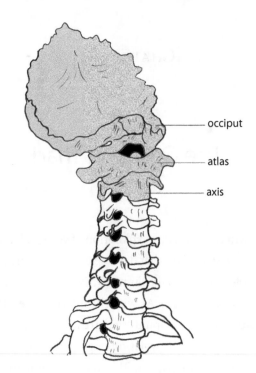

— occiput

— atlas

— axis

Figure 10.1. The occipital triad.

Occipital Triad Anatomy

Understanding and accurately visualizing the anatomical relationships of the occipital triad is an important starting point, so let's take time to clarify the specifics of this area.

We will orient to ligamentous anatomy and relationships from the most superficial to the most deep. Inertial issues can be found in any one ligament or in a combination of ligaments.

Superficial Relationships of the Occiput, Atlas, and Axis

The main ligaments that lie superficially in relationship to the deeper ligaments are the anterior atlanto-occipital membrane, the anterior atlanto-axial ligament, the posterior atlanto-occipital membrane, and the posterior atlanto-axial ligament.

- The *anterior atlanto-occipital membrane* is broad and dense and connects the anterior margin of the foramen magnum with the superior border of the anterior arch of the atlas. It is strengthened in the midline by a cord-like thickening that connects the basi-occiput with the tubercle of the anterior arch of the atlas.

This thickening is continuous with the anterior longitudinal ligament of the vertebral column. It is closely associated with the alar and apical ligaments.

- The *anterior atlanto-axial ligament* serves a purpose similar to that of the anterior atlanto-occipital ligament in that it connects the inferior border of the atlas to the superior border of the axis anteriorly. It is also strengthened by a rounded cord in the midline that is continuous with the anterior longitudinal ligament.

- The *posterior atlanto-occipital membrane* is also broad, but it is thinner than the anterior membrane. It connects the posterior margin of the foramen magnum to the superior border of the posterior arch of the atlas. Its most important relationship is to the dural membrane itself, where it is firmly attached anteriorly. Compressive forces in the occipito-atlanteal junction can be directly transferred to the membrane system via this relationship.

- The *posterior atlanto-axial ligament* posteriorly connects the inferior border of the arch of the atlas with the superior aspect of the arch of the axis. It serves the same purpose as the posterior atlanto-axial ligament above and the ligamentum flavum below.

The Deeper Relationships of the Occiput, Atlas, and Axis

The ligaments that directly connect the axis with the occiput are the tectorial membrane, the cruciate ligament, the two alar ligaments, and the apical ligament. These ligaments intimately interconnect the occiput, atlas, and axis, and generate a critically important unified system of triad dynamics. The tectorial ligament is superficial to the cruciate ligament, which is in turn superficial to the alar and apical ligaments

- The *tectorial membrane* can be thought of as a cephalad extension of the posterior longitudinal ligament of the vertebral column. A strong, broad band, it covers the ligaments of the dens and is in close relationship with its transverse ligament. The tectorial membrane connects the posterior surface of the axis to the occiput just anterior to the foramen magnum on the basi-occiput. It blends with the cranial dura mater where the dura mater attaches to the basilar portion of the occiput. Compressive forces in the cervical area and the spine generally can be directly fed into the dural system via this relationship. If the tectorial membrane is in contraction, the occiput, atlas, and axis will all become compressed together.

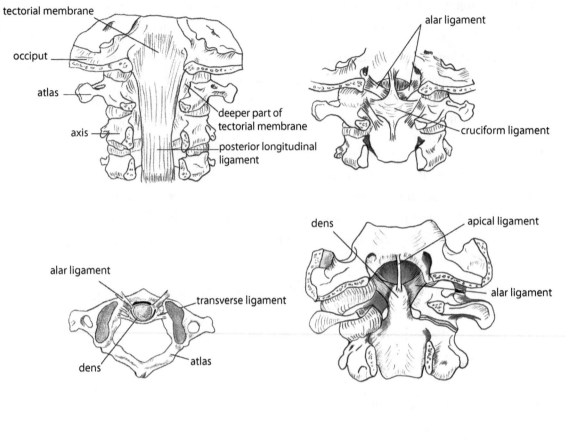

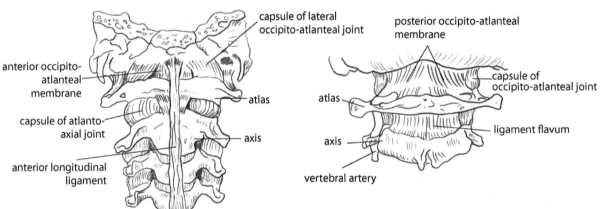

Figure 10.2. The layering of the membranes of the occipital triad.

- The *cruciate ligament* is composed of the transverse ligament and its extensions superiorly (crus superius) and inferiorly (crus inferius). Its center part, the transverse ligament, is a thick and strong band that arches across the atlas and straps the dens in place. There are synovial membranes around the dens that allow it to rotate in the space made by the anterior arch of the atlas and the transverse ligament, like a peg-and-socket joint. The superior extension of the cruciate ligament goes from the transverse ligament to the basi-occiput above, where its upper fibers merge with dura. Its inferior extension attaches to the posterior border of the body of the axis. The cruciate ligament helps bind the three bones into a single unit of function. Contractions held within it will obviously compress them together.

- The *alar ligaments* are strong cords that connect either side of the dens to the condylar parts of the occiput. They pass obliquely and laterally superior from the dens to the occiput. Along with the apical ligament, they help suspend the axis from the occiput.

- The *apical ligament* extends from the tip of the dens and connects it to the anterior aspect of the foramen magnum, suspending the dens from the occiput. The apical ligament can be considered to be a rudimentary intervertebral disc, and it contains traces of the notochord. It is thus closely related to both the early embryology of the system and to the midline expression of the Breath of Life in the system. Its fibers also merge with cranial dura (Figure 10.2).

Examples of Common Inertial Issues

Bones and ligaments are integrated in form and function. Thus joint compression and patterns of fixation will always involve the local ligaments that maintain the joint's stability. Inertial forces and related fulcrums and tensions can be held in any or all of the above bony-ligamentous relationships.

Joint capsule dynamics may be organized around compressive forces, along with contraction of the posterior atlanto-occipital membrane. Adhesion between it and the dural membrane will strongly compromise the motility and mobility of the dural tube. It is not uncommon for the alar and apical ligaments to be tense and contracted in their relationships, which can introduce compressive tendencies into the whole triad system. The cruciate and tectorial ligaments may also tense and contract due to the presence of inertial forces, and these contractions will often be coupled with bony compressions. Because their upper fibers merge with the dura mater and dural tube, compressive issues in the occipital triad can be transferred directly to the cranium—including reciprocal tension membrane and sutures—and to the vertebrae and sacrum below.

Many of these inertial forces, and the patterns they generate, can be traced to unresolved birth trauma. I once treated a thirty-two-year-old woman who came to see me for upper neck pain and lower back issues. In the third session her system began to organize around the occipital triad area. As I held her occiput, and we deepened into the forces at work, she became aware of very old feelings of resistance, fear, and lack of space. We found ourselves orienting to her birth experience, and she became aware of her scared little one within. As her system deepened into a state of equilibrium, she was able to hold her own inner birthing infant with love in a way that did not happen at the time of her birth, where she was shunted off to the side as the medical focus shifted to her mom. As she held her little one in awareness, the potency shifted in her system and the unresolved birthing forces were processed. This was a deeply moving experience for us both. The occipital triad area softened and a much more fluidic quality emerged in its interrelationships. Her midline then lengthened and the session shifted orientation to her lower back. Clinical work continued for a number of sessions and she reported that her upper neck issues had not come back and, even more important, she seemed to have an easier relationship to the ups and downs of life. She also noticed that her tendency to react to those around her when she felt a lack of interpersonal space had greatly softened, and she could maintain a more open relationship to others around her in times of stress.

Inertial issues in the occipital triad can thus have far-reaching consequences not just for structure, fluid circulation, and nerve function, but also for personal and interpersonal experience. This area thus serves as a concentrated gateway for the entire body-mind. Some further inertial issues are summarized in the sections below.

Structure

When exploring dural tube and spinal relationships, you may notice a sense of compression or congestion at the top of the spine. This area is very prone to compressive and torsional patterns due to birth trauma, traumatic experiences, and postural issues. If the occipital triad becomes inertial, the cranial base and dural motion may be strongly affected. The whole vertebral column will also be affected, and reflections will be found in all its other relationships. Compressive patterns at this superior pole of the spine will also be reflected in the lower lumbar area, especially at the lumbosacral junction. All sorts of symptoms can be generated by these conditions.

Fluid Circulation

Occipital triad inertia can also greatly affect fluid movement in arteries, veins, and cerebrospinal fluid. The vertebral artery threads its way through the transverse processes of the cervical vertebra and makes a nearly right-angle turn between the atlas and occiput, while the carotid artery is located at either side of the triad structure, and the basilar artery and Circle of Willis are just superior to the occiput. Compression in the occipital triad can compromise the blood supply to the brain stem (Figure 10.3).

The veins draining the head are similarly affected. The internal and external jugular veins and the vertebral veins can be compromised by occipital triad compressions. This can generate a backpressure in venous sinus drainage and a general sense of fluid congestion, producing a marked effect on the quality of fluid drive and potency in the system as a whole.

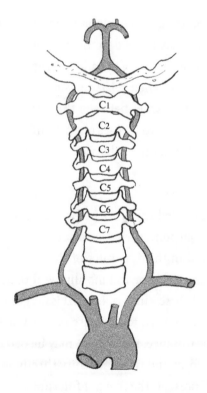

Figure 10.3. The vertebral artery and its ninety-degree turn.

Nervous System

Nerve function is similarly vulnerable to compression and congestion in the occipital triad area. The jugular foramina—passageways for the glossopharyngeal, vagus, and spinal accessory nerves—are particularly important. Intraosseous compressions in the occiput and compressions between the occiput, atlas, and axis will affect the jugular foramina and may cause impingement of the vagus nerve, with possible repercussions throughout the body, with potential impact on the function of the heart, lungs, digestive organs, and neuroendocrine-immune system. As introduced earlier and more fully discussed in Chapter 18, cervical tension can be related to the stress response, sympathetic nervous system sensitization, sensitization of the locus ceruleus—a major stress nuclei, and to sensitization of the social nervous system and orienting response. These territories are also discussed more deeply in our trauma chapters, especially Chapter 19.

Clinical Approaches

There are three basic areas of clinical exploration in this chapter. Our first approach focuses on the forces that may be held in the bony dynamics of the occiput itself (intraosseous issues). The dynamics of the atlas and axis will be strongly influenced by these unresolved forces and their related tissue effects. Our second exploration focuses on potential inertial issues between the atlas and the occiput (occipito-atlanteal junction), while the third focuses on the unified function of occiput, atlas, and axis and the essential relationship between the axis and occiput.

Intraosseous Occipital Issues

Inertial fulcrums can be located anywhere in the body. If they are located in the cells and tissues of an individual bone, then—as introduced in Chapter 6—intraosseous distortions are generated in the dynamics of that bone. These forces will affect the tissue of the bone and its form and motility will then distort in some way. It is not uncommon to find these kinds of inertial issues in the tissue of the occiput. The bone involved may be sensed to be dense or inertial and to be inwardly patterned in some way. For instance, the occiput may be perceived to be torsioned or compressed in its own form and tissue motility throughout the cranium may be organized around it. If present, the inertial fulcrum involved will also affect the unified dynamics of the occipital triad. For example, the atlas may become wedged between the condylar parts due to intraosseous forces located in the occiput.

Because intraosseous distortions commonly originate in prenatal and birth experiences, you can sometimes feel that you are holding an infant's head in your hands as you hold an adult skull. As this emerges, you must respect the infant's experience as you hold the adult skull. As described in the clinical vignette above, the client may also sense the wounded little one within and this can become an important aspect of the healing process. Respectful contact and patience are especially important in working with intraosseous distortions because these patterns generally arise from trauma. Discharge of shock affect, CNS activation, and similar phenomena can emerge as these patterns resolve.

The occiput is in four parts at birth: the squamous portion, the two condylar parts, and the basi-occiput (Figure 10.4). These parts can be forced into compressive and/or torsioned relationships during the birthing process. Common inertial patterns include rotations of the squama of the occiput relative to the rest of the parts, torsioning across the condylar parts and the foramen magnum, and compressive telescoping of the occipital structure toward the SBJ. The form of the occiput can distort because bone is living fluid tissue, not like the dry and hard examples of dead bone or plastic models used for anatomical study.

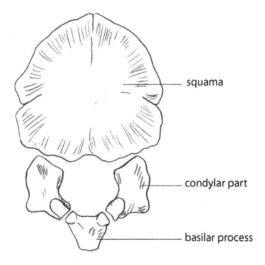

squama

condylar part

basilar process

Figure 10.4. The occiput at birth.

During the birth process, forces can be introduced into the occiput that cause its parts to compress, or telescope, together. As the parts of the occiput are forced to compress together, the tectorial membrane and the alar and apical ligaments will be pulled superiorly. This typically compresses the axis and atlas as a unit

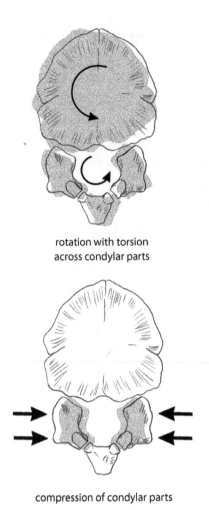

rotation with torsion
across condylar parts

compression of condylar parts

superiorly into the condyles of the occiput. You can thus end up with a common compressive picture in which the condyles of the occiput, atlas, and axis are all compressed together. These same forces can also generate medial compression in the condylar parts of the occiput. This will, in turn, wedge the atlas between its articulations and compromise both its motility and mobility.

Intraosseous distortions of the occiput will always affect the dynamics of the atlas and axis as they will be pulled superiorly by the intraosseous forces present. The atlas can become wedged in its articulation with the occipital condyles if there is medial compression generated by the telescoping or compression of structure (Figure 10.5).

Figure 10.5. Common intraosseous distortions of the occiput.

Augmenting Condylar Space

As session work unfolds, you may sense an inertial pattern clarifying around an intraosseous occipital fulcrum. This will be coupled with various kinds of patterns and compressive issues in the relationships of the occipital triad. For instance, as an inertial pattern clarifies, you may sense a narrowing and medial compression of the occipital condyles, and a wedging of the atlas into the condylar parts. If the forces involved seem intransigent, and the system cannot deepen into the state of balance, then one approach to the density of the inertial issues present is the augmentation of space in the parts of the occiput and across the foramen magnum.

The classic version of this process is called the *condylar spread*. In the next exploration, we will be emphasizing the natural expression of space in tissue relationships at the height of the inhalation phase of primary respiration. As space is accessed, potency will be expressed in the inertial fulcrums present, compressive forces and patterns in the occiput, and between it and the atlas, and then have the potential to be resolved.

Exploration:
Condylar Spread

After resourcing yourself and your client, and starting the session as usual, place your hands under the client's occiput in an occipital cradle hold. In your wide perceptual field, orient to the fluid tide and then include the tissues and their motility. See if a sense of compression and narrowing across the foramen magnum clarifies. If you sense density, restricted motion, or inertia between the condyles and atlas, you may want to orient to the condyles and their relationship with the atlas more specifically. In the following exploration you will relate to inertial occipital condylar issues and the possibility of the augmentation of space in their dynamics. This largely occurs via your resonance with what is natural as—at the height of inhalation—space is naturally generated in tissue relationships.

To do this, change your hand position from the occipital cradle to a classic condylar spread position. Spread the heels of your hands apart so that your fingertips point toward the occipital condyles. Orient to the condyles by imagining that you are extending your fingers toward them (Figure 10.6).

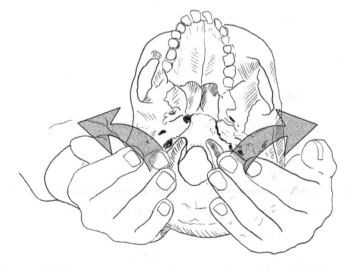

Figure 10.6. Augmenting space in occipital-condyle relationships.

Settle into your awareness of fluid and tissue motility in the cycles of primary respiration. Allow your hands and fingers to be soft and fluidic. Sense-imagine that they are suspended in the fluid body and, at the height of inhalation, allow them to be moved by the tidal surge and to take a deeper breath at its height—this is somewhat like kelp being moved by the tide in which the plants are suspended. As this occurs, your fingers will spread subtly apart, following the natural transverse expression of potency and widening at the height of inhalation. Again, if no tide is clearly present, allow your fingers, suspended in fluid, to take a deeper breath as though the tide is moving them.

As space is accessed, orient to expressions of potency. You may sense potency pulsating in inertial fulcrums, and/or a welling up or drive of potency in and around the area. Be open to any level of healing process that emerges.

When the conditional forces resolve, you will sense a softening and lateral spreading of the condylar parts and an expansion across the foramen magnum. You may also sense that the atlas softens—is released from the condyles—and settles inferior. Finish with appropriate integrative processes (sacral hold, sacrum-occiput hold, etc.).

Orienting to the Occipital Triad

In this section, we explore the occiput-atlas-axis triad and its dynamics. For study purposes, we first explore the occipito-atlanteal junction (referred to sometimes as the O/A junction) and then widen our view to include the axis. The first step will be to orient to the area and to see if any inertial patterns clarify. Please review your anatomy of the relationships if needed.

Exploration:
Orienting to the O/A Junction _____

In this exploration, we will learn a new hold, the *occipito-atlanteal hold* (O/A hold). With the client in the supine position, start the session as usual and orient to primary respiration and the holistic shift. Move to the head of the treatment table and cradle the occiput so that your hands curl around its squama with the pads of your fingers against the occipital ridge and the tips of your fingers pointing anteriorly, toward the atlas. Your hands should be close together supporting the occiput (Figure 10.7). See if you can sense the presence of the atlas at your fingertips. Ideally, it will seem as though the atlas is floating on

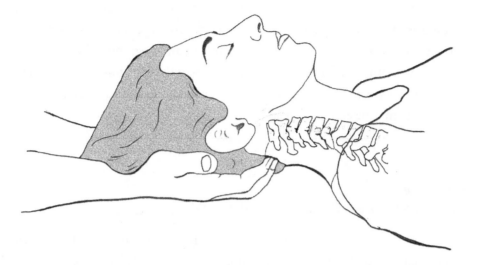

Figure 10.7. Occipito-atlanteal hold.

your fingertips. Orient to the physical and fluid bodies and mid-tide dynamics in your wide perceptual field.

See if you can perceive the motility of both occiput and atlas. As the squama of the occiput widens and settles footward in inhalation, its basi-portion rises at the SBJ. Likewise, in inhalation, you may sense the atlas subtly widening and rising. Note how the motility of occiput and atlas is oriented to the primal midline.

Settle into your orientation and see if an inertial pattern and its fulcrum clarify. You may sense qualities of compression, fixation, and resistance in occiput-atlas dynamics as this unfolds. Holding your wide perceptual field—physical body suspended in fluid body, suspended in tidal body—see if a state of balance emerges and deepens as the forces involved enter equilibrium. On a tissue level, you may sense that the tensions perceived in occipito-atlanteal relationships also access equilibrium. It may feel like the tissue field as a whole settles around the organizing fulcrum.

Deepen into the state of balance and see what level of work clarifies—local expressions/pulsations of potency, the shifting of potency in fluids, and/or the emergence of Long Tide phenomena. As these healing intentions manifest, you may likewise sense a processing of the conditional forces generating the compressive issues—commonly as heat and pulsation—and a sense of further settling, softening, and expansion of the tissue field. As this occurs, you may also sense softening of local tissues as the atlas settles and floats free in its relationship to the condyles of the occiput.

Orient to the reorganization of the relationships of the occipital triad and realignment to the primal midline. You may also sense that the atlas reorients itself between the axis and occiput. Finish with an integrative hold.

In some situations, if the compressive forces at the occipito-atlanteal junction are very deep and tissue affects very entrenched, more specific augmentation processes may be extremely helpful in resolving the inertial forces.

Exploration:
Augmenting Space in Occiput-Atlas Relationships _____

As we have seen, the atlas should ideally be free to float in its relationship with the occipital condyles. However, compression of the atlas into the condyles of the occiput is common. Compression of the occipito-atlanteal is also commonly combined with rotation and torsional forces. If the system cannot access a state of balance or equilibrium as inertial fulcrums and patterns clarify, then one clinical option is the augmentation of space between the atlas and occiput. Here again, the intention will be to augment the space that is naturally accessed at the height of inhalation.

In the O/A hold, orient to the atlas via the tips of your fingers. Settle into your perception of the fluid tide—add awareness of the motility of the tissue field—and notice how the occiput and atlas manifest their interrelated motility. You may become aware of compressive forces fixing the atlas in the condyles of the occiput. You may sense that the atlas cannot float freely in the condyles in the phases of primary respiration.

Again sense that your hands and fingers are suspended in fluid. At the height of inhalation, allow the heels of your hands and your fingers to be moved by the inhalation surge—to take a deeper breath with the tide—and as this occurs, the heels of your hands and your fingertips will subtly spread apart as space in the relationships is accessed. As you allow your hands to be suspended in fluid and orient to the inhalation surge, it feels like they are breathed or moved by the tide and its potency. As this occurs it is as though the cells and tissues of your hands and fingers are also taking a deeper breath in resonance with the action of potency in the fluids. Again, if no fluid tide is expressed, allow your fingers, suspended in fluid, to resonate with the natural space present and to take a deeper breath as though the tide is moving them (Figure 10.8).

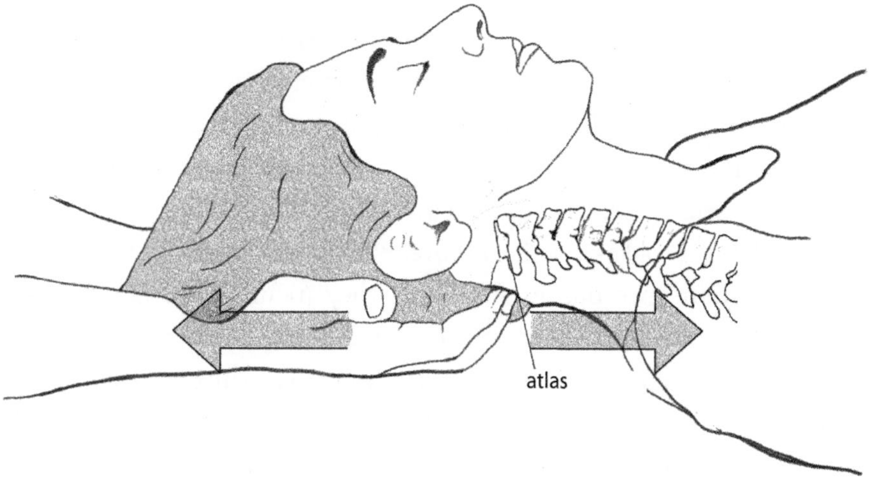

Figure 10.8. The augmentation of space in occiput-atlas relationships.

As space is accessed, listen for expressions of potency in and around inertial fulcrums and in local fluids and tissues. You may sense a deepening into the state of balance and/or more immediate expressions of potency accompanied by a softening and spreading of tissues.

When the inertial forces are resolved, you may sense that the tissue field as a whole settles, softens, and expands; the occiput-atlas relationship also softens, as the atlas floats more freely in the condyles and reorients to the midline. Wait for the completion of the reorganization and realignment stage and see how motility is now expressed. Note the quality of the fluid tide at the end of the session.

Exploration:
Orienting Holistically to Occipito-Axial Relationships _____

After exploring the specific patterns of the occipito-atlanteal relationship, we next take a wider approach where we will hold the whole triad in our awareness. I commonly start with this orientation in session work. As discussed above, the occipital triad is a holistic organization of bones, ligaments, and joint capsule fluids, where both atlas and axis are ideally floating in the joint relationships and hanging freely from the occiput.

In this exploration, we widen our inquiry to include the whole of the triad relationship by contacting the occiput and axis, spanning the atlas. In this position, you will orient to the motility and motion of the whole triad area, wait for a pattern to clarify, and orient to the emerging healing process.

Start at the side of the table and the feet of the client as usual. After the holistic shift clarifies and deepens, move to the head of the treatment table and again take up the O/A hold as described above. When settled comfortably into the O/A hold, slide your fingertips inferiorly until they are under the axis. We call this the *occiput-axis hold.* The first palpable spinous process inferior to the foramen magnum is the axis. Spread your fingers transversely along the posterior arch of the axis. You are still supporting the occipital squama in the palms of your hands. You will now be cradling the occiput with your fingers posterior to the axis (Figure 10.9).

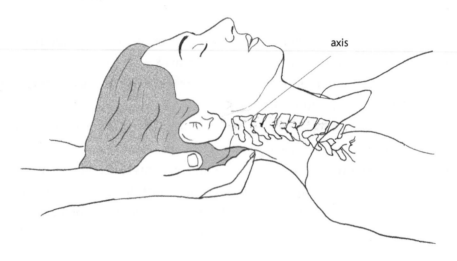

Figure 10.9. The occiput-axis hold.

In this position, first orient to the fluid tide, add the tissue field, and sense the motility of the whole triad in the phases of primary respiration. You will ideally sense a rising and widening in inhalation with clear differentiation between the parts of the triad (occiput, atlas, and axis) in their expression of motility. The atlas is also ideally sensed to be floating between the axis and occiput in the phases of primary respiration. Notice how the expression of motility is oriented to the primal midline.

Maintain your wide perceptual field and orient to whatever healing intentions emerge. As the system accesses a state of balance, notice expressions of potency, levels of healing processes that clarify, the resolution of conditional forces, the settling and expansion of the tissue field, and expressions of reorganization and realignment to the primal midline.

Exploration:
Holistic Augmentation of Space in Occipital Triad Relationships _____

If there are compressive issues in the triad as a whole, or in any aspect of its dynamics, you may sense a poor expression of motility or a block-like manifestation, where it is difficult to differentiate independent expressions of motility throughout the triad. You may likewise sense specific areas of compression and congestion, as when the atlas is compressed in the dynamics of the occipital condyles. The intention of this next approach is to augment space in the relationships of the triad as a whole.

In the occiput-axis hold, settle into your relationship to the fluid tide and tissue motility. Again, notice how this is expressed in the cycles of the tide, and the triad's relationship to the primal midline. Is the expression of the midline clear, or do inertial forces and patterns obscure it?

Orient to the inhalation phase of the fluid tide and the expression of the potency within it. Sense that your hands and fingers are suspended in fluid, and at the height of inhalation, allow the heels and fingers of your hands to be breathed, or moved by the tide. Allow your hands to take a deeper breath at the height of inhalation as the heels and fingers of your hands spread apart. Again, this largely occurs via resonance with the space naturally accessed through the midline at the height of inhalation. If no tide is expressed, allow your fingers, suspended in fluid, to resonate with the natural space present and to take a deeper breath as though the tide is moving them. Maintain your wide perceptual field as you orient to this, and note the expression of potency that emerges in the space accessed.

As healing processes emerge, orient to the action of fluids and potency and for the resolution of conditional forces, tissue softening and expansion, and reorganization of the triad relationships. You may sense the ligaments involved softening and lengthening and the bones dropping into a more fluid relationship to each other. Note how the occiput, atlas, and axis have reorganized their motility after these forces have resolved.

Augmenting Fluid Drive in the Cervical Area

Another clinical option—if the inertial forces in the relationships of the occipital triad are very dense—is the augmentation of fluid drive and the expression of potency in the area. In the occipital triad hand positions, you can augment fluid drive with the heels of your hands from the cisterna magna to the fulcrums and relationships below it. In this hand position—where the triad extends inferiorly below your occipital contact—this is commonly oriented to in the exhalation phase, where potency is returning to the midline and the fluid tide is receding. Similar to augmenting space, it is as though your hands are being moved by the tide and its potency in exhalation with an orientation to fluid and potency, rather than to space. You can also use your fingertips to subtly initiate lateral fluctuations in extremely dense situations. Again, the intention is to augment the action of potency in these inertial states in order to initiate healing processes. Remember Becker's admonition to orient to the action of the potency in the conditions present!

CHAPTER 11

Cranial Base Patterns

In this chapter, we continue our journey of exploration of tissue structures organized around the primal midline and orient to the cranial base, its motility and patterning. This chapter offers students and practitioners a clear framework for orienting more specifically to the particulars of inertial patterns and organizing fulcrums found in the cranium and body as a whole.

Classically, particular patterns of inertia in the cranial bowl were given names oriented to the cranial base and, more specifically, to the dynamics of the sphenoid and occiput at the SBJ. These patterns were commonly used as a primary point of entry both to cranial dynamics and to the entire system. Some of the most intransigent of these, and the inertial forces and fulcrums that generate them, are commonly introduced in connection with the birth process. As we have seen, the birth process introduces strong forces into the infant's system. These, if not resolved at the time of the experience, may generate inertial fulcrums and related tension and defensive patterns, not just in the cranial base and cranial bowl, but in the body as a whole.

Later in life, when a new trauma is experienced, the system will tend to default in its protective response in the same way it is centering unresolved birthing forces. Later experiences will then become layered and coupled to the original birth experience. Thus many of our deepest inertial issues originate in very early life experience. Prenatal and birth experiences can significantly shape the relationships of the cranium and body as a whole, and the patterns described below can be an important gateway into this material. Because of this, we commonly teach the patterns described in this chapter halfway through our foundation course along with the birth process and birthing dynamics. The following sections are geared to help you orient to their emergence as the inherent treatment plan unfolds.

The Cranial Base and the Sphenobasilar Junction

The cranial base and sphenobasilar junction (SBJ) are traditionally considered to be the functional heart of the cranium and a natural fulcrum for all bony motility. Indeed, Sutherland considered the SBJ to be a key fulcrum in the human system, allowing access to the entire history of the client. He considered the sphenobasilar junction to have functions similar to a joint with a disc. Hence, in osteopathic circles, it is sometimes also called the *sphenobasilar symphysis* (SBS). Sutherland reported seeing a number of fetal skulls with actual discs between the sphenoid and occiput, showing that embryologically the sphenoid and occiput can be considered to be modified vertebrae. The SBJ is located at the most superior pole of the embryological notochord. At birth, the joint is a synchondrosis—a cartilaginous bridge—making it more stable than a disc joint. It retains the function of a synchondrosis throughout life (Figure 11.1).

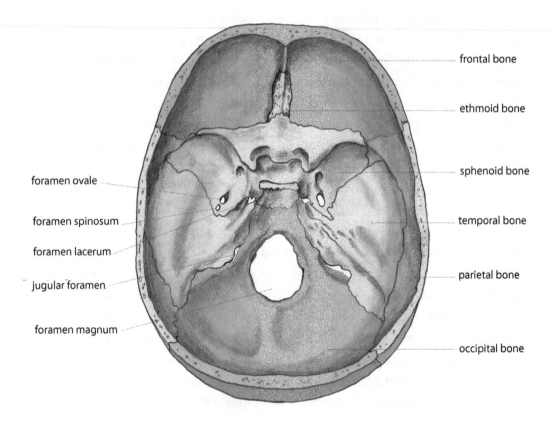

Figure 11.1. The cranial base.

In the traditional biomechanical concept, the sphenoid bone is considered to be the major gear of the cranium. As the sphenoid bone rotates and expresses its motion, the other midline bones are said to rotate in the opposite direction. This is like a child's game of gears in which there is one master gear that drives all other gears. As we have seen in Volume One, however, bones are not really gears, nor is their motility mechanical. Motility, when experienced in mid-tide dynamics, is seen to be fluid and holistic in nature (Figure 11.2).

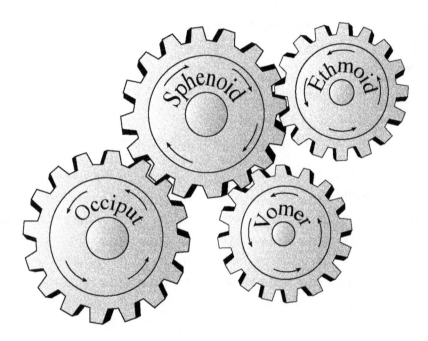

Figure 11.2. The gears of the cranium.

In a biodynamic context, the SBJ is the natural location for an embryologically derived automatically shifting fulcrum. This fulcrum is a site of potency that orients the motility of the cranial bones to the midline and bioelectric field that organizes the human system. Beyond the cranium, all bony motility will orient to the SBJ in some way. If there were no inertial patterns held in the system, then motility around the SBJ would be expressed with balance and ease.

Major cranial nerves pass through or near the cranial base via foramina in and between its bones. Impingement or stress along these nerves can generate nerve sensitization and affect nerve function with impact throughout the body. This is a common origin of respiratory and digestive issues in infants due to unresolved birthing forces. Major arteries and veins also pass through these foramina, and patterns of inertia held in the cranial base can affect the functioning of these blood vessels. The brain stem is located in the basilar portion of the occiput just below the SBJ, so inertial patterns here can also affect autonomic nuclei and the neuro-endocrine-immune system.

The pituitary gland, which controls many metabolic and stress response functions, is also located in the cranial base. It rests in the saddle of the sphenoid bone in the sella turcica. It is strapped into this saddle by dural membranes called the diaphragma sella. Patterns of inertia in the bones and membranes of the cranium may be fed into the pituitary via these relationships, again affecting the neuroendocrine-immune system. As you investigate the dynamics of the cranial base, you will sense how all tissue structures in the cranium are totally interdependent in their dynamics.

Sutherland's Fulcrum and Reciprocal Tension Motion

As we have seen, all cellular and tissue motility, including cranial bones and membranes, manifests natural reciprocal tension motion around embryologically derived fulcrums and the notochord/primal midline. In this context, we must again appreciate the suspended, automatically shifting fulcrum located in the straight sinus—Sutherland's fulcrum. Sutherland's fulcrum is an embryologically derived point of potency located in the anterior aspect of the straight sinus, where the falx and tentorium meet the great vein of Galen. Both the falx and the tentorium are naturally suspended around this fulcrum point. Sutherland's fulcrum is the natural, automatically shifting fulcrum for the reciprocal tension motion of membrane and connective tissue as these express their motility in the cycles of the tide. It is the intrinsic point of resolution for both the natural reciprocal tension motion of the membranes *and* for inertial forces that affect their dynamics. It is around this fulcrum that all forces are ideally resolved and balanced and through which ease of motion is maintained.

Bone is a connective tissue; the motility and patterns of motion of cranial bones are totally integrated with those of the reciprocal tension membrane—the falx and tentorium. If there were no inertial patterns in the system, then the membranous-articular motion of the cranium would be in lovely fluid balance both around Sutherland's fulcrum and the SBJ.

If the system is centering inertial patterns, then this point of resolution will shift away from its ideal midline location. This makes an awareness of its dynamics essential for practitioners. If this point of balance shifts closer to the midline, then

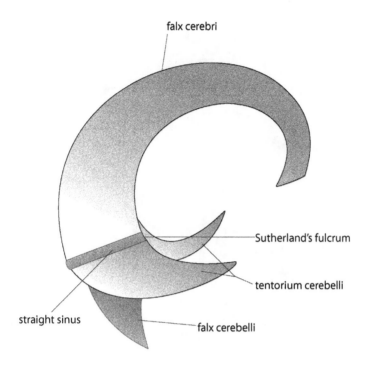

falx cerebri

Sutherland's fulcrum

tentorium cerebelli

straight sinus

falx cerebelli

Figure 11.3. Sutherland's fulcrum.

you know that something has really been resolved. This is crucial to appreciate when relating to cranial base patterns (Figure 11.3).

Motility of the Cranial Bowl and the SBJ

In the mid-tide, the motion around the SBJ is ideally sensed to be fluidic and integrated. In the inhalation phase of the tide, the SBJ, as an automatically shifting fulcrum, rises like the center of a flower. As it ascends, all of the other bones around it move like fluidic flower petals opening to the sun (Figure 11.4). As this occurs, the occipital squama and greater wings of the sphenoid dive caudal (footward). This diving is classically described as a rotation around transverse axes in opposite directions (i.e., the occiput rotates in the opposite direction to the sphenoid) (Figure 11.5). The reverse occurs in exhalation. As the SBJ settles footward, the flower petals close. This is not a mechanical motion. Bones are fluidic forms and motility is cellular, experienced as an organic welling-up and settling. As the SBJ shifts, the whole membranous-articular flower-like dynamic organized around it will also shift. This, in turn, all orients to Sutherland's fulcrum as a unified connective tissue dynamic.

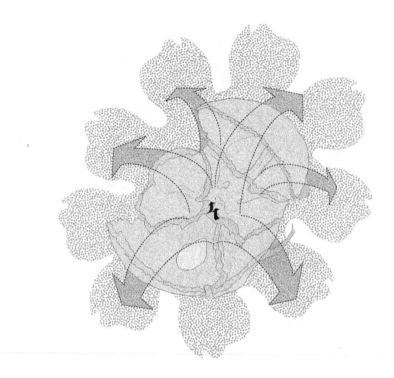

Figure 11.4. Flower-petal motility.

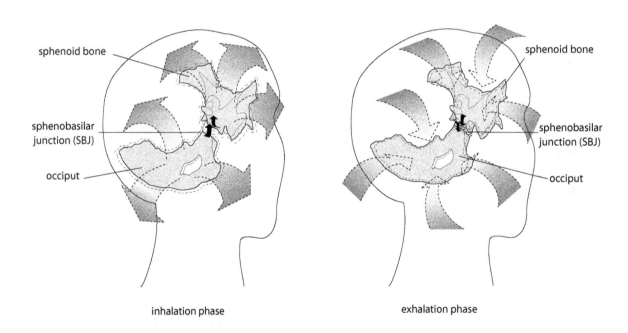

sphenoid bone

sphenobasilar
junction (SBJ)

occiput

inhalation phase

sphenoid bone

sphenobasilar
junction (SBJ)

occiput

exhalation phase

Figure 11.5. Inhalation-exhalation of the sphenoid and occiput.

The Cranial Base and Inertial Issues

Inertial patterns in the cranial base and cranium as a whole are patterns of fixation where the tissues of the cranium have become conditioned to express certain forms and motions due to the presence of inertial forces and fulcrums. These forces may be located in the SBJ itself, or may be an expression of inertial issues remote to its immediate dynamics. An inertial pattern in the cranial base may be formed as a result of local unresolved traumatic forces, or may be generated in compensation for inertial fulcrums found almost anywhere in the body.

As we shall see, these unresolved issues will be expressed around the SBJ in particular ways. Sutherland observed that inertial patterns in the cranium can be broken down into particular components and that these can be named and eventually directly perceived. He outlined six inertial patterns that are commonly expressed around and in the SBJ. In the following sections you will begin to explore these patterns and learn to perceive and orient to them.

Patterns of Experience

Inertial patterns organized around the SBJ tell a larger story than the tensile dynamic sensed. These patterns are expressions of a client's living history and show how life experience is being centered by the potency of the Breath of Life. In this psycho-emotional wholeness, deeply ingrained beliefs about self and the world the client inhabits may also be present. These may have their roots in our earliest experiences of life and can be held just as rigidly as any physical fulcrum.

These psycho-emotional-physiological patterns are expressions of the deeper developmental and traumatic schemas present in a person's life history and personality process, and must be approached with clarity and respect. The inertial fulcrums organizing any inertial pattern may thus hold the history of shock and traumatization and related emotional and psychological forms. It is thus imperative that practitioners understand the nature of traumatic activation and have the appropriate cranial and verbal skills to meet these as they arise in session work. We explore trauma resolution skills in some depth in later chapters.

It must be also remembered that inertial patterns are manifestations of health, and are patterns of containment and compensation for unresolved forces still present in the system. These are held in the best possible balance given the forces present in the dynamics of the whole. Common origins of cranial base patterns are the birth process, blows, falls, and accidents. Even strong emotional shock can generate tissue patterns in the cranium. Patterns originating in other parts of the body may also be expressed in some way around the SBJ as patterns of compensation.

Biomechanics and Biodynamics of the Cranial Base

Sutherland based his original model of motion and his terminology on the biomechanical concepts that prevailed at that time in the osteopathic profession. Thus the traditional description of cranial base motion is biomechanical in theory and language. The biomechanical approach states that bones move around axes of rotation, motion transfers mechanistically from structure to structure, and the whole system operates like a clockwork apparatus. This viewpoint is why paired terms like flexion-extension and internal-external rotation were used to describe bony motion and tissue motion in the body.

These concepts are transformed in a biodynamic understanding. Motility is sensed to be much more organic and fluidic in nature and is directly perceived as an inner breath that arises all at once in the whole person. Potency, or life force, is sensed to be the organizing and driving factor. *Axes of rotation* and similar biomechanical phrases are at best just approximations of reality. On a bone level, the deeper sense of motility and motion is that of a fluidic inner motility, a welling up in each structure during the inhalation phase yielding an expansion and widening of that structure. The subsiding of this surge is the exhalation phase, palpable as a settling in the tissues. Interosseous motion between structures is really an expression of this deeper inner motility. It is the drive of the potency in the fluids that naturally generates both intra- and interosseous motion. The qualities of these are organic and fluid when perceived through the slower tidal rhythms. Indeed, bones are part of a unified tensile tissue field, a living liquid crystalline matrix.

Perception and the Sphenobasilar Inquiry

In the following sections you will learn to perceive the classic patterns commonly found around the SBJ as the inherent treatment plan unfolds. You will maintain a wide perceptual field oriented to all three bodies—tidal, fluid, and physical bodies—and mid-tide dynamics. As we have seen, as you orient to mid-tide dynamics, the motility of individual structures, like the sphenoid bone and occiput, are perceived to be part of a wider field of action. Here you are not just orienting to individual structures, but are sensing a unified fluid-tissue dynamic. In this greater whole, you can still perceive the motion of the individual structures.

As the holistic shift deepens, and you hold all three bodies in awareness, you may sense that the fluid and physical bodies are suspended in the center of your perceptual field. As you settle into this awareness, you will orient to the sphenoid and occiput and, as the inherent treatment plan manifests, the particular motions and forms around and in the SBJ will clarify. In this context, orienting to cranial inertial patterns becomes an intuitive process of inquiry.

Classic Cranial Base Patterns

Sutherland's nomenclature is used below to describe the inertial patterns commonly sensed around the SBJ. Classically, there are two categories of inertial patterns found in the dynamics of the SBJ. These are called *physiological patterns* and *nonphysiological patterns*. Physiological patterns are those that are naturally allowable in the joint dynamics of the SBJ and include flexion-extension, side-bending, and torsion. Nonphysiological patterns are those that are not normally allowable in SBJ dynamics. These include lateral shear, vertical shear, and compression. In a biodynamic context, the distinction between physiological and nonphysiological patterns somewhat breaks down as you realize that all of these patterns are expressions of unresolved forces of experience.

In an ideally functioning system the only motion you would sense around the SBJ would be natural expressions of motility. The SBJ will have a sense of rising and sinking in the phases of primary respiration. Again, if we liken the cranium to a fluid flower, and its bones to petals, then we may have a more organic sense of motility. In inhalation, as the SBJ rises, the flower petals ideally open and widen in a symmetrical, fluid and organic manner and, in exhalation, as the SBJ settles, the flower petals likewise close and narrow in symmetry. However, everyone has conditional patterns present in their system and these will be expressed in some fashion as inertial patterns around the SBJ. The patterns described below are presented in the classic categories of physiological and nonphysiological. In these explorations we will use either or both of the classic vault holds—Dr. Becker's or Dr. Sutherland's (Figure 11.6).

In the following sections we also use the classic idea of axes of rotation to describe the patterns and help you orient to them. However, although the idea of axes may initially help you become familiar with these patterns, please don't take them too literally. In the mid-tide, these inertial patterns are perceived as fluid-tissue distortions in the physical and fluid bodies as a whole, rather than as mechanical rotations around set axes. It is also important to remember that these patterns

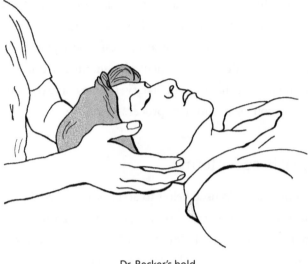

Dr. Becker's hold

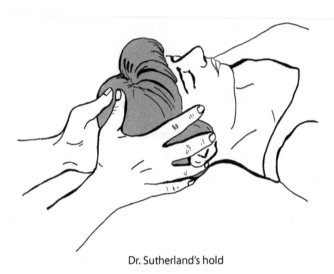

Dr. Sutherland's hold

Figure 11.6. Classic vault holds.

are patterns of fixation. The tissue field will still express its inhalation-exhalation motility in the best way possible, but in a compensated fashion given the inertial fulcrums and patterns present. Hence, in the natural cycles of motility, you may also sense particular conditioned forms of motion and organization.

Physiological Patterns

Physiological patterns are extremes of allowable motion in the dynamics of the SBJ that become fixed in place. In an inhalation or exhalation pattern, the system is held in one phase of primary respiration or the other. As the practitioner orients to the client's system, either inhalation or exhalation may seem to be clearer or stronger in the cycles of primary respiration.

Side-bending patterns commonly occur when one side of the cranium experiences strong medial forces, which generate a narrowing on one side of the cranium and a bulging on the other. Torsion patterns commonly occur when the sphenoid bone on one side is forced inferior or superior, generating a twisting motion at the SBJ. In the descriptions below, we have changed the classic flexion-extension nomenclature to inhalation-exhalation, as this is more appropriate in a biodynamic context. Let's look at these in some detail.

Inhalation and Exhalation Patterns

In an inhalation pattern, due to unresolved inertial forces, the SBJ is held in a superior position. This is its natural inhalation position. The flower petals of the cranial bones are then also held in inhalation, as are all other cranial structures. As the practitioner orients to tissue motility, the inhalation phase may be sensed to be more prominent. In an extreme fixation, the person's head may look widened and the cranium may have a rounded look with wide, prominent cheekbones and wide orbits.

In an exhalation pattern, the SBJ is held inferiorly. This is its natural exhalation position. All other cranial structures will then also be held in exhalation. In this case, as the practitioner orients to tissue motility, the exhalation phase may be sensed to be more prominent. In the extreme, the resulting patterns are basically the reverse of the above. In the front view, the cranium may appear narrow side-to-side and the face will seem narrow. You may also see a narrow forehead, sunken eyes, hollow cheeks, and a prominent sagittal suture.

Inhalation patterns are commonly introduced during Stage Three birth dynamics. As the baby moves through the pelvic outlet, strong anterior-posterior forces may impact the cranium, which may tend to hold structures in an inhalation position. Likewise, anterior-posterior compressive forces may be introduced into the SBJ area, forcing it superior into its inhalation position. Here the head may seem wider side-to-side than front-to-back.

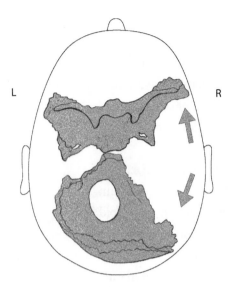

right side-bending

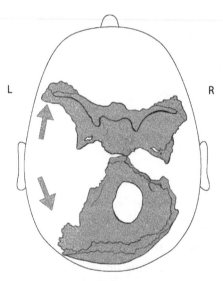

left side-bending

Figure 11.7 Sphenobasilar
side-bending

Exhalation patterns are more likely to be fed in Stage One or Stage Two, as more medially compressive forces impact the cranium, which may generate an exhalation position in the tissue field. Here the head may seem wider front-to-back and narrower side-to-side. Extreme exhalation patterns may be fed into the baby's cranium if the mother has a platy-pelloid shaped pelvis, which is very narrow front-to-back, generating strong medially compressive forces.

Side-Bending Patterns

In the physiological pattern called side-bending, the greater wing of the sphenoid and the squamous portion of the occiput have been forced together on one side. Structures on one side are crunched together and structures on the other side are widened apart. This widening can be perceived as a bulge on one side of the cranium, classically called the side of the *convexity*. The side of the narrowing is called the side of the *concavity*.

In the classic description, side-bending is said to occur around two vertical axes located in each bone. Due to a strong force of some sort, the sphenoid and occiput are forced to rotate in opposite directions around these axes and become fixed in this side-bent position. Please remember that tissues are really fluid-tissue—any pattern of fixation is a holistic physiological distortion organized around unresolved forces, not just a simple rotation around axes.

As the inherent treatment plan unfolds, and a side-bending pattern clarifies, you will sense a bulge on the side of the convexity. The pattern is classically named according to the side of the bulge. For instance, if you sense the bulge on the right side, it is called a *right side-bending pattern* (Figure 11.7).

Side-bending patterns may be fed into the cranium when strong medially compressive forces are introduced into its lateral aspects. This is most likely in birth Stage One or Stage Two, when the side of the baby's head may be pressed onto the maternal sacrum. Medially compressive forces may then be introduced into the cranium, generating a side-bending pattern, especially if one side of the cranium experiences stronger forces. These will be fed into the cranial base and a narrowing on the side of the impact will result, along with a bulge on the side opposite.

Torsion Patterns

As practitioners orient to a client's system via the vault hold, they may sense a quality of twisting between their hands. This may indicate the presence of a torsion pattern. In classical nomenclature, torsion is said to occur around an anterior-posterior axis from glabella to inion running through the center of the body of the sphenoid and SBJ. Due to strong forces, the sphenoid and occiput were forced to rotate in opposite directions around this axis, and torsion occurs in their tissues, especially at the SBJ. As the bones rotate in opposite directions, the synchondrosis distorts in a twisting fashion.

The torsion pattern is named after the high, or superior greater wing of the sphenoid bone. As practitioners sense a torsion pattern, it may seem as though their hands are twisting in opposite directions around a transverse axis between their palms. For instance, as a torsion pattern clarifies, practitioners may sense a twisting motion between their hands, and note that one greater wing is higher, or more superior, to the other. If the high greater wing was sensed on the left side, it is called a *left torsion pattern* (Figures 11.8 and 11.9).

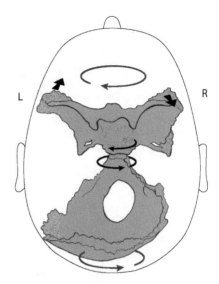

right torsion

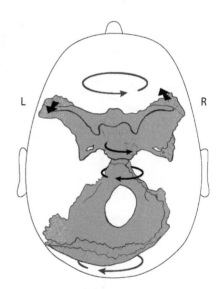

left torsion

Figure 11.8. Sphenobasilar torsion.

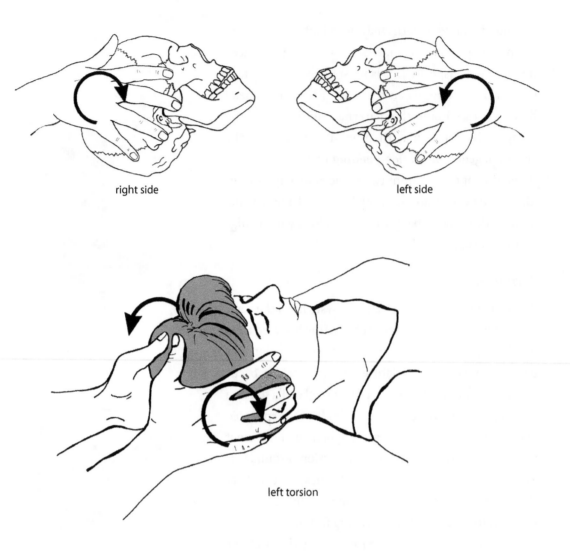

right side
left side

left torsion

Figure 11.9. Sensing left torsion as a twisting between the hands
with left greater wing superior.

Torsion patterns are commonly fed into the system in the same birth stages as
in side-bending—Stage One or Stage Two. The greater wing on the birth lie side is
commonly in conjunct with the maternal sacrum and may experience compressive
dragging forces as it moves through the birth canal. As this occurs, the greater wing
that meets the sacrum is commonly dragged inferior and the opposite greater wing
shifts superior. So if the baby's left side is conjunct with the maternal sacrum, then
the left greater wing would be dragged inferior as birth progresses, and the torsion
pattern generated would be named after the opposite greater wing, which is forced
superior on the right side (right torsion pattern).

Nonphysiological Patterns

Inertial patterns whose motion dynamics are not naturally allowable in the SBJ are called *nonphysiological patterns*. These are generally considered to have more serious consequences than the physiological ones discussed above, because they commonly generate strong resistances and tensions in reciprocal tension motion and inhalation-exhalation dynamics. Nonphysiological patterns tend to be more intransigent and symptoms tend to be more extreme.

Classically, in physiologically allowable motions, the bones are said to rotate around axes in *opposite* directions. In nonphysiologically allowable motions, the bones are forced to rotate in the *same* direction.

Nonphysiological patterns commonly arise during the prenatal period or the birth process, when sutures are not yet formed. The vault bones have space between them and the cranial base is flexible and resilient. The forces of birthing may compress and shear parts of the cranium. The bones are literally forced into positions not natural to their dynamics by the compressive and shearing forces present.

The classic nonphysiological patterns are lateral shear, vertical shear, and compression. In the two shearing patterns, the sphenoid and occiput are forced to shear in opposite directions at the SBJ instead of meeting precisely in the middle. This can generate strong resistance to motion in the SBJ, strongly affect motility, and create strong backpressures throughout the system. In compression, the sphenoid and occiput have been forced toward each other by a strong force, which then generates an inertial fulcrum in the SBJ itself.

Nonphysiological patterns are always the result of trauma of some kind, in which strong outside forces have impacted the cranium—through birth trauma, accidents, blows, or falls. They must be approached with this understanding. Compression patterns may also be generated by strong emotional shock and are commonly associated with chronic states of stress.

Sphenobasilar Lateral Shear

While orienting to a client via the vault hold, a practitioner may sense that one greater wing is laterally more prominent than the other. This may indicate the presence of a lateral shear pattern. One common origin of lateral shear is the birth process, during which pressures on one side of the baby's head may force the sphenoid bone to shift to the other side, generating a lateral shearing at the SBJ. As this pattern clarifies in session work, the sphenoid bone will then be sensed to be more prominent on the side it has shifted toward.

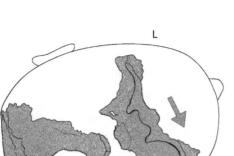

right lateral shear

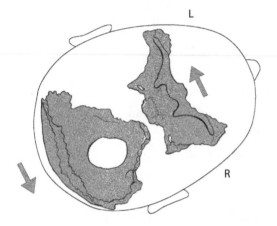

left lateral shear

Classically, lateral shear is said to occur around two vertical axes, one in each bone (sphenoid and occiput), and the two bones are said to have been forced to rotate in the same direction. In classical thought, if the two bones are forced to rotate in a clockwise direction (viewed from above), the body of the sphenoid will shear laterally to the left side of the cranium relative to the occiput. If the two bones are forced to rotate in a counter-clockwise direction around vertical axes, the body of the sphenoid will shear laterally to the right of the cranium relative to the occiput. Again, the idea of axes of rotation may or may not be helpful. It is simpler and, in terms of birthing forces, more accurate to orient to the presence of shearing forces in a more organic fashion.

Lateral shear is named after the side of the cranium that the body of the sphenoid has been forced to shear toward. Hence, if the practitioner senses that one greater wing has shifted toward, and is more prominent on, the right side, then it is called *right lateral shear* (Figure 11.10).

Figure 11.10. Lateral shear.

Lateral shear generates a parallelogram-like shape in the cranium when viewed from above. This can most easily be seen in infants when the pattern arises due to birth trauma. The frontal bone-forehead may be slightly shifted toward the side of the lateral shear. In the vault hold, if a lateral shear pattern clarifies, the practitioner may sense that the greater wing of the sphenoid has shifted laterally to one side of the cranium as the occipital squama shifts in the opposite direction. It may feel like a parallelogram shape in your two hands. For instance, in left lateral shear the greater wing on the left side will feel as though it is shifted to the left, while the occipital squama may be sensed to have shifted in the opposite direction (Figure 11.11).

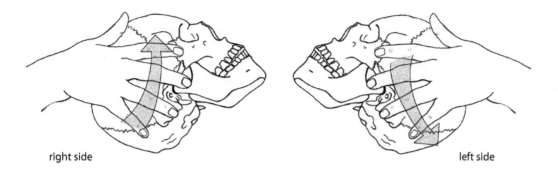

right side   left side

right lateral shear

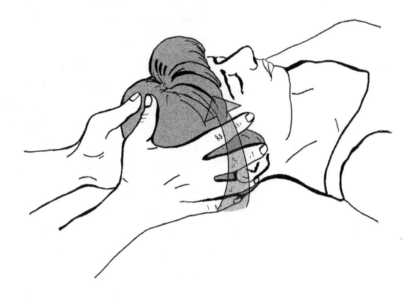

Figure 11.11. In left lateral shear the sphenoid will be sensed to be shifted to
the left, while the occiput is to the right.

Lateral shear patterns are commonly fed into the system in birth Stages One
or Two. The infant experiences compressive forces on the birth lie side conjunct
with the maternal sacrum. The forces introduced either by dragging forces, or by
prolonged pressures, shift the sphenoid to the opposite side, generating a lateral
shearing in the SBJ. Thus if the baby is a left birth lie, the left side of its head will be
in conjunct with the maternal sacrum and the sphenoid bone may be forced in the
opposite direction, yielding a right lateral shear pattern.

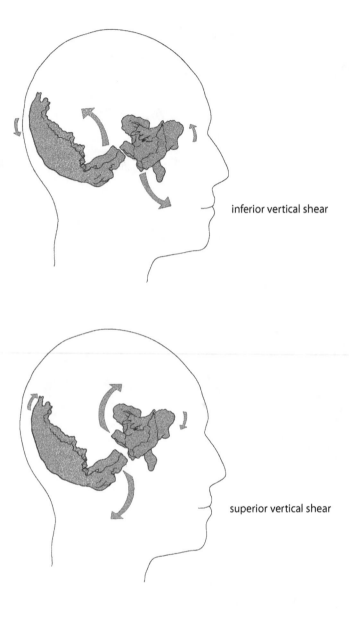

inferior vertical shear

superior vertical shear

Figure 11.12. Sphenobasilar vertical shear.

Sphenobasilar Vertical Shear

In the classic description of motility around the SBJ, the sphenoid and occiput are said to rotate around transverse axes in opposite directions. Vertical shear is generated when the two bones are forced to rotate in the *same* direction. It occurs when the body of the sphenoid has been forced to rotate either superiorly or inferiorly relative to the basilar portion of the occiput. This pattern commonly originates during later stages of the birth process when anterior-posterior pressures are placed upon the infant's cranium.

The presence of vertical shear may generate a paradox in inhalation-exhalation dynamics. In the natural way of things, as the fulcrum in the SBJ automatic shifts in inhalation and exhalation, the basi-occiput and rear of the body of the sphenoid follow. In the inhalation phase the SBJ rises, while in the exhalation phase it settles. In vertical shear, rather than a mutual rising of the basi-occiput and rear of the sphenoid in inhalation and a mutual settling in exhalation, each is held in opposite direction.

There are two kinds of vertical shear: *superior* or *inferior.* In superior vertical shear the sphenoid has been forced into a relative inhalation position, while the occiput is held in a relative exhalation position. Here the rear of the sphenoid is forced superior relative to the basi-occiput. In inferior vertical shear, the reverse occurs; the sphenoid is forced into an exhalation position, while the occiput is held in the inhalation position. Here the rear of the sphenoid is forced inferior in relationship to the basi-occiput (Figure 11.12).

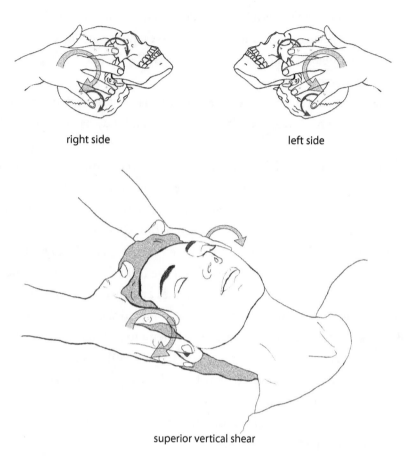

right side

left side

superior vertical shear

Figure 11.13. Practitioner experience of superior vertical shear.

To aid in your perception of this, imagine that there is a transverse axis through the palms of your hands while in the vault hold. If you sense both hands being rotated around this axis so that all of your fingers move anterior and inferior, then you are sensing a *superior* vertical shear. Here the sphenoid is held in a relative inhalation position, while the occiput is in relative exhalation. The rear of the sphenoid will be sheared superior relative to the occiput (Figure 11.13). Alternatively, if you sense that your hands are subtly rotated so that all your fingers rotate posterior and superior, then you are sensing an *inferior* vertical shear pattern. Here the sphenoid is held in relative exhalation, while the occiput is in relative inhalation. The rear of the sphenoid will be sheared inferiorly relative to the occiput.

In superior vertical shear, as the sphenoid is held in relative inhalation, the facial structures may follow this and have a widened look. In the extreme, this may yield a frontal bone with a prominent superior aspect, such as a bulging forehead. This is most prominent if the pattern is the result of birth trauma. At the same time, the occiput is held in relative exhalation and may have a narrowed look or feel. Viewed from above, the person's face may seem wide while the back of the head seems comparatively narrow.

In inferior vertical shear, as the sphenoid is held in relative exhalation, the facial structures are also held in an exhalation position, and may have a narrowed look. In chronic situations, the frontal bone may follow the greater wings posterior to the extreme and the forehead will look sloped at an acute angle, sometimes called a ski-slope forehead. This is obviously the reverse of the bulged look seen in the superior vertical shear pattern. Viewed from the front, the person's face may seem narrow while the back of the head seems comparatively wide.

Vertical shear patterns commonly have their origins in birth Stage Three, when anterior-posterior pressures are placed upon the infant's cranium. As the infant moves through the pelvic outlet, dragging forces are placed upon its frontal, sphenoid, and occipital bones, which may generate a vertical shearing of the sphenoid at the SBJ. In early Stage Three, the sphenoid will tend to be forced into an inhalation position as it is dragged over the maternal sacrum, while forces placed upon the occiput by the maternal pubic arch, may force the occiput into relative exhalation, generating a superior vertical shear pattern. In later Stage Three, when the infant's head moves into an extension position, the forces reverse and an inferior vertical shear may be generated.

Compression in the Sphenobasilar Junction

Compressive issues are common in cranial base relationships. Compressive forces may be fed into the SBJ and its surroundings during the birth process, especially birth Stage Three. In compression, inertial forces in the SBJ close down the available space and generate density in the tissues of the joint. During the inhalation phase, space cannot be accessed in the SBJ and ease of motility between the two bones becomes compromised.

Compressive issues are always generated by traumatic forces—birth process, accidents, overwhelming emotional shock, and blows to the head are likely origins. SBJ compression can also be generated by other chronically compressed relationships along the primal/notochord midline in the vertebral column and pelvis. Specific areas commonly coupled with SBJ compression include compression at the occipito-atlanteal junction, compression in the lumbosacral junction, and intraosseous distortions of the occiput such as condylar compressions and torsions. Severe compression held in the SBJ and cranial base can generate inertial conditions in the system as a whole. The fluid tide may seem sluggish, with low fluid drive. The cranium may seem very dense and the sphenoid and occiput may not be expressing much motility. In some chronic situations, it may feel like you are literally holding a very dense solid mass with little or no motion. The fluid system may also feel very dense and congested, as there may be much potency bound in centering the traumatic forces that generate the compressive pattern. Sometimes a general state of fluid stasis is sensed, which is always the result of overwhelming trauma of some kind.

The infant experiences compressive forces all through the birth process. The vertebral axis, pelvis, and cranium may all encounter strongly compressive pressures, and inertial fulcrums and tissue compression may result. As seen above, in the third stage of birth, the infant's cranium is commonly in an anterior-posterior position between the maternal sacrum and pelvic arch and may experience compressive forces along an anterior-posterior axis, which, in turn, may generate local compression in and around the SBJ. It is also common, due to unresolved Stage Three birthing forces, to see a telescoping of multiple structures in relationship to the SBJ. For example, the atlas and the squama, condyles, and basilar sections of the occiput may all become compressed and telescoped together as a consequence of the presence of unresolved birth forces through the midline. In our experience, these axial forces must be treated as a whole before individual fulcrums can resolve efficiently. We earlier discussed axial compression in our chapters on the vertebral axis and dural tube dynamics.

I have treated many babies with digestive issues, sleeping problems, sympathetic nervous system activation, and sensitized startle reflexes. In almost all cases, compressive issues generated by birthing forces were key orientations in their healing processes. These commonly involved a combination of compressive issues located in the SBJ, occiput, O/A junction, and jugular foramen. If these forces are not resolved in infancy or childhood, they will certainly manifest in the adult system in some way.

It must be remembered that working with babies is very different from adults. The holding environment ideally includes mother's presence and contact, and the practitioner's presence must be clearly negotiated with the infant so that permission to treat is given by the little one. The practitioner must be sensed as a secure and safe holding environment that includes mom and ideally dad if present. Please see our earlier chapters on the birth process.

Clinical Orientations

The following clinical explorations orient both to compressive issues in the SBJ and to the emergence of cranial base patterns in the natural unfolding of session work. Remember that cranial base patterns are expressions of many layers of history and past experience. These must be oriented to spaciously—with the knowledge that the client's system is accessing layers of experience, which uncouple and are expressed sequentially as the inherent treatment plan unfolds. Practitioner motion testing and analysis are unhelpful here as they may introduce new forces into the client's system, may activate many past life experiences all at once—including unresolved traumatic impacts—and will interfere with the natural unfolding of the inherent treatment plan.

As part of the learning process in foundation trainings, we generally teach students to orient to compressive forces and issues in the cranial base and SBJ before orienting to other patterns. This is due to the fact that compressive forces, and the resultant tissue compression they generate, commonly overlay other patterns, or fix them in place. Compression may also be the most obvious pattern to manifest in the SBJ. It can override the other patterns, and call for treatment first. Because of this, we will first explore compressive issues in SBJ dynamics, and then explore a more open approach where cranial base patterns emerge in the unfolding of the inherent treatment plan.

Exploration:
Augmentation of Space in SBJ Dynamics _____

This exploration is oriented to the augmentation of space in and around the dynamics of the SBJ and its surroundings. The intention will be to access space in the natural dynamics of the inhalation phase of primary respiration. This process is about augmenting the natural expression of space in the inhalation phase, not about releasing a physical resistance. Resistance will resolve when the forces organizing it resolve.

Start as usual and, after the holistic shift has deepened, move to the Sutherland vault hold. Settle into your contact and orient to the fluid tide in your three-body awareness. As the fluid tide clarifies, let the anatomy and dynamics of the tissues also come into your awareness. Notice how the sphenoid and occiput express motility in the cycles of the tide. If compressive forces are absent, the SBJ will rise with ease and the flower petals will naturally spread. No resistance will be sensed. If there is compression, you may sense pulling into the SBJ, density or lack of motion, or a block-like resistance. In extreme cases, the client's head may even feel like a solid mass.

From here, orient to an intention of the augmentation of space in the dynamics of the SBJ and cranial base in general. At the height of an inhalation phase, allow your fingers to be suspended in fluid and moved by the expression of fluid potency. Again, this is somewhat like kelp at the bottom of the ocean being moved by tidal forces. As your fingers are moved by the tide, they also take a deeper breath with the flower petals of the cranium as they open at the height of inhalation, thus also resonating with the natural expression of their motility. As this occurs, your fingers will subtly spread apart. This intention augments the natural expression of space in the inhalation phase of primary respiration at the SBJ and the cranial bowl as a whole. If no tide is expressed, allow your fingers to resonate with the natural space present and to take a deeper breath as though the tide is moving them. When space is accessed, remember Becker's admonition to orient to a change in state in the potency, not just to emergent tissue patterns or motions. Potency may be sensed to build in the relationship, to shift toward the SBJ in the fluids, or to permeate the area in some way (Figure 11.14).

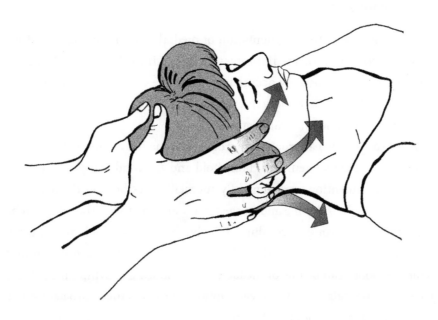

Figure 11.14. Augmentation of space in SBJ relationships.

Alternatively, when space is accessed, you may sense a settling into a deepening state of equilibrium emerging around the inertial fulcrum—physical body suspended in fluid body, suspended in tidal body, suspended in Dynamic Stillness. As this suspensory system deepens, listen for the healing process that emerges from the deepening stillness. In either case, wait to sense an expression of potency in the compressive fulcrum. This may be sensed as pulsation, a driving force in the fluids, or as a deeper, softer welling up and permeation of potency in the area. As this occurs, you may sense the inertial forces being dissipated back to the environment in some way—commonly via heat and pulsation or as a vector-like streaming.

As inertial forces are resolved, the sphenoid bone may be sensed to float anterior as part of a softening and expanding in the whole cranium. Wait for reorganization of the fluids and tissues to midline organizing principles—such as Sutherland's fulcrum and the primal midline. When the compressive forces are truly resolved, you may sense an expansion throughout the tissues of the cranium and the system as a whole.

Explorations:
Medial Compression _____

This exploration is the augmentation of medial space in and around the SBJ. It is very common for medial forces to be fed into the cranium during the birth process. This usually occurs in birth Stage One or Stage Two. Medially compressive forces can be very intense and will affect the motility of the SBJ, the temporal bones, and all local relationships.

I will suggest two alternative approaches to medial compressive forces—the first using the classic temporal bone hold and a second using a "temporal ear hold." These intentions will generally augment space both in the relationships around the temporal bone and in the temporal bone itself. The temporal bones can experience strong forces during the birth process, which may affect all of these inner and outer relationships. Unresolved birthing forces in and around the temporal bones can be one of the factors contributing to symptoms of tinnitus, trigeminal neuralgia, and glue ear. Option 1 below is the approach I generally teach in foundation courses. Option 2, however, can also be helpful in situations where the affects of inertial forces are very dense and intransigent.

Option 1: The Temporal Bone Hold—Augmentation of Space

In this option, the practitioner uses the classic temporal bone hold and augments space by deepening into inhalation as the temporal bones express their inhalation motility. Let's say, via a vault hold, that you sense a strong compressive issue that dampens down both SBJ and temporal bone motility—perhaps a strong inertial fulcrum was sensed in these dynamics. You will then change your hand hold to the temporal bone hold.

Using the temporal bone hold, settle into your relationship to primary respiration and orient to the expression of the motility of the two temporal bones. Orient to the inhalation phase of expression of the two bones. Again, at the height of inhalation—as your hands are floating on the tissues, suspended in fluid—allow your fingers and palms to be moved by the tide and to take a deeper breath in this direction. As you allow this, resonate with and augment the natural expression of the inhalation motility of the temporal bones. As described earlier, if no tide is expressed, allow your fingers, suspended in fluid, to resonate with the natural space present and to take a deeper breath as though the tide is moving them. This amplifies the natural expression of space in the sutural relationships around the temporal bones (Figure 11.15).

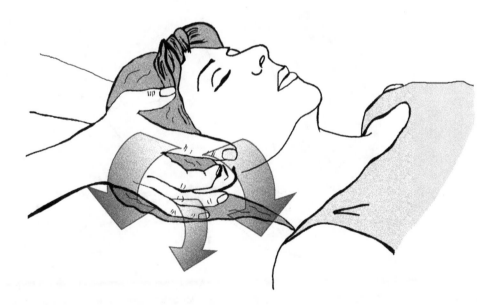

Figure 11.15. Augmentation of space via temporal bone hold.

Option 2: The Temporal Ear Hold

As discussed in Volume One, the temporal bones lie in the cranial base and their petrous portions point toward the SBJ at a 45-degree angle. The intention of this next option is to more directly relate to the petrous portion of the temporal bones as they sit in this 45-degree triangular space. Compressive forces in the relationships around the petrous portions are very common, usually due to birthing or later traumatic forces introduced into these relationships.

Start in the temporal bone hold as above, orient to temporal bone motility over a number of cycles, and then change to a *temporal ear hold*. To do this, place your fingers posterior behind and around the ears with fingertips at the temporal bones and thumbs over the ear canal. You are basically cupping the ears posterior with your fingertips where the ears meet the cranium, while you place your thumbs over the ear canals. Allow your hands to again float on the tissues, suspended in fluid (Figure 11.16).

At the height of inhalation, there is a natural expression of space in the sutures involved along the 45-degree angle. At the height of inhalation, as your hands float in fluid, allow them to be taken deeper into inhalation. As your fingers follow the temporal bones into inhalation, they breathe deeper along this 45-degree

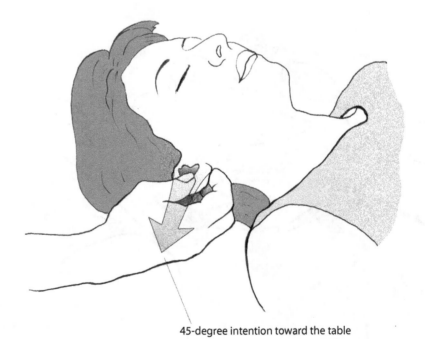

45-degree intention toward the table

Figure 11.16. Augmentation of space via temporal ear hold.

angle toward the treatment table. Again, this has a doing-not-doing quality where your hands are both being breathed and take a deeper breath in this direction at the height of inhalation.

As space is augmented and accessed in either hold described above, you may sense expressions of potency, pulsations, a sense of a driving force in the fluids, or a deeper, softer welling up and permeation of potency in the area. You may also sense the resolution of inertial forces as heat, force vectors clearing, further pulsations, and so on. When inertial forces are resolved, you may then perceive the whole cranial base reorganizing and much greater ease in inhalation and exhalation dynamics.

Exploration:
Cranial Base Patterns and the Inherent Treatment Plan _____

This exploration is used both in the learning of clinical skills related to cranial base patterns, and in preparation for everyday clinical practice. It is important that students familiarize themselves with these patterns on a felt-sense level, and learn to orient to them when they arise in the context of the inherent treatment plan.

There are a few things that may help in the early days of this exploration. The first imperative is to know the related anatomy. It is useful to study and use models of disarticulated bones to become familiar with these dynamics. In one exercise used in class, students connect the sphenoid and occiput at the SBJ with any pliable clay-like medium, and notice how the clay distorts, twists, bulges, and compresses as they move the bones in the patterns described above. They then see if they can visualize these patterns in their mind's eye.

Then one student holds the sphenoid and occiput from below, in the position he or she would be in if a person was lying on a treatment table. Then a second student holds the bones as though sitting at the head of the table holding a client's head in a vault hold. The first student moves the two bones in the relative positions of each pattern while the other student, with eyes closed, simply senses the dynamics that emerge in the hands. The intention is to begin to get a felt-sense of each pattern. We then do perceptual exercises in which students hold their hands in the space in front of them as though they are holding a cranium in the vault hold. Guided by a tutor, they move their hands in space to reflect the various patterns as though they were clarifying in session work.

In this clinical exploration, you will orient to the client's system in open enquiry. As the inherent treatment plan unfolds, you may sense particular cranial base patterns emerge that are not separate from the wider fluid-tissue field. Over time, you will also appreciate that these patterns will naturally be shown to you in the precise order in which healing processes need to unfold.

Start as usual. After the holistic shift deepens, move to the vault hold. Allow your relational field to again settle and orient to the physical and fluid bodies in the wider field. First orient to the fluid tide and then add the cranium as though it is like a flower opening and closing its petals in a fluid field. As the SBJ rises, the flower petals open, and as it settles, the petals close. As you orient to the inhalation phase, notice if space manifests between the tissue structures. Which sutures seem inertial, unable to access space?

Settle into your receptive state and allow the potency to show you its priorities. Have patience and wait for the inherent treatment plan to clarify and trust that the system will set its own priorities. As you maintain a wide perceptual field, a particular inertial pattern will commonly begin to clarify. This may be experienced as a distortion pattern in the wider fluid-tissue field. The organizing fulcrum for the inertial pattern may also clarify, located in the cranium or remotely. Let this fulcrum come into your awareness. The whole fluid-tissue field may seem to organize around it.

Orient to whatever inertial pattern comes to the forefront—see if you can recognize one of the patterns described above. As you hold your wide perceptual field, you may sense the deepening suspensory nature of the healing process—tissues suspended in fluid, suspended in Long Tide.

Orient to a deepening state of equilibrium in all fields and for Becker's three-phase healing awareness. Listen for action of potency in the stillness. As the process deepens, maintain a wide perceptual field and Long Tide levels of healing process may emerge and/or the system may deepen into Dynamic Stillness. Observe what emerges in these levels. When the process is completed, listen for the reorganization and realignment of potencies, fluids, and tissues to natural fulcrums and the midline.

The process may also include other fulcrums that are related or coupled to the inertial fulcrum generating the cranial base pattern. As these clarify, you may sense potency shifting through the fluids to attend to them.

The session described above is simply an open session within which the practitioner can begin to orient to cranial base patterns as they clarify in session work.

The Layering of Condensed Experience

The layering of our history is clearly seen in cranial base patterning. For instance, a particular pattern may be accessed in one session, perhaps a left torsion pattern. This torsion pattern and its organizing fulcrum may seem to resolve. Then, in a subsequent session, a new torsion pattern organized around a different fulcrum is perceived. These kinds of clinical experiences are expressions of various life experiences and related unresolved forces, which become layered and coupled in the system. All of these unresolved experiences are holistically centered by the action of potency as a unified field, and arise in session work in the order appropriate for that person's healing process. Again, this cannot be analyzed or motion tested for, but must be holistically received as one orients to primary respiration and the unfolding process.

Stanislav Grof has developed a beautiful way of discussing this kind of coupling. He coined the term COEX matrix, or COEX system (Grof 1993). COEX means *condensed experience*. In this understanding, all of our history is held in present time in a layered and condensed fashion. These layers of experience coalesce and generate various mind-body states and behavioral patterns. In the classic COEX system, a theme ties certain layers of condensed experience together. This theme has the quality of a life statement or life theme. For instance, various condensed experiences may resonate with a theme of abandonment, while another layering of condensed experience may resonate with a particular self-view, or sense of self-worth, and another may be organized around a loss of trust in intimacy and intimate relationships. We may be holding numerous COEX systems within us and they are, in turn, all coupled and condensed together as the Breath of Life acts to center all unresolved experience as a unified whole. Each torsion, side-bending, shearing, or compressive pattern that emerges is coupled with many layers of experience, and psycho-emotional processes and beliefs about self, intimacy, relational others, and the world we live in are all inherently coupled with each and every form.

Thus, when a present stressful experience resonates with a COEX system, a whole layering of life process, reactions, beliefs, and conditions may become activated. For instance, a recent car accident may resonate and become coupled with a deep fear of loss and abandonment held from earlier experiences. Many layers of unresolved experience may have been activated by the accident and flood the client's experience. He or she may become lost in emotional states—may find that all sorts of symptoms emerge and even engage in unskillful life decisions as these states are experienced. Any level of these may emerge in session work and it can be overwhelming for the client when it does.

I have worked with many people where recent trauma had touched off layers of past history, which emerged all at once. When this occurs, it is not just the present experience that clients are dealing with, but the whole of the coupled, condensed, layered, and unresolved forces still active in their systems. It is like striking middle C on a piano and all the other Cs vibrate. It is thus important to have established resources in a client's system, and for the holistic shift to be available in session work. It is also very important to understand trauma and trauma resolution, and to have clinical skills in place that help moderate and appropriately pace a client's arising process.

I once worked with a client who was in a motorcycle accident. As he was thrown off the motorcycle, his clavicle hit the pavement and was fractured. He was fortunate that this was the only physical damage done other than bruises. Beyond the shock of the present experience, he found himself entering a deep depression. This was a familiar childhood state. In session work, we discovered that a deeply seated COEX system was activated that held themes of abandonment and betrayal, which had its origins in birth experience and early childhood. The skill of the work was to help these condensed layers of traumatic experience uncouple in the resources of primary respiration. As this occurred, particular fulcrums and related inertial patterns emerged in a paced manner, and became the focus of the healing process without traumatic overwhelm being experienced. This is actually a natural process that, once resources are established, emerges in the context of the inherent treatment plan.

As cranial distortion patterns manifest and resolve, related life statements or themes may also emerge. Sometimes a process of insight ensues, within which clarity is attained and something let go of. Likewise, an emotional process may emerge like a wave and resolve. Sometimes shock affects will be expressed, autonomic energies engaged, and traumatic cycling completed. Again, appropriate trauma skills must be in place, and the pacing of the client's healing process is paramount. Ideally, the COEX system resolves its layered issues in a step-wise fashion. All of this can change that person's life. In this process, the practitioner must remember to allow space, to not judge the process, and to let go of any needs around the session work. We must remember to hold our work in a still, receptive, and respectful field of awareness. We must also remember that healing unfolds from within and, as Still stressed, this work and the laws governing it, are not framed by human hands.

CHAPTER 12

The Venous Sinuses

In this chapter we will learn to orient to the venous sinus drainage system of the cranium. In previous session work you may have sensed sluggishness in a client's fluid system, and an overall sense of low vitality even after resourcing work, stillpoints, ignition processes, and so on. In a classic cranial context, one approach to low fluid drive was to augment the flow of venous drainage in the cranium via what was called *venous sinus drainage*. The venous sinuses provide fluid drainage for the cranium and this system can become sluggish and dense; this drainage approach was intended to free up the flow.

Inertial forces and fulcrums in cranial dynamics—and their related cranial base and dural tension patterns—all affect the form and function of the venous sinuses, leading to stasis, fluid backpressure, and a reduction of the system's capacity both for fluid drainage and for the uptake of potency in cerebrospinal fluid. This will affect the quality of potency and drive of fluid fluctuation throughout the whole system. In a classic cranial context, orienting more directly to the venous sinuses helps facilitate space in the fluid system, encourages fluid drainage, and enhances fluid fluctuation and the uptake of potency in cerebrospinal fluid.

However, in a biodynamic context, as the inertial forces and related fulcrums generating lowered fluid drive resolve, related venous sinus congestion also resolves—so it is not really necessary to work biomechanically through the sinus system. Nevertheless, inertial forces may be located in a specific sinus area, and it is still useful to know how to relate to the involved sinus more directly.

The Venous Sinus System

The venous sinuses carry venous fluids and cerebrospinal fluid out of the cranium toward the heart. The venous sinuses are not true veins; they are spaces formed in dura that collect blood and cerebrospinal fluid for recycling via the circulatory system. They are an integral part of the dural membrane system.

Cerebrospinal fluid is produced in the choroid plexuses that line the ventricles of the brain. After bathing the brain tissues, CSF moves into the venous sinuses via the arachnoid granulations, found especially in the sagittal sinus (Figure 12.1). Venous blood and cerebrospinal fluid then flow through the sinuses to the main outlets from the cranium, the jugular foramina, and internal jugular veins, and on to the heart. Other smaller exit routes include the facial vein, the deep cervical vein, and the external jugular vein.

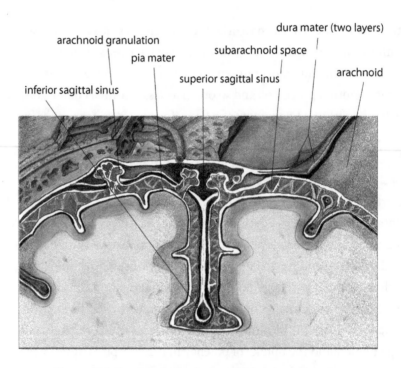

Figure 12.1. Section through the sagittal sinus showing
arachnoid granulations.

The major venous sinuses include the sphenoid-parietal sinuses, the superior and inferior petrosal sinuses, the cavernous and intercavernous sinuses, the basilar plexus, the sagittal sinuses (superior and inferior), the straight sinus, the transverse sinuses, the occipital sinus, the marginal sinus, and the sigmoid sinus. Again, in a classic context, effective venous sinus treatment requires a thorough knowledge of anatomy. I suggest that you trace or draw these channels in a number of views, to include the sinuses mentioned above (Figures 12.2a and b). This will give you a clear visual sense of their relationships.

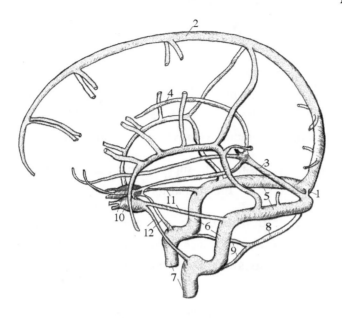

1 = confluence of sinuses
2 = superior sagittal sinus
3 = straight sinus
4 = inferior sagittal sinus
5 = transverse sinus
6 = sigmoid sinus

7 = internal jugular vein
8 = occipital sinus
9 = marginal sinus
10 = cavernous sinus
11 = superior petrosal sinus
12 = inferior petrosal sinus

Figure 12.2a. Major venous sinuses and the venous system.

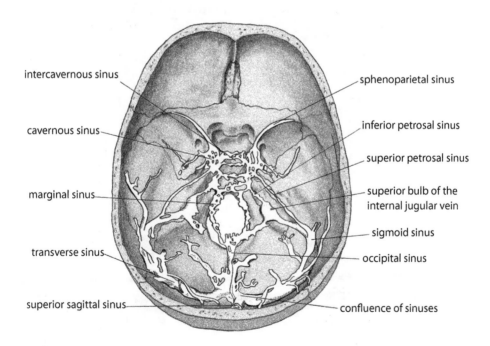

Figure 12.2b. Venous sinuses at the base of the cranial cavity, seen from above.

Venous flows are summarized below.

- From the superior cranial fossa, the venous flow moves from the sphenoid-parietal sinuses toward the middle cranial fossa via the cavernous and intercavernous sinuses. It then flows via the basilar plexus to the inferior cranial fossa and then to the internal jugular veins via the jugular foramina.

- The temporal area drains from the superior and inferior petrosal sinuses to the sigmoid sinuses and then to the jugular foramina.

- The parietal areas drain from the superior and inferior sagittal sinuses to the straight sinus and to the confluence of sinuses, to the transverse sinuses, and then to the sigmoid sinuses and jugular foramina.

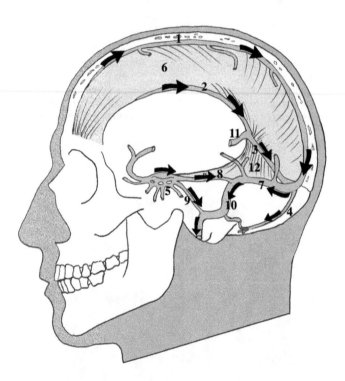

1 superior sagittal sinus	7 transverse sinus
2 inferior sagittal sinus	8 superior petrosal sinus
3 straight sinus	9 inferior petrosal sinus
4 occipital sinus	10 sigmoid sinus
5 cavernous sinus	11 great cerebral vein (galen)
6 falx cerebri	12 tentorium cerebelli

Figure 12.3. Direction of flow in venous sinuses.

- From the occipital sinus, the venous flow moves inferiorly toward the marginal sinuses, the sigmoid sinuses, and the jugular foramina and will also leave the cranium via cervical veins (Figure 12.3).

American anatomy texts usually state that the occipital sinus drains upward into the confluence. Most European texts state that the occipital sinus drains into the sigmoid sinus below (Clemente 2001, plate 768). My sense is that it can flow either direction and commonly drains inferiorly toward the sigmoid sinus during session work. I use that direction of flow here. Venous flow will seek the easiest way out of the cranium via these routes and always has an alternative route. Obstruction in one route can be partially accommodated by other routes.

Venous Sinus System and Inertial Issues

Venous sinus stasis is not uncommon. The fluids in the sinuses can become inertial due to the presence of unresolved inertial forces and the dural tensions they generate. Congestion in the sinuses can generate fluid backpressure in the cranium and inefficient drainage of blood, waste, and cerebrospinal fluid—contributing to low vitality and poor ignition of potency in cerebrospinal fluid. Venous sinus congestion is thought to contribute to tension and strain in the membrane system, hormonal imbalances, and pressure on cranial nerves, especially in the cavernous and intercavernous sinuses (Figure 12.4). The affected person may experience headaches, neck tension, and a sensation of congestion in the head, among other symptoms.

A cranium holding chronic fluid congestion and inefficient venous drainage may feel rigid and solid. Motility of tissues and fluid drive may feel sluggish or

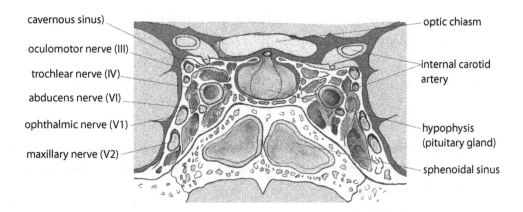

Figure 12.4. Section through the cavernous sinus.

dense as the potency becomes inertial and the fluid drive of the system is lowered. Orienting more directly to venous sinus drainage does encourage fluid movement throughout the cranium by at least temporarily decongesting the channels of flow that fluids must take to leave the cranium. However, the inertial fulcrums that generate the congestion must be resolved for any of this to have lasting effect.

Cranial Outlets

In our exploration of the venous sinus system, we will be taking a classic approach to our inquiry and view the venous sinuses as the plumbing system of the cranium. In this context, it makes sense to start with the lowest level of blockage so that higher congestion has an exit route when it is resolved later. Thus the first step in orienting to the venous sinus system is to recognize that its outlets from the cranium are critical in the drainage process. If the drain is blocked, fluids will back up through the rest of the plumbing system. Thus, we will orient to the outlets of the cranium first and then continue our exploration from the bottom up.

The thoracic inlet is the first area to consider. Inertial issues here may generate backpressure against venous flow. Pressure can be fed into the internal jugular vein and into the other venous outlet routes such as the external jugular vein, deep cervical vein, and the vertebral vein. Other potential relationships at the low end of the cranium that may generate backpressure include the cervical fascia, the occipital cranial base—including the axis, atlas, occipital condyles, foramen magnum, and intraosseous occipital issues—cervical vertebra, and the jugular foramina.

Thoracic Inlet Relationships

Our main discussion of the thoracic inlet is presented in Chapter 16 on connective tissues. If this area is not relatively free of inertial forces, work to encourage venous drainage above may result in discomfort for the client instead of renewed circulation. Discomfort may take the form of head congestion, heaviness, spaciness, headaches, and so on.

As you orient to the motility of the tissues of the thoracic inlet, be sure to include the related vertebra, including the cervicals and upper thoracics. Vertebral fixations in this area can also affect venous and cerebrospinal fluid flow. It may also be relevant to orient to the vertebrae more specifically with the explorations described in Chapter 8.

The thoracic inlet includes a continuous, multifaceted set of relationships that create the opening from the neck into the torso. Key structures include the manubrium, clavicle, and scapulae, plus the inner circle created by the articulations of the first ribs with the manubrium and first thoracic vertebra. Many important structures pass through this opening, including the jugular veins and arteries, and the vagus and phrenic nerves.

Exploration:
Thoracic Inlet

After starting as usual, and after the holistic shift has deepened, sit at the side of the table and place the palm of your cephalad hand under C7–T3, perpendicular to the client's body. After establishing a relationship with the client's system, place your other hand transversely over his or her clavicles and upper sternum holding the thoracic inlet in your awareness. In your wide perceptual field, establish a relationship to the fluid tide and tissue motility in the fluid and physical bodies. Allow your hands to float on the tissues, suspended in fluid, and orient to the tissue motility of the area (Figure 12.5).

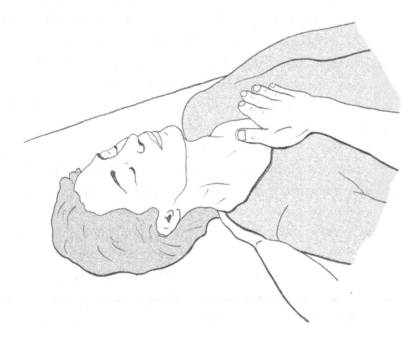

Figure 12.5. Thoracic inlet hold.

Settle into your still and receptive state and orient to whatever inertial pattern clarifies, to an emergent state of balance, to the deepening of the system into its suspensory nature, and to the expression of healing processes that may emerge from any level of action. As inertial forces resolve, you may sense the tissues of the thoracic area, and the tissue field as a whole, reorganizing to the primal midline. You may also sense an enhanced quality of drive in the fluid tide.

Occipital Base Issues

Next in sequence from the bottom up is the occipital triad area. Inertial issues here can strongly affect venous outflow. These issues may go back to birthing forces and birth trauma. If inertial issues are present here, explore the occipital triad and intraosseous occipital issues, as described in previous chapters. Occipital triad inertial issues directly affect the dynamics of the jugular foramina, internal jugular veins, external jugular veins, and the deep cervical veins.

Jugular Foramina

The jugular foramina are the narrowest points in the drainage system. Located in the occipito-mastoid suture, between the occiput and temporal bones, this important pair of openings is the path for the internal jugular veins, receiving the outflow of the major sinuses of the head (Figure 12.6). The transverse sinuses merge into the sigmoid sinuses as they pass through both jugular foramina to become the internal jugular veins. Obviously, compression or congestion in jugular foramen relationships can be a major factor in venous sinus congestion.

The jugular foramina are also important because they are passageways for important nerves: the vagus, glossopharyngeal, and spinal accessory nerves. Compression in jugular foramen relationships is commonly generated by birth trauma. The forces of whiplash injuries can also be held here, leading to puzzling visceral symptoms. Inertial fulcrums in, or affecting, the jugular foramina can generate digestive, respiratory, and sucking problems in infants, and digestive and respiratory issues in adults, as well as a wide range of other symptoms. Hypersensitivity or facilitation of these nerves often indicates impingement at the jugular foramina, and neuroendocrine effects may be far-reaching.

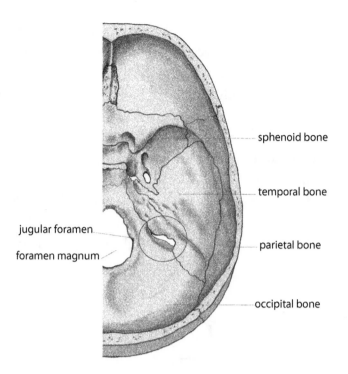

sphenoid bone

temporal bone

jugular foramen

parietal bone

foramen magnum

occipital bone

Figure 12.6. The jugular foramen.

Exploration:
The Jugular Foramen _____

In this exploration, we make a direct relationship to the jugular foramina via a new hold, the temporal-occipital hold. The intention is to facilitate the resolution of inertial forces by orienting more directly to these relationships. The first step will be to orient to the system via a vault hold, and to see if we are drawn to work with either jugular foramen.

After starting as usual, move to the vault hold. In your wide perceptual field, orient to the fluid and physical bodies and fluid tide and tissue motility. Then, in your wide perceptual field, orient to the jugular foramina using your knowledge of the area anatomy. As the system settles, see if an inertial pattern or fulcrum clarifies. See if you can sense an inertial issue in either jugular foramen. This may be sensed as a pull into the area or a motion dynamic organized around it. You may sense that the temporal bone and occiput move in a block-like fashion on the side of a compressive issue, without a sense of space or fluidity between them. See which jugular foramen you are drawn to first.

To relate directly to that specific jugular foramen, change your hand position. First place one hand under the occiput, cradling it in the palm with your fingers spread wide to give support. Be sure that the heel of your hand is not pressing against the client's head. This hand position will stabilize the occiput as you cradle it. Place your other hand at the temporal bone in the temporal bone hold. Here your middle finger is curved and placed lightly in the patient's ear canal. Your index finger rests anterior to the ear at the zygomatic process while your ring finger rests posterior to the ear over the mastoid portion of the temporal bone. Your index and ring fingers make a solid contact, though the pressure is very light. You now are in relationship to the two bones bordering the jugular foramen. In this position, the temporal-occipital hold, see if you sense the jugular foramen (Figure 12.7).

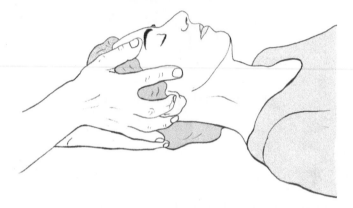

Figure 12.7. The temporal-occipital hold.

Settle into your awareness of motility at both occiput and temporal bones. As the occiput and temporal bones express their inhalation dynamic, is there a sense of space generated at the occipito-mastoid suture? What inertial pattern clarifies? Orient to Becker's three-phase process and the settling into a state of balance. As the system deepens into equilibrium, notice what level of healing process emerges. Orient to the expression of potency in the inertial fulcrum and for a resolution of inertial forces. Again, this may be sensed as pulsation, heat, shifts of potency in the fluids, and so on. Wait for a sense of softening and expansion in the tissues of the relationship.

This is often enough to resolve the inertial forces present. However, if the forces are very dense, then an augmentation of space in the relationships may be of great value.

Maintain your contact at both occiput and temporal bone. At the height of the inhalation of the fluid tide, allow your hands to be taken by the tide and breathe more deeply in the direction of inhalation motility. Your hand at the occiput follows occipital motility in inhalation, as your hand at the temporal bone follows temporal motility. Again this is as though your hands are both breathed more deeply by the tide and, at the same time, take a deeper breath in that direction. I sometimes also take a deeper physical breath as my hands orient to this intention. It really has the sense of your hands suspended in fluid being move by the tide like kelp in the sea. As before, if no tide is expressed, allow your fingers, suspended in fluid, to resonate with the natural space present in the sutural relationship, and to take a deeper breath as though the tide is moving them.

As space is accessed, the system may deepen into a state of balance, or potency may be directly expressed in the inertial fulcrum. Again notice the expression of potency in the relationships. Listen for a resolution of the inertial forces present. You may sense expansion and reorganization as the potencies, fluids, and tissues reorient to midline phenomena.

Clinical Highlight

Infants often present issues related to the jugular foramen. I have attended to many infants with colic, related digestive issues, respiratory issues, sleeping issues, and sucking problems, all due to the aftermath of the birthing process. As discussed earlier, infants must be approached with extra-sensitive negotiation and conscious contact. They will sense your intentions and will accept your contact if they feel safe and resourced in your presence.

Many years ago a young woman came to see me with chronic digestive issues including excessive acidity, headaches, and exhaustion. Her headaches had been a feature of her life from childhood onward, but the hyperacidity was a relatively new symptom. Orthodox investigations did not reveal any physiological etiology. She was diagnosed as having anxiety states and psychological tension, and her physician prescribed tranquillizers.

We initially oriented to stillness, stillpoints, and resourcing work, because her system was very depleted and inertial. As she gained resources over a number of sessions, her system was able to deepen into the holistic shift and the inherent treatment plan began to express itself. As sessions progressed, one of the important patterns that clarified was an intraosseous distortion of the occiput and a very compressed jugular foramen on the right side. There were also temporal bone issues on that side, coupled with cranial base compression. The sub-occipital area was tender to the touch. The compressive fulcrums organizing these effects were clearly located in and around the right jugular foramen and SBJ areas.

These issues were related to forces generated by birth trauma. There was also sympathetic nervous system activation and brain stem hypersensitivity present. Over the course of the sessions, as the birthing forces resolved, sympathetic shock affects cleared through the fluids, and emotional edges of fear and sadness also arose. These seemed to underpin her anxiety states, and the headaches were directly resulted from these forces at work in her system. Over a number of sessions, she was able to clear these emotional affects in a resourced and very present manner. The headaches were clearly related to the jugular foramen issue. Fluid backpressure was arising from the jugular foramen, and it was alleviated as the fulcrums affecting the jugular foramen resolved. We oriented to these issues over time. Resolving the inertial forces in the jugular foramen itself was a key component in the alleviation of her symptoms.

Explorations:
Orienting to the Venous Sinuses _____

After orienting to the outlets to venous flow, we now turn our attention to the sinuses themselves. We will again work in a bottom-up fashion—orienting to the lower sinuses first and then moving up to sinuses farther away from the outlets. In this process, we will use classic hand positions, which allow a direct relationship to some of the major venous sinuses. As we systematically work our way through these major sinuses, remember that although each sinus area has a particular name, you are really relating to a continuous space formed in the dural membrane.

In the following explorations, we are assuming that the client's system has already accessed the holistic shift, that while orienting to the system from the vault hold, you have sensed major fluid congestion in the cranium, and that you have first oriented to the venous outlets as described above.

Confluence of Sinuses
The confluence of sinuses is the meeting place of the major venous sinuses, including the sagittal, straight, transverse, and occipital sinuses. The confluence

of sinuses can be found just anterior to the inion, the external occipital protuberance.

With the client in the supine position, let the external occipital protuberance (inion) rest on your two middle fingers. Place your two middle fingers together and then support them by placing your index and ring fingers under them (Figure 12.8). Let the client's head rest on these two middle fingers, balanced on them by the thumbs and heels of your hands. Allow all the weight to be taken on your middle fingers. With the head's weight on your fingers, this contact becomes a new fulcrum for the system. Once the contact is well established, in your wide perceptual filed, orient to the confluence of sinuses anterior to your fingers.

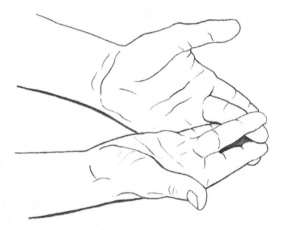

Figure 12.8. The confluence of sinus hold and occipital sinus hold.

If congestion is present, the occipital bone and the confluence may feel dense and rigid. The contact may feel sensitive or painful to the patient. Give the system space and allow the system to deepen into a state of balance and equilibrium. Wait here until you feel a distinct softening and expansion of the area. As inertial issues in the confluence resolve, you may sense a surge of fluid through the sinus. The occiput will also soften locally, and the sensitivity that the patient first experienced will be alleviated.

Occipital and Marginal Sinuses

After this first process, orient to the occipital and marginal sinuses. The occipital sinus lies below the confluence. It ends at the foramen magnum where it splits to form the marginal sinus around the foramen (see Figures 12.2a, 12.2b, and 12.3).

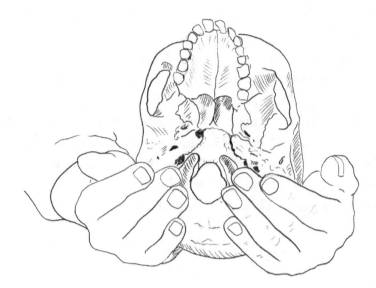

Figure 12.9. Marginal sinus hold.

For the occipital sinus, maintain the same hand position as above and move one finger width inferior (caudal) along the mid-line of the occiput to form a relationship to the occipital sinus. If you sense density there, repeat the above process. If there is congestion at the level of your contact, the tissues of the occiput may feel dense and rigid. With the weight of the head on your middle fingers, again orient to the state of balance and wait for a sense of softening, expansion, and fluid movement.

Continue to move down the occipital sinus one finger width at a time until you reach the foramen magnum. Whenever you sense density, orient to the state of balance, the resolution of inertial forces, and a softening and expansion in the local tissues. When you arrive at the foramen magnum, shift your intention from the occipital sinus to the marginal sinuses. At the foramen magnum, the occipital sinus divides into two sinuses on either side of the jugular foramen. To relate to these interior sinuses, use a condylar spread hand position similar to the one used for the occipital triad (see Figure 10.6).

Separate your middle fingers and point them toward the occipital condyles and foramen magnum. Your hands are slightly separated, and your middle fingers form a V-shape pointing toward the foramen magnum. The weight of the cranium is taken by the middle fingers and by your hands in general. Settle into this contact. From here you will orient to the augmentation of space in the occiput and marginal sinus areas, as learned in Chapter 10. At the height of an inhalation phase, allow your fingers to augment space in the marginal sinuses by breathing more deeply in the inhalation phase of occipital motility. Wait for a softening and spreading in the area (Figure 12.9).

Transverse Sinuses

Next we move superiorly, to the transverse sinuses. The two transverse sinuses move in opposite directions laterally from the confluence of sinuses across the occiput to merge with each sigmoid sinus. The sigmoid sinuses dive into the jugular foramina and are continuous with the internal jugular veins (see Figure 12.2a). If you have a skull model, look at the inner surface of the occipital bone. You will usually see narrow indented areas fanning out on either side of the confluence of sinuses. Dural membranes peel off from the lining of the cranium at these raised areas to form the transverse sinuses.

Place your little fingers at the external occipital protuberance (the inion) and line up the other fingers in a more or less straight line along the transverse sinuses. Your little fingers are touching along their outside edges. Your other fingers are touching each other and are lined up transversely under the transverse sinuses. Try to make your fingertips line up horizontally as much as possible (Figure 12.10).

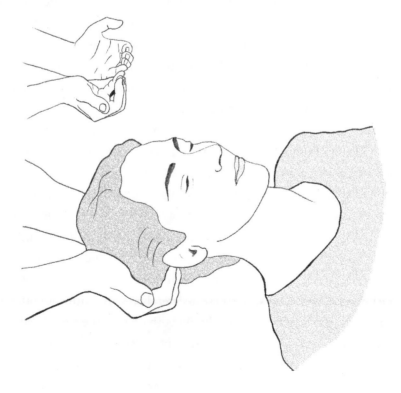

Figure 12.10. Tranverse sinus hold.

Again, take the weight of the cranium onto your fingertips. You may have a sense that you are subtly balancing the sinus system on your fingertips. As before, orient to a state of balance and the resolution of inertial forces, and wait until a softening and expansion in the tissues is felt. You may again sense fluids flushing through as the congestion resolves.

Straight Sinus

The straight sinus starts at the confluence of sinuses, anterior to the external occipital protuberance. It then moves anteriorly at about a thirty-degree angle. The anterior aspect of the straight sinus is the location of Sutherland's fulcrum, the suspended, automatically shifting fulcrum for all membranes and connective tissues. As it shifts in the cycles of the tide, the unified membranous-connective field shifts and is oriented to midline. You obviously can't physically have your fingers directly over the straight sinus because it extends interiorly from inion. In this process, you will have a relationship with its posterior pole via the inion and will contact its most anterior pole through your awareness. I will describe two processes; one is a classic contact, described largely for reference purposes, and the second is a modified version that is easier to use.

For the classic hold for the straight sinus, place your middle fingers at the external occipital protuberance as above, lift the client's head with your fingertips into anatomical flexion (forward-bending), and place your thumbs on top of the patient's head near or on the midline of the sagittal suture. You must really lift the client's head off the table into flexion to get your fingers in this position. Then let your hands settle onto the table and let the client's head settle into a position that rests balanced on your middle fingers. You now have your middle fingers at the confluence of sinuses and your thumbs as far along the sagittal sinus, and as close to the midline, as possible (Figure 12.11a).

Orient to the anterior aspect of the straight sinus in the cranium from your thumb contact, about one-third of the way in from the posterior of the head. This will place you in relationship to the anterior pole of the straight sinus at Sutherland's fulcrum. The weight of the cranium should be mainly placed on your middle fingers at the inion, while you balance the client's head with the rest of the fingers of your hands. Don't create lateral pressure with your other fingers. When you find yourself in relationship to both poles of the straight sinus, it may feel like you are literally holding the straight sinus between your middle fingers and thumbs. You may also sense the inion settling into your hands. Orient to a state of deepening equilibrium and balance, and wait for a perception of softening and expansion. This may be perceived most clearly at inion.

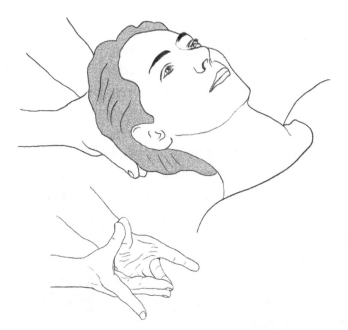

Figure 12.11a. Traditional straight sinus hold.

If your hands are too small, or if you find the classic hold uncomfortable, here is an easier-to-use hand position. While cradling the occiput with one hand, spread your fingers and place the middle finger of that hand at the inion and take the weight of the cranium largely on that finger. With your other hand, place your thumb at the sagittal suture on top of the cranium. Use this thumb to orient your awareness to the anterior aspect of the straight sinus and Sutherland's fulcrum (Figure 12.11b). Using your contacts via your two hands, orient to the whole of

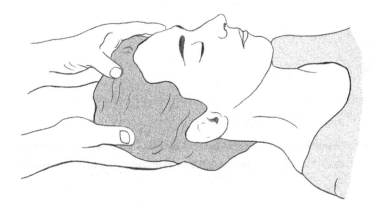

Figure 12.11b. Alternative straight sinus hold.

the straight sinus between your fingers. Again, settle into your wide perceptual field, orient to stillness, deepening equilibrium, and a processing of inertial forces and issues in the straight sinus itself. As this occurs, you may sense the cranium settling, a sense of softening at the inion, and a clearing of fluid through the area. You may even sense a *whoosh* of fluid through the area.

Augmenting Fluid Drive through the Straight Sinus

Sometimes the straight sinus can become very congested. In these cases you might also decide to orient to the augmentation of fluid drive through the area, via the use of a V-spread.

While cradling the occiput in one hand, place a V-spread at the inion. Use the index and middle fingers of the cradling hand to do this. The inion should be in the middle of your V-spread. Place the fingers of your other hand at the superior aspect of the frontal bone and orient to the fluid tide from that contact.

Orient to the expression of the fluid tide and the biomagnetic quality of potency driving it. As you sense an exhalation of the tide, potency is shifting caudal toward the fluid midline in the neural tube. As you sense the exhalation receding of fluid and potency, augment the action of potency and fluid drive through the straight sinus by simply orienting to it via your finger at the superior aspect of the frontal bone.

Notice a shift in potency toward and through the straight sinus. You may notice a sense of pulsation at the inion and a fluid release from the straight sinus through the confluence of sinuses and transverse sinuses. The straight sinus generally drains more into the left transverse sinus, and you may thus sense more of a fluid release on that side.

Explorations:
*Sagittal Sinus*_____

Next we move to the superior sagittal sinus. The sagittal sinus stretches from above the inion to the superior aspect of the frontal bone at the metopic suture. We will gradually move along the sagittal sinus in an anterior direction, from just above the inion to the beginning of the metopic suture, working in three steps.

Step One

Place the fingers of both hands together under the client's head along the midline above the inion. Your index fingers are just above the inion—almost touching—and the rest of your fingers are vertically oriented superiorly along the midline on either side of the sagittal sinus (Figure 12.12a).

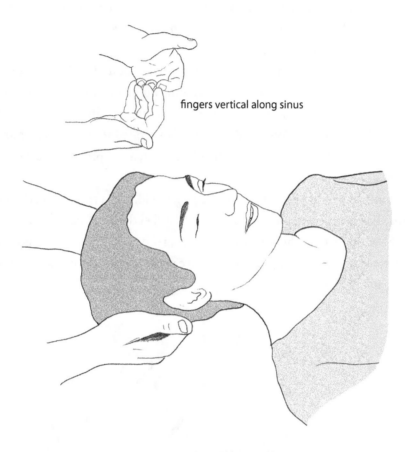

fingers vertical along sinus

Figure 12.12a. Sagittal sinus hold.

Take the weight of the cranium on these fingers and settle into a still and receptive state. Orient to a deepening equilibrium and softening of tissue, and a sense of fluid release through the sinus. If the sagittal sinus seems very dense and congested, you can augment space in its dynamics in the inhalation cycle of the tide. At the height of inhalation, allow your fingers to be taken by the inhalation surge and orient to the natural spreading apart of the suture and sinus. Allow your fingers to follow the inhalation motility of the tissues and to take a deeper breath at the height of inhalation. You may sense that, as you allow this, your fingers also subtly spread apart. Again orient to a softening of the tissues and a movement of fluids through the sinus. When this occurs, move anteriorly one finger width at a time along the sagittal suture with the same intention.

Step Two

When your hands come out from under the client's head, cross your thumbs and place them on either side of the sagittal suture just anterior to where you were last working. You will orient to the augmentation of space through the sagittal sinus via your thumb contact.

Again orient to the inhalation surge of the fluid tide and to the quality of tissue motility present. At the height of inhalation, you may sense a natural spreading or widening in the sagittal suture as space is expressed in its dynamics. At the height of inhalation, allow your thumbs—suspended in fluid—to be moved by the tide and to take a deeper breath at its height, also spreading apart as space is accessed.

Continue by moving anteriorly one finger width at a time along the sagittal sinus. Focus on the sagittal sinus areas that feel dense or congested. If, at the height of inhalation, the suture and sinus spread and widen easily, move to the next contact point. You can expect to have some areas feel congested while others do not (Figure 12.12b).

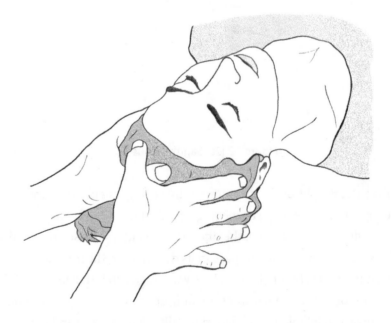

Figure 12.12b. Sagittal sinus hold (thumbs crossed).

Step Three

When you come to the top of the client's forehead, you will be in relationship to the metopic suture—the original space between the two parts of the frontal bone at birth. This suture is still present in about 10 percent of the population. The sagittal sinus continues here under the midline of the frontal bone. Change your hand position by aligning your fingers closely together along the midline of the frontal bone, as we did in step one, on either side of the metopic suture. Again orient to the inhalation cycle of the fluid tide. At the height of inhalation, allow your fingers to be breathed by the tide and to take a deeper breath both with its expression, and with the natural quality of space generated in the tissue field. Your fingers will spread apart in resonance with this at the height of its surge. Again orient to a sense of softening, expansion, and spreading in the area (Figure 12.12c).

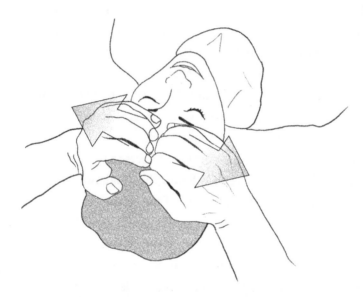

Figure 12.12c. Metopic suture and most anterior aspect of sagittal sinus.

Exploration:
Cavernous and Intercavernous Sinuses

The cavernous sinus and intercavernous sinuses are located in critical positions. The cavernous sinuses lie on either side of the sella turcica and the body of the sphenoid, and are connected by the intercavernous sinuses. They provide venous drainage for the pituitary gland area. Congestion in these sinuses can directly affect pituitary function. In addition, the internal carotid artery and its sympathetic nerve supply pass through the cavernous sinus. Cranial nerves also pass through the sinus, including the oculomotor, trochlear, opthalmic, and the maxillary branches of the trigeminal nerve. Congestion in the cavernous sinus can have direct effects on these nerves, causing entrapment neuropathy and nerve facilitation. We will use a contact with the greater wings of the sphenoid bone to engage these sinuses. If you look at a skull model, notice how the greater wings of the sphenoid merge with the lesser wings and take you to the sellae turcica and cavernous sinus.

In this exploration, you orient to the augmentation of space with the cranial base and SBJ. As space is accessed in these areas, the space in the deeper sinuses resting on the SBJ and pituitary area are also augmented.

Holding a wide perceptual field, orient to the fluid and physical bodies. Place your hands in a Sutherland vault hold. The Becker hold can also be used, but I find that the Sutherland hold gives the practitioner a wider orientation to the bones of the cranial base and to the space naturally generated in their relationships in the inhalation phase. Again allow your hands and fingers to float on tissues, suspended in fluid. In your wide perceptual field, orient to the SBJ area and the cavernous and intercaverous sinuses.

At the height of inhalation, allow your fingers to resonate with the expression of potency and space and to subtly follow the inhalation motility of the cranial bones in inhalation, especially those of the sphenoid and occiput, and to be moved deeper into the inhalation direction, as though they are taking a deeper breath in that direction.

As space is accessed, orient to the sinuses in the SBJ area and to any sense of fluid response. You may again sense this as a clearing through the sinus areas, and as a *whoosh* of fluid in the sinus system,

A classic completion process for venous sinus drainage is to finish with an exhalation stillpoint process. I would suggest that, if you do this, you move to the sacrum and orient to exhalation stillpoint and stillness from that contact as an integrative process.

Additional Considerations with Venous Sinus Processes

Low Blood Pressure

Low blood pressure is a commonly discussed contraindication for biomechanical venous sinus work. I have not seen this as a major issue in the gentle approach we take. However, this classic contraindication should be considered. In the reverse situation, high blood pressure, venous sinus drainage is positively indicated, along with exhalation stillpoint processes.

Autonomic Effects

With venous sinus processes, clients may experience autonomic effects such as nausea, other digestive symptoms, and heart palpitations. Unresolved jugular foramen compressive issues affecting the vagus nerve are the probable cause of these kinds of responses. Also, increased fluid flow can place temporary pressure on the vagus nerve, generating vagal responses from the viscera and elsewhere. Unresolved jugular foramen issues can also generate headaches and cranial nerve responses due to backpressure. Backpressure or change of pressure can even affect the orbital nerves passing through the cavernous sinus, leading to temporary visual distortions such as blurring. Autonomic effects may also relate to unresolved intraosseous occipital issues or nerve facilitation in brain stem autonomic nuclei that was activated and not resolved. All of these can be noted and treated in subsequent session work. Educate clients about these possibilities to help them understand their experiences.

Toxic Release

Increased fluid fluctuation and fluid flow, and a related intensifying of potency in the fluids, may encourage the processing of toxicity. Cleansing of toxic material can temporarily give rise to nausea, joint pain, and digestive issues. Tell clients to drink eight glasses of pure water each day for at least three days after this work. Reducing toxic intake, such as cigarettes and alcohol, is highly recommended.

First Aid

Venous sinus work, along with the use of stillpoints, is classically used as first aid for acute episodes of migraine, vertigo, inflammation, and fever. These processes can also be an important aspect of ignition of potency in the fluid system generally, and the third ventricle specifically, as described in Foundations Volume One.

CHAPTER 13

Facial Dynamics

The next few chapters explore the relationships of the face, the hard palate, and the temporomandibular joints. This completes our journey of exploration oriented to the tissues of the cranium. The face and hard palate are obviously not separate from the dynamics of the cranium and body as a whole, and their dynamics are deeply integrated with those of the cranial base and cranial bowl.

Introduction

The bony structures of the face and hard palate can be considered to be hanging off the cranial bowl, suspended from the frontal and sphenoid bones. The bones of the face and hard palate will mirror the sphenoid bone in motion and positioning (Figure 13.1).

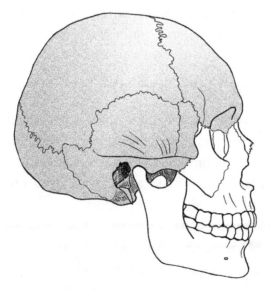

Figure 13.1. The facial structures are suspended from the cranial bowl.

The cranial bowl, face, and hard palate are a unified field. Inertial patterns found in the cranial bowl will be reflected in the face and hard palate. Similarly, inertial patterns in facial and hard-palate dynamics will be mirrored in the dynamics of the cranial bowl. There is thus a direct and interactive reciprocal relationship between the cranial base and the face and hard palate—what happens in one area will affect the other. For this reason, awareness of the dynamics of the cranial base, as explored in Chapter 11, is a prerequisite for approaching the face and hard palate.

To learn about the face and hard palate we will be using a series of clinical explorations designed to provide a clear experience of the relationships involved. These are not treatment protocols; they are explorations set up as a learning process. As you build experience and awareness of these relationships, they will naturally present themselves as the inherent treatment plan deepens and unfolds.

The frontal bone, sphenoid, ethmoid, maxillae, palatines, vomer, and mandible are all integral parts of the wider tissue field, which expresses its motility as a whole, and are thus part of a much wider dynamic. This becomes clear as the holistic shift deepens and the suspensory system—physical body suspended in fluid body, suspended in tidal body—clarifies. The facial structures are then clearly sensed to be part of a unified cellular-tissue field suspended in fluid, organized and moved by the tide.

As we orient to the particulars of the face and hard palate, please remember that—unlike sometimes taught—it is not that one bone moves another, or that the membranes move the bones, or that pressure changes move the bones, but rather that cells and tissues are simultaneously organized and moved by the potency in the body's fluids, as a unified, tensile field.

Dynamics Superior to the Hard Palate

We will first orient to the frontal and ethmoid bones. The frontal processes of the maxillae articulate with the frontal bone at the frontal-maxillary suture. The maxillae express their motility and motion as though they are hanging from the frontal bone (Figure 13.2). The maxillae articulate directly to the ethmoid bone and indirectly to the sphenoid via their articulations with the palatine bones and vomer. Inertial fulcrums in superior structures may generate distortions in facial, hard palate, and TMJ relationships because the maxillae cannot hang freely. As we found in previous clinical explorations, inertial fulcrums found in or between any of these structures will affect all others and may manifest as inertial patterns sensed throughout the tissue field.

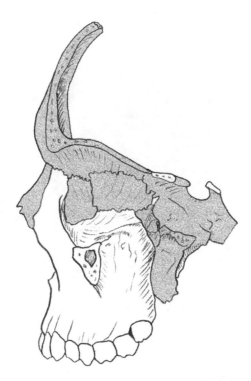

Figure 13.2. The maxillae hang from the frontal bone.

The relationships directly superior to the hard palate that can affect or reflect its dynamics include the sphenoid bone, reciprocal tension membrane, the frontal bone, the ethmoid bone, and orbital structures in general. We will first generally tune into the area above the maxillae. Then we will more specifically relate to the frontal bone, the falx cerebri, the ethmoid bone, and the orbital structures to get a clearer sense of their dynamics. Each orbit of the eyes is composed of seven inter-related bones (Figure 13.3):

- Frontal—"ceiling," or superior wall

- Sphenoid—back and lateral (outside) walls

- Maxilla—floor and part of the medial rim

- Zygomatic—parts of the lateral walls and floor

- Palatine—small part of the posterior floor

- Ethmoid—majority of the medial wall

- Lacrimal—part of the medial wall

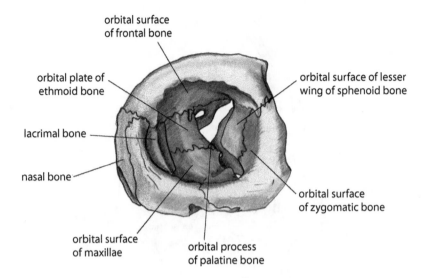

orbital surface
of frontal bone

orbital plate of
ethmoid bone

orbital surface of lesser
wing of sphenoid bone

lacrimal bone

nasal bone

orbital surface
of zygomatic bone

orbital surface
of maxillae

orbital process
of palatine bone

Figure 13.3. Orbital region.

Respectful Awareness

As we approach our exploration into facial structures, please hold respectful awareness for the rich implications of this region, as there may be many resonances of our earliest experiences held in its dynamics. Birth trauma may be reflected in inertial fulcrums and patterning in facial relationships—which must be empathetically held by the practitioner—as may the impact of our earliest prenatal experiences. The frontal-ethmoid area is the terminus of the embryological longitudinal axis, and it is thought by some to hold memory of the implantation of the fertilized egg into the wall of the mother's uterus. I have personally noted this connection to our earliest experiences in client work. Likewise, birthing forces may be fed into facial and hard-palate dynamics and emerge for healing purposes as facial structures are oriented to in session work. Indeed, as you hold the facial dynamics of an adult, it may sometimes feel like you are holding an infant or even a fetus in your hands.

Facial dynamics are also very much part of the polyvagal system, whose social engagement system, discussed in Chapter 19, mediates relational interchange throughout life. Facial structures are thus intimately related to early relational experiences and attachment processes, as discussed in Chapters 2 and 3. Facial structures will reflect our inner sense of self-worth, how we feel we appear to others, how we communicate to those in our relational world, and how we feel received and responded to in that interchange.

The pineal-pituitary axis through the third ventricle is also just posterior to this area, so inertia here may extend into the neuroendocrine-immune realm. The prefrontal cortex of the brain is posterior to the frontal bone, relates to present-time awareness, and is part of sophisticated stress responses.

Finally, more esoterically the area between the eyebrows is considered to be related to the sixth chakra or ajana chakra, relating to self-understanding and spiritual union. It is also where the primal midline exits the body as it spirals and merges with the wider ordering field. For all these reasons, this is an area that deserves to be approached with respect and sensitive negotiation.

Explorations:
Orbital Relationships _____

The intention of the following explorations is to attune to the motility of the orbital region and begin to appreciate both its specific dynamics and its relationship to the hard palate below. After negotiating your relationship to the client's system as usual, and after the holistic shift has deepened, you will first use the vault hold as a vantage point and then shift to a new hold, the orbital hold.

Starting the Session

Start the session as usual; stand at the side of the treatment table and orient first to primary respiration in your own system and then to the client's midline and primary respiration relative to his or her system. Then move to the client's feet; negotiate your contact and relational field and orient to the holistic shift. Remember: "Hands floating on tissues, suspended in fluid, with you and your client both suspended in a wider fluid field." Orient to the three bodies—physical, fluid, and tidal—and wait for the emergence and deepening of the holistic shift.

Vault Hold

With the client still in a supine position, move to the vault hold. Holding a wide perceptual field, negotiate your contact, orient to the physical and fluid bodies, and orient to the clarification of the mid-tide. Sense the fluid tide and its quality of drive.

Then include the tissues and their motility in your awareness. Sense the expression of motility in the cranial bowl, and then orient to the frontal and orbital areas anterior to your hold. Do not narrow your perceptual field as you do this. From this vantage point you may sense tissue motility and particular inertial fulcrums and related motion and tension patterns.

Orbital Hold

From the vault hold change your hand position to an orbital hold to sense the general relationships of the orbital area and its expression of motility and motion. Still sitting at the head of the table, place your palms over the client's frontal area and form a "V" with your thumbs gently touching the glabella area between the eyebrows. Spread your other fingers over the maxillae and zygomatic bones (the cheek bones) (Figure 13.4).

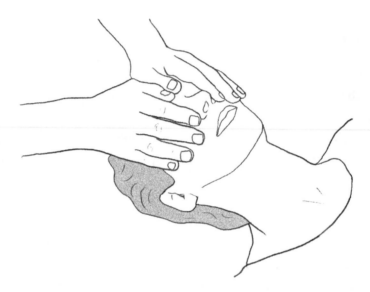

Figure 13.4. Orbital hold.

From this vantage point, orient to the motility of the tissues in the orbital area. Can you sense cells and tissues literally being breathed in the cycles of the tide? As you listen, you may sense a general widening and narrowing of the orbits in inhalation and exhalation. As the sphenoid expresses inhalation, the orbit widens obliquely and becomes shallower. The opposite occurs in exhalation.

Notice any inertial fulcrums and patterns that begin to clarify in your perception. Orient to any level of healing process that emerges. Remember Becker's three-phase awareness—seeking, settling/state of balance, and reorganization-realignment. Orient to a deepening stillness in the equilibrium accessed. Listen for manifestations of healing intentions in the stillness, such as expressions of potency, Long Tide, or Dynamic Stillness. Wait for a sense of softening and expansion of the relationships. Listen for reorganization of tissue structures and realignment to the primal midline and to natural fulcrums such as the SBJ and Sutherland's fulcrum. Notice how the tissues express motility and the quality of fluid tide now present.

Frontal Relationships

The orbital hold can provide a wealth of information about the frontal area. General information can include overall relational symmetry and orientation to the midline and how the tissues are expressing their inner breath, or motility. Any pattern of expression not clearly oriented to Sutherland's fulcrum, the SBJ, or the primal midline, is organized around an inertial fulcrum of some sort. You may have noticed inertial patterns such as tensile motions and forms, and/or fluid fluctuations organized around other areas of the cranium, the hard palate, or anywhere in the rest of the body. For example, orbital motility may generally move around a sutural relationship of the frontal bone due to a compressive force or inertial fulcrum located between it and another bone.

The frontal bone expresses its motility and motion as though it is two bones, reflecting its state at birth. The suture between the two parts is called the metopic suture. This suture gradually fuses to form a single bone although the metopic suture is still partially or wholly present in some adults. Again, as in all bony forms, the motility of the frontal bone has a fluid, flower-petal quality to it, oriented to the SBJ and Sutherland's fulcrum as part of the wider motility of the whole cranium. In the inhalation phase, the

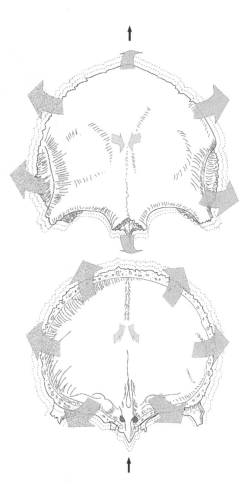

Figure 13.5. The motility and motion of the frontal bone in inhalation.

lateral aspects of the frontal bone move anteriorly while the glabella area moves posteriorly as though there is still a hinge at the fused metopic suture (Figure 13.5).

The frontal bone has a number of direct relationships that can affect hard-palate dynamics. Among others, these include its articulation with the maxillae and ethmoid bone. The ethmoid bone literally hangs from the frontal bone in its ethmoid notch. The ethmoid's crista galli anchors the falx cerebri through this notch. This relationship creates a direct link between the structures of the face and the dural membrane system, and inertial patterns and related tensions on either side can be reciprocally transferred. Both the frontal and ethmoid bones also articulate with the sphenoid bone and will reflect cranial base patterning. Because of this continuity of relationship, the dynamics of the frontal, sphenoid, and ethmoid bones will directly affect the hard palate below (Figure 13.6).

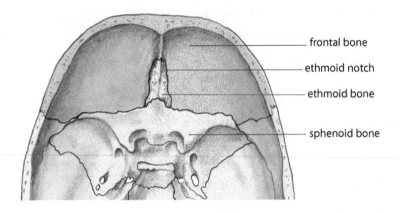

frontal bone

ethmoid notch

ethmoid bone

sphenoid bone

Figure 13.6. The relationship of frontal bone to the ethmoid and sphenoid in the cranial base.

Indirect relationships will also be a factor in facial and hard-palate dynamics. Inertial fulcrums and patterns located in other parts of the system can be transferred to the frontal bone, ethmoid, vomer, and hard palate in various ways. For instance, an inertia fulcrum in a sacroiliac joint may generate tension through the dural membrane system, which may then be transferred to the frontal-ethmoid area, generating compression in its relationships. As you orient to facial specifics, remember the wider context—the body is a holistic form suspended in a wider fluidic-tidal field. Also remember that the fulcrum organizing an inertial facial pattern may be remote to its local dynamics.

Explorations:
Frontal Bone Relationships _____

In these explorations, we will first orient to the frontal bone as described in Volume One, and then shift to a frontal-occipital hold for a wider sense of the relationships and dynamics of the area. The intention is to explore the relationships directly above and behind the ethmoid bone and facial structures in general—the frontal bone, falx, and occiput. Any inertial issues in these relationships will obviously affect facial motility and dynamics.

Frontal Hold

Start as usual at the side of the table and then move to the client's feet. After the holistic shift has deepened, move to the frontal bone hold, as discussed in Foundations Volume One. Place your elbows on the treatment table above the client's head. These serve as fulcrums that allow your hands to float on the tissues of the frontal bone. Then place your hands over the frontal bone with your thumbs crossed and your fingers in gentle contact with its anterior and lateral aspects—fingertips just overlapping the orbital ridge. Your thumbs are fulcrums for your palms and fingers, stabilizing each other where they are crossed and enabling both hands to function as one unit. Contact is all along the fingers and upper palm, not just at the fingertips.

With hands suspended in fluid, orient to primary respiration and motility of the frontal bone, the glabella area, and ethmoid bone. See if any inertial patterns clarify, involving any combination of frontal, ethmoid, and/or falx cerebri. Orient to healing processes as they emerge and to any reorganization that occurs.

Frontal-Occipital Hold

Shift your contact to a frontal-occipital hold. One hand holds the occiput, fingers spread and pointing caudal. Balance the occiput on this hand, without putting pressure on it with the heel of your hand. Your other hand is placed over the frontal bone with fingers spread, also pointing caudal, supported by your elbow on the treatment table. Your fingertips are just below the orbital ridges of the eyes. Your gentle contact is all along the fingers, not just at the fingertips. Orient to the physical and fluid bodies and mid-tide level of expression. First let the fluid tide come to you and then include the tissues in your awareness. Include the falx from the ethmoid all the way to the back and base of the occiput in your orientation (Figure 13.7).

From this vantage point, allow the reciprocal tension membrane to come into your awareness. Can you sense the reciprocal tension motion of the falx and the frontal and occiput bones? Do not overfocus; maintain your wide perceptual field and let these motions come to you.

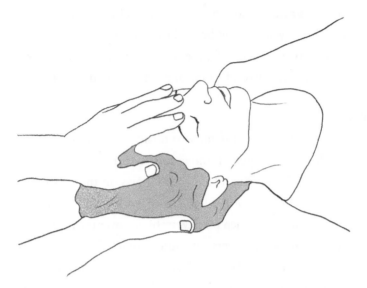

Figure 13.7. Frontal-occipital hold.

As you sense motility, does there seem to be a balanced relationship between the bones and membrane system? Does there seem to be a clear orientation to Sutherland's fulcrum? If an inertial pattern clarifies, orient to the emergence of healing intentions, and for a reorganization of the tissues and fluids to their natural fulcrums and the midline. How has the system responded to the work? Do you sense a shift to a more balanced relationship to Sutherland's fulcrum? Is the fluid tide stronger? Is there clearer organization of motility around the primal midline?

Augmentation of Space—the Ethmoid Notch

The ethmoid bone hangs from the ethmoid notch of the frontal bone and its crista galli passes through this opening to anchor the falx. If the falx is holding a contractive tension pattern, the ethmoid may become compressed into the notch. This may reduce the expression of motility of both ethmoid and frontal bones. Alternatively, if the ethmoid bone is compressed into the ethmoid notch due to trauma of some kind—birth trauma is an example—then a dragging force may be introduced into the membrane system that can affect the dynamics of the sacrum and pelvis below. The next hand position offers a more specific awareness of the ethmoid notch of the frontal bone and can be useful as a vantage point when deeply compressive forces are present. I find I rarely need to use this particular augmentation process, but in severely compressed circumstances it can be of use. Thus the intention of the following exploration is to access and augment space in the relationships of the ethmoid notch.

Let's imagine that, in the frontal bone hold or frontal-occipital hold, you sensed an intransigent compressive fulcrum in the ethmoid notch area. Change your hand position to an ethmoid notch hold. I find it easiest to work standing at the head of the treatment table while stabilizing my body against it. I also stabilize my arms by keeping my elbows in contact with my body. In this standing position, lightly place one thumb over the glabella area, just above the nasal bones. Place your other thumb over the first with your fingers along the lateral aspects of the frontal bone (Figure 13.8). Negotiate your contact with the client's system and orient to the physical and fluid bodies. Allow the fluid tide to clarify. Then orient to tissue motility and the dynamics of the ethmoid notch. Ideally, during inhalation, the frontal-ethmoid area will seem to settle posterior as the sides of the frontal bone widen out. As this occurs, the ethmoid notch subtly widens. As described in Volume One, in the mid-tide this feels like a fluid widening of the tissue-flower petals of the cranium.

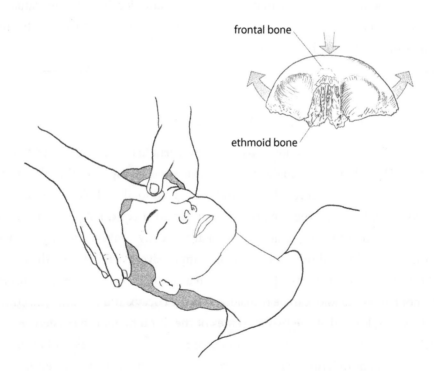

frontal bone

ethmoid bone

Figure 13.8. Augmentation of space in the ethmoid notch.

Allow your fingers and hands to feel fluidic and to be suspended in a wider fluid field. At the height of inhalation, allow your fingers—which are suspended in the fluid tide—to be moved or breathed by the tide. Basically your fingers are resonating with the tidal motion and the expression of tissue motility at the height of inhalation. Again, if no tide is expressed, allow your fingers, suspended in fluid, to resonate with the natural space present and to take a deeper breath as though the tide is moving them. This augments the tissues' relationship to the natural augmentation of space at the height of inhalation.

As space is augmented in the relationship, deepen into stillness and allow forces to enter equilibrium. In your wide perceptual field, be open to any level of healing process that emerges and listen for expressions of potency and forces at work in the area. As these are expressed, you may sense a processing of inertial forces and an expansion across the ethmoid notch. This may be perceived as a softening and spreading of the ethmoid notch and clearer ethmoid motility.

You may also sense a freeing up of the relationship between the frontal bone and the ethmoid bone. If the compressive issue was very dense and chronic, the ethmoid bone may not have been expressing much motility at all. As inertial forces resolve, you may sense a powerful surge during the inhalation phase and a clarification of the primal midline as it spirals anterior through the cranial base and glabella area. Listen for a reorganization of the tissues and a more balanced motility relative to the midline.

Relationships of the Ethmoid Bone

Having explored wider relationships, let's now orient to the ethmoid bone more specifically. Directly attached to the most anterior-superior aspect of the falx, ethmoid bone dynamics are integrated with, and connected to, the whole of the reciprocal tension membrane all the way to the sacrum and coccyx. Patterns anywhere in this continuum of bone, tissue, and fluid are directly conveyed to any other part of the system. Inertial fulcrums, such as compressive issues between the ethmoid and frontal bone, or inertial patterns, such as torsion and side-bending between ethmoid and sphenoid, can be transferred to the coccyx and sacrum. The ethmoid and coccyx, located at the two extremes of the dural membrane system, are also embryologically paired as the two poles of the primitive streak and notochord. Randolph Stone described a direct energetic relationship between the ethmoid and coccyx: each reflects the other (Stone 1999). The ethmoid is also the site of unusual properties relating to orientation in space, because it has one of the richest concentrations of biogenic magnetite in the body. This substance responds to the earth's magnetic field, and is thought to be a factor in orienting and homing instincts as well as sensitivity to electromagnetic fields in general (Kirschvink, Winklhoger, and Walker 2010).

In mystic traditions, the ethmoid bone is considered to have important esoteric functions. It is a very light and airy bone. Its lateral masses contain spacious air cells that are considered to be an important interface between the energies of the outside world and the life force within. The outer breath of the air meets the inner breath of primary respiration in the ethmoid. This brings the *prana* in the air into relationship with the prana of the sixth chakra located in the third ventricle, just posterior to the ethmoid. In many spiritual traditions, this area is a focus of meditative practices as a gateway to spirit and source. It is also the exit point of the primal midline as it merges into the wider bioelectric field. I point all this out to encourage you to treat this area with utmost respect and humility.

As introduced above, common inertial patterns related to ethmoid dynamics include compression in the ethmoid notch of the frontal bone, compressive patterns in relationship to the sphenoid bone, the maxillae, and vomer, and compressive orbital patterns. You may also sense patterns of torsion and side-bending in the ethmoid's relationship to the sphenoid bone. Traumatic forces generated by falls on the coccyx may also generate ethmoid bone compression. As potency spirals in to center traumatic forces in the coccygeal area, dural membrane is pulled inferior toward the inertial fulcrum being generated in the pelvis, and pressure is then created at the superior pole at the ethmoid notch. The traumatic force is laterally transferred to the ethmoid via the continuity of fluid and membranous relationship.

Ethmoid Bone Motility

Classically, the motility of the ethmoid bone is described as a reciprocal rotation and widening-narrowing around a transverse axis. As with all midline bones, its rotational motion mirrors that of the sphenoid. In inhalation, as the falx narrows front-to-back and the sphenoid rotates anterior-posterior, the ethmoid (1) rotates in the opposite direction to the sphenoid, (2) while its lateral masses and air cells widen, and (3) its anterior end shifts superior-posterior as part of the general anterior-posterior shortening of the cranium (Figure 13.9).

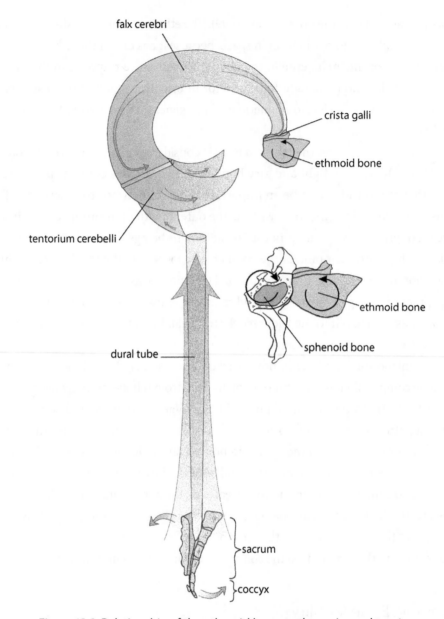

Figure 13.9. Relationship of the ethmoid bone to the reciprocal tension membrane in the inhalation phase.

Inertial Ethmoid Patterns

All potential inertial patterns in the cranial base (between the occiput and the sphenoid) can also occur between the sphenoid and ethmoid bone. Classically, these include patterns of fixation in five categories:

- Compression occurs when the two bones have been forced together

- Torsion occurs when two bones have rotated in opposite directions around an anterior-posterior axis

- Side-bending occurs when the two bones have rotated in opposite directions around vertical axes

- Lateral shear occurs when they have rotated in the same direction around vertical axes

- Vertical shear occurs if the two bones have been forced to rotate in the same direction around vertical axes (Figure 13.10)

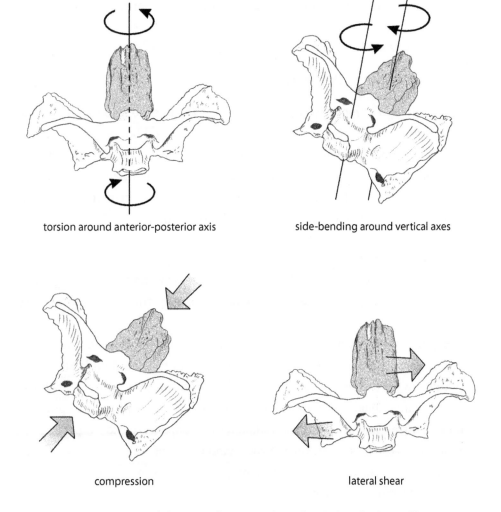

torsion around anterior-posterior axis

side-bending around vertical axes

compression

lateral shear

Figure 13.10. Inertial dynamics between the sphenoid and ethmoid bones.

All of these patterns of fixation are factors of the unresolved inertial forces still present in the system, affecting the relationships of bones, membranes, and connective tissues.

Patterns in the cranial base and between the sphenoid and ethmoid are fully interdependent. Patterns expressed behind the sphenoid—between it and the occiput—may also manifest in front of the sphenoid as sphenoid-ethmoid patterns, and in the hard palate below. Patterns may be generated in either direction—the ethmoid and hard palate below influencing the cranial base, or vice versa.

We are expanding our view of the ethmoid to embrace new relationships, including the maxillae and the nasal bones, in addition to continuing our interest in the frontal bone and the sphenoid. Sphenoid-ethmoid-frontal relationships need to be relatively fluid and free in their expression for the maxillae and the hard palate to hang with ease from the orbital processes at the frontal bone.

Explorations:
Sphenoid-Ethmoid and Orbital Relationships _____

In the next few explorations, we will contact the nasal bones to explore the relationships between the frontal bone, ethmoid, nasal bones, and maxillae. Please remember that these are not treatment protocols. The intention here is to become familiar with these relationships so that we can orient to them as the inherent treatment plan unfolds. We start with a general orientation and then narrow our inquiry to the sphenoid and ethmoid bones.

General Orientation

In this first exploration, the intention is to orient to and sense the general dynamics of motility expressed in frontal, sphenoid, ethmoid, and maxillary relationships.

Begin as usual with the client in the supine position; orient to the holistic shift at the feet, then move to the vault hold. Orient to the fluid tide and tissue motility. In your wide perceptual field, include an awareness of the frontal bone, ethmoid, and orbital area. Orient to motility in the phases of primary respiration. Take your time and see if any inertial pattern organized around the ethmoid or orbital areas clarifies. Then change your hand position.

Sit at the cephalad corner of the treatment table. Very gently contact the frontal bone at its lateral aspects with your thumb at one lateral aspect and the pads of the fingers of the same hand at the other. With your other hand's thumb and index finger, lightly hold the nasal bones near their articulation with the frontal bone. Elbow support can be very helpful for this (Figure 13.11).

In this position, orient to the overall motility of these tissues—the frontal bone, sphenoid, ethmoid, nasal bones, and the orbital processes of the maxillae. As the frontal bone expresses inhalation, you might also sense the nasal bones and maxillae doing the same. This may be sensed as a widening and filling in inhalation and the reverse in exhalation. You may also sense that, as the sphenoid bone expresses inhalation and dives anterior-inferior, the ethmoid expresses its motility in the opposite direction. Orient to any inertial patterns in these overall relationships that clarify. Sense the priority arising in the fluids and tissues. Orient to the state of balance and deepening equilibrium, the expression of potency, and whatever level of healing process emerges. As inertial forces are resolved, listen for qualities of softening, spreading, and reorganization of tissues in the area.

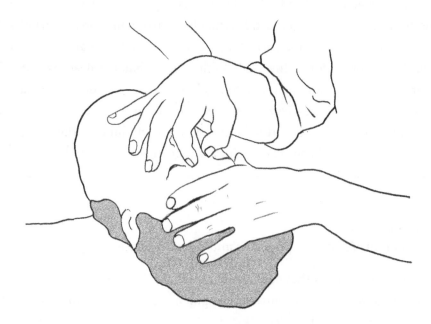

Figure 13.11. Frontal-ethmoid hold.

Specific Orientation to Sphenoid and Ethmoid Relationships

In this further exploration, you use a similar hand hold as above, but orient more specifically to the sphenoid and ethmoid bones, their motility, and any inertial issues or patterns that clarify.

Start as above and again move to the vault hold. First orient to the motility of the cranial bowl and then hold the sphenoid and ethmoid in your awareness. From here, gently place the thumb and index finger of one hand on either side of the nasal bones near their articulation with the frontal bone. Place your other hand over the lateral aspects of the greater wings of the sphenoid bone. If your hand is too small to actually reach the greater wings, you can still perceive the greater wings via the lateral aspects of the frontal bone, as in the hold above. Negotiate your contact and orient to the physical and fluid bodies and mid-tide.

In this position, orient to the motility of the sphenoid and ethmoid bones in the inhalation-exhalation phases of primary respiration. Settle into your listening and allow things to clarify. As above, you may sense that, as the sphenoid bone dives anterior-inferior in inhalation, the ethmoid expresses its motility in the opposite direction.

You may notice one or more of the patterns described above, including compression, torsion, side-bending, and shear. As any of these clarify, orient to the inertial fulcrum that generates it. This may be local or remote to its dynamics. As the healing process clarifies, orient to an emergent state of balance—a dynamic equilibrium of the forces involved. As the state of balance deepens, listen for expressions of potency and orient to any level of healing process that clarifies. As inertial forces are resolved, the tissue field will naturally soften and expand, reorganize, and realign to natural fulcrums and the midline. As this occurs, you may sense the ethmoid bone expressing a deeper and clearer motility and motion.

Exploration:
Augmentation of Space in Spheno-Ethmoid Relationships _____

If the inertial forces that generate compression between the sphenoid and ethmoid bones are very dense, the augmentation of space in their sutural relationship may be of service.

Maintaining the same hold as above, orient to the inhalation and exhalation phases of the mid-tide. At the height of inhalation, allow your fingers to be suspended in fluid and breathed by the tide and its potency. It is as though your hands and fingers are resonating with and moved by the rising of the tide, and your fingers at the nasal bones rise anterior—it's almost like they are moved anterior as they attune to the rising of the primal midline (Figure 13.12).

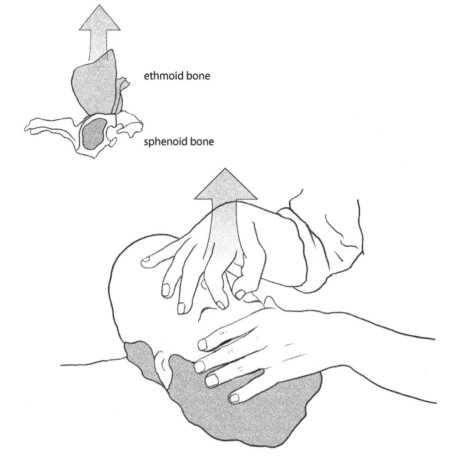

ethmoid bone

sphenoid bone

Figure 13.12. Augmentation of space in sphenoid and ethmoid relationships.

When space is accessed, orient to any level of healing process that emerges. Wait for a sense of softening, disengagement, and expansion in these relationships. The ethmoid may be sensed to float anteriorly toward the ceiling.

If the ethmoid seems chronically compressed and congested, you may sense a sudden surge of motion at the ethmoid and a sense of greatly improved motility throughout the whole system. The client sometimes perceives that a long-term sense of pressure is being resolved. This can have a revitalizing effect on the whole system due to the ethmoid's strategic position at the anterior-superior pole of the membrane system and the primal midline.

CHAPTER 14

The Hard Palate

Having explored the relationships superior to the hard palate, we are ready to approach the vomer, maxillae, and palatines. The maxillae make up the front of the hard palate and the palatines the rear. The sphenoid bone, vomer, maxillae, and palatine bones are mutually interdependent in their motility and dynamics. The phrase *spheno-maxillary complex* is commonly used to acknowledge this unified quality.

The Motility of the Spheno-Maxillary Complex

The maxillae and palatine bones articulate with the sphenoid at its pterygoid processes. The vomer articulates with the body of the sphenoid above and the maxillae below (Figures 14.1a and 14.1b). In gliding articulations, the palatine and vomer meet the sphenoid, protecting the cranial base from impacts of biting, chewing, and talking. Sutherland called the palatines and the vomer *speed reducers* because of this function. Think of them more as *amplitude reducers,* as their gliding articulations reduce the forces generated by the physical motion of the mouth (Figure 14.2).

Descriptions of individual bony motility are at best approximations of reality, giving practitioners a chance to break down a unit of function into its particulars. Traditionally, movements of this area have been described in terms of each bone's axis of rotation in flexion and extension phases. But bones don't really move around axes of rotation; they express a unified intraosseous widening and a unified narrowing in the phases of the tide and in relation to each other. As in our earlier metaphor, they are more like fluid flower petals manifesting an inner fluidic breath. The relatively free or restricted mobility of the bones relative to each other is a function of the space generated in sutures and joints in the inhalation phase of the tide. As the sphenoid expresses its inhalation, the following interdependent patterns of motility occur (Figures 14.3 and 14.4).

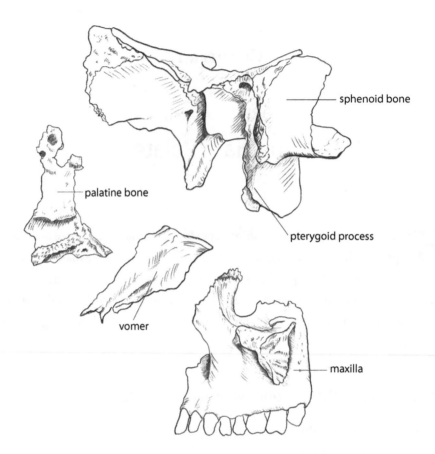

Figure 14.1a. Sphenoid bone, palatine bone, vomer, and maxilla (disarticulated).

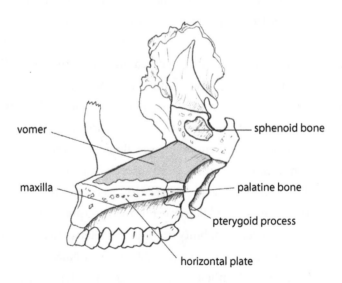

Figure 14.1b. The relationships of the hard palate.

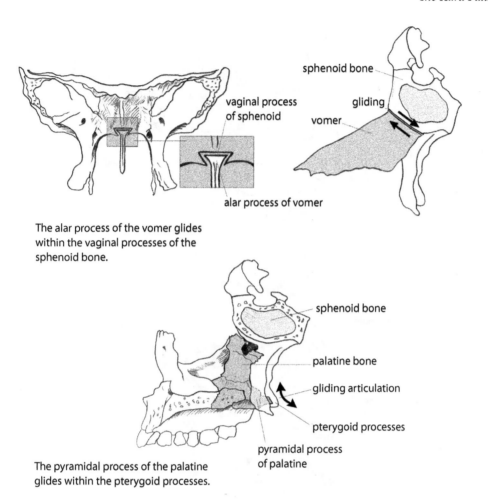

vaginal process of sphenoid

alar process of vomer

sphenoid bone

gliding

vomer

The alar process of the vomer glides within the vaginal processes of the sphenoid bone.

sphenoid bone

palatine bone

gliding articulation

pterygoid processes

pyramidal process of palatine

The pyramidal process of the palatine glides within the pterygoid processes.

Figure 14.2. Speed or amplitude reducers.

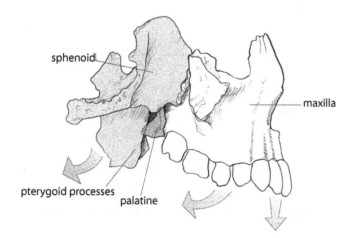

sphenoid

maxilla

pterygoid processes

palatine

Figure 14.3. Movement of the hard palate in the inhalation phase.

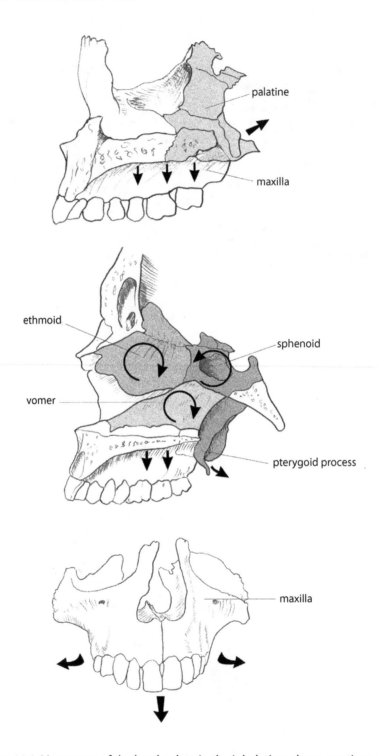

Figure 14.4. Movement of the hard palate in the inhalation phase, continued.

Motility of the Maxillae

If all articular relationships around the maxillae are relatively free, the maxillae express their motion as though they are suspended from the frontal bone. In inhalation, the horizontal plates of the maxillae drop inferiorly as the rear of the vomer descends at the interpalatine suture. The arch of the hard palate flattens and widens. The palatine bones mirror this as they move inferiorly and laterally at their horizontal plates.

Motility of the Palatines

The palatine bones lie between the pterygoid plates of the sphenoid at the rear and the maxillae at the front. The anterior aspects of their horizontal plates overlap the horizontal plates of the maxillae in shelf-like articulations. Posteriorly, their pyramidal processes articulate with the pterygoid processes of the sphenoid bone. Each palatine rests in the groove between the medial and lateral pterygoid plates. In the inhalation phase, the pterygoid processes widen apart and rotate in an inferior-posterior direction. As this occurs, the pyramidal process of the palatine bones glide between the pterygoid processes and move inferiorly and laterally as part of the lowering of the hard palate in inhalation. The inhalation motion of the palatine bone is integrated with that of the vomer as it descends inferiorly onto the hard palate.

The gliding action of the palatine bone between the pterygoid processes of the sphenoid is extremely important. Compressive issues between the pyramidal processes of the palatines and the pterygoid processes of the sphenoid can compromise the amplitude reduction inherent in the joint. This will generate inertial fulcrums directly affecting the cranial base and may also impact the spheno-palatine ganglion—an important ganglion with connections to the facial and trigeminal nerves, lying just anterior to the ptyergoid processes. I have treated clients who have had compressive issues in this area generating various kinds of pain, including headaches, facial pain, and trigeminal neuralgia.

Motility of the Vomer

The vomer articulates with the maxillae, the sphenoid, and the ethmoid bones. The alar surface of the vomer is flared open and articulates with the rails of the vaginal processes of the sphenoid. As the sphenoid expresses inhalation, the vomer rotates in the opposite direction in a gliding action. Chewing motions are absorbed and dispersed similar to the palatine-pterygoid process action. In inhalation, as the vomer rotates in the opposite direction to the sphenoid bone, its inferior-posterior aspect descends inferiorly at the rear of the hard palate. As the sphenoid expresses inhalation, the inferior-posterior aspect of the vomer descends toward the hard palate as the horizontal plates of the maxillae and palatines lower and widen transversely.

Contact and Intimacy in Intra-Oral Work

Orienting to the hard palate may involve finger placement inside the client's mouth. Here we are literally entering the client's body. We are venturing into an extremely sensitive psycho-emotional area, and due caution and empathy are needed. The mouth directly registers our experiences of getting our most fundamental needs met. Termed *oral needs* in neo-Reichian psychotherapies, these begin in the womb and are highlighted immediately at birth with the baby's securing of maternal bonding and protection through nursing. The baby may perceive lack of contact and bonding after birth as life threatening, so the oral impulses have a tremendous emotional urgency from the very beginning. Taste and smell are strong senses at birth, and babies and young children will constantly place things into their mouth as they explore their world. The experience of oral needs continues throughout life with essential nourishment both physically and psycho-emotionally.

The mouth is our life-preserving interface with the outside world, first with mother and with food as we get older. The mouth also plays a survival role as the vehicle for verbal communication, the baby's primary way to alert caregivers of needs and later the medium of social communication. The mouth plays crucial roles in eating for comfort, expression of feelings, and sexual contact and gratification. It may also be a focus for sexuality and abuse issues.

Problems with expressing our needs and emotions can show up as tension in the mouth area. Oral needs can become so charged that the issues involved may lead to eating disorders such as anorexia, bulimia, and obesity. The mouth is extremely sensitive, with a highly disproportionate supply of sensory and motor nerves in its tissues. Several psychology systems, especially neo-Reichian forms, note the reflex relationship between oral needs, the mouth, and the pelvis—a view also advanced in Stone's polarity therapy. Thus the mouth can hold tensions and emotional charge relating to sexuality, including traumatic experiences and abuse.

I know from clinical experience that issues of abuse, abandonment, and rejection can all generate tissue tensions and psycho-emotional charge in the mouth area. Tissues of the hard palate and jaw can hold memories of experiences that may not be directly related to the physical dynamics of the mouth. These include a whole range of factors that all relate to our ability to get our needs met and our sense of safety with intimate contact and close relationships.

Dental experience is another reason to approach intra-oral contact cautiously. Many people have had dental experiences that are unpleasant and even traumatic. These can be restimulated by having a practitioner's fingers inside a client's mouth.

When you need to place your fingers in a person's mouth, the first priority is to communicate what you are doing and why it is necessary. Approach the work delicately, with respect and slow pacing. Give the client power and control in the situation. Explain the work to the client before doing it and give a clear sense of choice and options. I also work out a code, such as a hand signal, so the client can easily indicate when to stop. The important thing here is to be conscious of the issues and to approach things slowly, with awareness of the full implications. As in all of our work, we are not imposing our will onto a person's system, but rather we are helping to open doors and windows that have perhaps been forgotten.

Surgical gloves or finger cots are used in all intra-oral work, including every application in this chapter. These are widely available at pharmacies, drug stores, or medical supply companies.

Tuning to the Dynamics

In the first exploration we simply orient to the motility of the sphenoid bone and hard palate to see if we can sense sphenoid-maxilla and sphenoid-vomer interdependent motility. We will use two different holds to approach these. The intention is to become familiar with this area generally, before moving to specifics. Repeated practice is highly recommended, using numerous study sessions to develop the capacity to accurately orient to and visualize this fairly complex set of interrelationships. By having lots of practice with this sensitive area, the practitioner will be able to more comfortably hold a neutral space for clients in actual clinical practice.

Remember, as we enter these clinical explorations oriented to motility, to hold all three bodies—physical, fluid, and tidal bodies—in your wide perceptual field. The tidal body is the overall field that the Long Tide generates, the fluid body is the field of body fluids and the potency within it, and the physical body is the interdependent form and motility of the cellular-tissue field. As you hold this wide perceptual field orient to the fluid and physical bodies and the fluid tide—as it manifests in the fluid body—and tissue motility as it manifests in the physical body. This is the territory of the mid-tide, the tidal phenomenon generated by the potency manifesting in the fluid and physical bodies. Notice the quality, form, and overall orientation of tissue motility to the primal midline. Remember also to use the metaphor of the bones as fluid-tissue flower petals suspended in a wider fluid field.

Also remember the delicacy of placing your fingers in another person's mouth. Tell the client why you are entering the mouth, work slowly, and empower the client to say no at any time. Orient the client to a hand signal that can be used to mean "take your fingers out of my mouth!" Give clients the option of not doing the work if it is initially too charged for them. Chapters on trauma, central nervous system activation, and related trauma skills are presented later in this volume and can be very important in all of our work. Commonly, skills such as slow pacing and cultivation of resources come into play when we work in this area.

In all of the following hard-palate holds, be sure that elbow fulcrums support both of your hands. These holds can be created in either a sitting or standing position. If I sit near the head-end of the table, I rest my elbows on small cushions placed on the table so that tension doesn't build in my hands as I work. If standing, I commonly place my caudal foot on a chair or stool near the head of the table, and place the elbow of my caudal hand—which will be placed in the client's mouth—on my thigh near to my knee, creating an elbow fulcrum for my hand. I brace the elbow of my cephalad hand—the one resting on the sphenoid-frontal bone—against my body, again creating elbow support. These elbow fulcrums allow my hands to float on tissues suspended in a wider fluid field, without generating tension in my hand or arm, and also clarifies my contact with the client's system and gives the client's system stable reference points

Exploration:
The Sphenoid-Maxillary Hold _____

Start as usual with the client in the supine position; move to the feet, and after the holistic shift deepens, move to the head of the table and the following hold. Place one hand over the frontal bone so that your thumb is over one sphenoid greater wing and your index or middle finger is over the other. If you cannot reach the two greater wings, you can still sense them from the lateral aspects of the frontal bone. Place the palmar surfaces of the index and middle fingers of your other hand so that they are touching the biting surfaces of the upper teeth. Be sure that you are over the rear molars. Your fingers form a V-shape as they span the alveolar arch. Place them as far back as possible without eliciting a gag response. Again, allow your hands—supported by your elbows—to soften, floating on the tissues, suspended in fluid (Figure 14.5a).

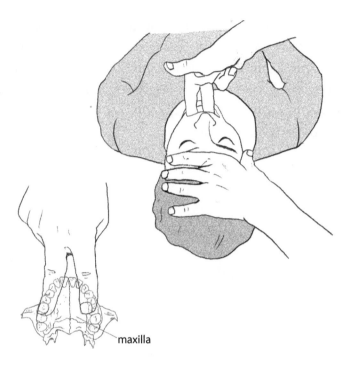

maxilla

Figure 14.5a. Sphenoid-maxillary hold.

Orient to a wide perceptual field, holding the physical and fluid bodies in your awareness. See if you can sense the motility of the sphenoid and the maxillae clarify in the mid-tide as a unified and integrated dynamic. In inhalation, the hard palate ideally lowers—especially at its rear aspect—and the alveolar arch widens apart. As your fingers contact the upper teeth, you may sense a widening between your fingers and lowering of the rear of the palate. Maintain a wide perceptual field as you listen to motility. Do not narrow your intention; let the tissues and their motility come to you.

If an inertial pattern clarifies, orient to its organizing fulcrum, to the state of balance, to the action of potency, and any level of healing process that emerges, and for the reorganization of tissues to the midline.

Exploration:
The Sphenoid-Vomer Hold

From the hold described above, remove your fingers from the client's mouth. Again orient them to your next hold, the sphenoid-vomer hold. With your cephalic hand still over the frontal area and greater wings, place the index finger of your caudal hand over the midline of the hard palate, touching the underside of the interpalatine suture. The inferior end of the vomer is directly above your contact. Some people have a bump at the roof of the mouth, where the vomer is pressing upon the suture. This is an expression of compressive forces and implies restricted motility (Figure 14.5b).

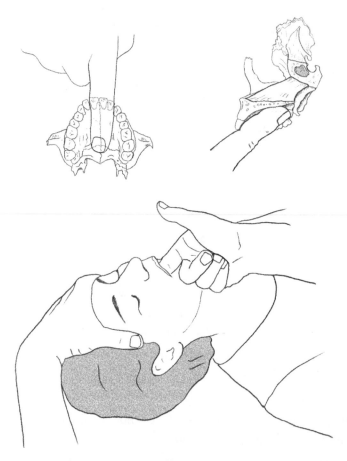

Figure 14.5b. Sphenoid-vomer hold.

In your wide perceptual field, orient to the fluid tide and tissue motility. See if you can sense the unified and integrated tissue motility of the sphenoid bone and vomer. In inhalation, the vomer descends upon the rear of the hard palate as the alveolar arch widens. You may sense this as a subtle pressure on your finger. Maintain a wide perceptual field as you do this. Do not narrow your intention; let the tissues and their motility come to you.

As above, if an inertial pattern clarifies, orient to the arising healing process, and for the reorganization of tissue structures to the midline. Finish with an integrative hold (sacrum, sacrum-occiput, etc.)

Compressive Issues in the Hard Palate

These next sections explore compressive forces and their impact on hard-palate dynamics. If compressive forces are present, they commonly mask other inertial patterns such as torsion or shearing patterns and/or bind them into fixed relationships. Compressive issues can also fix the amplitude reducers so that forces of eating and chewing directly impinge upon the cranium.

Compression in the sutures of the hard palate is quite common and usually generated by trauma. Origins can be diverse, from birth process to dental work, impact shock from accidents or sports, various forms of abuse, or other causes. Again, please clearly and sensitively negotiate entering the mouth of a client in all intra-oral sessions.

Key Relationships in Hard-Palate Compression

- The relationship of the inferior aspect of the vomer with the interpalatine suture

- The maxillae, vomer, and sphenoid relationships

- The relationship between the maxillae, palatines, and pterygoid processes of the sphenoid

---

Compression in Vomer-Interpalatine Relationships

We will first explore the inferior surface of the vomer as it rests on the interpalatine suture. The vomer can become compressed inferiorly into the interpalatine suture, generating inertia in hard-palate dynamics, affecting the cranial base and the whole system. Compression in the interpalatine suture is often coupled with compression between the alar surface of the vomer and the rostrum of the sphenoid. The two maxillae may also be compressed medially into each other at the interpalatine suture, transferring inertia to the vomer (Figure 14.6). These issues commonly have

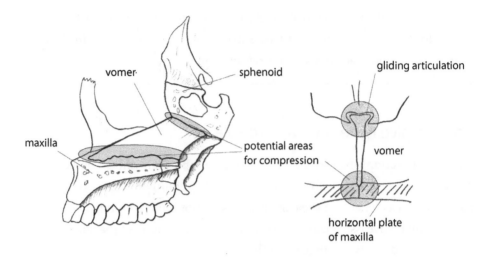

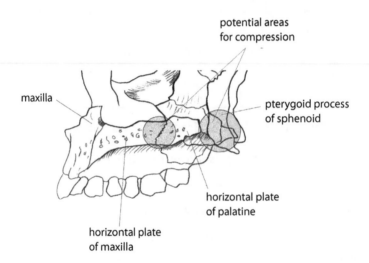

Figure 14.6. Sutural relationships and potential sites of compression.

their origins in the birth process, but may also be caused by any intense traumatic impact to the palate area.

Explorations:
Interpalatine Suture _____

In the following explorations we orient to the relationship between the vomer and maxilla at the interpalatine suture. In our first exploration we simply become aware of the motility present and any healing process that emerges. In the second exploration, we more specifically orient to compressive forces in this area. Again, placing your fingers in a client's mouth needs to be clearly negotiated before contact is made. We are assuming here that this area becomes highlighted as the inherent treatment plan unfolds.

General Orientation

Start as usual; make contact at the client's feet, wait for the holistic shift, and then move to the vault hold or an orbital hold as in Figure 13.4. In your wide perceptual field, orient to the fluid tide and tissue motility, including the hard palate in your awareness. See if you are drawn to the hard palate in any way. You will next move to an interpalatine hold. Place finger cots or a surgical glove on your fingers or hand before you do this.

Moving from the vault hold, sit or stand at the head of the table. Place both index fingers side-by-side on the roof of the client's mouth, one on either side of the interpalatine suture. I find the most comfortable position to be standing at the head of the table with my body leaning on its end for stability, and my elbows braced on the sides of my body, creating elbow fulcrums that allow my hands to float on the client's tissues (Figure 14.7).

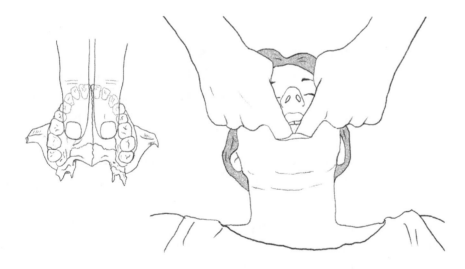

Figure 14.7. Interpalatine hold.

With your index fingers on either side of the interpalatine suture, orient to the motility of the vomer and the two maxillae in inhalation and exhalation. In inhalation, you may sense the palate lowering and widening. The rear of the vomer may be perceived to lower onto the hard palate while the palate itself lowers and widens.

As you settle into your listening, you may sense an inertial pattern clarifying. You may perceive distortions of motion and form in the tissue relationship, eccentric motions, tissue strains and pulls, general congestion, or even very little motion at all. Notice the inertial fulcrum that seems to organize this. Is there a specific sutural relationship that is involved? Do not narrow your perceptual field; orient to this area in the context of the whole tissue field suspended in the fluid body—let the tissues and their history come to you.

Settle into stillness and wait for the forces involved to enter equilibrium. In the state of balance, orient to any level of healing process that emerges. This may include the action of tidal potencies, a surge of potency into the area, dissipation of inertial forces (commonly perceived as a release of heat and pulsation), a sense of permeation of potency into the area, a deepening into Long Tide processes, or a further deepening into Dynamic Stillness as a ground of emergence for healing intentions. Wait for a general sense of softening and expansion in the area. Notice the reorganization phase and new alignment to Sutherland's fulcrum.

In many cases this may be all that is needed to help the system resolve compressive issues in these relationships. If there is still a sense of compression, it may be useful to explore the augmentation of space in the area.

Augmentation of Space in the Interpalatine Suture

In this exploration, we will explore the possibility of the presence of compressive forces and medial compression between the two maxillae in the interpalatine suture. The vomer and the two maxillae can become compressed or jammed together. This may have its roots in the birth process and is very common territory in clinical work with infants. The intention here is to orient to the natural space that is generated at the height of inhalation, and to resolve the compressive forces present. This intention commonly follows from the above work when very dense forces, compressed tissues, and little motility are sensed.

In the same position as above, orient to the inhalation phase of primary respiration and to the sense of fluid tide and tissue motility. Allow your fingers—suspended in fluid—to be moved by the tide at the height of inhalation like kelp in the sea, and take a deeper breath in resonance with the tidal forces (Figure 14.8). As your fingers and hands resonate with the action of potency in the fluids—and with the sense of widening and filling through the tissues—they subtly widen apart in that direction and sutural space is augmented via resonance. If

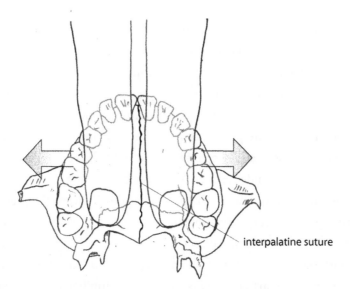

interpalatine suture

Figure 14.8. Augmentation of space with the interpalatine hold.

no expression of fluid tide is obvious, allow your fingers, suspended in fluid, to resonate with the natural space present in the sutural relationships and to take a deeper breath as though the tide is moving them.

Once space is accessed, listen for the action of potency, a deepening into equilibrium, and healing processes. Wait for a sense of softening of tissue relationships and reorganization and realignment to midline.

Augmentation of Space in Sphenoid-Vomer-Maxillae and Sphenoid-Palatine-Maxillae Relationships

As you saw above, the sphenoid, vomer, and maxilla are in intimate three-part relationship. The vomer hangs from the vaginal processes of the body of the sphenoid and meets the maxilla at the interpalatine suture. As you may also remember, the gliding articulation between sphenoid and vomer is one of the "speed reducers" that buffer the cranial base from the forces introduced by chewing food.

Spheno-vomer-maxillary compression: The vomer hangs at a 30-degree angle as it descends from the sphenoid to meet the interpalatine suture below (see Figure 14.6). As you were listening at the sphenoid-vomer hold above (in Figure 14.5b), you may have sensed a strong upward force pushing against the inferior aspect of the sphenoid along this angle. Alternatively, you may have sensed density, block-like motility, or very little motion at all. These all commonly indicate the presence of compressive forces in sphenoid-vomer-maxilla dynamics. These, in turn, may generate tissue compression between the sphenoid and vomer and may also indicate that both sphenoid-vomer and vomer-maxilla sutural relationships are affected. These patterns of compression can also be transferred into the dynamics of the cranial base as a strong pressure against its natural motility.

Spheno-maxillary-palatine compression: As described above, the sphenoid articulates with the palatines via its pterygoid processes. The relationship between the two is a gliding one and, as with the vomer relationship, also acts as speed or amplitude reducer. The force of chewing and talking is softened as the pyramidal processes of the palatines glide between the pterygoid processes of the sphenoid. If this relationship becomes compromised, the gliding action is lost and these forces are directly transferred to the sphenoid and cranial base. As with the vomer and sphenoid above, this will affect the whole of the system. Anterior to that articulation is the relationship between the palatine and the maxilla. The palatine articulates with the maxilla, and its horizontal plate rests on the horizontal plate of the maxilla in a shelf-like fashion. The palatine rests on the shelf of the maxilla (see Figures 14.2, 14.3, 14.4, and 14.6).

There are thus two sutural relationships to be aware of here. The first is the gliding relationship between the pyramidal processes of the palatines and the pterygoid processes of the sphenoid. The second is the articulation of the shelf of the horizontal plate of the palatines with the horizontal plate of the maxillae. Compression in any of these relationships may be sensed as a posterior pull into, or as an anterior-posterior jamming between, hard palate relationships. Alternatively, you may not sense much motility at all.

Exploration:
Augmentation of Space in Hard-Palate Relationships _____

In this exploration, you relate to either spheno-vomer-maxillae or spheno-palatine-maxillae compressive issues. We will use the same hand holds learned earlier—the sphenoid-vomer hold and the sphenoid-maxillary hold. These approaches are much more straightforward than those described in my older volume, which are more biomechanically oriented. In a biodynamic context, if the practitioner is really grounded in the three bodies—with an appreciation of the action of potency in the fluid body—then augmentation of space occurs via practitioner resonance with the tidal forces and space naturally generated in the tissue field at the height of inhalation. In either the spheno-vomer or spheno-maxillary hold explored above, you may have sensed strong compressive forces at work, generating intransigent tissue compression in hard-palate relationships. The following augmentation process helps the inertial potency in these fulcrums access space and resolve the inertial forces present.

While in the sphenoid-vomer hold, if compressive forces are present, you may sense a compressive pull superiorly along an angle of approximately 30 degrees, your lower hand being drawn toward your upper hand. Alternatively, you may sense very little motility at all, or a block-like locking between the structures as they attempt to express motility. Likewise, in the spheno-maxillary hold, you may sense a posterior pull, or resistance, on ether or both sides of the hard palate, a block-like density or very little expression of motility at all.

In either case, as the inherent treatment plan deepens, you will sense the tissues organizing around an inertial fulcrum in local hard-palate dynamics. You may very likely perceive an inertial fulcrum in one or more of the sutural relationships of the hard palate area. If you sense any of these compressive issues, the augmentation of the action of potency and space in the sutural relationships involved can be very helpful.

In either the spheno-vomer or spheno-maxillary hold, orient to the quality of the fluid tide and tissue motility present. Notice how the tissues are organizing around an inertial fulcrum in any of these relationships.

Remember that, at the height of inhalation—as potency shifts in the fluids—space is naturally generated in all sutural relationships. Again, maintain a soft contact—fingers floating on tissue, suspended in fluid. As you sense the fullness of inhalation, allow your fingers to be suspended in and moved by the tide, as though they are taking a deeper breath in the direction of the natural expression of potency and tissue motility.

At the height of inhalation, in the sphenoid-vomer hold, your fingers at the greater wings follow the sphenoid in its widening and footward motion, while the finger at the vomer follows the inferior deepening of the hard palate as the rear of the vomer moves inferior. In the sphenoid-maxillary hold, your fingers at the greater wings again follow the inhalation widening and footward motion of the sphenoid, while your fingers under the maxillae resonate with the widening apart of the hard palate as its posterior aspect settles inferior. Again, if no tide is expressed, allow your fingers to resonate with the natural space present and to take a deeper breath in the direction of inhalation motility as though the tide is moving them.

As above, once space is accessed, orient to any level of healing process that clarifies. Listen for the action of potency and wait for a sense of softening and space to arise in sutural relationships. You may sometimes sense the forces present in the sutures releasing in a ratchet-like fashion. Different inertial fulcrums may resolve in the different sutural relationships at different times.

In the sphenoid-vomer hold, as inertial forces resolve, you may sense an inferior and anterior softening and settling of the vomer and maxillae away from the sphenoid as compressive forces resolve, and a much clearer sense of motility in their three-fold relationship (sphenoid-vomer-maxillae).

Likewise, in the sphenoid-maxilla hold—where you are in a bilateral anterior-posterior relationship to the pterygoids-palatines and maxillae—you may perceive the tissues of the palate softening and expanding either bilaterally or more on one side than the other. The compression on one side of the hard palate may resolve before the other, and one articular relationship on the same side may soften before the other. Remember that on each side of the palate there are two separate articular relationships that may be holding compression (both a pterygoid-palatine and a palatine-maxilla suture on each side).

In the sphenoid-maxillary hold, as compressive forces resolve, you will ideally sense pterygoid-palatine-maxillae relationships soften and float anterior with ease (toward the ceiling with the client in the supine position). In either hold, as compressive forces resolve, listen for tissue reorganization and realignment to the primal midline. Is there now a greater ease and balance of motility in these relationships? Does the fluid tide manifest more clearly in the relationships (Figure 14.9 and 14.10)?

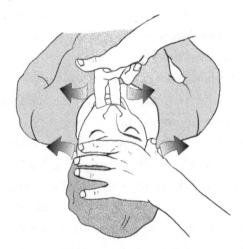

Figure 14.9. Augmentation of space in sphenoid-maxilla hold.

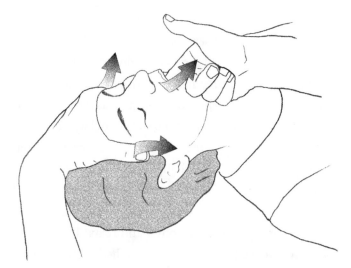

Figure 14.10. Augmentation of space in sphenoid-vomer hold.

Clinical Highlight

Compression in sphenoid-vomer-maxillae relationships can have many clinical repercussions. Inertia can be transferred throughout the hard palate, generating malocclusion and other dental problems. Compressive forces can also be transferred to the cranial bowl above. Compression between the vomer and the sphenoid bone is especially contentious, affecting the cranial base generally and the relationship between the sphenoid and occiput more specifically. I have worked with many cases of cranial base congestion and related tension headaches that originated in the hard palate. I have even seen neuroendocrine issues arise due to the backpressure generated in the hypothalamus and pituitary area by a severely compressed sphenoid-vomer sutural relationship.

A good number of years ago, a client was referred to me by her dentist. The client was experiencing trigeminal neuralgia coupled with low energy and exhaustion. After a number of sessions, the relationship between the sphenoid bone, vomer, and maxillae came to the forefront. A strong inertial force was present that seemed to have its origin in an accident that affected these relationships. It generated fulcrums in the field around her body, and vortex-like motions could be sensed around her cranium. This inertial issue was intensified by the dental extraction of two upper molars. The intensification of these forces affected the trigeminal nerve and seemed to generate inertia in the cavernous sinus that, in turn, affected pituitary function.

Her energy dropped and this also affected her motivation and self-esteem. The compensations that were maintained by her system in relationship to the earlier accident had been overwhelmed by the added forces introduced in the dental sessions.

These forces resolved over a three-month period. In one session I worked more directly with sphenoid-vomer-maxillae relationships as described above. As space was accessed in the relationships, a deepening state of balance and equilibrium was sensed. The vortex-like fulcrums in the field around her cranium seemed to still, and a gentle vibration or energetic interchange could be sensed. When the primary compressive force of the accident finally resolved, a force vector literally streamed out of her cranium. This occurred in a very resourced manner, and the client commented that her whole body seemed to soften and relax. In subsequent sessions, her central nervous system gently cleared its sympathetic activation and the venous sinus system resolved its related inertial issues. As these processes completed, her potency clearly reignited in the fluid system (see birth ignition in Volume One). Her sense of vitality was greatly enhanced and the fluid tide certainly seemed fuller and more present. She did not get tired as before, and sessions were ended at this point.

Clinical Repercussions of Compressive Issues in Hard-Palate Dynamics

Inertial fulcrums in hard-palate relationships will affect the whole system, and especially be reflected in cranial-base dynamics. Unilateral compression between one set of pterygoid processes and its related palatine bone can generate torsion patterns in the cranial base. Bilateral compression—between both sets of pterygoid processes and both palatine bones—can impinge on the motility of sphenoid and occiput and, even more poignantly, can affect the SBJ's ease of shifting in the cycles of the fluid tide. This will have repercussions throughout the physical and fluid bodies, damping down tissue motility in general, manifesting as poor fluid drive and lowered vitality. Likewise, bilateral compression can also generate either inhalation or exhalation patterns in the cranial base, depending on the forces present.

Compression between the pterygoid processes and the palatine bones can also generate entrapment neuropathy issues (nerve entrapment). The spheno-palatine ganglia rest in the sphenoid-palatine fossa on each side of the midline and pterygoid-palatine compressive issues can directly affect these ganglia. The maxillary branch of the trigeminal nerve may be especially affected by pressure on this ganglion. Sensory facilitation of this nerve may result in sensitivity in the maxillary sinuses, the maxilla generally, and the upper teeth. Trigeminal neuralgia can result (Figure 14. 11).

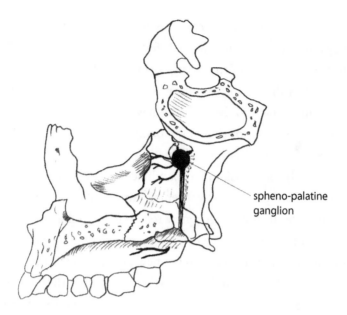

spheno-palatine
ganglion

Figure 14.11. The sphenoid-palatine ganglion.

Birth trauma is a common origin of compression for either the sphenoid-vomer-maxillae or sphenoid-palatine-maxillae groups. Thumb sucking can alleviate a sense of compression and jamming in these sutural relationships, especially with sphenoid-vomer compression. In treating infants and young children for these issues, relate to their system as if they are a membranous-fluid body, not firmly formed like adults. The holding field you generate, along with an awareness of family dynamics and attachment issues, is of critical importance. Base the work on perceiving the infant as a fully conscious, relational being, and negotiate your contacts accordingly. Infants can be very in touch with Long Tide, Dynamic Stillness, and Source, and your orientation to these primary territories is of the essence. Intentions of space, fluid skills, and augmentation of space in sutural relationships are common specific territories of clinical work that emerge, but your holding field, as a field of being-to-being presence and warmth, is of primary importance.

Temporomandibular Considerations

In the above work, you helped the system resolve compressive forces in the maxillae and hard palate. As these forces resolve, the maxillae may reorient to the midline and natural fulcrums and the position and motion of the hard palate may also be affected. For instance, the resolution of compressive fulcrums in pterygoid-palatine-maxilla relationships may allow the maxilla to shift anterior in its reorganization process, while the resolution of compression in sphenoid-vomer-maxilla relationships may allow it to shift in a more inferior-anterior direction. These shifts will also affect the occlusion of the biting surfaces of the teeth. As the maxillae shift, the upper teeth will also shift anterior and inferior. As the maxilla realigns to the midline, the mandible and the lower teeth will commonly also realign to come into relationship to the new position of the maxilla.

However, if other fulcrums are affecting the temporomandibular joints (TMJ), such as local TMJ compression, the mandible may not be able to reorient to the new position of the hard palate. It may then be important to orient more directly to the mandible in order to encourage a new relationship to the maxillae above. Orienting to TMJ motility and, if needed, augmenting space in the TMJs, can help the mandible realign in relationship to the new position of the maxilla.

The motility of the mandible is closely associated with the temporal bones. As described in Volume One, in the inhalation phase, the petrous portions of the temporal bones near the SBJ rise, as the rest of the bone organically flops out like fluid flower petals. The squama widen laterally and inferiorly, and their mastoid portions move medially and superiorly as they come closer together. The temporomandibular fossae follow this motion, rotating inferiorly and widening apart. In classical descriptions, the temporal bones are said to rotate around oblique axes through their petrous portions. The mandible also follows this motion and, in inhalation, moves inferiorly as its legs widen apart laterally. It has a natural orienting fulcrum along the midline at C2 (see Figure 15.2).

Explorations:
TMJ Motility and the Augmentation of Space _____

In these explorations, we make our first contact with the mandible and the TMJs. Although we discuss TMJ dynamics in more detail in the next chapter, the explorations here offer an introductory feel for the TMJs and their inertial issues. The intention here is to explore space in the joint dynamic and to encourage a resonance between the new position of the hard palate and the mandible in general. Here we are assuming that you start as usual and move to the TMJs after the holistic shift has deepened and, perhaps, after the hard palate has completed its realignment process.

TMJ Motility

Place the fingers of both hands just above the angle of the mandible (Figure 14.12a). Negotiate your contact—let the palms of your hands gently float on the tissues of the temporal bones and TMJs. Orient your perceptual field to the physical and fluid bodies and let the fluid tide and motility of the mandible clarify. In inhalation, you may sense the mandible subtly shifting inferiorly as its legs widen apart laterally.

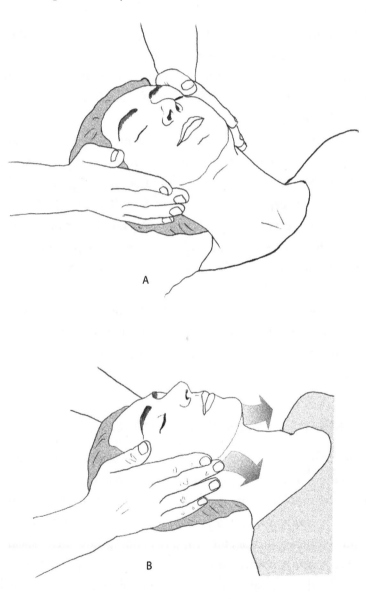

Figure 14.12. Mandible hold.

The TMJs and mandible may express almost any possible motion pattern, including compressive issues, circular motions, shearing motions, pulls in different directions, and so on. As an inertial pattern clarifies, orient to its organizing fulcrum and allow the state of balance to clarify and deepen. Orient to Becker's three-phase healing awareness and to any level of healing process that emerges. Wait for a sense of softening of tissues and realignment to the midline.

Augmentation of Space

As softening and realignment to midline occurs, this may be all that is needed for the mandible and TMJs to realign to the new position of the maxillae above. However, it is very common for the TMJs to hold compressive issues on either one side or bilaterally, and augmentation of space in these joint relationships may be very helpful.

At the height of inhalation, allow your palms and fingers—suspended in fluid—to resonate with the expression of potency, motility, and space accessed. Again, it is as though at the fullness of inhalation, your fingers are both moved by the tide and take a deeper breath in this direction (Figure 14.12b). As this occurs, the palms and fingers of your hands will subtly move inferior and spread apart. Likewise, if the fluid tide is not being expressed, allow your fingers to resonate with the natural space present and to take a deeper breath as though the tide is moving them.

As space is accessed, listen for the action of potency and orient to any healing process that emerges. As inertial forces are resolved, listen for the joint relationship to soften and for the mandible to float inferiorly.

Specific Patterns in Hard-Palate Dynamics

In the following sections, we explore further hard-palate inertial patterns. Birthing forces are a common origin of these, whose fulcrums will also be reflected in the cranial base and cranium more generally. Likewise, the unified dynamics of the hard palate may express similar patterns to those found in the cranial base—compression, inhalation-exhalation, torsion, side-bending, and lateral shear—and will mirror cranial base patterning.

Likewise, hard-palate patterns may reflect pelvic dynamics. The head and pelvis are two ends of a unified tissue field. We have already seen that the sacrum and occiput can reflect each other's patterns. Randolph Stone pointed out that, in a similar manner, the temporal bones can reflect the patterns of the ilia, the TMJs those of the acetabula (the hip joints), the mandible that of the pubic bone, and the occipito-mastoid sutures those of the sacroiliac joints. Thus cranial-pelvic dynamics are part of the unified tissue system and are reflective of each other's patterning, and ease or lack of ease of motion (Stone 1986).

In a classic context, sphenoid-maxillae patterns are said to occur around the same rotational axes as cranial base patterns. However, please remember that bones do not actually rotate around axes, but express a unified fluid-cellular motion, again more like fluid flower petals responding to shifts in the tide. The inertial patterns we are describing are not those of solid plastic bones, or dried-out specimens, but are literal cellular distortions in the wider fluid-tissue field. Thus descriptions that rely on axes of rotation are at best approximations of what is a very organic fluid-tissue pattern of organization. That being said, I will use axes of rotation to describe these patterns as they may make it easier to initially visualize the dynamics. These are consistent with the nomenclature generally used to describe cranial base patterns. This is so that you can appreciate how the cranial base and the sphenoid-maxillary complex is a unified field of action.

We describe these motion dynamics in text and diagrams, but working with plastic models is also a great way to become familiar with the possibilities, both visually and as a felt-sense in your hands. The more familiar you are, the more readily you can recognize them as they arise in your session work.

Inertial patterns found in the hard palate are an expression of the unified dynamic between the sphenoid bone, vomer, palatine bones, and maxillae. The sphenoid bone is a transition point for cranial-bowl-hard-palate patterns (Figure 14.13). Patterns behind it (such as sphenobasilar patterns) will reflect patterns in front and below it (such as face and hard-palate patterns), and vice versa.

The clinical explorations below are designed to encourage an intuitive relationship to these patterns. The patterns will clarify, along with their fulcrums, as the inherent treatment plan unfolds. It is simply a matter of recognizing them, orienting to the fulcrums generating them, and responding appropriately. The following sections here describe these dynamics as a unified sphenoid-maxillary complex in which the interdependent structures become fixed in relationship to each other in various ways.

Inhalation-Exhalation Patterns

In an inhalation pattern, the sphenoid bone is held in an inhalation position along with all of the other sphenoid-maxillary structures. The greater wings may seem to

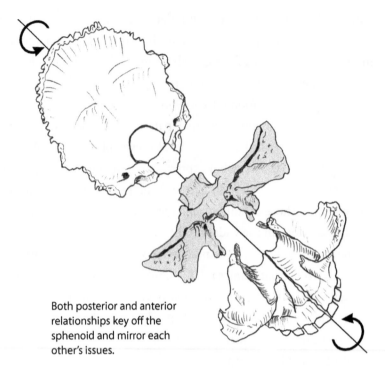

Both posterior and anterior relationships key off the sphenoid and mirror each other's issues.

Figure 14.13. The sphenoid keystone.

be rotated inferiorly. If you are also holding the vomer with a finger on the midline of the interpalatine suture, its posterior aspect will seem to be inferior, exerting a subtle pressure on your finger. The hard palate may seem inferior and wide. Holding the maxillae via the underside of the teeth, as described above, you may sense that the arch of the palate is wide and the maxillae are externally rotated (see Figures 14.3 and 14.4).

The exhalation position presents the opposite of all these, with the sphenoid bone relatively superior at its greater wings while the arch of the hard palate seems narrowed and high.

Torsion Patterns

Torsion is a relatively common sphenoid-maxillary pattern. Classically, torsion is said to occur around an anterior-posterior axis, just as it does in the cranial base. In torsion, the sphenoid bone rotates in one direction around an A-P axis as the maxillae are rotated in the opposite direction. This may occur due to dragging forces of birth introduced as the infant's face moves over the sacral promontory. As you hold the sphenoid bone at its greater wings, and the maxillae at the upper surfaces of the teeth, you may sense a torsioning between them. One side of the hard palate will seem to be higher (superior) relative to the other. The torsion is named after the high maxilla side. Thus in right torsion, you may sense the maxilla on that side to be relatively high compared to the opposite side. The vomer is commonly found bent into a C-curve (Figure 14.14 shows left torsion).

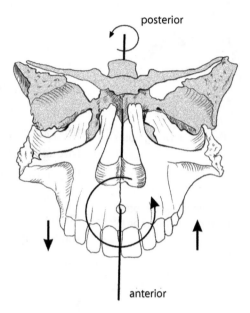

In left torsion the maxillae rotate around the A-P axis, with left maxilla high.

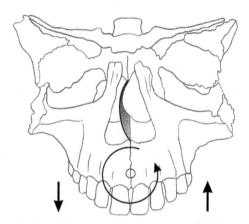

In left torsion of the spheno-maxillary complex, the vomer commonly is bent into a C-curve.

Figure 14.14. Torsion of the hard palate.

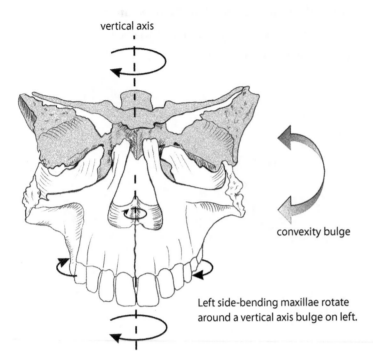

vertical axis

convexity bulge

Left side-bending maxillae rotate
around a vertical axis bulge on left.

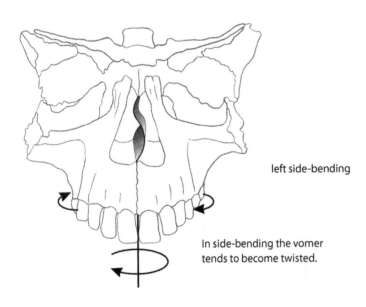

left side-bending

In side-bending the vomer
tends to become twisted.

Figure 14.15. Side-bending of the hard palate.

Side-Bending Patterns

Side-bending is also a common sphenoid-maxillary pattern. As with the cranial base, side-bending can be said to occur around vertical axes, as the maxillae is forced to rotate to one side or the other. Again, birthing forces are a common origin of this pattern. As the baby descends through the mid-pelvis and meets the sacral promontory, the maxilla on that side may encounter medial forces, which introduce a rotation of the maxillae relative to the sphenoid above.

This rotation can be sensed as you hold the sphenoid bone at its greater wings, and the maxillae at the upper surfaces of the teeth. As you orient to the tissues, you may notice that the maxillae seem to rotate more to one side than another. Side-bending is named after the side that seems to be bulging, so right-side-bending means the maxillae rotate away from the right side of the face. In side-bending the vomer commonly becomes twisted or torsioned between the sphenoid bone and maxillae (Figure 14.15 shows left side-bending).

Lateral Shear Patterns

In lateral shear, the maxillae are forced to shift laterally in relationship to the sphenoid bone. In the spheno-maxillary hold you may sense that the maxillae are shifted either to the right or left. Shear is named for the direction of movement, so right lateral shear means the maxillae are shifted to the right side of the face. The vomer tends to bend in an S-curve between them (Figure 14.16 shows left lateral shear).

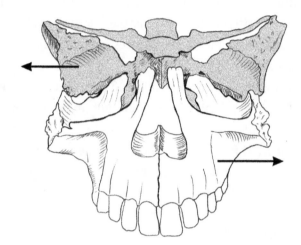

In left lateral shear the maxillae side-shifts to the left.

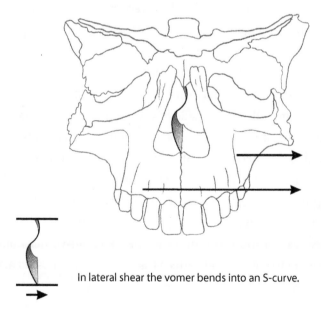

In lateral shear the vomer bends into an S-curve.

Figure 14.16. Lateral shear of the hard palate.

Explorations:
Sphenoid-Maxillae-Vomer Patterns _____

In these explorations, we are using both the sphenoid-maxillary and sphenoid-vomer holds learned above. You first sense whatever patterns arise in your sphenoid-maxillary hold, orient to the dynamics that arise, and then move to the sphenoid-vomer hold. The intention is to let the pattern manifest as you hold a wide and still perceptual field. Let the tissues communicate their history to you. As patterns clarify, orient to the inertial fulcrum involved, to the forces at work, and the state of balance as these forces enter equilibrium, plus any level of healing process that emerges.

Start as usual; deepen into the holistic shift and move to the vault hold. Orient to the general quality of the fluid tide, tissue motility, and potency of the system. Then include the hard palate in your awareness. From this vantage point you may sense specific inertial fulcrums around which the system has had to organize. You may sense motions or distortions that relate to the patterns described above, such as torsion or side-bending.

Sphenoid-Maxillary Patterns

Move to the sphenoid-maxillary hold. In your wide perceptual field, orient to the fluid and physical bodies and mid-tide. Orient to the motility of the sphenoid-maxillary complex. You may sense the alveolar arch widening transversely in inhalation as the sphenoid expresses inhalation. Notice if the system prefers one phase to the other.

Alternatively, as motility is expressed, you may sense a torsioned motion, where one maxilla will be sensed to be superior, or in side-bending you may sense a rotation of the maxillae to one side or the other. Likewise in lateral shear, the maxillae may seem shifted to one side or the other. Orient to whatever pattern clarifies—and to the inertial fulcrum organizing it—as the inherent treatment plan unfolds. Orient to the system deepening into equilibrium and to any level of healing process that emerges. As inertial forces are resolved, listen for the reorganization of tissues and for realignment to midline.

In the next exploration, you move to the sphenoid-vomer hold, described above, and orient to any inertial pattern that clarifies. The tissues may also show you one of the other inertial patterns described above.

Sphenoid-Vomer Patterns

Change your hand position to the sphenoid-vomer hold. Orient to the fluid tide and motility in inhalation and exhalation. See if an inertial pattern emerges and sense the shape of the vomer as it clarifies—is the vomer bent into a C- or S-curve, or twisted between the sphenoid and maxillae? Again, orient to the state of balance, and to any level of healing process that emerges. The resolution of inertial forces may be sensed as a release of heat, pulsation, and streaming of energy or force. Listen for a softening of the tissue relationships and for reorganization and realignment to the primal midline. Pay attention to the quality of the fluid tide and the drive of potency in it.

Specific Example: Sphenoid-Maxillary Patterns in Torsion

In the sphenoid-maxillary hold, orient to fluid tide and the motility of the tissues. As you listen—and a pattern clarifies—the position of the maxillae may indicate that the hard palate is in a torsioned position relative to the sphenoid bone. Torsion is named after the high side of the maxillae. For a left torsion pattern the left side of the hard palate is higher than the right side. You may also sense rotation of the hard palate around an anterior-posterior axis relative to the sphenoid bone.

Let the overall sense of this pattern—and the inertial fulcrum organizing it—come into your awareness. Orient to the state of balance, the dynamic equilibrium of the forces generating the torsioned form and to any level of healing process that emerges, for the action of potency and resolution of inertial forces. Orient to tissue reorganization and for the fluid tide to reassert itself. What are the qualities of tissue motility like now? How does the fluid tide express its potency?

Sphenoid-Vomer Patterns in Torsion

Now change your hold to the sphenoid-vomer hold. Again let the motility of the tissues come into your awareness in the phases of primary respiration. In a torsion pattern, the vomer is commonly held in a C-curve form.

Again, orient to the state of balance and for the action of potency in the area. Listen for reorganization of the tissues and for a new expression of motility in the relationships.

Other Considerations

The torsion pattern may reflect a similar cranial base pattern, or it can be the reverse. For example, a right torsion of the hard palate may reflect a right torsion in the cranial base. The maxillae may follow the sphenoid and be high on the same side that the sphenoid's greater wing is high. A torsion pattern may seem to move through all of the structures at once, with the origin in either the cranial base or the hard palate. Conversely, the high maxilla may be found on the side opposite to the high greater wing, showing torsion in opposite direction behind and in front of the sphenoid bone. I have found that reverse patterns of this kind are almost always due to unresolved birth forces.

Palatine Relationships

The palatine bones are connecting links between the pterygoid processes of the sphenoid and the maxilla. If palatine relationships are compressed, the gliding action in the pterygoid processes is lost, and motility dynamics can be severely affected. We have already explored compressive issues between the sphenoid bone, palatine bones, and maxillae. Compressive fulcrums in palatine-pterygoid relationships may severely restrict the sphenoid bone in its motility and may also generate a torsion pattern in the cranial base as the greater wing of the sphenoid is pulled down on the compressed side. It may also affect the sphenoid-palatine ganglion, generating pain and neuralgia. Sometimes these inertial forces are so strong—and tissue affects so ingrained—that the pyramidal process of the palatines can become chronically impacted into the pterygoid processes and it may then be useful to make a more specific relationship to the palatine and its dynamics. In this next set of explorations, we contact the palatine bone and orient to its relationship to the pterygoid processes of the sphenoid.

Explorations:
The Palatine Bone _____

Vault Hold

After starting as usual, move to the vault hold. Orient to the quality of the fluid tide and the drive of the potency in it and to the overall expression of tissue motility. Then allow the hard palate to come into your field of awareness. Orient to this area without narrowing your field of awareness and without overfocusing on the details of the client's system. Allow a sense of the tissues below your hands to clarify.

As the system deepens, specific inertial fulcrums may clarify. Tissue compression between the pterygoid processes and the palatine bone may feel like a strong pull into that relationship. The sphenoid bone may seem pulled inferiorly into the pterygoid-palatine area. Alternatively, you may sense a strong resistance or backpressure coming from the pterygoid area on one side or both sides. Start with the side that you sense to be more resistant.

The Sphenoid-Palatine Hold

Move to a sphenoid-palatine hold. Place one hand over the frontal bone on the greater wings of the sphenoid, as learned previously. Place the index finger of your other hand over the horizontal plate of the palatine bone at the rear of the hard palate. To do this, slide your gloved or cotted index finger along the upper molars past the last molar. Then slip your finger just medially to the rear of the hard palate. You are now on the horizontal plate of the palatine bone. Be sure that your elbows are comfortably supported on the table or on cushions, or stabilized on your own body (Figure 14.17). Again, let your contact be soft, floating on tissue suspended in a fluid field.

In this position, you are in direct relationship to the sphenoid and palatine bones. Orient to the fluid tide and tissue motility. Allow the motility of the sphenoid and palatine—as part of the hard palate—to come into your awareness. See if you can sense independent motion as they express their motility. If the motion seems block-like and rigid, there may be a compressive fulcrum in the sutural relationships.

As you settle into this awareness, maintain your wide perceptual field—physical body suspended in fluid body, suspended in tidal body of Long Tide—while oriented to the local dynamics. See if a particular inertial fulcrum and pattern clarifies. As these clarify, orient to a deepening state of balance and any healing process that emerges. As inertial forces resolve, you may sense a greater ease and independence in the motion between the two bones and fuller motility being expressed. Finish with an integrative hold—sacrum, sacrum-occiput, or feet.

This may be all that is needed to help the system resolve the compressive forces involved. If resolution does not feel complete, or if the forces are very intransigent, augmentation of space in the maxillae-palatine-pterygoid sutural relationships described above may be helpful. To intend this, with your hands suspended in the client's fluid body and tide, at the height of inhalation, allow your fingers

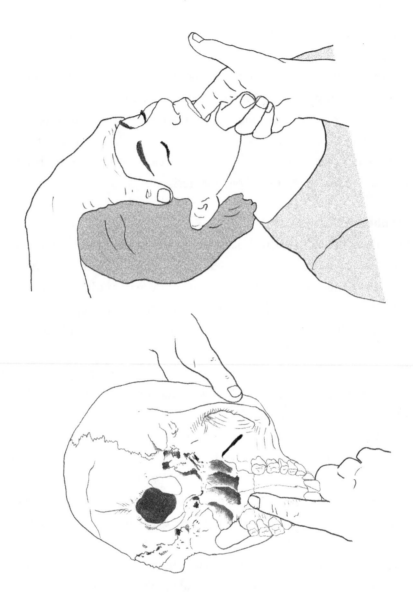

Figure 14.17. Sphenoid-palatine hold.

to resonate with the action of potency, tissue motility, and the natural space generated at the height of inhalation—again, this is like your fingers are being breathed by the tide, and take a deeper breath in the natural direction of inhalation motility. Note how the potency is expressed, note the resolution of inertial forces and reorganization of the tissue field. Return to the vault hold—how is tissue motility now expressed? Is there less of a pull into the pterygoid area? Is the motility of the sphenoid more balanced, with great ease?

Zygomatic Bones

The last facial bones to explore are the zygomatic bones. These connecting links fill the spaces between the sphenoid, frontal, maxillae, and temporal bones. They allow these bones to have an indirect relationship and function as a structural and motion link for the area. The zygomatic bones allow for the complex set of motility between the sphenoid, frontal, temporal, and maxilla bones to be reconciled as a unified system. The zygomatic bones also act as speed reducers and perform a protective role for facial structures similar to the function of the vomer and palatines. Inertial issues in the relationships of the zygomatic bones can therefore strongly affect the whole system. Fixations in the sutural relationships of the zygomatic bones are generally due to physical trauma such as accidents, falls, and blows to the face (Figure 14.18).

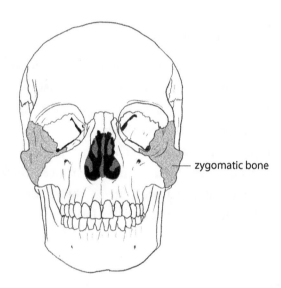

zygomatic bone

Figure 14.18. Zygomatic bones in skull.

Zygomatic Motility

In the inhalation phase, the zygomatic bones express a transverse widening by rolling anteriorly and laterally along an imaginary oblique axis. This rolls the orbital border laterally and increases the superior-medial/inferior-lateral diameter of the orbit (that is, the diagonal line from the superior-medial aspect of the orbit to the inferior-lateral aspect). This is part of the overall transverse widening of the orbit in the inhalation phase (Figure 14.19).

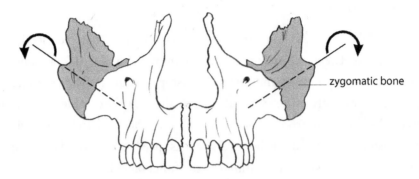

In inhalation the zygomatic bone widens
transversely around an oblique axis.

Figure 14.19. Motility of zygomatic bones.

Perceiving Zygomatic Patterns

Inertial issues in the sutural relationships of the zygomatic bones are usually perceived by sensing the motility of the bones that articulate with it. You may sense density or backpressure from a specific articular relationship, or a tissue pull into one of its sutural relationships. Alternatively, you may sense that the motility of another bone is organized around an inertial fulcrum related to the zygoma or one of its sutures. The zygoma may seem to be moving in an eccentric or block-like way in conjunction with one of its articulating bones. The sense of fluidity and continuity with the unified tissue field may seem to be lost.

Exploration:
Zygomatic Hold _____

Start as usual and move to the vault hold. Hold a wide perceptual field and sense the quality of the fluid drive and potency of the system. Then allow the zygomatic area to come into your field of awareness. Let the tissues of this area come to you in the wide perceptual field rather than narrowing your attention down to the area. From the vault hold, orient to the motility being expressed in the phases of primary respiration. See if eccentric tissue motions and/or fluid motions are organized around any of the zygomatic sutural relationships. Move to a zygomatic hold (Figure 14.20).

Place the index finger and middle finger of each hand spread obliquely over the zygomatic bones in a V-shape with fingertips pointing medially and inferiorly. Let your fingers float on tissues, suspended in fluid. In this position, see if you can perceive the motility of the zygomatic bones in inhalation and exhalation. Do you sense the zygomatic bones obliquely rotating and widening in inhalation? Do any inertial patterns clarify? Are you drawn to any specific sutural relationship?

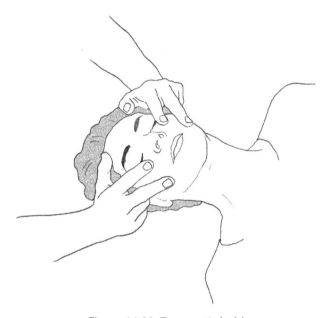

Figure 14.20. Zygomatic hold.

Orient to any inertial patterns that emerge, the fulcrums that organize them, and the state of balance as it deepens. As always, orient to any level of healing process that emerges, and for the resolution of any inertial forces present. Listen for softening and expansion of the tissues and for a reorganization and realignment to the midline.

Sometimes you may encounter strongly compressive forces in one of the sutures around a zygomatic bone. In these cases, you may want to orient to the augmentation of potency and space in the zygoma's sutural relationships. Using the zygomatic hold, at the height of inhalation, allow your fingers to be breathed/moved by the tide—again, as though they are taking a deeper breath in the inhalation direction. Note the response of potency with this resonance and for healing processes to be initiated. Note the response of the tissues to this and for resolution of inertial forces and reorganization/realignment of the fluid and tissues to midline.

CHAPTER 15

The Temporomandibular Joint

The intention of this chapter is to explore the temporomandibular joint (TMJ) and its dynamics. This will complete our tour of the face and hard palate.

As we have seen, the physical body is a holistic form. Inertial dynamics in any of its parts will affect the whole tissue field in some way. The temporomandibular joints are part of this unified field and will influence, and are influenced by, all other parts of the system. Inertial forces and related tissue issues found anywhere in the body may affect temporomandibular joint function in many ways.

Understanding the TMJs' multiple relationships begins with their relationship to the temporal bones. The condyles of the mandible sit in the temporomandibular fossa of each temporal bone. Temporal bone issues will thus directly affect TMJ motility and function. A direct connection also exists with the membrane system of the cranium because the tentorium is continuous with the temporal bone; therefore, the TMJs can be affected by membranous-connective tissue tensions and inertial fulcrums found elsewhere in the body.

This TMJ-temporal-tentorium complex, along with the pelvic diaphragm, sacral base, respiratory diaphragm and shoulder girdle, all express interdependent balance and compensation in relationship to gravity. For instance, the body will respond to a side-bent sacrum by balancing all other horizontal structures in relationship to it. The shoulders may compensate by slanting in the opposite direction, the atlas and cranial base may also shift in response to the sacrum, and the tentorium and temporal bones will follow by adjusting their position and mobility (Figure 15.1). Stone noted that the hip joints and TMJs have direct energetic, gravity line, and fascial resonances. He also noted that patterns involving the pubic arch and pubic symphysis would also be directly expressed in TMJ function and balance (Stone 1986). Nearby structures are also interdependent with the TMJs. For example, inertial issues in the face, hard palate, or cranial base can generate, or be affected by, TMJ patterns.

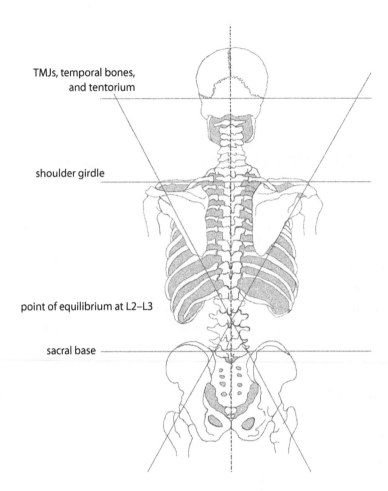

TMJs, temporal bones, and tentorium

shoulder girdle

point of equilibrium at L2–L3

sacral base

Figure 15.1. TMJs and horizontal gravity lines.

Muscular structures are particularly relevant to the TMJs. Chronic contraction of any of the muscles that move the mandible can generate inertia in TMJ function and affect the motility of the temporal bones and mandible. This is especially true of the temporalis muscle, which is very responsive to stress. Chronic tension in its anterior fibers can be transferred to the sphenoid and frontal bones, immobilizing the sphenoid bone and holding the condyle in a superior-posterior position. Chronic tension in its middle fibers can affect the temporal-parietal suture, generating an internal rotation of the parietal bone and mimicking an exhalation-type pattern. Chronic tension in the posterior fibers of the temporalis muscle can place traction on the lateral inferior-posterior aspect of the parietal and temporal bones, generating an inhalation pattern and maintaining an inhalation pattern in the cranium as a whole. Chronic temporalis tension can also generate compression in the TMJ itself, holding the condyle in a superior-posterior position and thus affecting TMJ function.

The TMJs can also reflect emotional tension. They often become tense when there is a need to hold back expressions of suffering or emotion that would be too dangerous or painful to allow. The TMJs are part of what is called the *oral segment* in neo-Reichian therapies. This is a horizontal band that includes the upper cervical area, occiput, the TMJs, and mouth. This whole segment can hold tension related to unresolved oral needs issues. These needs are commonly thought to be present from infancy and early childhood onward. They focus on the use of the mouth and jaw to get nutritional, nurturing, and contact needs met. In the adult, the oral segment may relate to generally getting one's needs met, as well as relating to sexual contact and sexual need and to comfort needs, such as eating and drinking. In terms of the nervous system, these needs directly relate to the social nervous system and early attachment processes, which can later manifest in TMJ tensions, along with face and hard-palate issues. We discussed attachment issues in Chapter 3 and describe the social nervous system in Chapter 20 on the polyvagal system.

Similarly, the TMJs may express other layers of nervous system activation. The trigeminal nuclei have connections to the sympathetic nervous system. Chronic tension and autonomic activation may be physiologically reflected via the trigeminal nerve at the TMJs, and anything that helps down-regulate CNS activation, such as stillpoints, resourcing work, CNS motility, and the work described in our trauma chapters, may provide TMJ relief.

Because the TMJs have so many interrelationships encompassing the entire body, holding a wide view of the whole system is particularly important. Do not narrow your perceptual field when orienting to the TMJ area; hold an awareness of the whole even while you are also simultaneously attending to local tissue relationships. As always, the effectiveness of the following explorations depends on the ability to perceive the inherent treatment plan as it unfolds. Fulcrums organizing TMJ motion and position may be located anywhere in the body, so treating TMJ issues may involve work elsewhere, as well as work with stress reduction, relaxation, and trauma counseling.

The Motility of the Mandible

In the inhalation phase, the mandible follows the temporal bones at its temporomandibular fossa, rotating inferiorly and widening transversely. Classically, as the temporal bones express their inhalation motility, they are said to rotate around an oblique axis through their petrous portions. As this occurs, the medial aspects of the petrous portions—near the SBJ—rises as the squama widen laterally and rotate inferior, while the mastoid portions move medially and superior. Sutherland described this motion as "wobbly wheels." We again must remember that motility is really organic and fluidic in nature and that the temporal bones manifest their motility more as fluid flower petals—with the SBJ as their natural fulcrum. As the squama move inferior and widen in inhalation, the temporomandibular fossa of each bone follow this, moving inferior-laterally and widening apart. The mandible as a whole also follows this inhalation pattern and tips inferiorly as its legs widen apart in the inhalation phase (Figure 15.2). Ideally, the condyles of the mandible should be floating in the synovial fluid of the temporomandibular fossa's joint capsules with an easy and balanced motion.

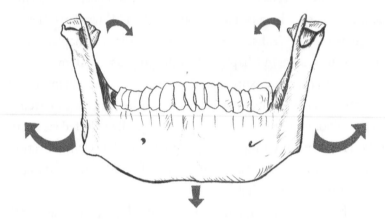

Figure 15.2. The motion of the mandible in inhalation.

In their motility and organization, the TMJs naturally relate both to the SBJ and to Sutherland's fulcrum as they shift in the cycles of the tide. These fulcrums orient them to the primal midline and midline functions in general. The TMJs also have a further orienting fulcrum in the system. According to Guzay's theorem, the fulcrum for ideal mandibular motion is located at the base of the dens of the second cervical vertebra. Guzay described this fulcrum in relationship to opening and closing the mouth, but it is equally true for mandibular motility in the phases of primary respiration. As the mouth is opened, the mandible maintains its balanced relationship to C2. The temporomandibular fossa on each side shift in position, but the relationship to the fulcrum at C2 is stable. The mandible should ideally express its motility and motion as if the second cervical vertebra is an automatically shifting fulcrum or balance point (Figure 15.3) (after Milne 1995).

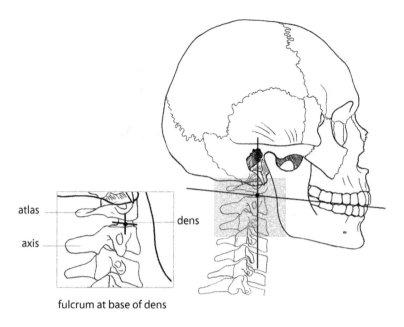

atlas

axis

dens

fulcrum at base of dens

Figure 15.3. The fulcrum for mandibular motion.

The position of the mandible reflects the position of the temporal bones. Hence the mandible will directly express its motility and position in relationship to the temporal bones and their motility and position. The mandible will obviously also express its motility dynamics relative to the nature of the forces present in the TMJs. The mandible will tend to shift toward the externally rotated temporal bone, held in the inhalation position. This will be overridden by compression in the TMJ, as the mandible will tend to pull toward the temporomandibular joint holding the most compression. Hence the client's chin may be seen to deviate toward an externally rotated temporal bone held in the inhalation position, or toward the most compressed TMJ.

Basic Anatomy and the Articular Motions of the TMJs

The TMJs are the most used joints in the body. They are paired joints composed of the relationship between the temporomandibular fossae of each temporal bone and the two condyles of the mandible. The TMJ is the only synovial joint in the cranial bowl, and it is actually a double synovial joint with a disc separating the two compartments (Figure 15.4).

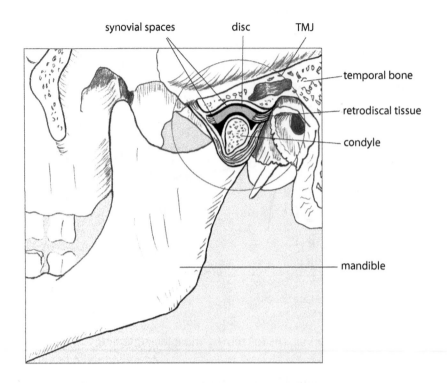

Figure 15.4. Anatomy of the TMJ.

Considering each compartment as a separate functioning unit, the upper compartment has a mainly gliding action and the lower compartment has a mainly hinged and rotational action. When the mouth opens, the mandible moves away from the upper jaw (maxilla) and the disc is drawn anterior. This is a gliding action as the disc and the condyle move forward on the mandibular fossa. The joint surface formed by the temporomandibular fossa and its articular eminence is an "S" shape. The shape of the disc follows this and has a biconcave configuration. The first movement in the joint as the mouth opens is an anterior and inferior gliding action with some rotation in its upper cavity between the disc and the fossa. The disc-condyle complex is drawn anterior and inferior as a unit.

As the mouth opens further, the condyle then moves on the disc with a hinge-like motion. Thus the disc becomes stabilized on the fossa and the condyle rotates on the disc like a hinged joint. The axis of rotation for this motion is located at about the center of the ramus of the mandible. The mandible is depressed (the mouth opens) by the lateral pterygoid muscles, aided by the digastric, mylohyoid, and geniohyoid muscles. The mandible is elevated (the mouth closes) by the temporalis, masseter, and medial pterygoid muscles (Figure 15.5).

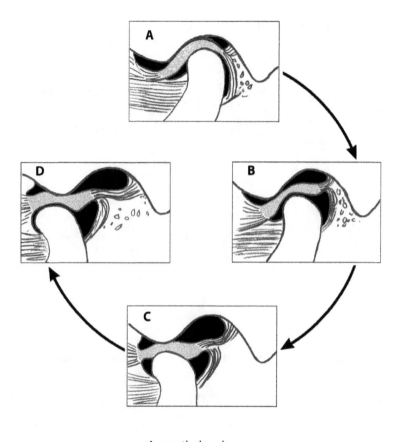

A: mouth closed
B–D: progressive motions as mouth opens

Figure 15.5. Motion of the TMJ as the mouth opens.

Disc and Ligaments

The disc, or meniscus, of the TMJ is an oval plate that sits between the condyle of the mandible and the temporomandibular fossa. It is thicker in its posterior aspect and can have a biconcave configuration that follows the "S" shape of the joint fossa. It is laterally attached to the joint capsule by connective tissue. Anteriorly it is attached to the tendon of the lateral pterygoid muscle and posteriorly to the elastic retrodiscal tissue (Figure 15.6). As the mouth opens, contraction of the lateral pterygoid muscle moves the disc and condyle anteriorly. This is opposed by the retrodiscal tissue posteriorly and by the thickened aspect of the disc itself. As the mouth closes, the lateral pterygoid relaxes and the retrodiscal tissue pulls the disc and condyle posteriorly. The disc and condyle function as one unit.

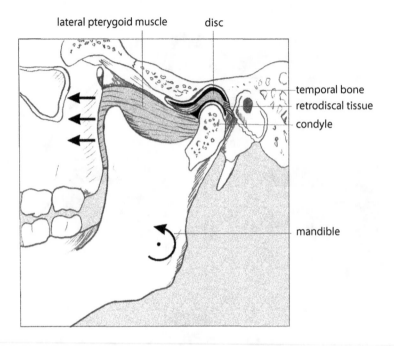

Figure 15.6. The lateral pterygoid muscle opens the mouth.

The important ligaments of the TMJ include the capsular ligament, the temporomandibular ligament, the sphenomandibular ligament, and the stylomandibular ligament. Inertial issues relating to either the temporal bones or sphenoid bone can be transferred to the TMJs via these ligamentous relationships. Likewise, inertial patterns and compressive issues in TMJ function can be transferred to either the temporal bone or sphenoid bone (Figure 15.7).

- *Temporomandibular ligament:* Attaches to the lateral surface of the zygomatic arch and then divides into two portions, one connecting to the lateral surface of the condyle and the other to the lateral surface of the upper aspect of the ramus of the mandible. The first portion prevents posterior dislocation of the condyle in the fossa and the second portion aids in the anterior movement of the condyle when the mouth opens.

- *Sphenomandibular ligament:* Attaches to the spine of the sphenoid superiorly and to the medial (inner) aspect of the ramus of the mandible. It commonly has some fibers that penetrate the petro-tympanis ligament and attach to the malleus of the ear. Tensions held in the ligament can thus give rise to hearing problems and tinnitus. The ligament generally stabilizes the mandible in its actions.

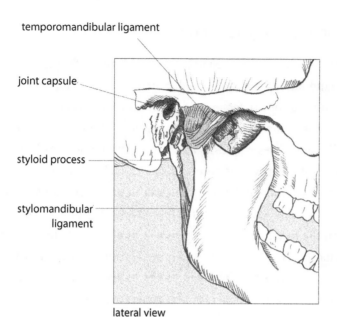

temporomandibular ligament

joint capsule

styloid process

stylomandibular ligament

lateral view

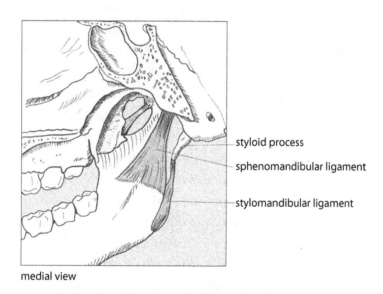

styloid process

sphenomandibular ligament

stylomandibular ligament

medial view

Figure 15.7. Ligaments of the TMJs.

- *Stylomandibular ligament:* Attaches superiorly to the styloid process of the temporal bone and inferiorly to the posterior aspect of the mandibular angle. This ligament is actually a specialized band of cervical fascia; tensions in the cervical area can be transferred to the TMJs here. It stabilizes the joint and helps prevent anterior displacement.

TMJ Syndrome and Dysfunction

TMJ syndrome is a general term used to describe a number of symptoms that involve the temporomandibular joint and related structures. This syndrome includes pain in the TMJs (either or both), facial pain, pain around the ears, pain in the skull, burning sensations in the nose, throat, and tongue, TMJ dysfunction such as lack of mobility, clicking noises, swelling, and ear symptoms such as hearing loss and dizziness. Other common symptoms include painful chewing, clicking and/or popping sounds when opening and closing the mouth, zigzag motions associated with jaw action, malocclusion, and other ear symptoms such as pressure or ringing, and finally pains in the facial area, skull, or even in the cervical area. TMJ syndrome may arise from the TMJs themselves—compressive force in the TMJs is commonly a factor—or the TMJ issue may be organized by patterns from almost anywhere in the body. As you can see, the term TMJ syndrome covers a wide range of symptoms and functional issues.

The temporal bones and tentorium are also commonly contributing factors in TMJ issues. Ease in temporal bone motility and balance in their relative positions are critical for properly functioning TMJs. TMJ function can also be affected by tension patterns in the cervical fascia and cervical muscles, in the muscular and connective tissues around the hyoid bone, cervical and occipital restrictions, atlas and axis inertial patterns and fixations, tension patterns in the reciprocal tension membrane system (especially the tentorium), and respiratory and pelvic diaphragm contraction. Hard-palate patterns can also feed into the TMJs and generate inertial issues and dysfunction. Obviously, many factors may affect TMJ function.

Trigeminal neuralgia has similarities to TMJ syndrome and their origins may be interrelated. In trigeminal neuralgia the trigeminal nerve is hypersensitive, leading to facial pain, burning sensations, and TMJ symptomology. The common features of trigeminal neuralgia are severe lancing or burning sensations in the face and jaw areas that may be initiated by chewing, talking, and cold weather. Trigeminal facilitation can also give rise to chronic tension in facial and temporalis muscles, and this may also generate TMJ symptoms. Furthermore, as noted above, there are collateral links between the nuclei of the sympathetic nervous system and the trigeminal nuclei. General sympathetic hypertonis and related stress issues must be addressed in cases of trigeminal neuralgia. Hyperarousal states in the neuro-endocrine system due to traumatization and chronic stress responses can generate trigeminal neuralgia.

TMJ Evaluation

When a client arrives with TMJ symptoms, it can be useful to establish a clinical baseline by assessing TMJ joint function to check the progress of treatment. Are compressive forces at work in the joint, and are external patterns affecting its function? The following approach, taught to me in osteopathic apprenticeship, is a traditional approach to analyzing TMJ function and is included here to present a complete picture of TMJ function.

For our purposes here, this evaluation process is mainly described to support initial learning in training courses, because it can help demonstrate effectiveness, and will show that biomechanical positional changes can occur as a result of biodynamic approaches. In an open clinical setting, the evaluation process is largely extraneous as the practitioner orients to a more holistic perception of the three bodies, the motility in the tentorium, temporal bones, and mandible, and the unfolding of the inherent treatment plan. However, it can at times help reassure clients that the work is progressing. Again, if you do explore the following, let your client know its purpose and negotiate any physical contact.

- *General alignment of facial structures:* Note any deviation from a straight line in the front of the face, running from the midline of the frontal bone, nasal bone, nose, and chin.

- *Alignment of teeth:* Using finger cots or surgical gloves, open the client's lips without physically opening the mouth. Look at the base of the teeth where they join the bone at the midline top and bottom. See if the lower and upper teeth line up at the midline or if there is a deviation.

- *Deviation from the midline:* With the client's lips open, ask him or her to bring the tips of the teeth together. Again note any deviation from the midline at the roots of the teeth.

- *Deviation in motion 1:* Ask the client to protrude the mandible forward as you watch the midline of the teeth. Note any deviation from the previous position during this movement.

- *Deviation in motion 2:* Ask the client to slowly open the mouth wide. Notice how the jaw moves. Is there any deviation from a straight route? Does the jaw take a circuitous route? Is there a jumping motion in the movement? As the client opens the mouth, are there audible clicks?

- *Space expressed when mouth is open:* Ask the client to open the mouth wide and see how many of his or her own knuckles can be fit in with the hand in a fist. A width of three to four knuckles is a normal range. If there is difficulty getting three knuckles into the mouth, there is a definite mobility restriction.

- *Posterior protrusion of condyles:* With the client in a sitting position, place your little fingers into his or her ear canals (external auditory meatus). Lightly press your fingers anterior into the ear canals. Ask the client to open and close the jaw. You can feel the condyles of the mandible in this position. As the client opens and closes the mouth, note synchrony of motion side-to-side. As the mouth is closed, do the condyles protrude posterior and press on your fingers—indicating a compressive pattern in the joint capsule? Or do you sense asymmetry in the motion of the two condyles—for instance, one condoyle may press more into your finger on one side, or shift sideways?

- *Hypertonicity in muscles:* Check for tension or hypertonicity in the lateral and medial pterygoid muscles by feeling around and under the mandible, from its angle to as far superior as you can feel. Feel for hypertonicity in the temporalis muscle above the joint and around the ears.

This procedure will give you a general clinical baseline and sense of the biomechanics of the TMJs. Remember that this picture may be arising due to intrinsic forces in the joint, or due to extrinsic influences from other parts of the cranium and body.

Relationships Inferior to the Mandible

Structures immediately below the mandible can affect TMJ function, especially the relationships of the hyoid bone and related connective tissue tracts. It is also useful to explore the relationships of the occiput, atlas, and axis, and the cervical area in general. Inertial forces and related tissue conditions, such as compression and adhesions, may generate connective tissue tensions that can affect cranial base, hyoid bone, and mandibular function.

Hyoid Bone Relationships

The hyoid bone is a floating bone that acts as a compression strut between the muscles and connective tissues of the anterior cervical area. There are important relationships above and below the hyoid that can directly affect the temporal bone, the mandible, and the TMJs. The hyoid is connected via muscles and connective tissues to the mandible, the temporal bone, the sternum, and the scapula. It is also directly connected to the cartilage of the thyroid gland and to the styloid process of the temporal bones via ligaments.

Superiorly, the hyoid is connected to the mandible via the geniohyoid and mylohyoid muscles. It is connected to the temporal bones via the stylohyoid muscle and the stylohyoid ligament. The digastric muscles and their fascia connect the mandible to the temporal bones via a ligamentous loop at the hyoid bone.

Inferiorly, the hyoid bone is connected to the cartilage of the thyroid gland via a membranous sheet of connective tissue and via the thyrohyoid muscle. It is connected to the sternum via the sternohyoid muscle and via the sternothyroid muscle, whose connective tissues are continuous with the thyrohyoid muscle mentioned above. Finally, the hyoid is connected to the scapula via the omohyoid muscle (Figure 15.8).

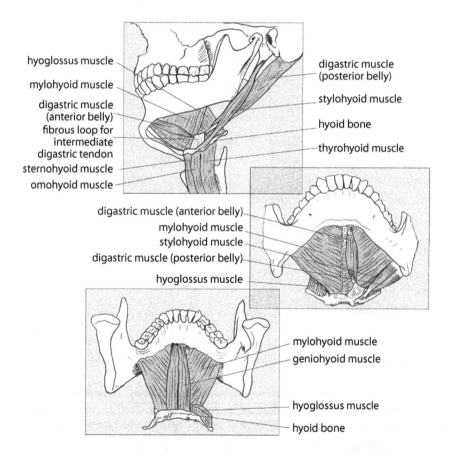

Figure 15.8. Major muscles relating to the hyoid bone.

Tension and contraction in any of these structures will affect the position, motion, and motility of the hyoid bone, the mandible, and TMJ above. These tension patterns may include the hyoid bone's relationship to the mandible, the temporal bones, the sternum, and the scapula. All of these relationships are continuous with the inferior aspect of the cranial base; the deeper vertical fascial tracts of the body literally hang from the cranial base. See Figure 15.9 for a diagram of some of the possible patterns of tension affecting the hyoid bone and its relationships (Figure 15.9).

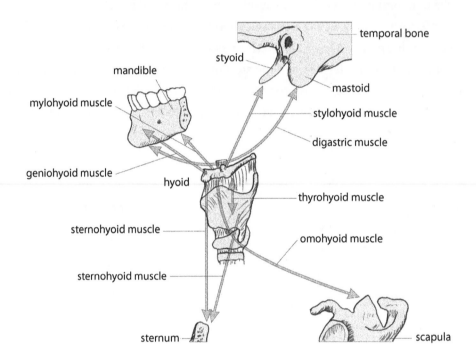

Figure 15.9. Tension patterns in hyoid dynamics.

Explorations:
Hyoid Relationships

The following clinical explorations orient to the dynamics around the hyoid bone. First you use a particular hold to become aware of the dynamics between the temporal bones, the TMJs, and the hyoid below. We then approach the whole of the dynamic between the hyoid bone and its superior and inferior relationships. Finally, you learn how to approach the specific tension dynamics between the hyoid bone and the structures that directly connect to it.

Temporal Bone and Hyoid Hold

Start as usual at the client's feet, and after sensing the holistic shift, move to a bilateral hyoid bone hold. Place your hands in relationship to the temporal bones and the hyoid bone by lightly resting your palms over the temporal bones, your fingers over the mandible, and your fingertips on either side of the hyoid bone (Figure 15.10). In your wide perceptual field, orient to the physical and fluid bodies and expression of the fluid tide and tissue motility. Let the motility and dynamics of these tissue relationships enter your field of awareness. As an inertial pattern clarifies, orient to whatever level of healing process emerges. Orient to the state of balance, to expressions of potency, for softening and expansion of tissue relationships, and for reorganization of potency, fluids, and tissues to the midline.

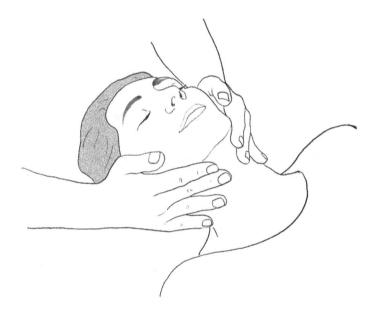

Figure 15.10. Bilateral hyoid bone hold.

Augmentation of Space

If the compressive fulcrums and inertial patterns present are intransigent, you can also orient to the augmentation of space in the tissue relationships. While still in the hyoid bone hold as above—and still oriented to the tissues and their motility—orient to the augmentation of space at the height of inhalation. To intend this, allow your hands and fingers to be suspended in fluid and, as they resonate with the tide and inhalation, allow them to be subtly moved apart. Again, it is as though your palms and fingers are being breathed and breathing more deeply in the fullness of inhalation. As the tide takes your fingers, they are subtly moved and spread apart. When space is accessed, orient to any level of healing process that emerges, listen for the action of potency and for reorganization of potency, fluids, and tissues to the midline.

Specific Hyoid Relationships

You may have perceived particular tension patterns between the hyoid bone and one of the structures with which it is connected. The hyoid bone sits under the mandible like a strut in a suspension bridge. It helps to balance all of the various tension patterns and pushes and pulls of the muscles and connective tissues in the anterior cervical area. The major relationships to think about include those of the hyoid bone to the mandible and temporal bone above (especially via the styloid processes) and to the sternum and scapula below. It might also be necessary to orient to the cervical area and C2 and C1 more directly.

If you become aware of any specific connective tissue tensions or pulls around the hyoid bone, you might want to make a specific relationship to them. From the general hyoid hold above, place the index and middle fingers and the thumb of one hand over the lateral aspects of the hyoid bone. Place the other hand over any of the structures that you are drawn to. These may include the mandible, the temporal bones, the sternum, the scapula, or the cervical area (Figure 15.11).

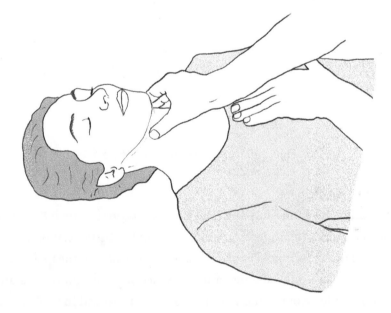

Figure 15.11. Hyoid bone connective tissue hold.

For instance, if you sense a tension pattern that relates to the mandible, you might hold the hyoid bone as described above and place your other hand cupped over the mandible. If a tension pattern relates to a temporal bone, then the other hand can be placed over the temporal bone on that side. If it is the sternum or scapula, place the other hand there. Finally, if it is the cervical area that you are drawn to, cup the area posterior to the hyoid bone in a general sense, or place the index finger and thumb of the other hand around a particular vertebra.

In any of the relationships above, the process is similar to what you have already learned. Orient to any inertial fulcrum and pattern that clarifies. Deepen into the ensuing state of balance and orient to any level of healing process that emerges. Listen for the resolution of inertial forces, and for the reorganization of the tissue relationships and reorientation to midline. Do this via your contact with the two poles of the relationship—hyoid bone to mandible, temporal bone, sternum, scapula, or cervical area. You can also orient to the augmentation of space, if appropriate, as described above.

Specific Approaches to TMJ Dynamics

In this section we begin to focus our attention more specifically on local dynamics in and around the temporomandibular joint. Please review the TMJ anatomy and motion dynamics sections above. First we will review the clinical explorations outlined in the chapter on the hard palate because these are good general approaches to TMJ issues. In the following descriptions we are assuming that you have been drawn to the TMJs as session work ensues and the inherent treatment plan unfolds.

Explorations:
Bilateral TMJ Hold Reviewed _____

After the holistic shift, a pattern oriented to the TMJs may clarify at some point in the session. In these explorations, you assume this and make a bilateral contact with the mandible and the TMJs as described and shown in the chapter on the hard palate. In the first process, you simply orient to motility and any inertial patterns that arise. In the second exploration, you explore the quality of space in the TMJs. As you orient to the augmentation of space in the TMJs, remember that space is naturally accessed in all joint relationships at the height of inhalation.

TMJ Motility

Perhaps you are listening from the vault hold and, as an inertial pattern clarifies, you are drawn to one or both TMJs. Move to the bilateral TMJ hold—as described earlier, place the fingers of both hands just above the angle of the mandible (see Figure 14.12). Let the palm of your hand gently rest over the temporal bones and TMJs. In your wide perceptual field, orient to the fluid and physical bodies, to the expression of the fluid tide, and to the motility of the temporal bones and mandible. In inhalation, you may sense the mandible shifting inferiorly as its legs widen apart laterally. As an inertial pattern and its organizing fulcrum clarify, allow the state of balance to clarify and deepen. Orient to any level of healing process that emerges. Wait for a sense of softening of tissues and realignment to the midline.

Augmentation of Space in the TMJs

It is very common for the TMJs to hold compressive issues on either one side or bilaterally, and an augmentation of space in these joint relationships may be very helpful in intransigent situations. We introduced this intention in the preceding chapter. At the height of inhalation, allow your palms and fingers—suspended in fluid—to resonate with the expression of potency, motility, and space accessed. Again, it is as though at the fullness of inhalation, your palms and fingers are both moved by the tide and take a deeper breath. As this occurs, the palms and fingers of your hands will spread apart. Again, if no tide is expressed, allow your fingers, floating on the mandible and suspended in fluid, to resonate with the natural space present in the TMJs and to take a deeper breath as though the tide is moving them.

As space is accessed, listen for the action of potency and orient to any healing process that emerges. As inertial forces are resolved, listen for the joint relationship to soften and for the mandible to float inferiorly.

Augmentation of Fluid Drive

The major ligaments around the joint respond to compressive forces by contracting. For instance, a chronically contracted sternocleidomastoid muscle can lock the temporal bone in an exhalation position and affect TMJ function. In this exploration, we augment the action of potency in the fluids relative to the ligamentous relationships around the joint and head of the sternocleidomastoid muscle.

Start from the vault hold and orient to the most compressed and inertial TMJ. You may sense a pattern of tissue organization around it, a tissue pull toward one TMJ, or fluid fluctuation that leads you to it. Start this process with the most dense and inertial joint.

Place your index and middle finger in a V-spread. One finger is on the ramus of the mandible just anterior to the TMJ and the other finger is in the hollow just posterior to the mastoid process of the temporal bone. The V should be placed at a right angle to the cranium and neck (i.e., the fingers are at right angles to the head and neck, and the fingertips are touching the tissues as described above) (Figure 15.12).

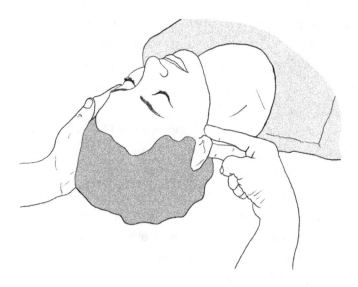

Figure 15.12. V-spread of TMJ ligaments.

Place the palm of your other hand on the opposite parietal bone. Maintain your wide perceptual field and orient to the inhalation phase of the fluid tide. Using the hand at the parietal bone, as you sense the fullness of inhalation, orient to the ligaments of the TMJs and the TMJ itself by subtly enhancing the felt-quality of potency in your monitoring hand toward your V-spread. This will have an electromagnetic feel to it and the intention in your hand is a very subtle amplification of the energetic drive toward the area. As you intend this, you may sense a shift in the action of potency in the fluids around and in the TMJ.

Wait for expressions of potency in the area—heat, pulsation, and/or fluid fluctuation—and for a sense of softening and expansion of the connective tissues and joint relationships. Wait for reorganization and a return to a clear sense of motility. Return to the vault hold and see if the felt quality of motility has changed.

Unilateral Augmentation of TMJ Space

It is very common for one TMJ to be more densely compressed than the other. In this exploration you orient to one TMJ at a time. You will be in direct relationship to the joint capsule of that TMJ and its local ligaments. Before and after this specific work you use the bilateral hold because it gives an overall sense of motility and joint dynamics and can help to balance TMJ function after specific unilateral work.

After settling into the holistic shift, move to a bilateral TMJ hold. Settle into your wide perceptual field and orient to the fluid tide and motility. See which TMJ you are drawn to. Does the motility of the mandible seem to be organized more around one TMJ than the other, or is there a compressive quality present, or sense of a pull into one side rather than the other? Move to the side that you are drawn to.

Sit to one side of the client's head opposite the TMJ being treated. With your caudal hand place your gloved or cotted thumb on the surface of the last molar tooth of the mandible. Place the fingertips of that same hand outside the mouth over the inferior aspect of the mandible. Rest your elbow on the table or on a cushion on the table so that the hand can float lightly on the tissues.

Then cradle the client's head with your other arm and place your cephalic hand at the temporal bone in the temporal bone hold—index finger over the zygomatic arch, middle finger in the ear canal, and ring finger over the mastoid area. You are holding a direct relationship to the TMJ on that side of the client's body. Again allow your hands and fingers to float on tissues, suspended in fluid (Figure 15.13).

Settle into your wide perceptual field and orient to the quality of the fluid tide and motility present. At the height of inhalation, subtly augment the quality of potency and space in the TMJ by allowing each hand to deepen into the inhalation expression of tide and motility, both at the temporal bone and at the mandible hold. The hand at the temporal bone resonates with inhalation (is moved by the tide and its potency) and follows the squama laterally and inferior and the mastoid area medially and superior, while the other hand follows the mandible inferior, especially via your thumb contact on the last molar. This has the quality of both hands suspended in fluid—being moved by the tide—and taking a deeper breath at the height of the inhalation phase. As described earlier, if no tide is expressed, allow your fingers to resonate with

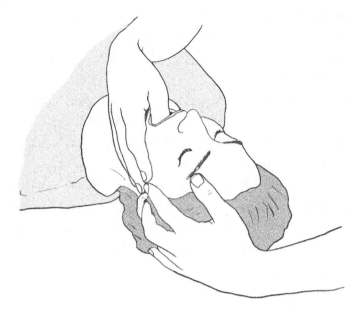

Figure 15.13. Unilateral temporomandibular joint hold.

the natural space with the TMJ, and to take a deeper breath as though the tide is moving them.

Orient to whatever level of healing process emerges. Listen for expressions of potency and for the resolution of the inertial forces involved. Wait for softening and expansion of the tissues, and for reorganization and realignment to midline.

After the above processes it is useful to again make a bilateral contact to both TMJs via the temporal-mandible hold. This can help you gain an overall sense of changes in motility and joint dynamics.

C2 and the TMJs

If there were not any inertial forces affecting TMJ motion and function, the mandible would naturally float in the synovial fluid of the TMJ joint capsules. Likewise, the motility of the mandible would be expressed as though it is floating in the TMJs around a natural fulcrum located at the second cervical vertebra (see Figure 15.3).

The upper cervical area and the mandible are in close proximity and intimately related. Remember that the stylomandibular ligament is a specialized band of cervical fascia and its relationships can be traced to the upper cervical vertebrae. C2 can be considered the location for an automatically shifting fulcrum that orients the mandible and the TMJs to the midline. This is, of course, a concentration of potency, not just an anatomical location.

Here we explore the relationship of the second cervical vertebra to the TMJs and mandible. This process can help the TMJs orient to the primal midline and also help resolve forces affecting their motion dynamic. It is a very useful orientation after the TMJ work above.

After starting as usual and being drawn to the TMJs, or after TMJ work as described above, place your hands in a modified occipital cradle. Place your ring fingers over the transverse processes and articular masses of C2, your little fingers at the base of the occiput, and your thumbs over the mandible. Allow your hands and fingers to float on tissues, suspended in fluid. Hold all three bodies in your wide perceptual field and orient to the fluid tide and tissue motility in the fluid and physical bodies. Your main orientation is to the motility of the temporal bones, TMJs, and to the mandible in its relationship to the upper cervical vertebrae (Figure 15.14).

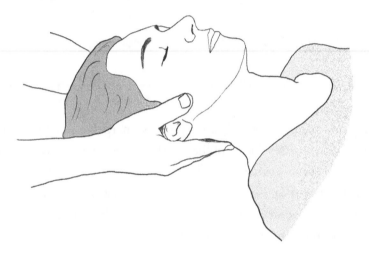

Figure 15.14. Modified occipital cradle hold (for orientation of mandible to C2).

Settle into a still and wide perceptual field. Orient to Becker's three-phase healing awareness. Listen for a settling into equilibrium and stillness; be open to any level of healing process that clarifies and for expressions of potency and the processing of inertial forces. Again orient to the reorganization phase and for a new relationship of the mandible to C2, the midline, and to Sutherland's fulcrum.

CHAPTER 16

Connective Tissues and Joints

As we have seen, the physical body is a unified fluid-tissue field. As we deepen into our work, we discover that the cells and tissues of the body are literally suspended in a field of fluid-potency, and are not separate from that wider field of action. Bone, membranes, fascia, and all other connective tissues are part of that field and are a functioning whole. The connective tissues of the body are totally interconnected and express motility and motion as a unified tensile field.

Rolfers are very oriented to connective tissues and fascia in their work. They discuss the nature of *tensegrity*, the natural tensions held in the tissue field organized in relationship to more stable bony structures. Buckminster Fuller, who developed the concepts around tensegrity, wrote:

> The word tensegrity is … a contraction of "tensional integrity." Tensegrity describes a structural-relationship principle in which structural shape is guaranteed by the finitely closed, comprehensively continuous tensional behaviors of the system and not by the discontinuous and exclusively local compressional member behaviors. Tensegrity provides the ability to yield increasingly without ultimately breaking or coming asunder.
>
> (Fuller 1975, 1979, p. 372)

Tensegrity is a structural principle developed by Fuller, based on the use of components in compression (such as bars or struts) inside a net of continuous tension (such as tension wires, cables, or tendons) in such a way that the compression members usually do not touch each other, and the tension members continually maintain a natural tension around the compression members, which delineates the form of the object, or built structure (Figure 16.1).

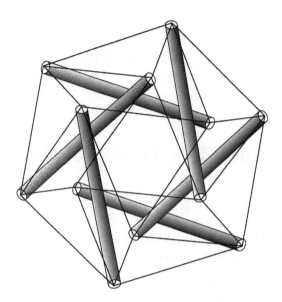

Figure 16.1. Simple tensegrity structure.

The connective tissue field of the human body is a unified tensegrity form organized by deeper forces at work. Bones—relatively denser than other connective tissues—are considered to be the compression members around which the rest of the connective tissue field maintains a natural tension. There are many corollaries to this concept in our work. As we orient to the physical body's motility, we directly perceive that its connective tissues express a natural rhythmic *reciprocal tension motion* in the cycles of the tide, ideally oriented to the primal midline. The natural tensegrity and reciprocal tension motion of connective tissues is a factor of the bioelectric ordering field and the tidal expression of potency in the inhalation and exhalation cycles of primary respiration.

As we have seen, embryological form is founded upon shifts in bioelectrics (Tufts University 2011), not genes and genetic interplay. Shifts in the bioelectric field set up tensions, flow, and motion in the fluids and cells of the embryo, which literally molds the embryo into a natural tensile form. The tissue field and its natural tensegrity are thus organized in wider bioelectric and fluid fields. Remember that the tissue field is naturally suspended in the fluid body—a body of fluid and potency—all suspended in an even wider tidal field. Tissue organization and tensegrity are maintained by the presence of the wider bioelectric field and by the expression of ordering potency in it. The bioelectric field generates the natural tensegrity of the tissue field, as potency in the fluids maintains its overall organization. As potency shifts in the fluid body, a natural reciprocal tension motion is generated in the tensegrity-tissue field. Tissue tensegrity and natural reciprocal tension motion are thus a factor of field phenomenon and the tidal expression of potency and fluid within which the tissues are suspended.

As you hold a client's feet and orient to the whole tissue field—suspended in the fluid body—you may sense this natural reciprocal tension motion throughout the body, which will be oriented around the primal midline and Sutherland's fulcrum—natural field phenomenon—and around any inertial fulcrums that also affect its motility. Likewise, as we hold this awareness and maintain a wide perceptual field, we may sense an inertial pattern clarifying around a particular fulcrum. For instance, you may be holding a client's head or feet as you orient to the fluid and physical bodies and mid-tide. As the holistic shift deepens, a pattern may clarify and the whole tissue field may be sensed to organize and distort around a particular fulcrum. Perceptually, you may sense tensions organized around the fulcrum, or a tensile pull into it, or around it. Likewise, you may sense a drive of potency toward the fulcrum, pulsations and fluid fluctuations related to it, and a distortion of the tissue field around it. We can sense this because the body is whole and is suspended in a wider field of action. The connective tissues in the body are a truly unified field, and information will be holistically communicated to the sensitive listener.

Connective Tissues and Liquid Light

As discussed above, connective tissues include fascia, ligaments, tendons, membranes, and bones. There are even connective tissue components in each cell, called microtubules. Connective tissue is composed of hollow collagen tubes and other fibers intermeshed in matrixes and sheets. These are held in a fluidic *ground substance* that has varying qualities dependent on the nature of the particular connective tissue. Ground substance is a viscous fluid similar to the interstitial fluid that surrounds all cells and tissues of the body. Ground substance can vary greatly in quality and density, from a watery state to a more gel-like state, to a more solid state. A wide variety of tissue types can manifest, depending on the fluidic nature of the ground substance, its constituents such as elastin and reticular fibers, and the quantity and arrangement of the collagen fibers (Figure 16.2). Fluid is also found in the hollow collagen fibers themselves, so connective tissues are essentially fluid passageways. The composition of the fluid in collagen tubes is essentially the same as cerebrospinal fluid. Fluid is also present between fascial sheets. Sheets of fascia are lubricated by serous fluid and can thus glide in relationship to the surrounding tissues.

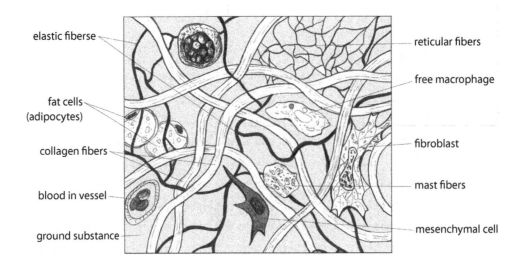

Figure 16.2. Components of connective tissues.

The organization of connective tissue is basically energetic in nature. Recent research shows that the fluids in collagen fibers are connected by hydrogen bonds that create a unified and cohesive fluid field. Collagen fiber itself is made up of triple-helix tripeptides. The peptides are wound around each other in a helical manner. There is clear evidence that the fluid in the collagen fibers forms coherent molecular bonds with these peptides. The fluid-cellular matrix that results forms a unified and ordered field throughout the body (Figure 16.3). Due to this, collagen fiber and its ordered fluid field have been likened to liquid crystal. The fibers assemble into coherent sheets that form an open, liquid crystalline, fluid-tissue meshwork throughout the body. This meshwork has been found to be continuous and whole. There is also evidence that the fluid-tissue matrix is a field of rapid communication, much faster than the nervous system, and that this occurs in a coherent, quantum-level bioelectric field of action. Communication throughout this field is organized as a whole in coherent quantum waveforms, perhaps at near the speed of light! (Ho and Knight 2000).

There is thus a unified liquid crystal matrix expressed as a whole throughout the body. This matrix is a unified field of communication. It has been postulated that states of consciousness are quickly communicated throughout the body as coherent waveforms that mobilize the cells for various kinds of activity. In essence, there is a quantum level unified field of action that organizes form and allows for rapid communication throughout the body via a unified and coherent bioelectric-fluid-tissue field. It is interesting that in biodynamics we orient to forces in the fluids

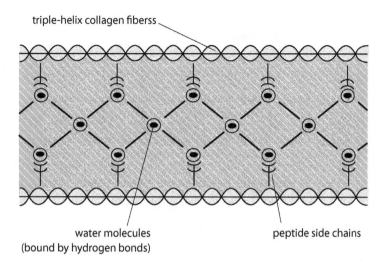

Figure 16.3. The collagen fluid-tissue matrix.

that organize the tissue field, and that this is being discussed in scientific circles as a unified field of action (Ho and Knight 2000).

Furthermore, Russian scientists have discovered that light photons are concentrated in cerebrospinal fluid and move in coherent waveforms throughout the body via its fluid systems—including the fluid-collagen matrix. An extremely rapid communication occurs throughout the body via coherent waveforms of liquid light in cerebrospinal fluid and the fluid-collagen matrix. In a wider context, Dr. Mae Wan Ho, in research with microscopic invertebrate animals, has discovered that these animals are organized in a quantum field of light and that this field is intelligently responsive to environmental impingements (Ho 1998). Sutherland's perceptual insight of cerebrospinal fluid as *liquid light* is being borne out by scientific inquiry. All of this has huge implications for the healing arts, no matter what framework or modality. In craniosacral biodynamics we consciously work with this unified bioelectric, fluid, and cellular matrix. This is one of the strengths of our work.

Connective Tissues and Stress

Connective tissues have great tensile capacity, reflecting reciprocal tension in response to pressure or load from any source. Even relatively inelastic bones and membranes have this ability. The whole potency-fluid-tissue matrix has tensile qualities in the cycles of primary respiration. As we have seen, each inhalation and exhalation cycle is expressed in all three layers as reciprocal, interactive, and perceptible motion—called reciprocal tension motion. This unified field responds to any stressor that impinges on its action.

One way to imagine this is to visualize two sheets of transparent plastic film or wrap. Between these sheets, imagine water with colored oil mixed in it. Imagine that these sheets are taut or tense, and that the oil-and-water mixture is in some way bound to the sheets, like the peptide-hydrogen bonds mentioned above. As you press on the sheets, they distort and the colored water-oil shifts and responds to your touch. As you remove your touch, the sheets return to their original position, as does the water-oil field between. As long as your touch continues, the transparent sheets with their water and oil will respond to your force in some way. Your touch is like the presence of an unresolved inertial force of some kind. When it is removed, or resolved, the unified field—organized by an energetic principle—naturally returns to its original state.

Thus, as a force impinges on the potency-fluid-tissue matrix, it responds as a whole—and the inertial forces entering the system are centered in the wider matrix in some way. In a biodynamic framework, this centering action is seen to be a function of the potency in the fluid body. As inertial forces impinge on the system, potency responds by condensing and becoming inertial to contain and compensate for the forces. This can be likened to a quantum-level bioelectric field of action in which the ordering matrix acts as a whole to meet forces that enter its domain. As the unified field of potency responds to the added force via coalescence, so does the tensile fluid-connective tissue matrix. Its fluidic ground substance responds by densifying, and its inner fibers—collagen, elastin, and reticular fibers—respond via densification and contraction. This occurs both locally and throughout the field as a whole. Tension or strain patterns in the connective tissue field are then generated.

Crystal Memory and Liquid Gel

Mae Wan Ho elegantly describes *crystal memory* (Ho and Knight 2000). Crystal memory is based upon the continuity of the quantum-bioelectric field with the fluid-tissue matrix. Memory is not simply a function of cells and tissues; it is expressed in the bioelectric-fluid-tissue matrix as an energetic principle. The concept of tissue memory, described by some in the cranial field, is seen to be basically energetic in nature, occurring totally in present-time. When forces are still active in the fluid-tissue field, the patterns and responses they generate will be present until these forces are resolved in some way. It is a function of the unified field, not just of the tissues per se. Tissue and cellular memory is thus not about the past. It is about unresolved forces that are currently maintaining disturbances in the present. Patterns of tensile and compressive distress will be retained by the system as a whole and will not resolve until the inertial forces that originate and organize them are processed in present time.

Connective tissues will respond to the presence of inertial fulcrums in various ways. Remember that connective tissues are formed in a fluidic ground substance. The gel-like state of the ground substance of connective tissue is maintained by the ease of relationships of the tissues and fibers in and around it, and by the thermodynamics of its immediate area. Gel-like substances tend to become denser in the presence of stasis in a process called *thixotrophia*. If inertial forces are present in the collagen-fluid matrix, its ground substance will be affected by the formation of crystallizations and adhesions, while its local thermodynamics will also change. The gel-like ground substance then tends to solidify, becoming denser, less resilient, less fluidic, and more inelastic—yielding a subsequent reduction in the ease of glide and movement of connective tissues, both locally and in the wider tissue field.

Densification and rigidity can also occur between sheets of connective tissue. The ability of fascial sheets to glide freely is called *fascial glide*. Inertial forces affecting serous fluid can cause the fluid to become denser and even dry up, leading to adhesions between connective tissue sheets. The fascial sheets resist movement instead of gliding easily. Connective tissue adhesions can generate inertial issues throughout the tissue field. The motility and motion of the tissues become organized around these fulcrums, with loss of mobility and the generation of fascial tension patterns.

Introduction to Transverse Structures

In this section we will explore the relationship between the dural membrane system and the connective tissues of the body. Fascia compartmentalizes the body, integrates the motions of its structures, connects tissue structures—and allows these to express independent motion. Most fascial tissue exists in vertical sheets in the body. These vertically oriented connective tissues meet transverse divisions in the body such as the pelvis, respiratory diaphragm, and thoracic inlet. At these significant horizontal divisions, connective tissues form transverse bands—such as the pelvic floor and respiratory diaphragm—or they attach to transverse structures—such

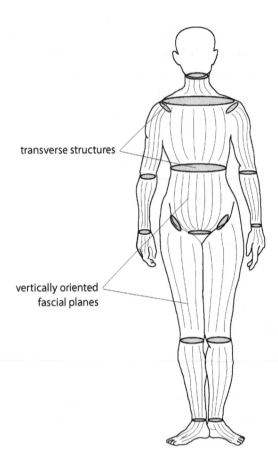

transverse structures

vertically oriented
fascial planes

Figure 16.4. Longitudinal fascia and transverse structures.

as the clavicles, sternum, and scapulae (Figure 16.4). These transverse structures all attach to the pelvis and spine. Inertial issues in their fluid-tissue matrix can therefore be directly fed into vertebral and dural dynamics and generate fixations or adhesions in the vertebral column and dural tube.

We have already encountered the effects of transverse connective tissue relationships. For example, in working with the dural tube we discussed the effects of tension arising from the respiratory diaphragm. Similarly, a transverse diaphragm may have been the location of an inertial fulcrum affecting vertebrae. As you orient to the client's system from any vantage point, you may sense a fulcrum located at a transverse structure—like the respiratory diaphragm or pelvis—perceived as a connective tissue pull or a distortion through the tissue matrix. In the explorations described below, we will place our hands in an anterior-posterior relationship to the transverse structure and orient to its motility (Figure 16.5).

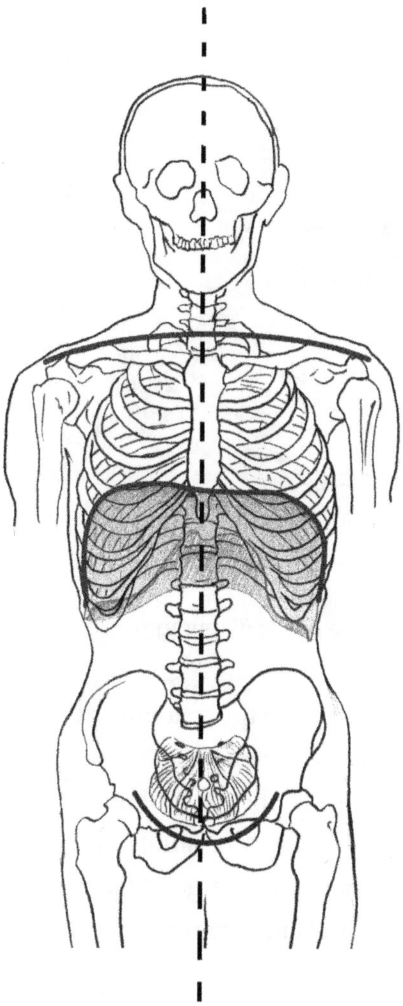

Figure 16.5. The transverse structures and the vertebral axis.

Exploration:
The Pelvic Diaphragm _____

Let's start with the pelvic diaphragm. We are arbitrarily beginning with the pelvis as the inferior pole of the system for learning purposes, but in open practice we allow the inherent treatment plan to unfold and work appropriately. The fascial and muscular relationships of the perineal floor are sometimes called the pelvic diaphragm in recognition of their transverse orientation. The pelvic diaphragm is composed of the levator ani—including the pubococcygeus, iliococcygeus, and coccygeus muscles—and the fascia covering their internal and external surfaces (Figure 16.6). The pelvic diaphragm is directly continuous with the other fascial

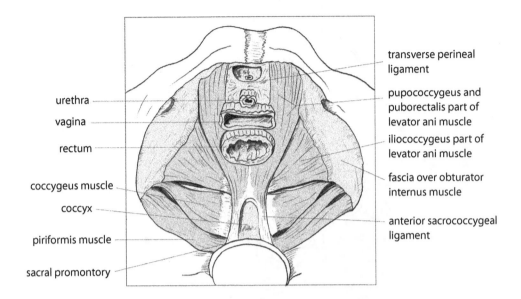

urethra

vagina

rectum

coccygeus muscle

coccyx

piriformis muscle

sacral promontory

transverse perineal ligament

pupococcygeus and puborectalis part of levator ani muscle

iliococcygeus part of levator ani muscle

fascia over obturator internus muscle

anterior sacrococcygeal ligament

Figure 16.6. The pelvic diaphragm.

relationships of the pelvis. Familiarity with the anatomy of the pelvis, both male and female, is essential for effective treatment.

As we move into this work, please hold the whole of the person in your awareness and remember that he or she is a unity of mind, body, and spirit. As discussed in Chapter 9, the pelvis can hold very charged personal issues. Issues relating to sexuality, self-worth, value, and abuse may be held in its tissue patterns. As usual, negotiate your contact with the pelvis with respect and clarity. Let the client know your intentions and why you are making contact there. Give clients the power to say "no" when it is necessary for them to do so.

Start as usual. We will assume that you have been at the client's feet, the holistic shift has deepened, and you are drawn to the client's pelvis. Here, you will move to a pelvic diaphragm hold. Sit at the side of the treatment table. First place one hand under the sacrum in a transverse position across the client's sacroiliac joints. Use the hand in the cephalic relationship to the client's body to do this. When you have established a relationship at the sacrum, place your other hand over the lower abdomen with the edge of your hand just over the client's pubic symphysis. To find the pubic symphysis in the least invasive way, have your client show you where the "pelvic bone" is and/or place your hand on the client's abdomen and move slowly inferiorly by firmly pressing down on the abdominal tissues, finger-width by finger-width, until you are finally just over the pubic symphysis. Let the client know your intentions before you do this. The pubic symphysis should lie under your hand at the level between your little and ring fingers (Figure 16.7). An alternative to this common hold is one I generally use: Instead of placing your hand transversely under the sacrum, use your caudal hand and place it in a normal sacral hold. Then place your cephalic hand over the pubic symphysis, keeping your thumb close to your other fingers, not straying past the client's pubic bone (see Figure 9.13).

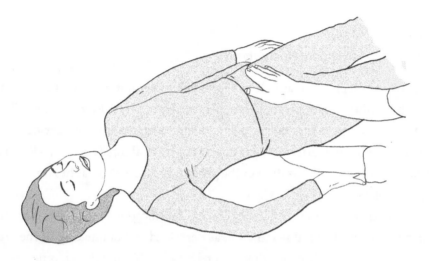

Figure 16.7. The pelvic diaphragm hold.

The hand over the abdomen should be very gently floating on the pubic symphysis and lower abdomen in a firm yet gentle touch. Do not apply any pressure at all; float on tissues, suspended in fluid as usual. The hand under the sacrum should not be grasping it any way. Imagine that your hand is floating under the table, still floating on tissues. Orient to the fluid and physical bodies, fluid tide, and tissue motility. Remember that the tissues you are holding are part of the wider fluid-tissue matrix and that you are in relationship to the three fields of potency, fluids, and tissues.

In this position, listen to the motility and dynamics of the pelvic tissues. Allow things to clarify. See if you can sense the presence and subtle motility of the pelvic diaphragm. Allow your upper hand to float and orient to the motions under it. Include the lower hand and include sacral and spinal motility in your wider awareness. As the system settles, orient to whatever inertial fulcrum and patterns clarifies. Orient to Becker's three-phase healing awareness, the settling into a state of balance—a dynamic equilibrium in all of the tension and force factors present, and to any level of healing process that emerges.

You may sense a drive or permeation of potency into the area, pulsations of potency and forces in the pelvic diaphragm and pelvis generally, a setting into deepening stillness, Long Tide phenomena, and so on. You are waiting for a resolution of the inertial forces and for a softening and expansion in the fluid-tissue field. The pelvic diaphragm may be sensed to soften, settle, and expand. Finish with a sacral-occipital side-lying hold, or return to the feet to allow for a period of integration.

Exploration:
Augmentation of Lateral Fluctuations _____

The pelvic diaphragm, as a fluid-tissue field, may not be able to express very much motility or motion at all due to a density of inertial forces. The collagen-fluid matrix that makes up the pelvic diaphragm may also be very dense—an expression of qualitative changes due to the inertial forces present—leading to thickening and crystallization of the ground substance and adhesions in pelvic fascial relationships.

Another way to orient to a strong inertial densification in the pelvic diaphragm area is the use of lateral fluctuation, as described in Volume One. If the area is very dense, with little expression of potency available and little motility sensed, you can initiate a lateral fluctuation of potency and fluid between your hands. This may activate the inertial potencies in the pelvic area and allow the system to begin to seek a state of balance and deepening equilibrium. This again, is a subtle doing-not-doing intention that has a very bioelectric-biomagnetic feel to it.

Really allow your hands to be suspended in fluid, even your hand under the sacrum. Sense the bioelectric-energetic quality of the potency between your hands in the fluid body. Subtly intend an energetic push from one hand to the other, until a shifting of potency in the fluids is sensed. This is, again, much more of an intentional process than a doing—you are not physically pushing on fluids or tissues, but more simply bringing the intention to your hands. This can be of help in very frozen, inertial areas.

Clinical Highlight

A woman came to see me with menstrual problems. She also was having difficulty in conceiving a child. In one of her sessions I made contact with her pelvis using the methods described here. Her whole connective tissue matrix began to distort around her broad ligament. The fulcrum for the pattern of strain throughout the pelvis seemed to be located in the broad ligament, on the left side near the ovary. As her system settled into a state of balance, a memory arose from her adolescence. She had been in a car accident and was not wearing a seat belt. Her pelvis twisted and was smashed against the door. As this memory came up, the shock in her system also was expressed. Strong emotions arose, mainly fear.

As I helped to slow the process down, there was a sympathetic discharge from her spine and pelvis through her legs, and shock literally poured out of the fluids and tissues of her pelvis. The inertial fulcrum in the broad ligament area resolved and its inertial forces literally streamed out of her body along the original vector path. I experienced it as a welling up of potency and as streaming of energy out of the pelvis, dissipating back to the environment. She experienced strong sensations of heat and pulsation. After this settled, the fluid tide strongly surged, there was a comprehensive tissue reorganization and realignment to the midline, and her pelvis and pelvic diaphragm expressed clear motility again. Her menstrual problems eased over the next few sessions. She contacted me a few months later to let me know that she had conceived.

Exploration:
Respiratory Diaphragm

The respiratory diaphragm is a key transverse structural relationship. It is a dome-shaped muscle with large sections of tendon. Its muscular parts can be separated into the sternal, costal, and lumbar parts. The sternal part arises from the dorsum of the xiphoid process, the costal part from the cartilage of the ribs, and the lumbar part from the lumbocostal arches and from the lumbar vertebrae via the crura. The central tendon of the diaphragm is a large and strong aponeurosis that is continuous with the pericardium of the heart. The diaphragm thus stretches right across the middle of the trunk of the body from the lower ribs to the lowest thoracic vertebrae (Figure 16.8). Keep this continuity in mind when approaching the respiratory diaphragm and its patterns.

Embryologically, the pericardium of the heart arises from the solar plexus area and is intimately related to the connective tissues of the respiratory diaphragm. Thus the connective tissues of the respiratory diaphragm are deeply involved in heart-centered protection. When there has been a need to protect one's heart, the respiratory diaphragm, along with the pericardium of the heart and its pericardial ligaments, will go into protector contraction and one's breath

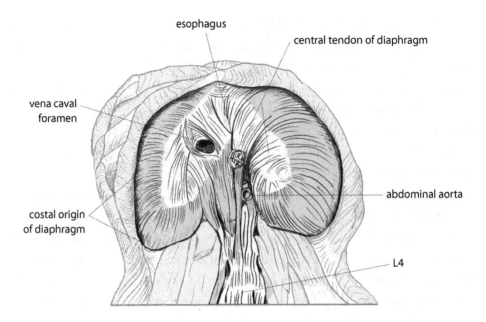

Figure 16.8. The respiratory diaphragm.

will shorten. These issues are always coupled with autonomic activation and the stress response, and may be involved in cardiac dysfunction.

Starting as usual, we are assuming that you have been drawn to the respiratory diaphragm as the inherent treatment plan unfolded. Sit at the side of the table; place your cephalad hand under the client's spine at the level of T10–L1. Place this hand so that the vertebrae are cupped in the heart of your palm. Your hand

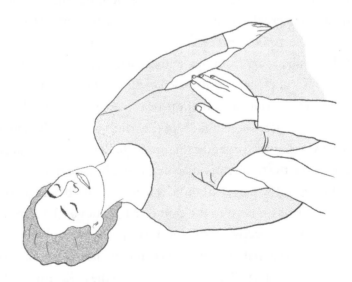

Figure 16.9. Respiratory diaphragm hold.

is transversely placed (at a right angle) relative to the client's body. After establishing your contact, place your other hand over the client's lower ribs, sternum, xiphoid process, and upper solar plexus area. You are now in relationship to the respiratory diaphragm and all its related structures (Figure 16.9).

Allow your hands to float on the tissues, suspended in fluid. In your wide perceptual field, orient to the fluid tide and the motility of this area. Orient to whatever pattern clarifies, the deepening into the state of balance, and to whatever level of healing process emerges. Work as described above for the pelvic diaphragm, applying the same principles.

Clinical Highlight

Many important structures pass though openings in the respiratory diaphragm, including the digestive tract, the arterial and venous blood supply, and the vagus nerve. I once treated a newborn baby who was having severe bouts of colic. She had a seemingly gentle water birth. In listening to her system, I noticed that her cranial base and the osseous structures in the cranium were not holding compressive forces to any great extent. Her vagus nerve did not initially appear to be compromised in any way.

Settling into our relationship, I sensed that her system was organizing around her respiratory diaphragm. As I gently negotiated a contact there, her eyes met mine and she smiled at me. I had the sense that she was telling me, "Yes that's it!" In a short time she communicated some fear, and some tissue shock was processed. Her diaphragm softened and her fluid tide became apparent. Her parents later communicated to me that the colic attacks had ceased. It seems that even though it was a gentle birthing process, she got a little scared along the way, and was holding that fear in her diaphragm. This had compromised the vagus nerve supply as it passes through the diaphragm, leading to her colic symptoms.

Exploration:
Thoracic Inlet

The thoracic inlet is the opening into the thoracic area created by a continuity of structural relationships. These include the manubrium, clavicle, and scapulae, and the inner circle created by the articulations of the first ribs with the manubrium and first thoracic vertebra. Many important structures pass through

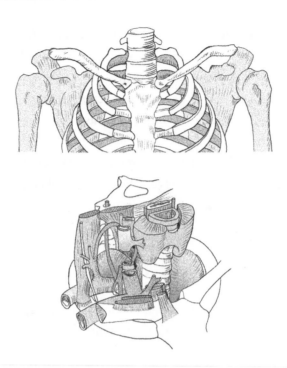

Figure 16.10. Thoracic inlet.

this area, including the jugular veins and arteries, and the vagus and phrenic nerves (Figure 16.10).

Again, we are assuming that, as the holistic shift has deepened, or as the session ensues, you are drawn to the thoracic inlet area. We will use the same approach previously applied to the lower transverse structures. Sitting at the side of the table, place your cephalad hand under C7–T3, transversely oriented to the

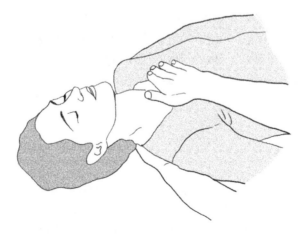

Figure 16.11. Thoracic inlet hold.

client's body. Once you establish a relationship with the client's system, place your other hand transversely over the patient's clavicles and upper sternum. Orient to the three bodies, fluid tide, and the motility and motion of the tissues that you are in relationship to (Figure 16.11).

Allow your hands to float on the tissues, suspended in fluid, and orient to any inertial pattern that clarifies. Again, orient to the inertial fulcrum that clarifies, to a deepening equilibrium, and to any level of healing process that emerges. Finish via a sacral-occiput hold, and/or at the client's feet to allow a period of integration.

Clinical Highlight

Tension held in the thoracic inlet can generate backpressure against fluid flow in and out of the cranium and can contribute to venous sinus congestion. This can lead to varied symptoms such as headaches, dizziness, and low vitality. Many years ago, I treated a construction worker. He had been off work for some time. His main symptom was dizziness. Neurological tests did not reveal anything to account for the symptoms. I was first drawn to the temporal bones and listened for any intraosseous issues or cranial base patterns, but compressive forces around the thoracic inlet proved to be the key factor. The tissue field began to organize around the thoracic area, manifesting as a tension pattern around his upper chest, compressed upper thoracic vertebrae, and much lateral fluctuations of fluid in the area. A clear backpressure in the fluid tide could be sensed as fluid echoing and lateral fluctuation in the vertebral and dural axis.

The thoracic inlet and upper thoracic vertebrae were the primary areas to emerge as the inherent treatment plan deepened. Potency began to shift in the fluids toward these relationships as I oriented to his system. As I supported the inherent treatment plan, I attended to the thoracic inlet and related vertebral fulcrums. We later discovered that this was coupled with an occipito-mastoid issue and related venous sinus congestion. Over a three-month period, his dizziness cleared up and he was able to return to work. The key was the initial highlighting of inertial forces around and in the relationships of the thoracic inlet.

Vertical Continuity of Major Fascial Tracts

We turn our attention now to the vertical arrangements of fascia, looking at the major connective tissue tracts from the top down, as all of these relationships should ideally function as though they are hanging from the cranial base. Incredible as it may sound, the major fascial relationships can be tracked superiorly to the cranial base and be perceived to literally hang from it.

Let's first look at the cervical area. The connective tissue tracts that descend from the cranial base and mandible can be thought of as a series of tubes that are continuous with the connective tissues below. The anterior tract begins with the pretracheal and buccopharyngeal fascia. The pretracheal fascia descends from the mandible and hyoid areas to cover the anterior aspect of the trachea. The buccopharyngeal fascia descends from the cranial base and pterygoid processes of the sphenoid bone to enclose the trachea and esophagus, and it is continuous with the pretracheal fascia anteriorly. This tube descends inferiorly to merge with the pericardium of the heart.

Posteriorly, the sheaths of fascia surrounding the internal carotid artery, internal jugular vein, and vagus nerve are called the *carotid sheaths* and are connected medially by a sheet of fascia called the *alar fascia*. The alar fascia merges anteriorly and inferiorly with the buccopharyngeal fascia and the pericardium. The carotid sheaths are loosely continuous with the most posterior tube of fascia, the prevertebral fascia. The prevertebral fascia forms a tube around the cervical vertebrae and the deep cervical muscles. Inferiorly it is continuous with the longitudinal ligaments of the vertebral column (Figures 16.12a and 16.12b).

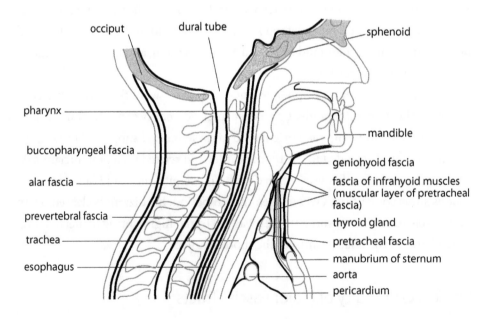

Figure 16.12a. Fascial tracts.

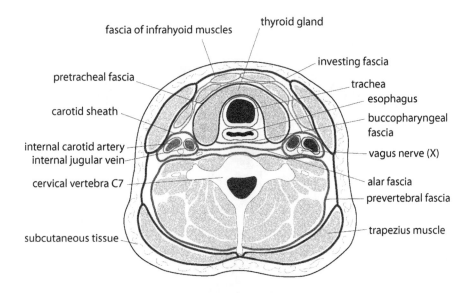

Figure 16.12b. Fascial tubes.

These tubes of the cervical area are continuous with the fascial relationships below. This is extremely important. The anterior tube is continuous with the pericardium and diaphragm below. The carotid sheaths also merge with the pericardium and are connected to the prevertebral fascia. The alar fascia merges with the buccopharyngeal fascia and pericardium. The prevertebral fascia is continuous with the connective tissue of the vertebral column all the way inferior to the sacrum. There is an important space between the alar fascia and the prevertebral fascia called the retropharyngeal space. This space allows ease of glide between the cervical tubes. It is continuous all the way down to the thoracic area and, in some cases, all the way to the respiratory diaphragm.

All these sheets of fascia are an integral unit. The pretracheal, buccopharyngeal, and alar fascias and the carotid sheaths all merge with the pericardium and diaphragm below, and the carotid sheaths are continuous with the prevertebral fascia and therefore with the connective tissues of the vertebral column (Figure 16.13).

Following the major fascial tracts inferiorly, we find more continuity below the diaphragm. One important vertical tract to emphasize is the continuity from the diaphragm to the falciform ligament of the liver, to the round ligament and the umbilical ligament, and on down to the pubic arch. We thus have a continuous connective tissue tract from the cranial base anteriorly down to the pubic arch, and posteriorly down to the sacrum.

The connective tissues of the visceral and organ systems show a similar continuity. Fascia covering the organs and muscles of the body can also become inertial,

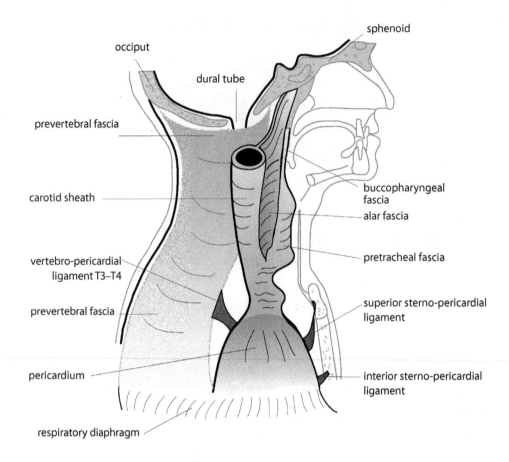

Figure 16.13. Cervical fascia and their continuity.

with adhesions between facial layers and tracts. The viscera have double layers of fascia, lubricated in their gliding action by serous fluid, so all the principles described for fascial tracts also apply to viscera and muscular systems.

Orienting to the Connective Tissue Tracts and Fascia in Sessions

As you include an awareness of connective tissue tracts and fascial relationships as part of the unified fluid-tissue field, inertial fulcrums in its dynamics will come to the forefront. By holding a wide perceptual field and truly having a sense of orienting to unified fluid-tissue matrix, the information naturally emerges. With patience, the inherent treatment plan clarifies and treatment decisions are made by the Breath of Life—not by our clinical analysis or technique. As inertial fulcrums clarify, the connective tissue matrix will distort as a whole around the fulcrum.

Let's imagine that you are standing at the foot of the treatment table holding a client's feet. Your hands are floating on tissue, suspended in fluid. In your wide perceptual field, the holistic shift has deepened and you begin to perceive a unified reciprocal tension motion throughout the body. The whole connective tissue field, a liquid-crystal matrix, manifests this motion in the cycles of the fluid tide and you may sense this natural motility as a truly unified fluid-tissue motion.

As you settle into your wide perceptual field, orient to this unified dynamic and an inertial pattern may begin to emerge. Perhaps you perceive a drive of potency toward an area in the body. You may then sense the whole connective tissue field literally distort around this area. For instance, from the feet, you may sense a drive of potency toward the right hip joint. You may then sense a literal distortion of the whole fluid-connective tissue field around that particular fulcrum in the hip. Awareness of the wholeness and natural tensegrity of the connective tissue field, and the unity of its reciprocal tissue motion in the cycles of the tide, is incredibly helpful in all session work.

Orienting to Joints

As an inertial issue clarifies, it is not uncommon for the connective tissue-fascial matrix to organize around inertial fulcrums in a joint. Knowing the specific anatomy of each joint is essential for effective treatment. Use whatever methods are necessary to gain deep knowledge of each site, including studying textbooks and videos, cadaver studies, tracing or drawing each joint from a number of positions, or constructing models from clay. Include all ligaments and joint capsules in your drawings or constructions. It is important to have visual images of the relevant anatomy in your mind's eye. Once you know your anatomy, let it recede into the background as you orient to the living anatomy and embodiment of that person's life history.

As you orient to a joint, the quality of its motility—and its ability to access space at the height of the inhalation surge—is critical. As you hold a joint, orient to the inhalation phase and notice the quality of space that manifests in its dynamics. If no inertial forces are present, the space generated will seem expansive and the inhalation motion of the joint will feel easy and open. If inertial issues are present, you may sense resistance, eccentric motions, density and fluid fluctuation, to name just a few possibilities. When inertial issues are present, proceed as normal. The first step is always to listen, orient to the fluid tide and motility, and follow the unfolding process.

Peripheral Joints and Automatically Shifting Fulcrums

Like any tissue form in the body, the motility of peripheral joints orient to the primal midline and a natural automatically shifting fulcrum. L5 is the midline fulcrum for the lower limbs, while the upper limbs orient to C7. These are embryologically derived: the limb buds extend from these fulcrums in the embryo, and C7 and L5 remain the suspended automatically shifting fulcrums of the limbs throughout life. When first holding a joint, as you sense its motility, see if there is a clear relationship to these fulcrums and to the midline (Figure 16.14).

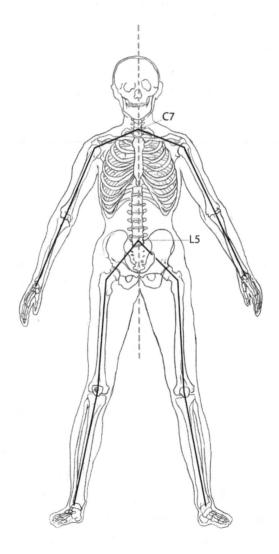

Figure 16.14. The midline of arms and legs orient to automatically shifting fulcrums located at C7 and L5.

Exploration:
Peripheral Joints and Suspended, Automatically Shifting Fulcrums _____

In this exploration we assume an inertial fulcrum has clarified at a knee, but the same general approach can be applied to any peripheral joint. You first hold the client's knee and orient to the local fulcrum involved, and then contact both the knee and its natural fulcrum at L5.

Hold the knee in both hands. As always, the first priority is to settle into a negotiated relationship, to orient to primary respiration relative both to your own system and to the client's and to settle into a still and receptive state. Maintain a wide perceptual field, orient to the fluid tide and motility of the knee, and listen for the generation of space in the joint dynamics in the inhalation phase of the tide. Note expressions of potency and fluid fluctuation in the joint and related tissues.

Orient to any inertial pattern that clarifies and to the fulcrum that organizes it. Again remember the first two of Becker's three-phase awareness—the seeking of a state of balance, and the settling into that state as the forces involved access a deeper equilibrium. Again, this is a systemic neutral, where the physical body is sensed to be suspended in fluid body, suspended in tidal body—all three bodies entering a deeper equilibrium, as the inertial fulcrum is suspended in their midst. As the state of balance deepens, orient to any level of healing process that emerges, to expressions of potency, and for the processing of inertial forces. Wait for a sense of space and expansion in joint relationships and for reorganization and realignment to the primal midline.

The forces in the inertial fulcrum may not easily attain a state of balance/equilibrium. The forces may be exceptionally dense and the effects of the forces—fluid congestion, tissue density, connective tissue adhesions, and so on may also be very entrenched. For instance, you may sense a very inertial joint with fluid congestion, density, and tissue adhesion. Other clinical skills—such as the use of lateral fluctuation, of space, and/or fluid drive—might then come into play as you meet the inertial situation.

If potencies and fluids have really become inertial and there is a state of parasympathetic immobility in the knee area, you might initiate or enhance lateral fluctuations of fluid and potency in the area. This can help activate the expression of inertial potencies in the organizing fulcrum. In this case, you might initiate a lateral fluctuation between your hands as they hold the knee. Again, this is done via your intention, is more bioelectric-biomagnetic than physical, and is not done via pushing into fluids and tissues or generating pressures in the area.

You might also choose to augment fluid drive toward the site of an inertial fulcrum. This, again, is more an intentional process than a "doing." Deepen into a relationship to the bioelectric quality of potency in the fluids, and at the height of inhalation one hand orients more to the inertial site, which augments a drive of potency toward it.

Likewise, you might choose to augment space in the joint relationship at the height of inhalation, by allowing your hands holding the knee to be moved by the tide and to take a deeper breath in the direction of the natural motility of the joint. If you are holding a knee joint, as your hands breathe with the tide, that would be sensed as a filling, widening, and cephalic rising. Again, if no tide is expressed, allow your hands to resonate with the natural space present in the joint relationships, and to take a deeper breath as though the tide is moving them.

When there is a sense of space, expansion, and reorganization in the knee, you can then orient the joint to its natural fulcrum in the midline at L5.

Place your caudal hand under the client's knee posterior to its popliteal area. Place your cephalic hand under the vertebral midline at L5. You can place the palm of this hand under the L5 vertebral area, somewhat overlapping the superior aspect of the sacrum.

As you hold this bipolar relationship, orient to the motility of the joint relative to L5 and the midline. You may sense a rising and widening in relationship to the midline in inhalation. Maintaining a wide perceptual field—still oriented to all three bodies—settle into the relationship and, as the two poles enter a state of equilibrium, you may sense a reciprocal action of potency at both these poles—perhaps as pulsation and a clearing of any further inertial forces present.

As this occurs, you may then notice a strong surge of potency rising through the fluids. The joint then may express a clearer relationship in its motility to its natural fulcrum at L5 and to the primal midline generally (Figure 16.15). The same process can be used for any peripheral joint. For example, if you are holding an elbow, relate it to its fulcrum at C7.

In Chapter 21, we describe the sensorimotor relationships that may also affect joint function, as these are commonly sensitized. In that chapter we suggest that, after the inertial fulcrum in a joint is resolved, practitioners should make a relationship to the sensorimotor nerve supply to that joint area. To do this, you hold the joint with one hand while placing your other hand under the spinal cord area that serves that joint with innervation. In the case of a lower limb, that

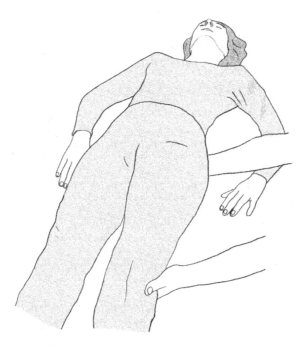

Figure 16.15. Orienting the knee to its natural fulcrum at L5.

would be at the level of T12–L2, the lower end of the spinal cord. A rough guide is that T12–L2 is the vertebral-spinal cord level for lower joints (pelvis and legs), and C7–T4 is the spinal cord level for upper limbs (joints, shoulders, elbows, and wrists). You might want to orient to nerve facilitation before moving to the knee-L5 relationship above. See Chapter 21 for more detail.

Clinical Highlight

An elderly woman diagnosed as having a calcified right ankle joint was referred to me. Her orthopedic consultant wanted to fuse the ankle with the hope that the pain would be reduced and the joint stabilized. The woman was afraid of having this surgery and was very motivated to explore alternatives. She had to travel a long distance for each session and the journey was difficult. As I held her ankle area in our first session, there was still some mobility present, with a decent expression of motility and potency. She was a very resilient person and a fighter. She had stress patterns that manifested as worry, anxiety states, and sleeplessness.

I saw her over a six-month period. During this time we worked with her ankle locally for many sessions, also orienting to its nociceptive sensorimotor nerve innervation, and to its natural fulcrum at L5. Most sessions were oriented to accessing the holistic shift and allowing the inherent treatment plan to unfold. We worked via accessing states of balance, and augmenting space and fluid drive in the area. Sometimes we both entered Dynamic Stillness in a state of darkness, or timelessness. I can remember one session where both she and I came back to a present awareness together and realized that something special had happened. Her overall stress symptoms softened after that session.

Pelvic issues soon clarified and her right hip joint was highlighted as a critical site of inertia. Her pelvis was very inertial; it was as though her ankle had supported her all these years and finally given way. Many sessions were focused on her hip and its very compressed forces. Vertebral and cranial base issues also arose, as did some issues that went all the way back to birth. In each session I always checked in with her ankle and finished with some specific work in relationship to it. She needed to be held at the ankle each session, or she would feel anxious and not met. Although each session was not necessarily oriented to the ankle, it was always important to touch base with it. It allowed her to feel contacted at her perceived issue.

Session work was slow, but I saw gradual progress. Although the major inertial forces organizing the tissue changes in her ankle were remote, the ankle showed deep changes in tissue form and function. In one session while I was holding her ankle, we again entered a deepening stillness, and something dramatic seemed to occur. There was stillness, a sense of rhythmic balanced interchange between the stillness, potency, and the tissues of her ankle, along with a settling and lengthening throughout her system. This felt like a rhythmic vibrancy in my hands within a depth of stillness. She terminated sessions soon after that and I received a simple thank-you note with a comment that her situation had changed and she could not come any more. I assumed that she had become discouraged or had decided to opt for surgery.

A year later a young woman came to see me. She said she was a friend of the woman's daughter. A few months earlier the elderly woman's daughter had returned from a year abroad and had found her mother dusting kitchen shelves, balanced on her ankle. Her ankle issue had resolved through our sessions and I had never known it!

On Unwinding and Macro-Motions

During session work, parts of a client's body may express both micro- and macro-motions. An arm may begin to move in a certain way, or a leg begins to express some motion, or a client's head may move or rotate rhythmically, perhaps in relationship to unresolved birth trauma. Perhaps as you are holding a knee, hip, or shoulder joint as explored above, the client's limb begins to move in some way. These motions are sometimes called unwinding motions. *Unwinding* has the connotation that something is releasing or being processed. However, when tissues and tissue structures move, they are not necessarily releasing or resolving anything. Macro- or micro-motions, whether they arise spontaneously or by practitioner initiation, may be patterns of organization around unresolved inertial fulcrums.

Macro-motions are commonly expressions of traumatic experience and are manifestations of trauma schemas. They are the shape of an experience, not the organizing factor itself. In essence, tissues do not really unwind; they show a pattern of motion and organization around a fulcrum. As we have oriented to over and over again, the fulcrum, and the forces within it, organize the motion. This kind of motion is thus a factor of unresolved forces in the client's system. To understand the motion, you must orient to the fulcrum and the forces within it that generate the motion.

Furthermore, during Stage Three of the Becker three-phase healing process, micro- and even macro-tissue motions may arise. These are also not "unwinding" motions. When inertial forces and fulcrums resolve, tissues are freed to seek their natural fulcrums, and a period of reorganization and realignment to the primal midline and suspended, automatically shifting fulcrums occurs. These motions must be given space so that a new organization can be accessed and expressed. If you treat these motions as unwinding of tissues or as new tensile strain patterns and engage them in any way, you will get in the way of the completion of a healing process.

Macro-motions may also be a manifestation of a frozen need to protect. When a motion like this is expressed, it may be a sign that a frozen fight-or-flight intention is beginning to surface. For instance, a client's arm may begin to move and an intention to guard, to strike out, or to protect, may begin to surface. Or the client's head may begin to rotate rhythmically, attempting to express the orienting response. I find this commonly happens as part of a clearing of hypersensitivity from the nuclei of the brain stem.

Macro-motions may shift into a particular position expressing an unresolved experience such as birth trauma. Almost any kind of motion can arise with almost any kind of origin. See Chapters 18–21 for skills around trauma and the stress response. These skills largely have to do with accessing the intention of the motion, slowing the process down, and helping the client to physically prepare to do whatever is being expressed before he or she actually, slowly, does it. The preparation phase mobilizes the muscle and joints and resets the nervous system to help complete the intention present. The idea is to mobilize the system in a resourced manner to complete the frozen fight-or-flight intention. Rather than continually repeating the need to protect through the cycling of the sympathetic nervous system, the energies of the intention can actually be completed.

If macro-motions arise, the intention is to access the forces at work that are generating the form of organization and the motions being expressed. One way to approach macro-motions is to follow the form of the motion and to sense its organizing fulcrum. As the form clarifies, gently slow the motion down until a state of balance relative to the inertial fulcrum is accessed. The principles are the same as in all of our work. Stillness is accessed, and this enables an expression of potency and a deepening of the healing process.

Traditional ways to initiate macro-motions include countering gravity as you hold a limb, or placing compression into a joint or tissue structure to initiate motion. For example, you might be holding a client's arm and sense motion arising. You might then subtly lift the arm in such a way as to counter the force of gravity. This can be a delicate process of balancing the motion, the weight of the arm, and the intention to support the arm. This process can allow a motion to arise as a pattern of organization around whatever fulcrum is being accessed. As this motion arises, the art is then to help the arm access a state of balance, a stillness, as an integral part of the whole tensile tissue field. I find that I do not need to initiate these kinds of motions. If they arise, I simply listen and help slow the motion down without getting in the way of it, until stillness and a deepening state of balance is attained. The important thing here, as always, is to access a stillness within which the forces and fulcrums that generate the motion clarify and resolve.

CHAPTER 17

Visceral Dynamics

Due to the origins of cranial work in osteopathic practice, traditional cranial courses focused on the relationship of bones and membranes to primary respiration. However, we incarnate in a holistic body and visceral-organ relationships are pivotal in the experience of our lives. Visceral dynamics are an essential aspect of all biodynamic approaches. The visceral world is our world of sensation, feeling, and emotion. In this chapter we look at the basic motility of each organ and its embryological origins, the mind-body-psycho-spiritual issues that may be associated with each organ, and how pre- and perinatal experiences may be held in the cells and tissues of the organs, including developmental trauma and attachment issues. Thus, as we make a relationship to a client's organ, we are not just touching an anatomical-physiological form, but are touching essential aspects of the client's felt-world, psycho-emotional history, and sense of selfhood.

Our visceral states of "knowing" are essential in our interpersonal experience of others and the world we live in. As we meet other people's organs, as we do in this chapter, we are meeting their inner world of feeling and beingness—which includes resonances with their earliest experiences, personal and interpersonal experiences of caregiving, primary others, love, joy, acceptance, rejection, trauma, personality development, and self-view. It may seem to be a lot to take in as practitioner, but our essential state of presence—and orientation to primary respiration and the underlying forces at work—has the potential to be extremely healing. Let's look at some of the basic neurology involved and then begin our journey into visceral experience—an exploration into the living state of another.

Attunement, Interoception, and Emotional Resonance

We introduced the concept of attunement and felt-resonance in Chapter 4, when we discussed babies' ability to attune to their primary caregivers via felt-experience.

Please review those sections, as felt-experience is very much viscerally oriented. In that chapter, we explored the neurology of mirror neurons and how perceptual experience—seeing, hearing, touching—becomes direct felt-knowing for the little one. This embodied knowing of experience—as feeling-tone, sensation, and emotional tone—is present throughout life. As we have experience, that experience resonates in our soma and viscera and—especially at a visceral level—gives us the ability to sense, know, and respond to our experience at a felt-level. The organs hold the resonance of all these experiences throughout life, and as we meet clients' visceral system, we are meeting the whole of their felt-experience and any unresolved trauma, fear, and anger that may still be cycling in their body-mind.

As we have seen, mirror neurons fire in response to our perception-experience of the intentional actions and states of other people, especially significant others, and events. This information goes to various areas of the cortex and, most tellingly, is directed downward into our body. Our outer experiences then become inner felt-experience via sensation, feeling-tone, and emotion. Our perceptual input of others then becomes a felt-body experience, which helps us sense and know the actions, states, and intentions of others very directly. Sensory nerves called interoceptors relay these feeling states back upward to our prefrontal cortex, which mediates present-time awareness. This generates a direct "felt-knowing" of both our internal states and the actions and states of others, which then become the ground for our internal organization and response to our external relational world. This felt-knowing builds up throughout our life, and we continue to know the felt-nature of our world in this way. The presence and impact of relational others and the experience of our activities—our joy and sorrows, highs and lows—and the possible resonances of past overwhelm and traumatic experience—are all present as direct felt, visceral knowing.

As we meet the viscera in this chapter, we are meeting all of this. The viscera are pivotal in our felt-experience of emotion and relationally mediated feelings. We feel our way into our relational world, and this world of feeling is held in our visceral dynamics. As the viscera resonate with our perceptual experience of the world, emotional states becomes felt-experience, and the resonances of these experiences will become held in the organs as feeling-tone and emotion. Unresolved painful and traumatic experiences, our self-view, our sense of inner security and self-worth—and the need to defend against further pain—may all come to the forefront as we meet organ motility and patterning.

For instance, when we place our hand on a client's liver, we may be also meeting the client's felt-sense of self and others, and feelings of sadness, anxiety, frustration, and loss may emerge, all reflections of how he or she has been seen and received in life. Likewise, as the liver area is pivotal in prenatal umbilical blood supply, we may also be meeting the felt-experience of the little one in the womb, or in the birthing experience and even umbilical shock if the cord is cut too soon. This may be mirrored in the umbilical area as contraction, sensitivity, and emotional states. As we meet the client's viscera and visceral dynamics, we thus need to be settled in our fulcrums and state of presence, oriented to the client's process in a state of resonance and true empathy. As we resonate with the arising conditions, our own process of interoception and feeling-response to the client's state will be initiated, which in turn, is the ground for our empathetic response to the arising process (Figure 17.1).

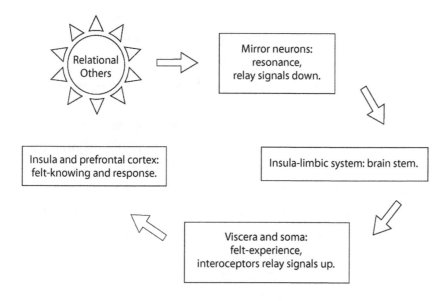

Figure 17.1. Relational experience and interoception.

Pre- and Perinatal Resonances

Pre- and perinatal experience may also be reflected in visceral dynamics. Dr. Frank Lake, a psychiatrist who is one of the fathers of pre- and perinatal psychology, was very aware of how early experience can be held at a felt-level in organ dynamics. He wrote of the intimate relationship between fetus, infant, and mother, and how resonances of umbilical experience can permeate the organs. He discussed what he called *umbilical affect*—the fetus and infant's direct felt-experience of mother's emotional life and world. He called this territory the *womb of spirit*—a period of time from conception to nine months after birth—where the infant is directly attuned to mother's states.

Lake believed that, for nine months after birth, the infant still directly senses mother's states as though he or she was still attached via the umbilical cord. Lake noted that, as fetuses and young infants directly sense mother's inner states via the umbilical connection, they cannot differentiate these from their own state. The direct infusion of mother's inner states, plus experience of her world via the umbilical cord, become theirs. Thus mother's emotions and inner feelings are also theirs. Lake believed that these umbilical affects set the baseline for ego development and secure or insecure ego systems (Lake 1979). These ideas are similar to those of Ronald Fairbairn, the early father of a full object relations theory of ego development. He believed that infants are in a state of *immature dependency*, in which they cannot differentiate their feelings and needs from those of mother or other primary caregivers (Fairbairn 1994a).

Lake categorized infants' felt-experience in terms of the intensity of umbilical affect—as positive, negative, and strongly negative. Hopefully, the prenate and infant experience a good-enough relational field, where negative affect can be experienced in the context of continuing trust in the holding field. The more negative the affect, especially strongly negative affect, the more likely it is that the young child will have to enter defended states too early and a defended personality with insecure attachment processes will be generated. Lake also discussed the primitive defenses of prenates and young babies. This is where it becomes very interesting in terms of organ and visceral work. Lake noted that prenates and infants do not have ego defenses to fall back on. Their modes of defending are very body-centered and visceral in nature. He discussed three basic ways that prenates and infants defend against intrusive or overwhelming input—*withdrawal, displacement,* and *dissociation.* If there is uncomfortable input, such as loud noise, quarreling, or inappropriate caregiver interventions, infants will withdraw by turning away, disengaging their attention, or in the extreme by dissociating.

The third mode of protection, dissociation, is very important in organ development and feeling-states. Here the prenate in the womb, or a very young infant who is experiencing his world as though the umbilical connection is still present, will displace the incoming bad umbilical feelings into other areas of his body, commonly organs. Thus incoming experiences of strongly negative affect may be displaced into the liver, stomach, intestines, and so on. So, as you meet the liver or intestines of a client, for instance, strong feelings, defensive needs, and self- and worldviews may also emerge. Also negative heart-centered relational experience—like inconsistent, intrusive, or abusive caregiving—will cause the infant's heart center to close down as the connective tissues around the heart contract to protect from further wounding as the soma takes on defensive tensions.

As we have seen in earlier chapters, there has been much research into prenatal experience and a good number of studies have shown that mother's psycho-emotional state clearly affects the infant due to the direct placenta-umbilical connection. High levels of maternal cortisol—an important stress hormone—clearly affect prenate and infant cognitive development and attachment processes (Bergman, et al. 2010). The abstract to an important research study (Field, Diego, and Hernandez-Reif 2006, p. 445) states:

> A review of research on prenatal depression effects on the fetus and newborn suggests that they experience prenatal, perinatal and postnatal complications. Fetal activity is elevated, prenatal growth is delayed, and prematurity and low birth weight occur more often. Newborns of depressed mothers then show a biochemical-physiological profile that mimics their mothers' prenatal biochemical-physiological profile including elevated cortisol, lower levels of dopamine and serotonin, greater relative right frontal EEG activation and lower vagal tone. Elevated prenatal maternal cortisol is the strongest predictor of these neonatal outcomes.

Thus, as we meet the organs in our work, we may also be meeting the resonances of these very early experiences, negative umbilical affect, early developmental trauma, and an overriding need to protect. Sometimes, as you meet an adult's viscera, it may even feel like you are holding an infant in your hands. I commonly ask clients to become aware of any sensations and feeling-tone in the area and help them resolve any emerging emotional or traumatic impacts in resources, primary respiration, and appropriate pacing. Please see chapters on trauma resolution later in this volume. The main point here is that as you meet an organ, you are meeting the whole of a client's life process, relational feeling states, emotional history, and past traumatic experiences.

Organ Motility

We will next orient to the basic motility of each organ and offer a basic approach to meeting organ fulcrums, inertial patterns, and unresolved developmental issues. We will contextualize this in the "being nature" of each organ, the emotional tendencies that may be present, and wider felt-sense of selfhood and worldview that may also be present. The motility of each organ—as in all tissue motility—is oriented to the primal-notochord midline and is grounded in the particulars of its embryological development. Let's look at each organ in turn, and then outline a basic clinical approach to organ motility and healing process, which will include motility, personal process, and CNS issues. We will start with the chest cavity and work our way downward to the pelvis and pelvic organs.

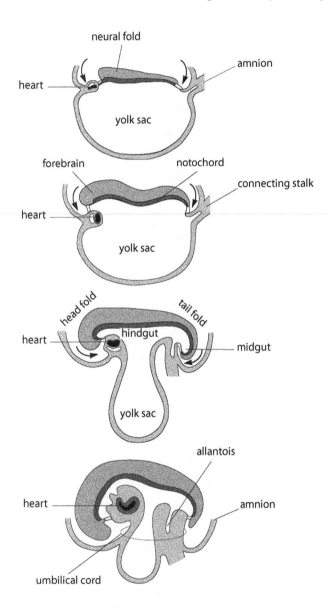

Figure 17.2 The folding of the heart into the body space.

The Heart

The heart is a wonderful organ—it is the first organ to begin to function in embryonic development, and will be functioning until our last breath. It pumps our lifeblood around our body and is pivotal in the oxygenation and sustenance of our cells, in the removal of carbon dioxide and waste products, and in our relational experience of life. It has unique embryological origins. It is the only organ to form outside of the body space. It forms at the superior pole of the embryonic disc, while the primitive streak emerges at the inferior pole near the connecting stalk. In the fourth week post-conception—when the embryo folds into a body tube—the primordial heart folds into the body space via a spiraling motion. The folding process takes three days, and during this time, the heart continues to grow as it spirals toward the midline of the embryo and becomes enfolded in form (Figure 17.2). The motility of the heart reflects this journey. In inhalation you will sense the client's heart diving and spiraling anterior-inferior from the client's right shoulder toward the left hip, and in exhalation the reverse will be sensed (Figures 17.3 and 17.4).

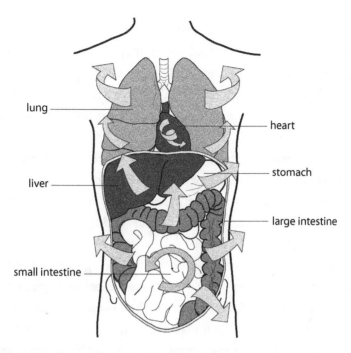

Figure 17.3. Organ motility 1 (after illustrations in Stone, C., 2007).

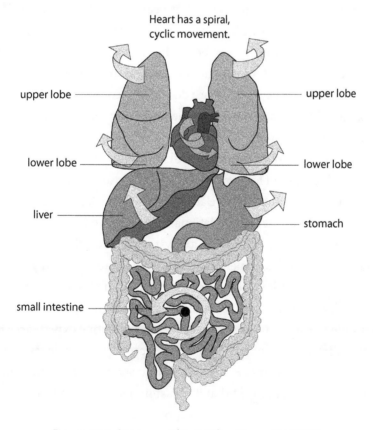

Figure 17.4. Organ motility 2 (after Stone, C., 2007).

The beingness of our heart manifests in love and relationship—the heart is our primary spiritual and relational center. If one has had the fortune to directly experience the presence of the Breath of Life, one discovers that it is a heart-centered experience of loving compassion. One's heart is cast open and one is filled with the bliss of love and loving kindness—this is not personal, but rather a universal quality of connection and direct knowing of our spiritual ground.

We sense and reach out to our relational world from our heart and heart center. The Heartmath researchers (www.heartmath.org) have discovered neurons in heart tissue and that the heart literally serves as our "relational brain." In Chinese philosophy, the word for heart is "heart-mind" and the heart is believed to be the center of our incarnating spirit.

The psycho-emotional and psycho-spiritual being-qualities of the heart have many facets. The heart center is one of our centers of primary ignition. As discussed in Volume One, Chapter 20, heart ignition occurs when the enfolding heart meets the quantum midline in the fourth week after conception. As the heart folds into the body space, it meets the embryo's energetic midline and heart center, and heart ignition occurs. In many spiritual traditions this is the moment that spirit—our most basic being-state—embodies in form. Thus heart ignition is about the ignition of being-in-form, or embodiment. Trauma at this level can leave the incarnating being only partially embodied and life then begins in a dissociated and disconnected state.

The heart relates to both the air and fire elements in Ayurveda. In the movement toward or away from relationship, like a doorway to connection with others, it can be open or closed relative to our experiences of being received or not in our love. As our relational center, it manifests the fire of our feelings of love and connection, and the living strength of purpose and will. The heart, which is naturally open to expressions and feelings of love and belonging, can also hold deep qualities of sadness, grief, frustration, and anger related to loss, to our feelings of our love being received or not, and to a depth of relational wounding and pain.

Ronald Fairbairn, the pioneering analyst mentioned above, understood that infants' hearts are inherently open and that they are naturally loving beings, whose greatest need is for their love to be seen and received. If this need is overridden via inconsistent, disconnected, cold, or abusive caregiving, then a deep wounding that Fairbairn called *primary trauma* may occur. The little one experiences relational trauma, withdraws from contact, and experiences insecurity, separation anxiety, and a loss of being at its core. Frank Lake wrote about the possibility of the little being becoming so traumatized that it is cast into a state of extreme stress where its very being is sensed to be lost, connection to Source is obscured, and the little one is cast into the terrible experience of nonbeing and heart-centered emptiness. He called this state *transmarginal stress*—a state of such deep overwhelm that the little one is pushed beyond the margins of what is tolerable or manageable. As these children then experience their early life, they may meet their world in this state and develop a dissociative and possibly depressive personality system. Insecure attachment is common here as the little ones cannot fully resonate with primary caregivers or sense the inner state and intentions of others. Their neurology is thus affected, where they cannot easily orient to others via the social nervous system and cannot clearly sense the mirroring of others' states internally. This is truly heart-centered wounding and a great sense of loss can be felt at the core of being.

If we need to protect our heart and heart center, our diaphragm will contract. The pericardium—called the heart's protector in Chinese medicine—will also contract, as will the pericardial ligaments, which suspend the pericardium from the thoracic vertebrae. A tense diaphragm, protected rib cage and chest cavity, and a dense and compressed mid-thoracic area (T3–T5), may result. A client may come in with thoracic vertebrae compression and pain, a tight diaphragm, and shortness of breath—all related to deeper heart-centered issues that have generated a need to protect the heart from further pain.

As we place our hand over a client's heart, we may thus also be touching feelings of loss, sadness, grief, low self-esteem, pre- and perinatal trauma, early relational trauma, and layers of heart-felt relational stress. This is no small thing and must be negotiated heartfully and clearly, again with appropriate pacing, relational awareness, and resonance, and clear orientation to primary respiration.

The Lungs

The beingness of the lungs traditionally relates to the air element in Ayurveda, which is about motion, life breath, and ease or lack of ease of movement in life. The lungs can be strongly affected by our heart's need to protect. As we are overwhelmed in life, our diaphragm may contract and tighten, breath becomes restricted, and lung mobility and motility reduced. The connective tissues around the lungs and pericardium may also tighten and inertial fulcrums affecting ease of function and motility will result. In Chinese medicine the lungs are associated with grief and anxiety, again very connected to heart-centered, relational suffering.

The lungs, in their embryological development, bud off the trachea and their motility reflects this budding process throughout life. The lobes of the lungs express their motility relative to the position of the trachea—in inhalation, the upper lobes of the lungs rotate externally and widen apart around vertical axes, while the lower lobes do a similar motion, but around oblique axes (Figures 17.3 and 17.4). As you sense the motility of the lungs, you may find some common inertial patterns and related fulcrums. For instance, you may sense rotational movements around the tip of the upper lobe where it lies under the clavicle, or where the lobes of the lungs meet each other, or, not uncommonly, at the base of the heart where its pericardium is continuous with the diaphragm. All this will yield eccentric qualities of lung motility, commonly expressed as tensile, rotational motions.

The Liver, Stomach, Pancreas, and Spleen

The liver, stomach, pancreas, and spleen again have unique qualities of beingness and motility. It is common to verbally acknowledge the deeply held feelings in these organs. The English language has many colloquial phrases that mirror this: "He hasn't the stomach for that," "I am feeling liverish today," "You have a lot of gall," or "He vented his spleen." All of these represent fiery feelings of some kind. In Ayurveda, these organs are related to the fire element—they manifest fiery energies related to motive power and transformation and—in relational wounding—may hold feelings of frustration, anger, and rage. In the extreme—as in transmarginal stress—this may be coupled with terror and overriding fear, and may also be expressed in relationally wounded states of shame, guilt, and blame. Lake notes that the prenate in the womb may experience strongly negative umbilical affect, as an inflow of cortisol and other stress hormones from mother's system; this may be felt and displaced into the liver or gallbladder and held as fear and anxiety, generating a deeply felt need to protect, coupled with frustration and anger, which may later generate insecure attachment and issues around one's empowerment and self-worth.

In a recent post-graduate course on the viscera, I had the group brainstorm the feeling qualities of each organ. When we oriented to the spleen, some very interesting sharing emerged. People talked about the polarity between strength and weakness, between empowerment and vulnerability. In Chinese medicine the spleen is an organ of transformation, where chi is transformed and life energy is enhanced. It can manifest feelings of pensiveness and worry and, as the participants in our visceral course described, can be the focus for vulnerable feelings. Overwhelming experiences can thus generate spleen-mediated feelings of vulnerability, worry, and fear, with a loss of empowerment and will to transform our lives when needed.

All of these states are literally felt in our guts, and color our sense of the world as our interoceptors relay these felt-qualities to our prefrontal cortex. These reinforce the contextualization of our historical wounds via the temporal lobe, and push the system into limbic mediated anxiety states, coupled with fear and depression. These traumatic feelings continue to infuse our world until we can slow down our process, orient to immediacy of felt-experience, orient to others—and the world we live in—from present-time felt-awareness, and allow the natural resources of primary respiration to come to the forefront.

The whole abdominal cavity and the organs within it—liver, stomach, pancreas, spleen, and intestines—all organize their motility in relationship to the umbilicus. In general, in inhalation the digestive organs, including the intestines, rotate and widen away from the umbilicus.

As discussed in Volume One, the umbilical center is a center for umbilical ignition that occurs after birth. Ideally, after the umbilical cord has stopped pulsing and the baby takes its first breath, an ignition occurs in the umbilical center behind the navel, which intensifies the expression of potency in the fluids and prepares the infant to be an independent physiological being. Umbilical ignition is commonly damped down, either by strongly negative umbilical affect, traumatic prenatal or birth experiences, medical interventions, or later experiences of overwhelm and shock trauma. Orienting to umbilical ignition issues was first developed by Randolph Stone and passed on to Dr. Robert Fulford, who brought it into the osteopathic community, and is covered in some detail in Foundations Volume One. Umbilical ignition issues—coupled with the trauma that may have affected the ignition process—may manifest as low energy and low motivation, and may be expressed as tension, contraction, fear, anxiety, worry, and low self-esteem in the digestive organs and intestines.

The motility of these organs again mirrors their developmental processes. The liver, pancreas, and spleen bud off from the primitive digestive tube, while the stomach forms within it. All three rotate into their positions as they develop (Figure 17.5). Their motility continues to express this rotational motion. In inhalation, the liver and stomach rotate around an oblique axis away from the umbilicus, widening and rotating superior-laterally as they widen apart. The pancreas develops by budding off the gut tube in two sections, while also rotating into position. In inhalation, its motility is expressed as a lengthening laterally, while its tip moves slightly anterior, which expresses its original rotational developmental motion. It is noteworthy that the spleen does not bud from the gut tube endoderm. Instead, it forms in the mesoderm behind the stomach and follows the rotation of the stomach into its final position on the left side. In keeping with the pathway it followed during development, the spleen expresses motility as an external rotation around a relative vertical axis, while also dropping slightly inferior (see Figures 17.3 and 17.4).

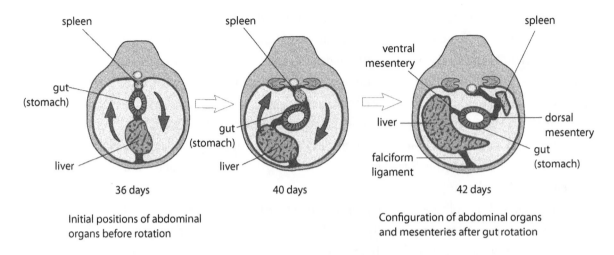

Figure 17.5. Embryo gut rotation.

The Kidneys

In Ayurveda the kidneys are air element organs whose beingness holds the dichotomy between fear and courage. They are intimately related to our adrenal glands and anxiety states, relate to available energy in life, and are very attuned to the stress response. In Chinese medicine they are the site of primordial chi (life force) and are organs of transformation manifesting our potential in life. The kidneys can cycle trauma and shock states and resonate deeply with prenatal and early transmarginal stress and the obscuration of being. In transmarginal stress our most basic sense of spirit and beingness becomes obscured due to developmental shock coupled with the fear of personal annihilation. The kidneys can resonate with these conditions, hold states of fear and anxiety, and need careful and compassionate holding by the practitioner. The afflicted person may suffer from states of anxiety, poor sleep, depressive processes, and low self-esteem. When clear and grounded, the kidneys manifest strength and are an emotional ground for courage in the presence of adversity.

In embryonic development, before the kidneys properly develop, there were two earlier sets of primordial filtering organs—the pronephros and mesonephros, which later give way to the metanephros, which forms the adult kidney. The metanephros forms in the lower pelvic region and ascends to the lower lumbar region in the sixth to ninth week in utero to form the kidney. As the developing kidney ascends, it also rotates 90 degrees into its final position. This ascending and rotational motion is mirrored in its motility. In inhalation, the kidney externally rotates around a relative vertical angle and also subtly descends. In some ways this rotating-descending

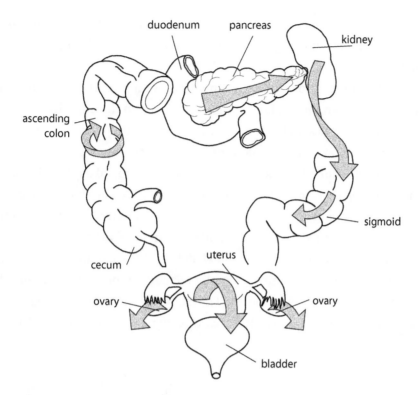

Figure 17.6. Organ motility 3.

motion is a settling back into its embryological origins and is very interesting in its expression (Figure 17.6).

The Small Intestine and Colon

In Ayurveda the intestines are fire and earth organs—they process our food, extract the nutrients we need to survive, and eliminate the wastes from that process. The beingness of these organs relates to principles of sustenance, getting needs met, and grounding our energies and lives. The small intestines resonate both with the fire and earth elements—fire in its relationship to the umbilical center, fiery motive energies, and the processing of nutrients, and earth in its grounding of the digestive process. The colon is governed both by air and earth elements—air in its filtering functions and earth in its eliminating functions. The intestines, like the kidneys, can cycle around fear and courage. In shockingly overwhelming circumstances we may lose our ground, be inundated with fear, and suddenly defecate—the intestines can hold feelings of fear, anxiety, and a loss of foundation and ground in life. Issues surrounding safety, security, and welfare can be held in the intestines, coupled with the states of autonomic fight-flight—fear, anxiety, and contraction. Solar plexus or sympathetic nervous system activation can be part of this picture. The person may suffer from sleep difficulties, gut-felt anxiety, poor digestion, constipation, and/or diarrhea.

The embryonic development of the intestines is unique. At around thirty-two days after conception, the midgut begins to extend into the umbilical coelom as the umbilical loop, and spirals out into the umbilical cord to lengthen and grow. At around forty-four days, the extension reaches its fullness and the intestine begins to spiral back into the embryonic gut, which completes around day 56 (Figure 17.7).

This spiraling developmental motion in the umbilical cord is expressed in the intestine's motility in various ways. The large intestine mostly expresses its motility as a widening-rotating away from the umbilicus in inhalation and a narrowing-rotating back toward the umbilicus in exhalation. The small intestine's motility more directly mirrors the spiraling developmental motion. In inhalation, while looking at the client's abdomen, the small intestines spiral around and expand away from the umbilicus in a counter-clockwise direction (see Figures 17.3 and 17.4).

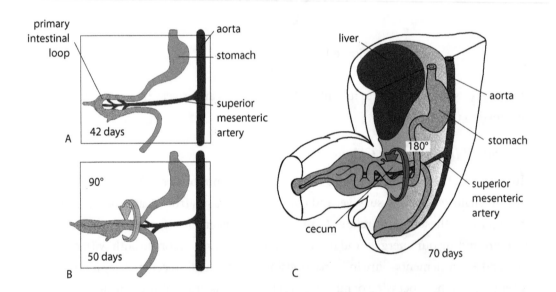

Figure 17.7. Embryo intestine rotation.

The Pelvic Organs

The pelvic organs are organs of elimination and procreation—the rectum and bladder, the uterus, ovaries, and vagina in women, the prostate gland, testicles, and penis in men—all manifesting a felt-quality of life, a beingness. In Ayurveda, the pelvic organs are supported by the water element—water seeks the lowest level—so issues of grounding and completion may be held in the pelvic area. Classically, the water element also orients to the unconscious—to our dream world, archetypal knowledge, and intuitive knowing. It governs deeply held unconscious emotions and feelings, and the watery organs of the pelvis can mirror all of this.

The pelvis expresses the sensual and sexual aspects of our lives. The organs of procreation—uterus, ovaries, prostate, and testes—can hold deep issues around self-worth and self-image. In woman, issues about fertility, miscarriages, abortions, sensuality, and self-image may be held as feeling-tone in the pelvic organs. The practitioner must also be sensitive to the possible presence of abuse issues, even early abuse or perceived abuse from infancy and childhood. This can all be very delicate to hold and are deeply relational in nature. The establishment of a safe holding environment is—as always—pivotal.

Both kidneys and bladder hold the dichotomy between fear and courage described above. Sudden danger can make one urinate in fear, and the bladder can hold issues cycling around insecurity and self-doubt. The bladder is also deeply connected to mammalian issues of boundary and nesting. Male mammals urinate to mark and protect the boundaries of their territories and females classically are involved in nesting and maintaining the family. Issues around personal and inter-personal boundaries, safety, security, and quality of home space can all generate fear and anxiety, held in the kidneys, bladder, and pelvis.

The embryology of the pelvic organs is complex. The urogenital system develops in close association with the urinary system. The ovaries and testes develop from identical primordial cells in both sexes—called the undifferentiated stage—where the embryo has the potential to develop into either a male or female. The differentiation into male or female is determined by the testis-determining factor on the Y chromosome. When present, testes develop. When two X chromosomes are present, ovaries develop. Both ovaries and testes descend into place—the ovaries into their position in the pelvis in relationship to the uterus and the testes to hang outside the pelvis.

The motility of the pelvic organs is more or less organized around the umbilicus. The rectum, bladder, prostate, and uterus all manifest a similar motility. In inhalation, they rotate anterior-inferior away from the umbilicus. The ovaries also express their motility relative to the umbilicus—they rotate anterior-inferior, but around oblique axes (see Figure 17.6).

Treatment Approaches

The clinical approach to organ issues is not different from any other. As the inherent treatment plan unfolds, visceral fulcrums and inertial issues will manifest over the course of treatment. As these emerge, the practitioner presence, orientation to the three bodies and primary respiration, and appropriate relationship to the arising process have the same importance.

Orienting to organs and their inertial issues has a number of basic components:

- Creating an appropriate contact to the organ involved with your footward (caudal) hand, by settling into a still and receptive state with hands floating on tissues suspended in fluid. Your hands themselves are ideally sensed to be fluid entities suspended in a wider fluid field.

- Orienting to the organ's motility and deepening into a relationship to the felt-quality of the person's being-state. This is a process of openness and attunement to the resonances of feelings and emotional tone, which is mostly about being heart-centered, nonjudgmental, and fully present.

- Helping the client orient to the feelings and sensations that may arise as session work continues, and to the felt-quality of the visceral area being attended to in the session. An appropriate verbal dialogue, oriented to mindfulness and felt-inquiry, can be very helpful as feelings and sensation arise.

- Settling into the unfolding of the inherent treatment plan as usual—orienting to the suspensory nature of system, to the inertial fulcrum and forces organizing it in your wide perceptual field, to the state of balance or dynamic equilibrium as it clarifies, to the level of primary respiration that emerges in the healing process, to the action of potency in the fluid body, and to the ground of Dynamic Stillness from which it all originates.

It is also helpful to orient to nociceptive issues that may be affecting organ function and generating CNS sensitivity. We discuss this in great detail in Chapter 21. Inertial issues in organ dynamics can sensitize the dorsal horn neurons of the spinal cord, which can set up hypersensitization in the related sensorimotor nerve loop and maintain organ sensitivity and inertial issues. To orient to this, place your other hand under the spinal cord area associated with that organ. While the footward (caudal) hand is placed over the organ, the other hand moves under the client with palm and fingers spread, palm or fingers under the appropriate vertebral level of the spinal cord. For organs below the diaphragm, this is at the lower level of the spinal cord at T11–L2. For organs above the diaphragm, your other hand is placed at the level of C7–T4, where the nerves, which serve the thoracic organs, emerge. Settling into a still state, the practitioner waits for the sensorimotor nerve loop and dorsal horn area of the spinal cord to enter equilibrium. Chapter 21 describes this in detail and explains how this work can be followed through other levels of neural processing.

Hand Positions

Your hand is placed on the various organs depending on their position in the body and their developmental motility. There is no firm rule on how to contact an organ—I make some suggestions here. In all of the hand positions described, I recommend that you use your footward (caudal) hand to make contact with the organ so that your arm is not in the way of your visual contact with the client's face—face-to-face contact may be important in the relational aspect of the work, and verbal sharing and inquiry may become crucial.

You might hold the client's heart from the right side of the body, with your hand spread over the heart area. With women, you must negotiate a contact that does not touch the breasts in any inappropriate or threatening manner. Place your hands over the lungs as appropriate, upper lungs in a transverse fashion and lower lungs in a slightly oblique manner, again negotiating appropriate contact.

When placing your hand over the liver, you might stand or sit on the left side of the treatment table, and place the heel of your caudal hand over the gallbladder area with your fingers spreading obliquely over the liver, pointing laterally. You can do this from the right side of the table also. You might hold the stomach in a similar manner. You might hold the pancreas from the right side of the table, with the heel of your lower hand over the solar plexus-duodenal area, fingers pointing laterally and slightly superior.

To place your hands over a client's kidney, you can work either supine or side-lying. With the client in the supine position and sitting at the side of the table, place your hand under the client's body spread under either the right or left kidney at the appropriate level. The right kidney is lower than the left—your hand is placed 50 percent under the lower ribs and 50 percent below, while your hand under the left kidney is placed higher up—mostly under the lower ribs.

Making contact with pelvic organs must be negotiated in a clear way. Remember the psycho-emotional and possible abuse issues that may be held there. Also remember that the pelvis is a vulnerable area to make contact with even if these issues are not critical in the client's process or life. I always tell clients at the beginning of session work that they can ask me to withdraw contact or stop the session at any time.

Ask the client to show you where the pubic symphysis is. Then make a negotiated contact, placing the heel of your hand over the superior aspect of the pubic bone, with your fingers spread out superiorly. You now have a relationship to all of the organs held in the pelvis. Maintaining a wide perceptual field, you can orient to the motility of any organ in the pelvic bowl from this position. To sense the ovaries, place your hand or hands obliquely over the ovary areas, again clearly negotiating your contact.

Another good way of orienting to the pelvic organs is via a sacral-pubic bone hold—this is very useful in general practice when you want to orient to sacral-pelvic issues. Start with your sacral hold, allow yourself to settle into your wide perceptual field, and then place your other hand over the pubic symphysis more or less as described above. You are now directly in relationship to the whole pelvic bowl—all of its bony, ligamentous, connective tissue, and organ relationships are between your hands.

Please remember to maintain a wide perceptual field, with fluid hands suspended in a fluid field, and allow the system to deepen into the healing process as the inherent treatment plan unfolds.

Clinical Example

Start at the side of the table as usual. First orient to the three bodies—the physical, fluid, and tidal bodies—and to primary respiration relative to your own system. Then orient to the client's system, midline, and three bodies.

Allow the relational field to settle, and move to the client's feet. Again first orient to your midline and three bodies, and then place your hands on the client's feet and orient to his or her midline, three bodies, and primary respiration relative to the client's system. As the system settles into its suspensory nature—physical body suspended in fluid body, suspended in tidal body of Long Tide—orient to the emergence and deepening of the holistic shift. In this example, let's say that,an inertial fulcrum clarifies in the liver area. You might sense the whole tissue field, now suspended in the fluid body, organizing around some issue in the liver area.

You might then make contact with the inertial site by placing your caudal hand over the liver as described above—imagine-sense that your hand is fluid and is floating on tissue, suspended in a wider fluid field. Settle into your wide perceptual field—physical body suspended in fluid body, suspended in tidal body—and orient to the motility of the liver. Work as usual; allow the system to access the state of balance or dynamic equilibrium and orient to whatever level of healing process emerges.

As inertial forces in the fulcrum are resolved, you might also orient to the nociceptive loop as described above—spread your other hand under the spinal cord at the level of T12–L2 and again settle into your wide listening. As the system settles into a state of equilibrium relative to the sensorimotor loop, you may sense a synchronous expression of potency both in the spinal cord and liver. You may sense a synchronous pulsation at both poles, with heat and autonomic clearing expressed. You may sense an electric-like streaming down the client's spine and legs as the autonomic cycling clears. Finish the session as appropriate.

Conclusion

This chapter is meant as an introduction to visceral motility, issues, and practice. In class situations, I set up sessions in which students explore each organ relationship in sequence for their learning purposes. The intention is to begin to attune to the presence, motility, psycho-emotional issues, and clinical potential of the organs so that they can be seamlessly incorporated into ongoing session work.

CHAPTER 18

Trauma Resolution 1: The Stress Cascade and Neuroendocrine Relationships

S tress and traumatic experience are part of everyday life and comprise a huge area of inquiry in all healing modalities. Study of stress and trauma has become a field in itself called *psycho-neuro-immunology*. Much of the suffering seen in clinical practice is generated by the unresolved cycling of the stress response and its neuroendocrine and autonomic nervous system processes. Indeed, in many ways, how we manage stress and trauma throughout life shapes and reshapes our personality system, its defenses, and our psycho-physiology.

Many clients will manifest anxiety, depression, and/or various states of autonomic activation and overwhelm as sessions progress. These may be coupled with personality forms and tendencies, emotional states, various feeling-tones, defensive processes, transference, and projections. These cycling processes may also cast the affected person into existential crisis, with coupled experiences of emptiness, meaninglessness, loss of being, and existential angst. It is imperative that the practitioner can recognize these states and can draw upon appropriate clinical skills to help clients negotiate them without again becoming overwhelmed or retraumatized. The following sections look at the nature of stress, its basic neurobiology, and appropriate clinical skills and responses.

Traumatization Is Physiological in Nature

In clinical practice, the practitioner will inevitably be confronted with the effects of traumatic experience, traumatization, and related suffering. These might manifest in many ways including emotional flooding, anxiety states, freezing or immobilized states, dissociation, trembling, rapid breathing, hot and cold sensations, sweating, and shaking. These arising states may have their roots in early prenatal and birth experiences, overwhelming early childhood experiences, or may be expressions of later one-off or repetitive traumatic experiences. The potential for trauma is with us from our earliest moments of life. Trauma in early life strongly affects bonding and attachment processes, and can be a major fulcrum in personality formation. Prenates, infants, and young children are more easily overwhelmed by intense experience than older children or adults and their stress response can likewise engage more quickly. Young children will also default to dissociative protective processes more quickly than older children and these states may even be the roots of Attention Deficit Disorder (ADD) and Attention Deficit Hyperactivity Disorder (ADHD) (Perry and Pollard 1998). Later trauma may quickly destabilize affected people's functioning and shift their personality processes from normal coping strategies to survival mechanisms, fight-or-flight, and states of overwhelm, freezing, and dissociation.

Traumatization has physiological foundations that are important to appreciate in session work and a somatic understanding of trauma is essential in this context. If a practitioner doesn't understand these, he or she might inadvertently encourage or collude in processes that are really not healing and may actually be retraumatizing. For instance, as a session progresses, a client's process speeds up and there is a flood of emotions. The practitioner might assume that this emotional release is part of a healing process, when in fact the client may actually be in a dissociative state coupled with escalating emotional and autonomic activation. The client's central nervous system, in this case, may register the current activation as a response to a newly overwhelming situation. In this scenario, emotional flooding may actually reinforce and intensify underlying patterns of traumatization and maladaptive states, and the client may then become retraumatized by the session experience.

Top-Down, Bottom-Up Processing

The first step in understanding trauma and traumatic response to overwhelming experience is to outline how the human brain is organized. The brain is basically set up in a hierarchical, triune fashion, with three levels of processing: (1) cortical, (2) limbic-emotional, and (3) brain stem sensorimotor-autonomic processing.

The top level, cortical processing, relates to the ability to hold meaning and context, to inquire into current circumstances and deduce from past experience, to rationally think things through, and to regulate one's affect and feeling states. An important area of brain function related to this process is the ability to be present and hold current experience in the light of present-time awareness. The area of the cortex that mediates this territory is the medial prefrontal cortex. It has connections to all major stress and autonomic nuclei. The process of mindfully orienting to present sensation and experience engages the prefrontal cortex, and helps the nervous system down-regulate the stress response if it has become hypersensitized. In traumatized individuals the ability to top-down process is largely lost, along with the ability to be in present time, to regulate affect, contextualize one's experience, and rationally orient to one's world of experience.

The next level is limbic-emotional processing, our emotional feelings and affect responses to both positive and negative experiences. In terms of the stress response, this level also mediates the central nervous system's response to novel or dangerous situations, a very important territory in traumatization. Limbic dynamics can become hypersensitized, generating hyper- or hypoarousal states, coupled with oversensitivity to sensory input and loss of orientation to present experience.

The lowest level is sensorimotor-autonomic processing, which is about survival needs and internal homeostasis. Ideally, we do not have to think about breathing, cardiac regulation, digestion, and the like. This level of processing also works without thought; it is pivotal in our response to novel and dangerous situations, initiating survival responses to perceived danger, along with defensive and dissociative processes. In traumatization, survival responses may become overactive and the person may experience hyperarousal states, or the person may find him- or herself lost in freezing states and/or dissociation.

In an untraumatized individual, a fluid homeostatic relationship of top-down, bottom-up processing is available. The person can hold meaning, concentrate, make decisions based on inquiry and past experience, and regulate his or her affect and responses to situations. At the same time, appropriate emotional responses to present-time situations are available, while the sensorimotor system takes care of basic internal needs. Likewise, survival responses are also fluidly available, as novel or possibly dangerous situations are met.

When a person is overwhelmed and left traumatized by experience, this situation may drastically change. The system can become locked in survival mode and the ability to top-down process may be largely lost. The person may be left cycling the stress response, where cortical processing is much less available. One cannot think through situations or regulate affect when one's emotional life cycles around survival emotions like fear and anger, while cortical memory processes throw up images of past trauma (flashbacks), and a person is locked in survival mode, hypervigilance, freezing states, dissociation, and inappropriate responses to current situations. The system becomes hypersensitized and stuck in bottom-up processing (Figure 18.1).

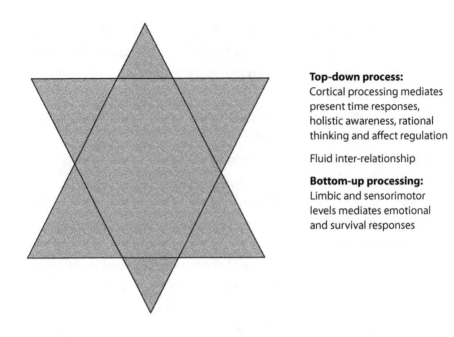

Top-down process:
Cortical processing mediates present time responses, holistic awareness, rational thinking and affect regulation

Fluid inter-relationship

Bottom-up processing:
Limbic and sensorimotor levels mediates emotional and survival responses

Figure 18.1. Top-down, bottom-up processing.

Stress and Adaptation

Stress is an integral part of our human experience. Almost any aspect of life can be experienced as stressful and we inevitably find ourselves under varying levels of stress, even in ideal circumstances. Family situations, close relationships, our work and finances, challenging experiences of almost any kind, or even just the pace of modern life all present us with stress. Going to work on the underground or subway, driving our car, meeting new people or forming new relationships—indeed, just walking down the street—all may have impact. Our relationships may become stressful, tension with partners or workmates may emerge, or tensions may develop in new situations. We may experience a wide range of traumatic events like accidents, falls, abuse, violence, crime, losing loved ones, losing one's work or home, and all kinds of shocking news. In a wider context, our prenatal, perinatal, and early childhood experiences of stress and traumatization may strongly organize central nervous system functioning, attachment systems, and personality formation. These may be compounded by later interpersonal encounters of almost any kind. Indeed, the response to any subsequently overwhelming experience will be added and layered onto the fabric of selfhood.

In response to all of these, our neuroendocrine system naturally shifts to what is known as an *adaptive state*. This means that it physiologically gears up to meet the stress. This response is orchestrated by certain nuclei (groups of neurons) in the central nervous system (CNS) and related hormones and neuroactive chemicals. There are many nuclei and brain areas involved in this response, all of which prepare us for action. This global shift in body-mind physiology is commonly called the *general adaptation response*. This global response is intended to mobilize us to meet the danger, stress, or challenge successfully. Once the stress is removed, or successfully dealt with, the body physiology then ideally shifts back to a more baseline state of homeostatic balance. We will discuss the general adaptation response in general terms in this chapter, and look more specifically at its neuroendocrine interactions in the next chapter.

The general adaptation response is mediated by the neuroendocrine system, whose parts and functions are completely interdependent. This system keeps our survival mechanisms running. It orients us to the external physical and interpersonal environment; it monitors internal responses and processes, maintains internal homeostasis, helps us to discern and respond to danger, to find food and mates, to repair internal damage, and a host of related functions. It runs in the background all the time. Indeed, this system can be considered the command headquarters for all homeostatic and survival processes.

When we encounter stressors, the neuroendocrine system gears up to meet the stress with almost instantaneous surges of neuroactive molecules that trigger responses throughout the body. Muscles, circulation, respiration, digestion, and other systems all respond in a symphony of complex interactions so that life can be sustained. If the stress is repetitive, chronic, or prolonged, or if the traumatic incident overwhelmed the system and was not able to be processed at the time, then the body physiology may not be able to shift back to homeostatic balance. The fluidity of the system may be reduced or lost and replaced by a quality of fixation. Stress nuclei may become hypersensitized to input and cycle a stress response inappropriately even though the danger has actually passed. The ability to self-regulate in the normal way is then lost. The system may literally become fixed in this state, with an elevated set point for an indefinite period of time. This is called a *maladaptive state*. Chronic maladaptive states can lead to both physiological and psychological dysfunction. In my clinical experience, these may include a whole range of dysfunctional states, including immune deficiency, autoimmune states, anxiety, depression, dissociative states, sleeping and eating disorders, somatic dysfunctions of all descriptions, chronic pain syndromes, and psycho-emotional breakdown. It can have vast mind-body repercussions.

The Stress Response

The general adaptation response is also called the *stress response*, as it is our psycho-physiological response to stressful or potentially dangerous situations. The response to danger is largely mediated by the limbic and autonomic nervous systems. The limbic system alerts us to possible danger and the autonomic system mobilizes us to meet it. The autonomic nervous system is classically divided into two aspects that are meant to function in reciprocal relationship. These are the *sympathetic* and *parasympathetic nervous systems*. The sympathetic nervous system relates to arousal states, vigilance, the musculo-skeletal system, and action, while the parasympathetic system relates to vegetative functions like digestion and elimination and rest and repose, and is the system that is involved in meditative and contemplative states. These two systems normally function in homeostatic balance, unless maladaptive states are present due to unresolved traumatic and overwhelming experiences. As we shall later see, the autonomic nervous system can also be divided into a triune system of social, sympathetic, and parasympathetic systems, which yields a clearer picture of what is occurring in both relaxed and stressed states. I describe this in more detail in Chapter 20.

There are four basic stages to the stress response: (1) the ideal or *resourced state*, (2) *orienting response*, (3) *fight-or-flight,* and (4) *overwhelm-shock*.

The Ideal or Resourced State

The resourced state is a fully resourced, relaxed, and present-time state. We can calmly walk in the forest and appreciate the sunlight and smells, can peacefully digest our food, and relate to our friends, and can use what is known as the *social nervous system* to get our needs met, while our neuroendocrine and autonomic nervous systems are poised in fluid homeostatic balance.

Orienting Response

If novel or potentially dangerous sensory input is perceived, then the neuroendocrine system rapidly shifts to the orienting response and a state called *active-alert*. In this state we momentarily freeze and orient to the environment. You may have experienced this recently. A loud noise occurs and you find yourself momentarily freezing as you orient around you—seeing, hearing, sensing for danger. This is not a fear state, but rather a calm state of heightened awareness and mental clarity whose intention is to orient to the possibility of danger. This is mediated by certain parasympathetic nuclei and by other CNS nuclei, such as the amygdala and locus ceruleus.

Fight-or-Flight

If danger is sensed to be present, the system dramatically shifts to the fight-or-flight response. This term was coined by Hans Selye in the 1930s and is our most basic response to stress, danger, and overwhelming situations. Here the sympathetic nervous system, which mediates arousal, vigilance, and action, surges along with increases in certain hormones, especially norepinephrine (noradrenaline) and epinephrine (adrenaline). Energies move to the periphery and our body is mobilized for action. We fight or flee.

Vegetative activities like digestion and reproduction are down-regulated, while the cardiovascular system, muscles, and limbs are geared for action. Concurrently, an up-regulation of what is called the *H-P-A axis* (hypothalamus-pituitary-adrenal axis) occurs, yielding a surge in the hormone cortisol. This mobilizes energies and helps maintain the adaptive response over time. This global response is intended to mobilize us to meet the danger, stress, or challenge successfully, and can occur instantaneously as novel or threatening input is sensed. Once the stress is removed, or successfully dealt with, the body physiology is designed to shift smoothly back to a baseline state of homeostatic balance.

Overwhelm-Shock

If our intentions to protect are overwhelmed and the fight-or-flight process is thwarted, then we may be cast into a deeply protective shock response. In this state the parasympathetic nervous system surges, overlays the fight-or-flight response, and sends the person into a state of immobilization, disconnection, dissociation, and shock. He or she is cast into protective, dissociative, freezing states where the psyche disengages from the overwhelming experience in order to protect the organism from further pain.

Commonly, during this state of immobilization, powerful sympathetic energies are still cycling underneath. This is important to understand both personally and in clinical practice. These energies have to be mindfully discharged and resolved in some way. Ideally, as a person comes out of shock states, he or she has the opportunity to resolve the underlying traumatic cycling. The sympathetic charge may be mobilized and cleared by trembling, shaking, and emotional expression, while the person ideally remains resourced in present-time awareness.

In everyday experience, this process of trauma resolution is commonly thwarted, as the trauma may be too overwhelming to process in the immediacy of the experience. Later, our minds, and the meaning we give the experience, may get in the way, while the cycling of past traumatization may prevent the resolution of current traumatic experience. The upshot of it all is that we may be left with some of these energies still cycling within us. This can lead directly to chronic autonomic arousal, the inappropriate initiation and cycling of the stress response, classic anxiety and depressive states, immune disorders, and the loss of our ability to fluidly respond to life.

The Stress Response in the Mammalian World

Let's make the above ideas more concrete. In this section we will look at the stress response by imagining the actions of an antelope on the African plains. It is important to remember that humans are mammals and the stress response is a basic mammalian defensive process. Although human cortical responses to stress may be more complex than other mammals, understanding an antelope's response to trauma still helps us understand much of our own human response. Below are five scenarios that are commonly observed in the wild and that illustrate aspects of the human stress response. Imagine you are safely sitting in a Land Rover, viewing the scene.

Scenario One

Let's imagine an antelope grazing on the African plains. I'm sure that you have seen scenes like this in TV documentaries. In our visualization, it is grazing at a short distance from the rest of the herd. At first there is no sign of danger and the antelope grazes in a relaxed fashion with no tension or fear obvious, oriented to present-time homeostasis and appropriately getting its needs met—the *ideal resourced state.* The antelope is grazing in a fully present state, without any neurotic tensions held over from past experiences of trauma or stress.

The antelope suddenly smells a micro-amount of lion spore. "Hint of lion" on the wind! The antelope will momentarily freeze, stop grazing, and become vigilant. It will stop its activity and enter the active-alert state of heightened awareness. It will also express what is called *orienting responses.* It will orient to the environment by turning its head, moving its ears—looking and listening for possible danger. It will scan the environment for clues. If there are no further clues that danger is present— say, that the lion is not in the area and its spore is not obvious—then the antelope will settle out of the active-alert stage and return to relaxed grazing. It returns to its resourced state and is not traumatized or stressed by the process.

Scenario Two

Let's imagine another scenario. Now a lion *is* in the area and is stalking the antelope. The lion is hiding behind a bush and the danger is clearly present. The antelope smells lion spore and goes into its active-alert state. This time, let's imagine that the lion jumps out of hiding and runs toward the antelope. The antelope will instantly and dramatically engage its *flight-or-fight* response. Its sympathetic nervous system will surge and become highly charged. Its metabolism dramatically increases, blood is directed to the periphery for muscular use, and the neuroendocrine system floods its body with stress hormones such as norepinephrine, adrenaline, and cortisol.

This is called a *mobilization response*. There is clear and present danger; the antelope's system surges and it flees. In this case, let's imagine that this survival flight is successful. The antelope mobilizes its flight response and successfully flees the lion. The antelope runs, jumps, and soars through the bush and the lion is left in the dust. There will be a point when the lion knows that it is not successful and it will stop the chase and even may express what, from the outside looking at the lion, may be called dejection. When the antelope knows it is successful, other hormones, such as endorphins, may flood its system. The antelope may experience exhilaration, euphoria, and even altered states of near ecstasy in its successful flight. It will keep running and jumping until its sympathetic nervous system charge is completed and cleared. When the antelope is free from danger, it will slow down, come to a stop, return to its active-alert state, and reorient itself to the environment. If no further signs of danger are present, it will naturally return to the relaxed, ideal state, look for its herd, and resume grazing. The important thing to note here is that the antelope successfully expressed its response to danger—it successfully fled and *was not traumatized by the experience*. It had the resources to meet the experience and could mobilize those resources with success. It was not overwhelmed by the experience; it was able to return to its relaxed state. It may even come out of the experience a stronger and more confident antelope!

Scenario Three

Let's look at a different scenario. Let's say that the lion has managed to stalk the antelope successfully and is quite close as it pounces. The antelope instantaneously engages its fight-or-flight response. It flees. This time, however, the lion is more successful. Perhaps there are a number of lions involved in the chase—lionesses usually hunt as a pride, or pack of hunters. Now the antelope's flight response is not successful. It is surrounded and trapped. Its flight-or-fight response has been overridden and overwhelmed by the lions. It cannot express the energy of mobilization in successful flight. If its flight-or-fight response is thwarted, the antelope will still try to protect itself. It does this by going into shock. If the antelope is really successful, it may go into shock before it is even touched by a lion. The parasympathetic nervous system surges and other neurohormones are released. The antelope may then suddenly collapse. This is a critical survival ploy to understand. Shock is part of our natural survival mechanism; it is a natural response to an overwhelming situation.

In shock, the antelope will go into a dissociative state. Its psyche will disconnect from its soma and sensations. This dissociative process is of extreme importance to understand in the therapeutic setting. Along with dissociation, the body will also enter an immobilized or frozen state. Its vital signs may become almost impossible to detect from the outside. Hence, it becomes *immobilized* and *frozen*.

The important thing to realize here is that this frozen state is a highly charged state. In the shock response, the normal balance between the sympathetic and para-sympathetic systems is upset. As the sympathetic charge is thwarted, the para-sympathetic system surges. The parasympathetic charge overrides the original sympathetic surge, strongly down-regulates the cardiovascular system, and the animal is catapulted into a catatonic state. Now both systems are surging, that is, are expressing greatly heightened activity. The huge charge in the sympathetic nervous system cannot be discharged in physical flight from the lions. This energy has to go somewhere. In this case, when the animal goes into shock, it literally implodes inward. The sympathetic charge, rather than being expressed and discharged in action, implodes and keeps cycling.

If the shock response is successful and the antelope is deeply dissociated and immobilized, then, from the outside, it will seem as though all vital signs have ceased and the antelope is dead. *This is all part of the antelope's survival mechanism.* The lions, when they reach the antelope in this state, may think that she is dead. They may smell the antelope, nudge it, and then, amazingly, if they are not famished, leave it alone! I have seen this happen in a wildlife documentary where the lionesses dragged the seemingly dead antelope over to their cubs to play with. Lions have learned in their own evolution, that eating dead animals may leave them very sick and is dangerous. The shock mechanism may then have actually saved the antelope's life! If the lions do eat the antelope, it is spared the pain of its death as its psyche is dissociated from physical sensations. There is a beautiful compassion to all of this. It is again important to note that the antelope may appear frozen or dead, but inwardly it is in a highly charged state.

Let's look at what happens to the antelope's system if the lions go away and it is not eaten. The antelope will gradually come out of the shock response. Its psyche re-associates with its body and its energies begin to shift and move. Its parasympathetic system down-regulates and the sympathetic nervous system discharges. If you were there, you might notice color and size changes in the antelope's lips and pupils. It then does something that is again clinically important to note. Its body begins to tremble and shake as the imploded sympathetic energies discharge. You may see this kind of response emerge in your own session work. The antelope may then express this discharge by standing up, bucking, running, or jumping. In this process it shifts out of its parasympathetic frozen state, clears the cycling sympathetic energies by action, and completes its fight-or-flight response. After this, it may then return to the active-alert state, reorient itself to its environment and to possible danger, and if none is perceived, it will then go back to its resourced, ideal state.

The powerful thing to note is that the antelope has survived, has successfully come out of shock, has discharged its imploded energies, and was not traumatized by the experience! It went through the stages of its defensive strategies and, although it had a traumatic experience, it was not necessarily left traumatized by it. *Traumatization occurs when the antelope cannot, for whatever reason, process the cycling energies of its shock response.*

Scenario Four

Let's look at a different possible ending for the above scenario. Let's say, for instance, that you are sitting in your Land Rover and have witnessed the whole event. You have seen the chase and have seen the antelope go into shock. You feel sorry for the antelope, the lions have left, and you rush over to the animal while it is still in shock. The antelope starts to come out of its shock response and begins to tremble. It is starting to express the natural discharge of its imploded energies. But in this case, you feel so sorry for the antelope that you begin to comfort it, perhaps placing a blanket over it, or stroking it. This seemingly compassionate act may actually stop the antelope from processing its shock. By intervening, you may have stopped its cycling parasympathetic and sympathetic energies from being discharged and prevented it from clearing both its shock response and the underlying fight-or-flight energies. Its hormonal system is also left unbalanced with a high volume of stress hormones still cycling. Peter Levine calls the inappropriate cycling of these energies *trauma-bound energy* (Levine 1997).

The antelope is now left in a state that is hypersensitive to new input, cannot appropriately respond to new stressors, and might even manifest what we would call anxiety or depressive states. When it next meets a lion, due to these cycling energies, it may not be able to orient to danger. As danger is sensed, instead of clearly entering an actively alert and oriented state, it may freeze in fear as the unresolved shock state floods its system. Hence, its natural survival mechanisms are now compromised, its resources are lowered, and its ability to meet traumatic or stressful situations is also compromised. This is a very dangerous situation for an antelope to find itself in, as it may become more easily overwhelmed by a dangerous situation, and may not be able to quickly or efficiently mobilize its resources.

Thus traumatization occurs when the cycling energies of the stress response become trapped and frozen in the body physiology. It is as though the system becomes frozen in time and has to react to present situations while it is still holding onto past experience. This may occur for many reasons, but the bottom line is that the shock, and the experience that it relates to, is entrapped in the system. The powerful energies of the flight-or-fight response continue to cycle and frozen and immobilized states may more easily be expressed in inappropriate ways.

Scenario Five

Another aspect of this process is that the antelope's limbic-emotional system may also become actively engaged. Let's imagine another scenario. The antelope is again grazing and the lions pounce. The antelope engages its flight-or-fight response. As above, in this new scenario, the lions are hunting in a pride and have the antelope surrounded. In this case the antelope is surrounded, is deeply in its flight response and is cornered. In this scenario, the antelope may express strong emotions like anger or fear. There may be some survival value in this. The added energy of anger can be instantly channeled into fight-or-flight, as it may buck in anger, hit a lion, and find a way out.

This is a risky strategy on two counts. First, the antelope can't hope to beat a lion at its own game—that is, trying to fight the lions. This is, however, a strategy of desperation. Second, if the antelope is cornered and overwhelmed as it enters its shock state, these strong emotional energies may implode along with the sympathetic surge. This may make its freezing response less effective and be dangerous to the organism. If it survives, when it comes out of the shock response, the antelope may not clear the emotional charge that also imploded in shock. When it next sees a lion, emotions like rage or terror may inappropriately arise and get in the way of its flight response, or fear may cause it to go into an immobilized state too early.

Our Human Dilemma

Our modern life may encompass factors that have only recently arrived in our experience, but the sophisticated physiological equipment that we employ in defense arises from ancient systems proven over long periods of time, all based on the survival imperative. It evolved over the course of our human development to meet challenges of evading predators, find food, and compete with each other for survival and species perpetuation. This has been so successful that we have come to dominate the planet and, ironically, now threaten our own survival with this success through overpopulation, stripping the world's resources, pollution, and global warming. It seems we as a species have a hard time working cooperatively rather than competitively in our survival needs. This may partly be due to the very physiological mechanisms that mobilize us for action and survival. They tend to be oppositional and confrontational in nature. This is especially true in male stress responses. Interestingly, women under stress tend to initially produce oxytocin, which calms their system and orients them to cooperative interaction and social contact. However, women's nervous systems will also engage the stress cascade when placed in overwhelming situations, and traumatization is not unique to any gender.

Human beings are more complex than antelopes in their response to stress and trauma. Levine points out that human beings aren't as successful in processing traumatic experience as other mammals tend to be (Levine 1997, 2010). This is due to a number of factors. Some relate to the complexity of human cortical development and nervous system dynamics; others relate to the strength and intricacy of human family and cultural conditioning.

In overwhelming traumatic experience, implicit emotional memories may become coupled with various feelings and emotional states, and explicit memories also become linked with the meaning we give to experience and our family and cultural conditioning. Due to all of these factors, as we experience new stress, our thinking mind may kick in too quickly and override natural defensive responses, or traumatically bound emotional states may inappropriately be expressed. Thus our thoughts and memories—and family, cultural, and societal imperatives—may undercut our natural processing of traumatic experience.

We are also generally conditioned from an early age not to show our shock and/or our feelings during or after a traumatic process. "You should be able to handle that" or "pull out of it" are common imperatives. We also tend to stop people processing their shock by interfering with their attempt to discharge it by shaking and trembling. Likewise, as human beings, we have an ambiguous relationship to our flight-or-fight processes. We are both predator and prey. The lion knows that it is predator and the antelope knows that it is prey and they act out their part of the drama clearly. Humans are both predator and prey. We have ambiguous responses to danger and our neocortex seems to kick in much faster than in other mammals. This is perhaps a major aspect of our difficulty in processing stress and trauma.

Another important aspect of this process is the strong relationship between fear, rage, and the dissociative process. In stressful or dangerous situations, a strong emotional charge of fear and/or rage can become coupled with processes of dissociation and immobilization. Just before the person enters a shocked state, strong feelings of fear or rage may arise as part of the natural mobilization response to the traumatic situation. As we shall see in the next chapter, this is a limbic stress response mediated by the amygdala. When threat is perceived, the amygdala— a major stress nucleus—mobilizes the system for action. If a limbic response is elicited, a mixture of rage and fear may arise. If the person is traumatized by the experience, these emotions can become associated or coupled with the charge held in the central nervous system. Later, under stress, the cycling energies in the central nervous system may become expressed as inappropriate rage or terror.

Thus traumatization can lead to inappropriate emotional responses in times of stress or overwhelm. How often have you seen a person in everyday life expressing inappropriate emotions such as anger or fear with little provocation? Your boss flies off the handle for no obvious reason, someone shouts at you while you are trying to help, or you freeze when someone says something to you? Likewise, we humans, in our roles of parent, teacher, or mentor, may not be sensitive to the needs of others in stressful situations. This is poignantly the case in early childhood. I have seen parents unhelpfully making their young child stop crying when he or she really needs to complete a fear response, or make them get up and get back on their bicycle after falling off, while they really need to process the trauma of the fall. Or even worse, making little ones wrong or bad for their behavior, without differentiating their actions from their basic OK-ness. It is hugely different to say to a child: "What you did was dangerous, you might hurt yourself and you scared me! Don't do that again!" as opposed to: "You idiot, you are impossible, an imbecile for doing that!" What may be the repercussions of these kinds of interventions in early childhood when the young person's attachment and ego system are still in development?

In the therapy setting, a client may transfer these kinds of feelings or processes onto the relationship and the practitioner may encounter a barrage of anger, or defensive personality process. The basic thing to understand here is that these emotional and psychological reactions also have physiological roots and that the energies of these processes can be resolved and healing can occur at that level.

Mobilization and Resources

Whether or not people are traumatized by an experience depends on the resources they can bring to bear and whether these resources can be mobilized at the time of the experience. As we have seen, fight-or-flight is a systemic defensive mobilization response. The mind-body will try to mobilize its resources to deal with a perceived threat or stress. The sympathetic nervous system surges and various neuro-active hormones flood the system. If this response is not resolved at the time of the event, these neuro-active chemicals and responses can be left cycling in the system. The person is then left in a traumatized state. The more traumatized a person is, the more his or her resources become bound up and the more difficult it is to express them. When this occurs, the ability to respond to stress becomes compromised. A person whose resources are low may be more easily overwhelmed by new situations—he or she may not be able to mobilize resources and may more easily enter into shock and dissociative-freezing states.

When a person is overwhelmed by an experience, the parasympathetic nervous system surges and a dissociative and frozen state results. Vital signs may become erratic or be drastically reduced and the pain response is lowered. These people become disconnected from present-time and are protected from painful sensations and experiences. This is part of the body's natural self-protective mechanism. If these cycling processes are not resolved in the context of the event, then, when people later meet stressful or challenging circumstances, their system may defer to the dissociative response. The traumatized person begins to live in trauma time, and all present encounters begin to refer back to past traumatic experience. People may live their lives in dissociation and freezing, in anxiety states, and be prone to experience inappropriate fear or anger.

In the therapeutic context, the concepts of mobilization and resources are thus important to grasp. When clients present trauma states, it is essential to recognize these and know how to relate to them. Emotional states that arise in session work may be direct expressions of the cycling of traumatic energies and unresolved traumatic experience.

Traumatic Experience and Traumatization

An experience that may be strongly traumatizing to one person may not be traumatizing to another. Whether a person will be traumatized by an experience depends on that person's resources and the ability to mobilize them. One person may have the constitutional, psychological, and emotional resources to process an experience, while another may not. One person may be severely traumatized by an event, while another may be able to respond to it and process it over time. To one person, life is an ongoing stressful process holding much anxiety, while to another, life is full of challenges that can be met as appropriately as possible, in current resources.

There are two important factors in stressful situations:

- A person may or may not have the resources to deal with the situation

- The person may or may not be able to express or mobilize the resources

  An experience may be potentially traumatizing if:

- The person does not have the resources to deal with the circumstances

- The person's resources become overwhelmed by the nature of the experience

- Shock affects of past traumatization arise and override the natural adaptation response (these may include emotional affects like rage or fear, anxiety states, or dissociation and freezing)

- The person goes into shock and can't process the experience

Trauma, Shock, and Traumatization

There are three totally interrelated aspects of the stress response. These are trauma, shock, and traumatization.

- *Trauma:* A traumatic experience arises due to a situation or event that is physically or emotionally stressful, challenging, or threatening to the integrity of that person.

- *Shock:* Occurs when a traumatic experience overwhelms the resources of that person and his or her ability to mobilize a defensive response. In overwhelm, a parasympathetic surge is especially important in initiating a dissociative response along with a flooding of particular neurohormones.

- *Traumatization:* Occurs when the shock response cannot be processed by the system. The person ends up cycling both sympathetic and parasympathetic energies with a high volume of stress-related hormones in the system. These continue to cycle until they are resolved in some way. Psychological, emotional, and pathological processes will become coupled with these energies.

If a person's resources are overwhelmed, layers of past traumatization may be restimulated and will become coupled to the new traumatization. As an example of this, a number of years ago, a friend of mine had a motorcycle accident. He was thrown off his motorcycle and his body slid along the road until his clavicle struck the pavement and was fractured. This was a very traumatic event. He was fortunately not badly injured beyond the fracture, but many processes were touched off for him. There was the immediacy of the present trauma. He had knowledge of trauma work and processed the immediate experience quite well. Then something happened. He started to feel anxious and depressed. He experienced low energy and anger at the same time. He felt stuck. He was wise enough to pay attention and discovered that unresolved birth trauma had been touched off by the event. The nature of the accident, where he slid along the road and was suddenly stopped, echoed his own birth process. He was able to work through this and learned a lot in the process. A recent trauma had activated a very early traumatic process and he was able to skillfully take advantage of it.

Common Repercussions of Traumatization

Traumatized clients will present with a wide range of symptoms. Any stage of the stress response may manifest in inappropriate ways as people lose the ability to cortically process new information in present time. The ability to top-down process is lost. They may be locked in survival modes, anxiety, fear, and dissociation without the ability to hold their present condition, with its sensations and feelings, in awareness or to inquire into its nature. The ability for affect regulation and mental inquiry is lost in the cycling of past trauma and its repercussions in the nervous system. Common symptoms are associated with each stage of the stress response:

- *The active-alert/orienting level:* People cannot orient to their inner or outer world; they may startle easily and be locked in confusion, fear, and anxiety states, or may live life in a frozen, immobilized state, stuck in parasympathetic cycling. There may be a clear inability to concentrate or orient to current tasks, novel stimuli, or life situations, and be unable to respond to everyday life.

- *The fight-or-flight response:* People may exhibit stress and sympathetic arousal states, including anxiety, depression, fear states, psychological tension, body tension, inappropriate responses and behaviors (overcontrolling, anger, withdrawal, fleeing, attacking, etc.). They may exhibit physiological symptoms like sweating, feeling hot/cold, rapid or irregular heartbeat, dizziness, or pain. They may have a tendency to withdraw from others or to inappropriately attack others.

- *Dissociative states:* People may exhibit frozen states, dissociative states, immobilized depression, may feel disconnected and numb (some clients report that they are living in a fog or cloud, feel "other-worldly," feel trapped behind a glass screen, can't focus or concentrate, feel foggy, "far away," etc.). Clients may not be able to orient to current situations or relationships, may experience numb or immobilized limbs, experience confusion and an inability to concentrate—all coupled with the inability to orient.

Common *Emotional* Symptoms of Trauma

Shock, denial, or disbelief

Anger, irritability, mood swings

Guilt, shame, self-blame

Feelings of grief, sadness, or hopelessness

Confusion, difficulty concentrating

Anxiety and fear

Withdrawing from others

Feeling disconnected or numb

Common *Physical* Symptoms of Trauma

Insomnia or nightmares

Being startled easily

Racing heartbeat

Aches and pains

Muscle tension

Fatigue, exhaustion

Difficulty concentrating

Edginess and agitation

Difficulty sleeping, waking up too early, inability to get back to sleep, etc.

CHAPTER 19

Trauma Resolution 2: Neuroendocrine Relationship and the Stress Response

In this chapter, we explore important aspects of the central nervous system directly involved in mediating the stress response, and also introduce clinical approaches that help down-regulate sensitized states of the CNS.

The Stress Cascade

I call the totality of the stress response and related traumatization processes the *stress cascade*. The stress cascade is a nonlinear network of interconnected cycling and cascading processes. All aspects swirl and loop together in an integrated and intricate process of mobilization and response, which is essentially about survival.

The neuroendocrine-immune system is a unified system with totally integrated and interdependent parts and functions. When we encounter stressors, this system naturally gears up to meet the stress with almost instantaneous surges of neuro-active chemicals that trigger responses throughout the body. Muscles, circulation, respiration, digestion, and other systems all respond in a symphony of complex interactions so that life can be sustained. This response generally originates in certain nuclei in the central nervous system and is mediated by their production of stress-related chemicals. Our primary orientation in this chapter is to explore the interrelationships of a number of specific CNS areas and nuclei—the amygdala, hippocampus, hypothalamus, locus ceruleus, and prefrontal cortex, among others (Figure 19.1).

We introduced the concept of the general adaptation response in the last chapter and looked at its related stress response in some detail. In these sections and the following chapters, we discuss important neurophysiology, and how the biodynamic craniosacral practitioner might orient to states of activation in session work.

The initial response to stress involves two interrelated actions. First is the activation of the sympathetic nervous system in the form of increases in norepinephrine

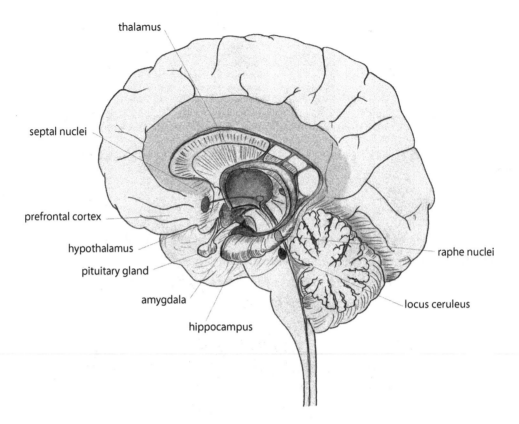

Figure 19.1. Important stress-related areas of the brain.

(noradrenaline) and epinephrine (adrenaline). Concurrently we experience an up-regulation of the H-P-A axis (hypothalamus-pituitary-adrenal axis) with a surge in cortisol. This global response mobilizes us to meet the danger, stress, or challenge successfully. Once the stress is removed, or successfully dealt with, the body physiology is designed to shift smoothly back to a baseline state of homeostatic balance (Figure19.2).

If the stress is repetitive, chronic, or prolonged, or if traumatic incidents overwhelm the system and are not able to be processed at the time of the event, then the body physiology may not be able to shift back to homeostatic balance. The stress response may stay active even though the danger has actually passed, and the fluidity of the system in its top-down, bottom-up processing may be reduced or lost. If this occurs, we will then lose the ability to self-regulate in the normal way. Our system may literally become fixed in this state for an indefinite period of time. This is called a *maladaptive state*, and it can be disturbing, debilitating, and even crazy-making.

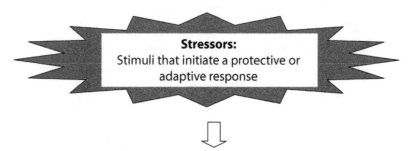

Stressors:
Stimuli that initiate a protective or
adaptive response

In response to stressors, the neuroendocrine-immune system shifts to
an adaptive state.

This shift is mediated by the amygdala, hypothalamus, locus ceruleus, and
other brain stem nuclei.

Sympathetic nervous system surges, H-P-A axis surges, with increased
norepinephrine, epinephrine, and cortisol.

Increased glycogen and mobilization of energy stores.

Increased arousal, vigilance, awareness, readiness for action.
Nonadaptive pathways are suppressed (e.g., digestion, reproduction).

Figure 19.2. The general adaptation response.

There are a number of interrelated cycles to be aware of as the stress cascade unfolds:

- Cortical processes mediating such things as present-time awareness, affect regulation, contextualization, and meaning

- Limbic processes mediating our emotional responses to experience

- Autonomic, sensorimotor responses largely mediating our internal environment and survival responses

- The H-P-A axis mediating and regulating many body processes including baseline levels of energy, energy expenditure in stress or trauma, energy expenditure in general, and energy storage

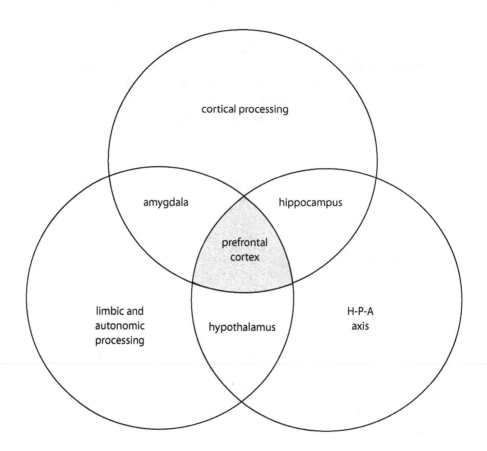

Figure 19.3. Interrelated cycles of adaptation and emotional regulation.

These cycles are largely coordinated by the interactions of the prefrontal cortex, hypothalamus, amygdala, hippocampus, and brain stem. In the following sections we will look at some of their important interactions and interrelationships in more detail (Figure 19.3).

The Role of the Hypothalamus

The question is where to start in describing all of this. The human body and its responses are nonlinear. The stress response is a cyclical, holistic process, in which multiple feedback loops inform each other. Given all of this, we will begin our discussion with the hypothalamus, which—in terms of homeostasis and neurological interaction—functions much like the conductor of a symphony orchestra. First, we look at the role of the hypothalamus and its basic inputs and outputs related to the stress response. Then we look at important nuclei and relationships, such as the amygdala, H-P-A axis, and hippocampus, in more detail.

The hypothalamus is a collection of nuclei located in the floor of the third ventricle. Its main role is to help the body maintain homeostatic balance and fluidity, and to coordinate physiological responses to arising conditions. In this interplay, it can be considered to be the hub for the interchange and coordination of top-down, bottom-up processing. In order to do this, it receives inputs from numerous areas of the body and sends regulatory outputs in return. Among its functions, it orchestrates and coordinates autonomic function, skeletal muscle contraction, visceral functions, hormonal secretions, emotional processes, the interface between voluntary and autonomic function, behavioral drives like hunger and thirst, and body temperature.

Most important in our inquiry, the hypothalamus orchestrates the overall nature of the stress response. It does not do this alone; it works in conjunction with input from many brain areas such as the amygdala, hippocampus, brain stem nuclei, and prefrontal cortex, and garners voluminous sensory information from numerous areas of the body via interoceptive input from nociceptive, kinesthetic, proprioceptive, vestibular, and visceral inputs. It monitors many levels of input from sensory receptors throughout the body and via the special senses. It receives the majority of this via the thalamus, which can be thought of like a major Internet server of the brain, from which a multiplicity of input is directed to appropriately related brain areas.

Let's first look at the major inputs to the hypothalamus that help it coordinate the stress response. These include biochemical neurotransmitter transmission (messenger molecules) as well as direct synapse connections. The hypothalamus receives input from: (1) the limbic system, especially the amygdala and hippocampus, (2) the cortex, (3) the special senses, (4) sensorimotor-brain stem areas, and (5) the body's nociceptors (pain receptors) as sensory input.

The Amygdala and Hippocampus

The amygdala is a set of bilateral nuclei located in the anterior-inferior portion of each temporal lobe. These nuclei function like sentries on a fortress, constantly scanning for novel or potentially dangerous activity. The amygdala quickly assesses whether current experience is threatening or perilous, gives emotional tone to new experience based on past experience, and mediates implicit emotional memories related to stress and trauma. When novel or potentially dangerous activity is sensed by the amygdala, it rapidly signals the hypothalamus and major stress nuclei that danger is present. If hypersensitized and not down-regulated, the amygdala can keep the stress response running far beyond the time of the experience.

The hippocampus, also bilateral, is located just inferior and posterior to the amygdala, inferior and parallel to the dorsal horn of each lateral ventricle. It coordinates the processing of memory and—with the temporal lobe of the cortex—integrates past memories with present sensory input, maintaining an integrated and cohesive sense of present-time experience. Likewise, together with the amygdala, the hippocampus mediates certain memory processes important in chronic stress processes and in everyday life. In research, it has been discovered that the functioning of the hippocampus is affected by the chronic cycling of stress hormones, where the person may experience fragmentation of present-time experience with a loss of integration and cohesion, both of the experience and of sense of selfhood. This is common in Post-Traumatic Stress Disorder (PTSD) (Finkelstein, et al. 1985; Sapolsky, et al. 1989).

In addition, the hippocampus has receptors for cortisol, a major regulatory and stress hormone. High levels of cortisol can keep the stress response running well past the original trauma. With the uptake of cortisol into its receptors, the hippocampus sends signals back to the hypothalamus to down-regulate the stress response. If these receptors are overwhelmed, they stop functioning properly and the feedback loop from the hippocampus to hypothalamus is broken, which makes it much harder to reset the nervous system and down-regulate the cycling of cortisol and the stress response. Hippocampal receptors will recover when the stress response is down-regulated via both mindfulness-based trauma resolution processes (as described in the verbal skills sections of Chapter 22) and craniosacral biodynamic approaches to the nervous system and its cycling (Willard and Patterson 1994).

The Cortex

The cortex provides interpretive functions and meaning to orchestrate a sophisticated set of responses. In top-down processing, the cortex maintains rational thought processes, gives context and meaning to present-time experience, coordinates long-term memory, and mediates affect regulation. As we shall later see, the long-term memory of stressful experiences, and the meaning we give them, can also keep the stress response running.

Cortical processing also relates to present-time awareness, which is mediated by the *medial prefrontal cortex,* an incredibly important area of the brain. It coordinates present-time awareness, integrates past experience in present time, and communicates to all major parts of the brain involved in emotional responses to current experience and to stressors, and is pivotal in cortical-limbic-sensorimotor homeostasis. In response to danger and stress, the ability to top-down process may be largely lost as the system shifts to defensive processes. Cortical processes of rational thinking, contextualization, and affect regulation may be down-regulated by the hypothalamus to allow for a rapid protective response largely mediated by the limbic and sensorimotor systems.

Mindfulness practice, which helps down-regulate the stress response and return the system to more fluid homeostasis, is founded on a person's ability to access present-time sensory awareness based upon the medial prefrontal cortex. The hypothalamus and prefrontal cortex are directly connected, allowing all cortical, limbic, and sensorimotor experiences to be held in present-time interrelationship. In mindfulness practice, as the traumatized person accesses present-time sensory experience via the prefrontal cortex, the limbic-sensorimotor systems get the message that there is no danger here anymore, and the cycling of the stress response then has a real opportunity to down-regulate and return to homeostasis.

Special Senses

The hypothalamus receives input from the special senses (the five external senses plus the internal proprioceptive sense) via the thalamus. As we shall see in more detail below, these senses have two pathways to the hypothalamus, a "fast" path via the amygdala and a relatively slower pathway via the thalamus. The hypothalamus mobilizes the system either way, but the fast path via the amygdala allows for an instant reaction and is really necessary for survival. For example, we might jump when we see a curvy stick on the ground even before we have actually had the time to identify whether it is a dangerous snake or just a piece of wood, or we might jump away from a sound before we identify the oncoming car in our pathway.

Sensorimotor-Brain Stem Processing

Brain stem-sensorimotor processing is about survival. Brain stem nuclei orchestrate and coordinate internal functions, maintain baseline functioning of visceral activities like cardio-respiratory and digestive functions, and allow these metabolic processes to be maintained without the need for constant awareness of them. The hypothalamus monitors, maintains, and coordinates the homeostasis of the body via these connections and interrelationships. In its regulatory function, the hypothalamus receives crucial input from many brain stem areas and nuclei, including sympathetic, parasympathetic, and social nervous system nuclei, and other key areas such as the reticular formation, the raphe nuclei, and the locus ceruleus—whose roles in the stress response will be discussed below.

Sensorimotor processing comes to the forefront in potentially dangerous situations, and its activities may become hypersensitized in overwhelming and traumatic experience. If this occurs, the traumatized person may then lose his or her ability to maintain baseline homeostasis and may be cast into constant vigilance and sympathetic and parasympathetic survival modes. The key factor in healing these levels of hypersensitivity in the stress response is to help resource the traumatized client both in felt-resource and in primary respiration, and to help the central nervous system complete its cycling stress response. We present various approaches below—and in following chapters—that help in the down-regulation of these levels of cycling via biodynamic cranial approaches, resourcing processes, client empowerment to mediate one's own process, and the use of appropriate verbal skills.

Nociceptive Input

Very importantly, the hypothalamus receives visceral and somatic input from the body itself. Much of this relates to input from nerves called nociceptors, also known as pain receptors. Nociceptors are nerve endings that detect internal danger; there are many millions of them in the body. The topic of nociception is underappreciated in the trauma literature, and is so important that we have devoted a separate chapter to it (Chapter 21). Traditionally, it was thought that the hypothalamus received somatic and visceral nociceptive input via the thalamus alone. But research has shown that the hypothalamus also receives input directly from nociceptors via the spinal cord. Some researchers have named this the *spinohypothalamic tract* (SHT) of the spinal cord. This tract has important repercussions for the stress response (Giesler 1994),

Chronic stress responses can be generated by ongoing low-grade nociceptive input from somatic or visceral origin. In other words, states of anxiety, depression, and chronic fatigue are not just based on external traumatic experiences; they may also be set off by internal, chronic nociceptive activity. Due to the connection of nociceptive fibers to the hypothalamus, chronic nociceptive input can directly initiate and maintain the general adaptation response and the whole of the stress cascade (Giesler 1994).

Nociceptive input from the body ascends to an important relay center in the brain stem—the periaqueductal gray cells (PAG)—which signals the raphe nuclei, also in the brain stem, to down-regulate the pain response via the release of serotonin. When this occurs, serotonin is released in volume transmission through cerebrospinal fluid, to sensitized levels of the spinal cord and beyond. The PAG also sends signals to the amygdala and autonomic nervous system to warn of potential internal danger, which can initiate the stress response and keep it running, and to the hypothalamus, which likewise may initiate the stress response and elevate cortisol levels, and will signal the release of endorphins to try to mitigate the pain experience in some way.

All of the above is part of the natural self-balancing processes of the body, but chronic nociceptive input can shift the system from homeostasis to a chronic cycling of sympathetic, parasympathetic, and dissociative processes. For instance, chronic nociceptive input to the hypothalamus may sensitize the amygdala, trap the system in an active-alert state, maintain high levels of cortisol in the system, keep fight-or-flight hormones cycling, and maintain high levels of endorphins and serotonin, which, in turn, supports ongoing dissociative processes.

Outputs from the hypothalamus that regulate homeostasis and autonomic activity are complex. Three outputs or responses are particularly important in stress responses. These are the H-P-A axis, the relationship of the hypothalamus to the locus ceruleus (a pair of brain stem reticular nuclei), and the autonomic nervous system response. We look at these three territories in more detail below (Figure 19.4).

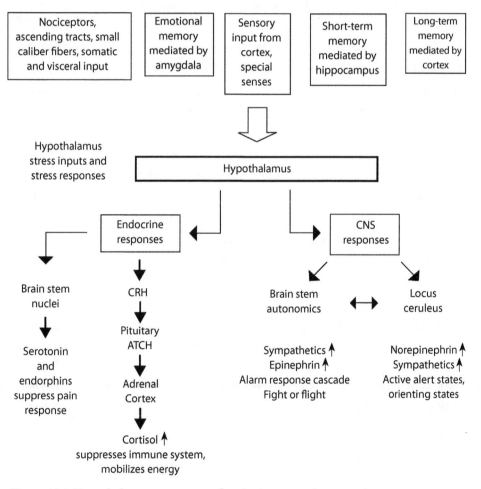

Figure 19.4. Hypothalamus: summary of major inputs and outputs in stress response.

The H-P-A Axis

The hypothalamus-pituitary-adrenal axis is of critical importance to understand as part of the stress response. The specific area of the hypothalamus especially involved in stress responses is called the *paraventricular nucleus*. It receives input from many areas of the brain, helping it to maintain homeostatic balance and modulate the stress response in the body. When the hypothalamus receives communication that there is internal or external danger, it releases a neurohormone called *corticotrophin releasing hormone* or *corticotrophin releasing factor* (CRH or CRF). In chronic stress conditions, either the hypothalamus continually receives these inputs, or the ability to down-regulate the CRH response is lost. CRH goes to the pituitary gland, which responds by producing *adrenocorticotrophic hormone* (ACTH). This enters the bloodstream, goes to the adrenal glands, and triggers the release of adrenal cortical steroids, especially cortisol. Cortisol stimulates the release and metabolic processing of energy needed for mobilization surges in the fight-or-flight response and suppresses the immune system.

Baseline levels of cortisol help maintain alertness during daytime and maintain a natural brake on the immune system that peaks during the night. This braking keeps the immune system from overreacting or attacking healthy cells and tissues. In hyperarousal states with high sympathetic activation, the H-P-A axis can become overactive, leading to high levels of cortisol, which inhibit the immune system and lead to immunodeficiency. This is a critical link, connecting chronic stress states with reduced immune function, and it is one reason highly stressed or traumatized people are more vulnerable to infections. In hypoarousal states, in which there is a high parasympathetic tonus, the H-P-A axis is commonly underactive, leading to low levels of cortisol, which can lead to autoimmune diseases in which an over-charged immune system may become self-destructive and attack the body's normal cells and dis-regulate homeostatic processes. The immune system depends on the right level of cortisol, as either too much or too little causes problems.

Cortisol has a further important function. It flows from the bloodstream into the cerebrospinal fluid around the brain and finds its way to the hippocampus, which has receptors for cortisol. When these receptors are filled, the hippocampus tells the hypothalamus to down-regulate the production of CRH, putting a brake on the H-P-A axis and the stress response it mediates. This is a feedback loop that down-regulates the stress response and helps the system to return to homeostasis. It has been found that chronically high levels of cortisol can overwhelm the cortisol receptors in the hippocampus, and they can then lose their ability to down-regulate the stress response. It has also been found that high levels of cortisol may damage the cells of the hippocampus, which can actually shrink in size. Remembering that the hippocampus is involved, along with the temporal lobe, in the integration of past experience with current experience, damage to the hippocampus and its receptors can also lead to a fragmentation of present-time experience and the loss of ability to contextualize current experience based on past processing. This alone can lead to chronic cascading of stress responses and the maladaptive states (Sapolsky, et al. 1989; LeDoux 1998). All of these dis-regulated states are commonly present in PTSD.

Figure 19.5 outlines the H-P-A axis. The locus ceruleus is included in this figure even though it is not technically part of this axis. It has an important role to play and is discussed below. The amygdala is also included, as its input is critical in setting the axis into play when danger is perceived. It is important to remember, however, that many factors can set the axis into motion, such as images and traumatic memories held in the cortex, implicit emotional memories mediated by the amygdala and hippocampus, and nociceptive input via the SHT spinal tract mentioned above.

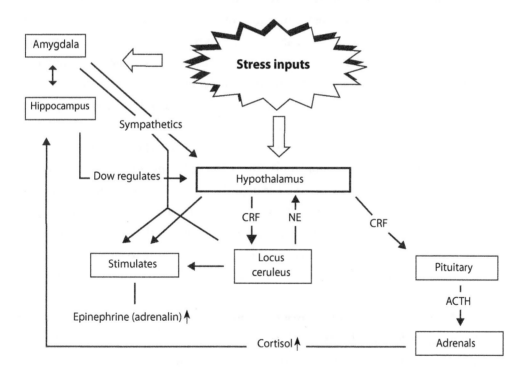

Figure 19.5. The H-P-A axis.

The Locus Ceruleus

The locus ceruleus is composed of two bilateral nuclei and is located at the superior floor of the fourth ventricle in the posterior aspect of the brain stem. The locus ceruleus has projections to just about every part of the nervous system. It has ascending fibers to the hypothalamus and amygdala and to virtually all of the brain and its cortex. It has descending fibers through the spinal cord and its interomediolateral cell column, to the preganglionic sympathetics, and to the sacral preganglionic parasympathetics.

The locus ceruleus produces norepinephrine (noradrenaline), a key arousal system neurotransmitter. Norepinephrine has wide-ranging effects in the mind-body system. It wakes us up in the morning and, as part of the stress response, it facilitates heightened awareness, orienting, and active-alert states, stimulates the sympathetic nervous system, and is prominent in hyperarousal states. In maladaptive states, the locus ceruleus may be chronically turned on, shifting the system from its normal orienting response to a state of chronic hypervigilance, coupled with sympathetic hyperarousal and hypersensitivity to sensory input. The chronic cycling of the locus ceruleus also leads to poor sleep patterns, in which the anxious, depressed person wakes up in the small hours of the morning, overwhelmed with anxiety and depressive feelings. In the extreme, the affected person may collapse into disorientation and dissociative disorders. These can be dangerous times when suicidal feelings may also emerge. Hypervigilance, chronic anxiety, depressive states—all coupled with sympathetic and/or parasympathetic activation—are again classic aspects of PTSD.

A further important consideration relates to how the locus ceruleus and hypothalamus communicate with each other. When activated, the locus ceruleus sends norepinephrine to the hypothalamus. This induces the hypothalamus to produce CRH and activates the H-P-A axis. The hypothalamus also sends CRH to the locus ceruleus, which induces it to send out more norepinephrine, creating a two-way, positive feedback loop that augments the stress response. If this loop does not down-regulate, the stress response keeps cycling. The locus ceruleus can be chronically stimulated by the amygdala and by chronic nociceptive input from the visceral and somatic systems, keeping all of this running.

Another interesting territory to highlight is that, as part of the orienting response, the locus ceruleus receives sensory input from neck muscles. Tense neck muscles are associated with a need to orient and defend, and can keep the locus ceruleus sensitized as though danger is still present (see Figures 19.4 and 19.5). We explore the down-regulation of this particular feedback loop in later sections.

The Role of the Amygdala

The amygdala is a key nucleus in the initiation of arousal responses, active-alert states, and the fight-or-flight response. It has direct connections to both the hippocampus and the hypothalamus. Like a sentry, one of its roles is to signal the hypothalamus that danger is present. The amygdala also signals the locus ceruleus, along with other brain stem nuclei, to quickly activate a sympathetic nervous system mobilization. Let's look at how this might occur.

Signs of external danger are taken into the brain by the special senses. These include seeing, hearing, touch, and smell. These signals first go to the thalamus before processing the information. As introduced above, these signals can then take two routes to the amygdala. The first is a relatively slow route. Signals go from the special senses to the thalamus and then to the cortex for processing. The cortex makes appraisals of the input, and, if the signals are registered as danger, or challenging to the system, a signal is then sent to the amygdala to initiate the stress response. By the time this all occurs, however, the snake would have bitten you and the damage would have been done.

There is a shorter and faster route to the amygdala, in which cortical processing is not involved. In this route, the sensory signals go from the thalamus directly to the amygdala. Joseph LeDoux calls it a *quick and dirty processing pathway* (LeDoux 1998). The internal representation of the object or situation is crude compared to cortical processing, but allows for a much faster response to danger or threat. Thus you find yourself running from the tiger before you actually see it, and jumping away from a snake only to find that it is a curved branch of a tree. If you had to wait for the cortex to process the sensory information, you might have been bitten by the time you realized there really was a snake. Cortical processing can override this quick response so that you realize that the curving figure is a branch and not a snake. This is an aspect of top-down processing. Then your stress response would not be set off, or would be quickly down-regulated. This quick response is important in sudden, dangerous situations. However, if this fast route is sensitized or facilitated, as in chronic stress states, we may find ourselves jumping and running from every sound or every twisted branch. Indeed, in post traumatic stress states this is exactly what happens (Figure 19.6).

Once the amygdala is aroused by internal or external danger signals, a cascade of processes ensues. It signals the hypothalamus to stimulate the H-P-A axis to produce cortisol, it stimulates the locus ceruleus to flood the system with norepinephrine, and it mobilizes a sympathetic nervous system surge. The amygdala, like

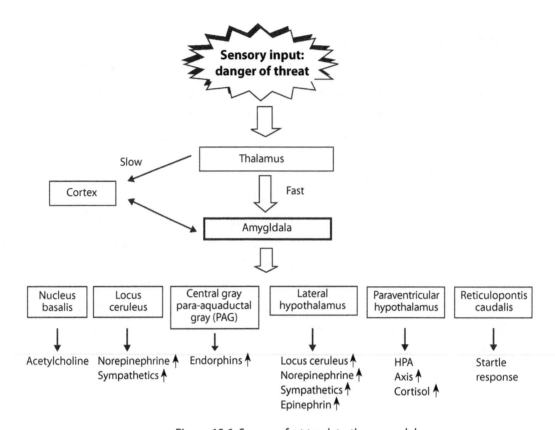

Figure 19.6. Sensory fast track to the amygdala.

the hippocampus, also has receptors for cortisol. In the presence of high levels of cortisol, the amygdala intensifies its signal to the hypothalamus, which, in turn, produces more CRH. This will keep the stress response running. Once again, the cortisol receptors on the hippocampus, which also feed back to the amygdala, are critical in the down-regulation of this response (see Figure 19.5).

Finally, the amygdala stimulates the nucleus basalis to release acetylcholine (ACh). This neurohormone generally arouses the cells of the cortex and makes them more receptive to incoming signals. Norepinephrine generally places the person into a hyperalert state and ACh makes the brain more responsive to the signals coming in. However, like norepinephrine, if this neurohormone is present in chronically high levels, hyperarousal and anxiety states will result.

Another interesting aspect of amygdala activation is the amygdala's relationship to another nuclei, the *septal nucleus*, which lies just anterior to the amygdala and is believed to be involved in the facilitation and coordination of pleasant feelings in the body. The amygdala, septal nucleus, and hypothalamus all communicate to each other via feedback loops. As it does not generally help to feel pleasant in dangerous situations—where you need to shift into flight-or-fight and protective responses—when the amygdala is sensitized it sends signals to the septal nucleus that down-regulates its activity, and it then becomes much more difficult to generate and feel pleasant sensations in the body, and to feel good in one's experience of life. Thus traumatized people have a hugely difficult time feeling good and orienting to the good things in their life, even when these are obviously present to those around them. An important aspect in healing trauma is the down-regulation of the amygdala's signals to the septal nucleus, which are also relayed to the hypothalamus, so that traumatized people can again access pleasant sensations and feel good about themselves and their world. As we shall see, a growing ability to rest in present-time sensory awareness, an ability to again access pleasant, resourced sensations and feelings—with the gradual down-regulation of the stress nuclei and CNS cycling—and a shift from traumatization to primary respiration and stillness are all essential ingredients in the healing process (Figure 19.7).

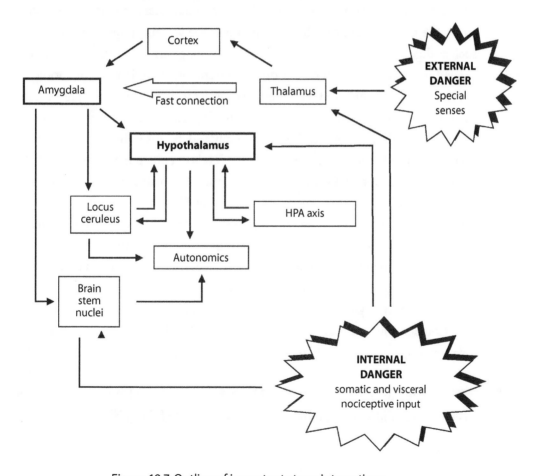

Figure 19.7. Outline of important stress interactions.

The Sympathetic Nervous System

All of the above processes intercommunicate with the autonomic nervous system, whose sympathetic activation is a crucial aspect of mobilization and defense. The sympathetic nervous system prepares and mobilizes the musculoskeletal system for action. It surges strongly during fight-or-flight processes. The sympathetic nervous system keeps surging until the danger is passed and the mobilization response is down-regulated. This process is largely mediated by the hypothalamus, with input from the amygdala and locus ceruleus. The sympathetic nervous system, among other affects, accelerates the heart rate and flow of blood to skeletal muscles and to the brain, while generally restricting the flow of blood to the digestive organs. It stimulates the release of glycogen from the liver for energy.

Very importantly, it also has fibers that directly connect to the adrenal glands, signaling the adrenals to release *epinephrine* (adrenaline) into the system. Epinephrine reinforces the action of the sympathetic nervous system in many ways. It constricts the smooth muscle of the skin and the blood vessels in the core of the body, such as digestive organs, and generally inhibits nonessential activities not directly needed for immediate survival. It dilates the smooth muscle in the arterioles of skeletal muscles to enhance their ability to contract in response to the fight-or-flight impulse. It excites cardiac muscle, increasing the rate and force of contraction. It also mobilizes the glycogen reserves in the body and increases the amount of energy that is available for action. Chronically high levels of epinephrine/adrenalin helps maintain anxiety states, exhaust the system, and lead to all kinds of symptoms.

Finally, the sympathetic nervous system has fibers that end in the immune system. All primary and secondary immune glands and lymph nodes, as well as the immune tissue lining the digestive tract, have a sympathetic nerve supply. The sympathetic system helps modulate immune responses. In general, a high level of sympathetic input to the immune system has an inhibitive effect. Thus, chronic stimulation of the sympathetic nervous system tends to inhibit the immune system. Coupled with the high levels of cortisol present in stress states, this can have a devastating effect on the body's defensive systems. Chronic stimulation of the sympathetic nervous system can lead to all sorts of mind-body issues, including anxiety states, depression, cardiac problems, respiratory problems, muscle tension, sleeplessness, undereating, immune suppression, and physical breakdown.

Memory Cycles

Memory can play an important role in the maintenance of chronic stress states and is mediated by at least four different processing systems: (1) explicit memories about stressful and emotional experiences, (2) implicit emotional memories, (3) long-term memory mediated by the cortex, and (4) short-term memory mediated by the temporal lobe and hippocampus. All of these come into present awareness via connections to the prefrontal cortex, the focus of present-time working memory. All of these memory loops can help drive chronic stress responses (Figure 19.8).

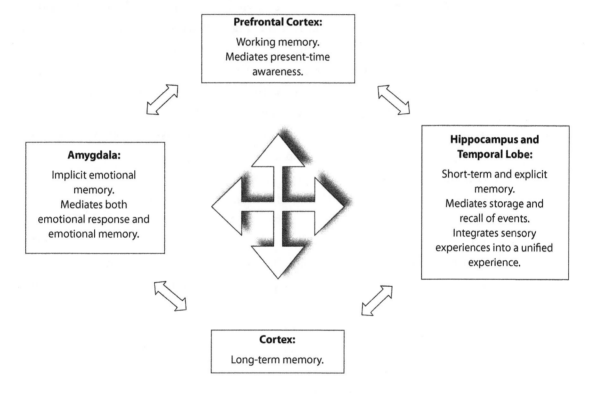

Figure 19.8. Some memory loop relationships.

Explicit memories relate to both short-term memories mediated by the temporal lobe-hippocampus system, and to long-term memories that are spread throughout the cortex. The hippocampus has a number of roles to play both in how we perceive our experiences and how we remember those experiences. The sensory inputs of an experience (sound, sight, touch, taste, or smell) are sent by the thalamus to the parts of the cortex that process each particular sense. Then these parts of the brain send their representations of these inputs to the hippocampus via the temporal lobe area of the cortex. This temporal area is called the *transitional cortex*. The hippocampus then integrates these various sensory inputs into a unified experience. Thus we can sense and perceive the sounds, smells, and sights in a room as a unified experience. Experience is initially held in the hippocampus-temporal lobe system as short-term memory, and, over time, these explicit memories are stored in other parts of the brain as long-term memory. The temporal lobe-hippocampus system stores explicit memory for up to two years, then the sensory components are transferred to other parts of the cortex for storage. In either case, it is the hippocampus that integrates the different aspects of memory into an integrated and cohesive experience (LeDoux 1998). That is why some researchers feel that dysfunction of the hippocampus arising from chronic stress may underlie the fragmented and confused states found in both post-traumatic stress disorders and in chronic fatigue states.

Implicit emotional memories are mediated by the amygdala. These are memories of the emotional component of a stressful or challenging experience. It is the amygdala that both initiates an emotional response to an experience and maintains an emotional memory of it. These are the charged, defensive emotions of fight-or-flight, and may be expressed in a spectrum from fear and anger to terror and rage (LeDoux 1998).

These memory cycles all have connections to the amygdala and hypothalamus. Thus a memory of a trauma can set off the stress cascade and related dissociative processes. Let's say I had an accident that involved a bright flash of light. In the future, if I again encounter a bright flash of light, the amygdala may interpret the flash as threatening based on prior experience. I begin to sweat, my heart pounds, and I can hardly breathe. The physiological responses are all coupled with the light. Even more confusing, I may not consciously remember the flash of light from the original accident—it may not be held as an explicit memory. So when I encounter a flash of light, no direct memory of the accident arises, but the emotional memory does. I end up sweating and afraid, but do not know why. I may feel anxious and become fearful, yet have no recognition of an event and no sense of what my fear is about. An experience of this kind can be really crazy-making and confusing.

Interpretive meaning provides another factor in memory processing. Human beings give meaning to experience. These are called *life statements* or *schemas* in psychotherapy, and they can have great impact. For instance, perhaps we experienced early childhood trauma of some kind in relationship to a close caregiver. We might be left with a felt-sense of fear coupled with a meaning such as "I will be destroyed by intimacy." This will be further coupled with flight-or-fight responses manifesting in defensive patterns of withdrawal or attack. Later, this schema may become transferred onto close relationships. The more intimate the relationship becomes, the more engaged the life statement and its feeling-tones become, and the more the stress response is activated. We may find intimate relationships hard to maintain as we become more and more anxious, fearful, and angry without ever really knowing why. Fight-or-flight processes kick in and we run away from the relationship or become angry and confrontational. This is the ground of insecure attachment processes and is a maddening loop. The very thing that is wanted— intimacy—is sensed as dangerous and suffocating. This is a simple example of how meaning, mediated by the cortex, will keep the stress response running. The amygdala again plays a role in this scenario, since some sensory experience of intimacy that was once associated with real threat can be perpetually interpreted as new danger, erroneously subverting or amplifying the whole interpretive meaning process (Figure 19.9).

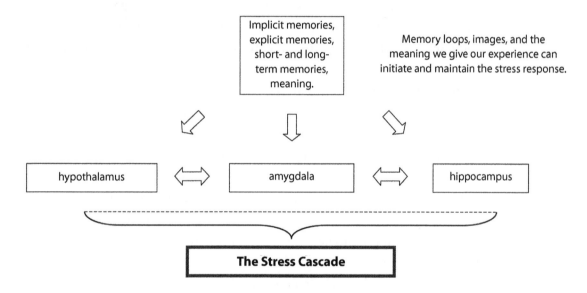

Figure 19.9. Cortical stress connections.

The cortical processes that give meaning to an event also have connections to the amygdala. The meaning we give to traumatic experience can keep the amygdala running and prevent the processing of the experience. We have to somehow recognize and let go of the given meaning and process the experience, but this is very difficult to accomplish via any rational process. There is a way out of this loop, however, and that has to do with present time. Healing is only accessed in present time, which is mediated by the medial prefrontal cortex. When a person can access present-time awareness via the medial prefrontal cortex and orient to present felt-experience, signals are sent to the major stress nuclei that there is no tiger out there anymore. Over time, with continued orientation to present experience, the stress response will be down-regulated. This is the core principle of Buddhist-influenced mindfulness practices, such as mindfulness-based stress reduction and mindfulness-based cognitive therapy now used in many orthodox health services.

The Prefrontal Cortex

The medial prefrontal cortex mediates and integrates present-time experience. This is called *working memory* and is a little like the RAM in a computer. Working memory is an extremely short-term memory system, which holds the present-time awareness of experience. All sensory areas of the cortex have inputs to the prefrontal cortex, as do long-term memory systems, the hippocampus-temporal lobe area and amygdala, so the prefrontal cortex receives all short- and long-term memories and their implicit emotional tone or charge. The prefrontal cortex can also send signals back into these areas, setting up a fluid interface with our past in the true here-and-now. Emotional memories mediated by the amygdala and explicit memories mediated by the hippocampus can be recalled in our present experience, and present experience can then be incorporated into both (Figure 19.10).

In this context, the medial prefrontal cortex plays a major role in mediating and down-regulating the stress response. It sends the amygdala information about the present nature of experience, about present time. It has the ability to say to the amygdala, "Hey, that experience is not happening now, cool it!" In other words, present-time awareness can help down-regulate the emotional cycling of the amygdala and thus down-regulate the stress response running in the system. I believe that Peter Levine's *somatic experiencing* method derives a major part of its effectiveness from this prefrontal cortex role (Levine 1997). The emphasis on present-time awareness in some psychotherapy forms, such as core process psychotherapy and mindfulness-based counseling, also keys into the regulatory role of the prefrontal cortex. Similarly, Eugene Gendlin's *focusing* process is very helpful in accessing the felt experience of an arising process in present time. This alone can help down-regulate the stress response (Gendlin 2003). Buddhist mindfulness practice also keys into the primacy of the prefrontal cortex in present-time awareness and the possibility of establishing witness consciousness, a state that helps the meditator see into his or her self-system. There is a realization that "I have a self, I am not the self; self is process and I am not an entity or thing." As

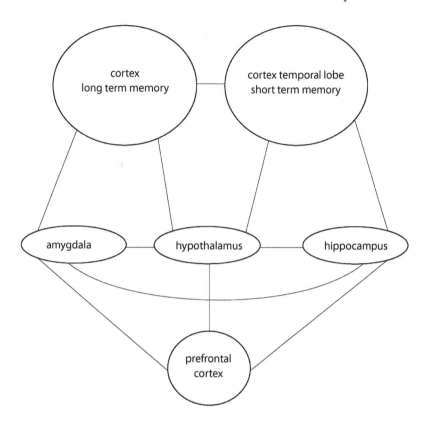

Figure 19.10. Interconnections for stress and emotional affect regulation.

the person deepens into present-time sensory awareness, the stress cascade is down-regulated and space may be accessed in his or her self-needs, fears, and projections.

Likewise, therapeutic processes that work through the body in present time, mediated by the prefrontal cortex, give access to real healing. Simply paying attention to sensation in the body can have this effect. Practitioners working with trauma ideally work to help clients come into a present-time relationship with their experience. This means helping a person to be present in a non-dissociative way, through all of the senses in the immediacy of present experience. Awareness of inner sensations and feeling-tones is especially useful as they give access to the nature of our inner experience. Present-time awareness helps down-regulate sympathetic activation and related stress hormones. As the prefrontal cortex communicates to the amygdala the present nature of experience, the amygdala has the opportunity to down-regulate its emotional response.

This is not as easy as it might sound. It takes repeated journeys into the present to let go of the past. Negotiating the stress responses as they arise in the present needs sensitive management and accurate practitioner recognition of the stages of processing, or the responses can become overwhelming and even retraumatizing. The client's process may need to be moderated for the safe discharge of the sympathetic arousal and down-regulation of the stress response. Some key points are: accessing and developing resources, accessing present-time awareness, orienting to sensation and embodied experience, accessing the felt-sense to help negotiate the felt meanings of experience, uncoupling memories and meanings from the sensations of the immediate experience, slowing down emotional processes, and/or sensitively mobilizing frozen states. We have to develop a resourced framework within which both parasympathetic and sympathetic nervous system cycling can safely clear and the system can return to homeostatic balance (Figure 19.11).

The amygdala gives the prefrontal cortex an emotional context for present experience, while the prefrontal cortex gives the amygdala the context of present time. Present-time awareness can help down-regulate the stress cascade.

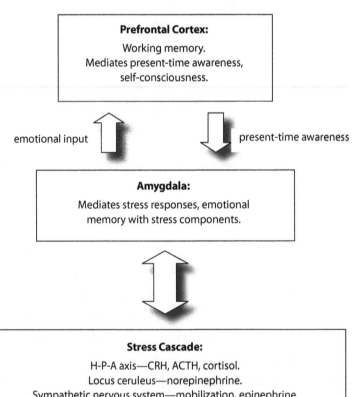

Figure 19.11. The prefrontal cortex and present time.

Summary of the Stress Cascade

Let's summarize the salient points here.

Input to the Amygdala and Stress Response System

Signs of external danger come in through the special senses and go to the thalamus. From here signals reach the amygdala by a slow route or a fast route. The amygdala initiates the stress cascade and the system is mobilized for action. Signals about internal danger can also reach the hypothalamus, amygdala, and locus ceruleus from nociceptors. Chronic nociceptive input can elicit both a chronic pain response and the general adaptation response.

Response of the Stress Cascade

Once the amygdala and hypothalamus are alerted to danger, the sympathetic nervous system is engaged; the adrenal glands release epinephrine/adrenaline into the blood system, the H-P-A axis produces cortisol, and the locus ceruleus pumps norepinephrine/noradrenaline into the system. The system is flooded with norepinephrine, epinephrine, and cortisol.

The norepinephrine released by the locus ceruleus also goes to the hypothalamus and augments its release of CRH, which, in turn, also loops back to the locus ceruleus to facilitate its release of norepinephrine. Both the hypothalamus and locus ceruleus thus reinforce each other's action, and both receive input from the amygdala. The amygdala continues to signal danger in the presence of implicit and explicit memories, high levels of cortisol, and chronic nociceptive input. This keeps the stress response running until it is down-regulated.

Cortisol in the blood stream also goes to the hippocampus, which has receptors for it, and the hippocampus then down-regulates the production of CRH. This down-regulates the whole stress cascade. These receptors can become overwhelmed, and the feedback loop to the hypothalamus is then compromised. The stress cascade can also be down-regulated via present-time awareness mediated by the medial prefrontal cortex. The prefrontal cortex maintains overall control over stress responses via top-down processing, and affect regulation in general. The prefrontal cortex sends information to the amygdala and hypothalamus about present experience and can tell them "there is no tiger here" (Figures 19.12 and 19.7).

All of this is not about the rational mind; it is physiologically driven and body oriented. That is why craniosacral biodynamics, with its emphasis on embodied

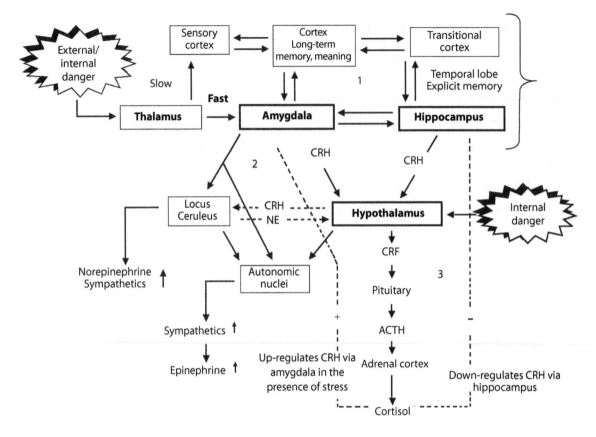

Figure 19.12. Major connections in the stress response.

forces and the manifestation of these in form and motion, can be so effective in the healing process. In a cranial context, states of balance and equilibrium in the nervous system can dramatically help in down-regulation and healing processes.

Clinical Presentations

Repercussions of chronic stress-related activation can present as active hyperarousal states within which everything seems to speed up, or as hypoarousal states within which everything seems to freeze or become immobilized. Clients in a hyperarousal state will be cycling norepinephrine, epinephrine, cortisol, and CRH. They may appear to be tense, excitable, and nervous. They may present with anxiety states, anxiety depression (exogenous depression), depressed immune function, poor appetite, and sleeplessness. These are all clinical indicators of chronic stress states such as PTSD.

The opposite of these states, hypoarousal, is equally common. Clients may report coldness and immobility in a part of the body. For instance, they may share that they are losing sensation in their legs and feel cold in the core of their body. This is an expression of unresolved parasympathetic cycling masking a frozen and incomplete protective response such as running or kicking. These states may need to be gently mobilized so that a shift to the sympathetic nervous system occurs and the underlying sympathetic cycling can resolve. Likewise, clients may exhibit listlessness, lethargy, sleep a lot, eat a lot, and be constantly tired or exhausted, with low energy, autoimmune issues, and true depression (atypical or endogenous depression), with low energy and low motivation. Again this is an indication of parasympathetic cycling, coupled with low cortisol, with a concurrent inability to marshal resources, and a frozen need to protect in some way. Furthermore, due to how the stress response may become compromised in overwhelming experiences— where the expression of the sympathetic nervous system is overlaid by a parasympathetic surge—a client may cycle from one state to another—from hyperarousal to hypoarousal, even in the same session.

Orienting to the Stress Cascade in Craniosacral Biodynamics

Nervous system hypersensitivity may be perceived as perturbation in the cerebrospinal fluid and fluids in general, as nerve and nuclei electric-like discharges and as tissue activation such as subtle trembling or more obvious shaking. Likewise, a frozen, stuck quality may be perceived, with little sense of potency, tide, or CNS motility present. It may be difficult to access the fluid tide or Long Tide, and the CRI (cranial rhythm) may be all that is apparent, or a more general state of inertia may be perceived. This is an indication that much potency is bound systemically in an attempt to center the stress conditions.

A chronically activated stress cascade is a systemic process and tends to be globally centered by the potency through the fluid system. Hence, the fluid tide may seem sluggish, low in vitality, or dense; the fluid drive of the system may seem low, the availability of potency will be lowered, and the motility of the CNS will be affected. Likewise, potency is commonly bound up around the primal midline (notochord midline) in a protective response to global traumatization. There may be a sense of a depressed or dense quality at the core of the client's system, yet there may be activation and perturbation cycling throughout the system at the same time.

Sympathetic activation and/or clearing is commonly sensed as an electric-like discharge through the fluids and tissues. For instance, you may be holding the sacrum and sense an electric-like streaming coming from the sympathetic ganglia. This streaming may be perceived to move through the buttocks and stream down the legs. This kind of discharge may be sensed when working with any tissue or tissue system. For instance, you may sense a sympathetic discharge when orienting to a vertebra, the cranial base, or an organ. This is commonly an indication that potency is processing the sympathetic cycling and its energy is being cleared. The client may sense heat, tingling sensations, or muscular trembling. If the client becomes overactivated in a sympathetic discharge (for example, the person may express an emotional flooding, or breathe more quickly, or begin to tremble), it may be important to give supportive verbal contact and slow pacing to help the cycling energies complete. A simple encouragement to allow the emotion "to wave through" and to slow the breathing may be an essential starting point in a practitioner's verbal suggestions. Exhalation-oriented stillpoints and orientation to Long Tide and Dynamic Stillness are also key cranial skills here.

In hypoarousal states you may perceive opposite kinds of processes. Little or no sympathetic discharge may be sensed. You may instead sense immobilized, depleted states with a density of potency throughout. The client may experience coldness, numbness, or a seeming paralysis. There may be dissociative processes involved (these may also be present in the sympathetic cycling described above). Dissociation may be sensed as a vacancy and "thinness" in the client's system, as if "no one is home," or as a sense that the client is very distant and unable to verbally communicate. Indeed, the client may seem entirely nonexpressive—seeming to be split off from a sense of embodiment and disconnected from sensations. However, with these hypoarousal states, be aware that these may be overriding and concealing a hyperarousal state underneath, so the treatment may show a progression from hypo- to hyperarousal processing, reflecting the sequential deployment of autonomic strategies. Pure parasympathetic states, in which there is no underlying sympathetic charge, may also present.

To work with traumatization and nervous system activation, the biodynamic craniosacral practitioner must be able to:

- Orient to the Dynamic Stillness

- Orient to the Long Tide and its tidal body

- Perceive the fluid body and the dynamics of potency and the fluid tide, and orient to states of dynamic equilibrium in all three bodies

- Perceive central nervous system motility

- Orient to the interrelationships of cortical processing, limbic processing, and sensorimotor processing—i.e., top-down, bottom-up processing

- Orient to the various aspects of the nervous system and its hypersensitivity—the H-P-A axis, the polyvagal system, CNS activation, and important stress-related nuclei

- Orient to nociceptive issues, nerve sensitization, and the facilitation of levels of CNS functioning—peripheral nerve facilitation, spinal cord facilitation, brain stem and higher center facilitation

- Use appropriate verbal skills, which empower the client to self-regulate and resolve traumatic cycling

Clinical Approaches

Craniosacral biodynamics offers very effective approaches that help down-regulate and moderate chronic stress responses. The holistic shift, states of dynamic equilibrium, and an orientation to CNS motility and the manifestation of potency in the fluid body are great starting points that can initiate autonomic clearing and a return to homeostasis. An orientation to the Long Tide is also essential as it is the root of primary respiration, is never in shock, and is the basic underpinning and support for the body's organization and homeostasis. The use of exhalation stillpoints is a traditional way to help lower the hypertonicity of the system and restore access to resources.

As we discuss in Chapter 22, helping clients to slow down their process, by taking a deep breath and becoming more aware of sensations and feeling-tones in their body, is also useful. In the case of frozen and immobilized states, augmentation of lateral fluctuation may stimulate potency locally and initiate a clearing of the cycling energies. For instance, a client may experience numbness in the legs and the practitioner may augment lateral fluctuations at the location where the numbness is felt to start in the body. If dissociative states are coupled with the stress process, inhalation-oriented stillpoints can help reintegrate the psyche with the soma and help access potency bound up at the core of the system. With clients who present traumatization and activation, it is imperative that the practitioner maintains the fulcrums, and can orient to both Long Tide and Dynamic Stillness relative to the practitioner's own system. Over a few sessions, the client's system will begin to resonate with this level of resource and session work can unfold with containment in the context of primary respiration.

Exploration:
CNS Motility and Dynamic Equilibrium _____

The clinical application described here offers options in relating to the central nervous system, particularly the brain stem and the structures in the limbic system. Again, it is essential to know the anatomy of the central nervous system. Review the anatomy of: (1) the brain stem and the location of major nuclei—such as the locus ceruleus, raphe nuclei, nucleus ambiguus, and dorsal motor nucleus; (2) the diencephalon—composed largely of the thalamus and hypothalamus; (3) the limbic structures—especially the location of the amygdala, hippocampus, and the temporal lobe area; and (4) the location of the prefrontal cortex and the organization of the cortex in general. Then put these images aside and let the living anatomy speak to you.

Start as usual at the side of the treatment table. First orient to primary respiration relative to your own system, then orient to the client's midline, biosphere, and primary respiration relative to the system. Move to the client's feet and wait for your relational field to settle. Wait for the holistic shift to clarify. As the holistic shift deepens, you will sense that you are holding a unified potency-fluid-tissue field. You may also sense clarity arising in the expression of primary respiration. Have patience here and give the holistic shift time to deepen. If the holistic shift cannot deepen, work with resourcing processes (such as orientation to felt-resources) and stillpoint process as appropriate.

Then move to the head of the table and use either Sutherland's or Becker's vault hold.

Again negotiate your contact to the client's system and orient to primary respiration. Orient to the fluid tide and to the motility of the CNS. As described in Foundations Volume One, the motility of the CNS is largely sensed through the ventricle system with the lamina terminalis (anterior wall of the third ventricle) as its natural fulcrum. The tissue of the nervous system generally widens side-to-side and shortens toward the lamina terminalis in inhalation. The ventricle system expresses a ram's horn-like motion relative to the shifting of the lamina terminalis.

Maintain a wide perceptual field and orient to the ventricles and their motion, including an awareness of the motility of neural tissue. As you are listening, over time, an inertial fulcrum and pattern may clarify. It may be sensed as an eccentric form and/or motion, a place of restriction, or as density in neural tissue. You may even sense a quality of agitation, or perturbation in areas that are running a chronic stress response, or electric-like discharges from areas of nervous system nuclei, especially those that relate to the stress cascade. Alternatively, you may sense density and inertia in particular areas. Do not look for anything; let the tissues and fluids express their history as you wait for primary respiration to express its priorities.

As an inertial pattern clarifies, maintain your wide perceptual field and orient to its organizing fulcrum. Do you sense a locus of stillness around which the motion or form is organized? Remember your anatomy. Is there a fulcrum in the brain stem or limbic structures? Do you sense activation or density in the hypothalamus, amygdala, or hippocampus?

As the state of balance deepens, maintain your wide perceptual field. Healing intentions may emerge from any level of action. The tidal potencies in the fluid body may shift and healing processes may clarify in the fluid and physical bodies at a mid-tide level. Alternatively, the process may deepen further and Long Tide phenomena emerge as healing processes clarify at that level, or the process may deepen into the Dynamic Stillness as a formative ground of emergence. Simply be open to any level of process.

Listen for the action of potency in the fluids, and for the processing or dissipation of inertial forces. You may sense various processes of clearing and discharge in the tissues of the central nervous system. For instance, you may sense sympathetic ganglion clearing as an electric-like discharge, which the client may experience as tingling and clearing through the arms and legs. Or you may sense localized clearing from various CNS nuclei in the brain stem, diencephalon, and limbic system.

When the healing process completes, listen for processes of realignment to midline and natural fulcrums, and for tissue and fluid reorganization. Does the motion of the CNS seem to be more aligned with its natural fulcrum at the lamina terminalis? Does the motion of the ventricles seem more balanced in inhalation and exhalation? Wait for the period of reorganization to complete. You may sense a surge in the fluid tide as this occurs and a new level of tissue organization in relationship to the midline and the lamina terminalis.

This general treatment orientation is a real starting point in resolving stress response-activation issues. You may also find that various augmentation skills may also be of service in states of chronic congestion and density.

Exploration:
Working with the H-P-A Axis

As described above, the H-P-A axis is a pivotal dynamic in the stress response and the system in general. The H-P-A axis is commonly hypo- or hypersensitized in chronic stress states. In this clinical application, we will orient to the dynamics of the H-P-A axis in order to help down-regulate the stress cascade and bring the system back to homeostasis. You use a vault hold to first get a general sense of CNS motility, with an orientation to the hypothalamus and pituitary areas. Then you move to an occipital cradle hold with an orientation to the brain stem (especially the fourth ventricle and locus ceruleus) and hypothalamus-pituitary axis. You then hold the occiput and adrenal gland on first one side of the body, and then the other.

Start the session as usual. Once the relational field and holistic shift have deepened, move to the vault hold. Negotiate your contact there and orient as above to CNS motility. Include an awareness of the hypothalamus and pituitary areas. See what clarifies, wait for a settling into a state of balance or equilibrium, and see how primary respiration manifests healing intentions.

Move to an occipital cradle hold and again orient to CNS motility. You may sense the brain stem rising, widening, and shortening in the inhalation phase. Include, in your wide perceptual field, an awareness of the hypothalamus, the fourth ventricle, and the locus ceruleus nuclei. Again wait for the system to deepen into a state of balance and see what level of healing process ensues.

Now again shift your orientation. Move from the occipital cradle hold and sit at the side of the table. Cradle the occiput with your cephalad hand. Make sure that the client's head feels comfortable and evenly balanced in your hold. Then place your other hand under the adrenal gland-kidney area on that side of the treatment table. This can also be done in the side-lying position.

As you settle into a wide perceptual field, orient to the hypothalamus-pituitary-adrenal gland axis. Again wait for primary respiration to clarify, for healing priorities to manifest and for forces to resolve in states of balance and dynamic equilibrium. You may sense clearing discharges both from the hypothalamus-pituitary areas and brain stem, and from the adrenal gland. Sometimes you may sense a synchronization of this clearing at all locations. This may be sensed as an expression of potency at work via synchronous pulsations in all areas of the H-P-A axis. Wait for the process to complete and move to the sacrum. Orient to the primal midline (notochord midline) and tidal and fluid bodies. Wait for an expression of the fluid tide to clarify and note any changes in the quality of the fluid tide, CNS and tissue motility, and organization in general (Figures 19.13a and 19.13b).

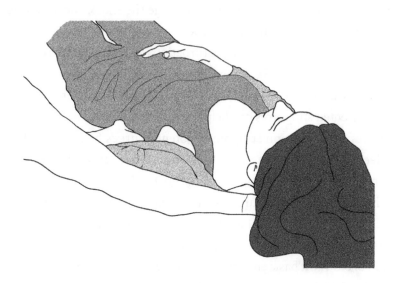

Figure 19.13a. H-P-A hold, with client on her back.

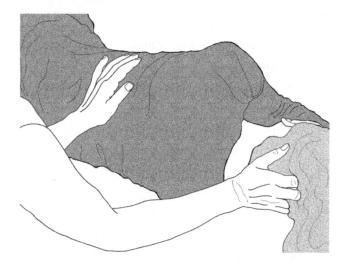

Figure 19.13b. H-P-A hold, with client side-lying.

The Use of Stillpoints in States of Activation

In hyperarousal states, exhalation stillpoints can help settle the system, slow things down, access stillness in the activation, down-regulate the central nervous system in general, help build resources, and access potency that has become locked in centering conditional forces in the system. Exhalation stillpoints can help shift the set point of the autonomic system from fixity to a more fluid response to the environment, and can help the system discharge the shock affects of trauma in a resourced state, as potency in the fluids acts to resolve the traumatization. As this occurs, the practitioner may sense perturbations and electric-like clearing in the fluids and tissues as the CNS cycling is processed.

In hypoarousal states, where the system is running a different physiology, inhalation-oriented stillpoints can help the system come out of frozen and immobilized states. In inhalation stillpoints, potency surges from the midline as the system deepens into stillness in the inhalation phase, and this augmentation of potency helps mobilize and process parasympathetic states. Inhalation stillpoints can also help manifest the resources of the system from the center out and may help in dissociative processes. In inhalation stillpoints, potency is expressed from the core and midline of the system to the periphery. The surge of potency accessed is an expression of our most basic empowerment to be here, and as potency is augmented in the fluids of the body, the dissociated psyche may be helped to reassociate and find its way back to embodiment.

Thus exhalation and inhalation stillpoints are specific in their effects and must be used appropriately. Inappropriately used inhalation stillpoints can exacerbate a hyperaroused state, as potency surging from the midline may intensify existing activation. Likewise, exhalation stillpoints can exacerbate a hypo- or dissociative state. Let the system guide you to the appropriate strategy, with exhalation stillpoints as the general approach for hyperarousal and inhalation stillpoints as the general approach for hypoarousal and dissociative conditions.

Exploration:
Sacral-Ethmoid Hold _____

The sacral-ethmoid hold, where you have the whole primal midline in your field of awareness, can also be used to good effect in states of nervous system activation.

With the client side-lying, and your arms comfortably placed on the treatment table, place one hand over the sacrum, fingers pointing caudal with the middle finger over the coccyx. Bring your other hand around the top of the client's head; with your elbow settled on the table, place your index and middle fingers in a "V" over the forehead-glabella area anterior to the ethmoid bone. This hold can help the client feel contained and held. Orient to the client's primal midline, bioelectric ordering field, and tidal body-Long Tide.

Allow the relational field and holistic shift to deepen and settle as you maintain orientation to the primal midline. Let the priorities of the system manifest and also notice how potency is expressed in the fluid body and CNS. You can also use your hand at the sacrum to orient the system to either exhalation or inhalation stillpoints, dependent on the arising process.

Clinical Highlight

In my clinical practice, a young woman had low-back and sciatic pain, and anxiety states that manifested as a general everyday tension, sleeplessness, and constant worry. In the first few sessions, the most pressing clinical intention was to find a way into contact and relationship because she initially experienced touch as painful. Contact intensified her discomfort. I began with resourcing processes and was able to help her find some sense of resource in her body sensations after a number of sessions. Her system was in a very activated and seemingly confused state. Pain tended to shift around and her system moved quickly from fulcrum to fulcrum without any healing processes being engaged. There was a high sympathetic tonus present and a sense of density in the fluids and tautness and dryness in her membrane system. It was very hard for her system to shift out of the CRI level and access the holistic shift. After a number of sessions oriented to establishing safety and contact, we began to work with exhalation stillpoints via a sacral hold. It took about seven sessions for her system to be able to access the holistic shift. Once this happened, the inherent treatment plan could begin to unfold.

In a number of sessions her system processed levels of sympathetic cycling and expressed some clearing in brain stem nuclei. Then, in one session, potency shifted toward her pelvis and there was a clarification of patterning around her right sacroiliac joint. She shared how her sensations and feelings seemed to be coupled to an old car accident. This was an extremely frightening experience for her. She was in the hospital for nearly a month after the accident. Some more sympathetic cycling was cleared, and I was able to help her stay with a coupled fear response. Both seemed to move through her body and dissipate, and a more settled state arose. Over the next sessions, her system shifted to vertebral issues, cranial base patterns, and more central nervous system resolution. The cranial patterns that then presented seemed to relate to birth trauma and early childhood issues. The main intention in this phase was to help her system manifest potency and reorient to midline phenomena and natural fulcrums. I also introduced her to the focusing process, in which one orients to an embodied felt-sense of an arising process, which she found very helpful. She managed to process some very deep patterns in a resourced and paced manner.

In one session in particular, her potency shifted deeply in her ventricle system, and the motility of the central nervous system came to the forefront. Here, I worked largely as described above, first from a vault hold and then from an occipital cradle. The session work oriented to deepening states of balance, stillness, and Long Tide phenomena. Again, there were periods of sympathetic clearing, especially from the brain stem.

In a few further sessions her system shifted to a more parasympathetic immobilized state. This seemed to relate to her car accident and hospitalization, and was also coupled with birth trauma. We worked with inhalation stillpoints to help mobilize her system. I also encouraged her to gently mobilize her legs by slowly tensing and releasing her leg and pelvic muscles, which helped her shift from the parasympathetic state of freezing and immobilization to a further clearing of sympathetic nervous system cycling. All of this helped her system process the immobilized state (see Chapter 22).

Her low-back issues were alleviated after the first ten sessions, and after fifteen sessions, her sleep patterns normalized and her anxiety levels were lowered. We continued to work with focusing sessions and table work. Orienting to Dynamic Stillness over a number of further sessions was especially important. Her system seemed to be moving to a more fluid and homeostatic state. Her autonomic tonus was regularized and seemed much less prone to activation. In the twenty-fourth session (over an eight-month period), she stated that she felt empowered enough to hold her process in ways that were not possible before, and sessions were terminated at that point. We had a follow-up session a number of months later, and her system had indeed stabilized and she was able to hold her personal process with much more space and equanimity.

In our next chapter we will more specifically orient to the autonomic nervous system in a context called the polyvagal concept, developed by Stephen Porges PhD, and learn to specifically relate to its dynamics.

CHAPTER 20

The Polyvagal Concept

The polyvagal concept is an important understanding of the autonomic nervous system, developed by Stephen Porges, whose work holds tremendous implications for the health fields because it refines our recognition of the processes at work in the stress response beyond the currently prevailing model. In the years since I first encountered Porges's concepts, their validity has been repeatedly confirmed in clinical contexts. His work is now receiving more and more acceptance in the worlds of psychology, neurology, and trauma resolution.

Autonomic Nervous System

The autonomic nervous system is pivotal in the regulation of survival functions. Its importance cannot be overstated. The entire field of post-traumatic stress disorder certainly falls in its scope, along with most degenerative diseases, all stress-related situations, autoimmune diseases, and many others. Classically, the autonomic nervous system is considered to have two branches, parasympathetic and sympathetic, which are thought to operate in a generally reciprocal and homeostatic manner: when one is up, the other is down. These two are thought to work synergistically to regulate crucial functions and physiological homeostasis, including the coordination of cardio-respiratory function and many other key survival tasks such as digestion, reproduction, and elimination. It is directly involved in all survival processes, maintaining muscle tonus, coordinating rest and repose, and fight-or-flight and protective responses throughout life.

Trauma theorists have naturally focused on autonomic functions in understanding the stress response. Great interest has been placed on the fight-or-flight response of the sympathetic, and the freeze response of the parasympathetic. Similarly, the control centers of autonomic function have been studied deeply. As we have seen, the hypothalamus provides higher-level control and regulation, and the amygdala initiates fight-or-flight processes via connections to the hypothalamus, locus ceruleus, and sympathetic system. Porges has developed further important clarifications in relationship to the autonomic nervous system, mammalian defensive responses, and social activities that have to do both with how the autonomic system has evolved and how its anatomy is organized.

In this orientation, also called the polyvagal theory, Porges realized that the parasympathetic system actually has two distinct sets of nuclei, which facilitate very different neurological processes. Both send nerves fibers through the vagus nerve, hence the term *polyvagal*. He realized that each set of nuclei really should be separated out in the description of autonomic function, and the polyvagal-triune autonomic nervous system is the result of his research (Porges 1995, 2001, 2011).

Triune Nervous System

Porges thus proposes a new model, the *triune autonomic nervous system*. This idea was originally based on his understanding of the hierarchy of the nervous system's phylogenic relationships. Phylogeny is the study of the evolution of life forms' functions, from ancient simplicity to modern complexity. Porges's three-part system is summarized below.

- The first level is an evolutionarily more primitive unmyelinated *parasympathetic nervous system* that sets a metabolic baseline for survival. Originating in the distant past, when creatures were passive feeders in a liquid environment, the parasympathetic has a small range of responses to novelty and stress, in the form of adjustments in metabolic rate, including death feigning or freezing via down-regulation of heart rate. Examples of parasympathetic-dominant animals are invertebrates and worms. The anatomy of this system consists of the nerves that operate heart-lung, digestive, and reproductive organs, particularly the vagus nerve and the cervical and sacral plexuses. Some authors also place the enteric nervous system (the gut brain) in the parasympathetic category, although the enteric nervous system operates with significant independence and has also been described as separate from the central nervous system.

- The second component is a more recently developed *sympathetic nervous system* that adds mobility and therefore a much more robust set of survival options. These later animals, including vertebrates all the way up the evolutionary ladder to mammals, have much wider survival options for finding food, finding mates, and escaping from predators by virtue of their striated muscle-driven appendages. The anatomy of this system consists of nerves that modify the parasympathetic system and operate muscles involved in mobilization activities and fight-or-flight. Particularly notable are the double chain of sympathetic ganglia running along either side of the spine, connecting with the spinal cord at thoracic and upper lumbar levels.

- The third level in this new scheme is a most recently developed myelinated system called the *social nervous system*, which advances survival repertoires even further by enabling sophisticated information processing and group behaviors. This new capability, exhibited in mammals and highly developed in primates, tremendously increases survival chances. The anatomy of this part includes nerves that operate facial expression, voice, hearing, mouth and head-turning, particularly cranial nerves V, VII, IX, and part of X and XI. The social nervous system enables many important social behaviors, but perhaps none is more important for survival than the mechanisms that generate maternal bonding.

As brain size increases, babies need enough time to mature and become independent. Structures and functions to secure this protected time are not a luxury; they are essential. The responses involved are not voluntary; they are too important for that, so they are hard-wired into autonomic-level functioning. The solution is a complex set of structures and functions that together create a neurophysiological-biochemical phenomenon whereby the newborn baby can orient to mother, get her attention, vocally communicate, manifest appropriate facial expressions, find her breast, nurse, coordinate sucking, breathing, and swallowing, and elicit profound caregiving motivations that endure for decades or even a whole lifetime. With this set of functions, ample time for sophisticated cortex development is secured and the ultimate survival machine, the human being, is enabled.

These three systems are highly interactive and overlap substantially. Most organs are directly innervated by at least two of the three, and indirectly affected by all three. But in that interdependent complexity, they generally operate in sequence. The newer systems operate by inhibiting and modifying the older, so the parasympathetic sets a baseline, the sympathetic acts on the parasympathetic, and the social acts on the sympathetic. In the presence of threat or novelty, this sequential scheme unfolds. We use our most sophisticated equipment first (social), then we try the older strategy (sympathetic), and if that fails we default to the oldest (parasympathetic).

For babies, the social strategy is really the only viable option, since they are too small and dependent to fight or flee. The archetypal defeat of the social nervous system is perceived betrayal by a caregiver, whether intentionally or through ignorance or through the baby's inability to contextualize their experience. A baby experiences its world directly as felt experience. So if its outer world of caregivers and conditions is not optimal, the little one may experience abandonment or betrayal, even if that is not actually the case.

If social relating is ineffective, the baby devolves to its next option, a sympathetic fight-or-flight response. If the sympathetic is not successful, the system will then shift to parasympathetic responses of immobilization and dissociation. Indeed, the primal defensive strategy of a baby is withdrawal and dissociation. Fight-or-flight has little use if you cannot move or protect yourself, so infants tend to readily move to their most primitive strategy. These autonomic processes also underpin the evolving ego-form and defenses of the young child and can energize defended self-systems and strongly influence attachment processes (Figures 20.1 and 20.2).

The Triune Autonomic Nervous System and Survival Mechanisms

Social nervous system: Social communication, orienting, self-calming

Sympathetic nervous system: Mobilization, fight-or-flight

Parasympathetic nervous system: Immobilization, freezing, death feigning

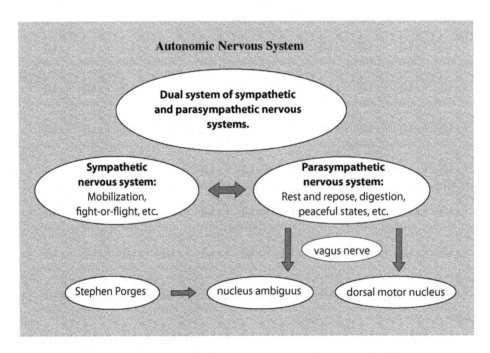

Figure 20.1. Old concept of autonomic nervous system as a dual system.

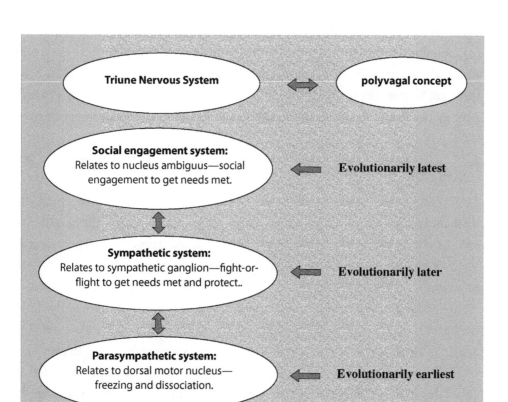

Figure 20.2. New concept of the autonomic nervous system as a triune system.

The Vagus Nerve and Its Nuclei

As introduced above, the term *polyvagal theory* originated with Porges finding that the traditional understanding of the parasympathetic system's key pathway, the vagus nerve, did not account for some anatomical and physiological subtleties. Rather than being a single system, the vagus nerve has been clearly demonstrated to have multiple nuclei—*dorsal motor nucleus, nucleus ambiguus,* and *nucleus solitarius.* These nuclei are all long, bilateral brain stem fibers at the level of the foramen magnum; they exhibit variations in structure and function that do not conform to conventional parasympathetic classification rules.

The ventral (anterior) or pharyngeal branch of the vagus (ventral vagal complex) arises from the nucleus ambiguus (NA). These fibers do not meet the normal criteria for classification as part of the parasympathetic branch of the autonomic nervous system. This system does have inputs to the heart and bronchi, appropriate for parasympathetic function, but it is myelinated, not unmyelinated as is the norm for the parasympathetic. Similarly, the ventral vagal's association (via the corticobulbar tract) with the nerves and structures controlling the face, neck, and throat also disqualifies it from classification as purely parasympathetic, because these are voluntary muscles. Nonconformance of these fibers serves as Porges's basic evidence that the vagus is not all parasympathetic, as previously assumed.

Dorsal Motor Nucleus

The dorsal (posterior) branch of the vagus (dorsal vagal complex) arises from the *dorsal motor nucleus* (DMN), descends to the torso, and innervates the heart-lungs and the viscera below the diaphragm. These are classic unmyelinated parasympathetic fibers. The parasympathetic DMN innervates the heart and lungs and viscera in general, coordinates digestion and elimination, and is in precedence in rest and repose and nighttime resting-sleep modes. Under stress, the DMN mainly slows the heart and lowers oxygen consumption to generate an immobility state. This system is associated with freezing and dissociative states in humans. In prey animals, this down-regulated state ("playing possum") has great survival value in that a predator may lose interest due to evolutionary programming against eating old meat that may be spoiled or infected. In human babies, the down-regulated state can make the baby less conspicuous, but may be dangerous as lowered heart rate and oxygen levels can compromise autonomic function and baseline metabolism. Extreme parasympathetic down-regulation can be fatal (Figure 20.3).

Nucleus Ambiguus

The *nucleus ambiguus* (NA) has significantly different functions, and coordinates many interrelated socially oriented tasks. It projects to the heart and bronchi, but it also goes to the muscles of the face, scalp, and neck. The projections to the heart and bronchi coordinate breathing with heart rate, allowing the heart and breath to speed up and remain in synchronization as we walk faster. It provides a vagal brake on the sympathetics to the cardiovascular system and is involved in self-calming processes. As the vagal brake is reduced, the sympathetics take over, and heart rate and breathing increase. When this NA-vagal brake is removed in threatening situations, a rapid response to danger is allowed as the sympathetics can take over without having to engage the sympathetic-adrenal system first. This is a typical mammalian response.

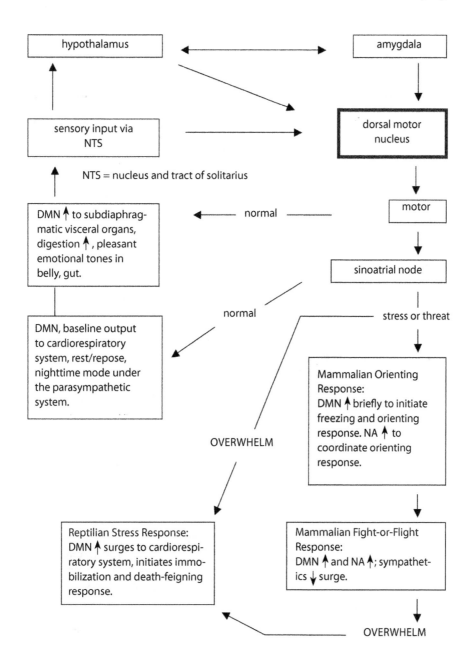

Figure 20.3. Polyvagal responses: dorsal vagus complex and dorsal motor nucleus.

In its social nervous system function, the NA coordinates head and neck motion in the orienting response and, in conjunction with its cardiovascular supply, mediates the relationship between chewing, swallowing, sucking, and breathing, controls the intonation of vocalizations, and is involved in the communication of emotional states and needs, and related facial expressions. All of these have direct bearing on

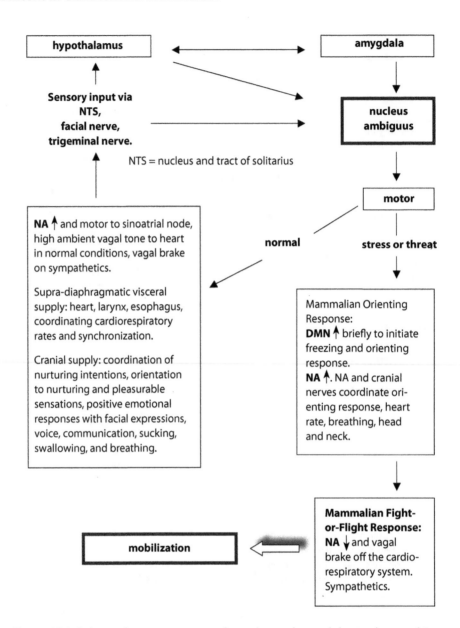

Figure 20.4. Polyvagal responses: ventral vagal complex and the nucleus ambiguus.

infants' survival engagement with their mothers and function in social activities and communications throughout life. Thus infants can orient toward the sight and sounds of mother, vocalize their needs, and show their related emotional states through facial expression. They can make sounds of joy, smile at mom, nurse, and breathe all at the same time in an integrated and coordinated way. In terms of defensive strategies, the NA also coordinates the orienting response, which allows mammals to calmly scan the environment for danger (Figure 20.4).

Signs of Autonomic Activation

As we have seen, signs of autonomic nervous system activation are very common in clinical practice. Various expressions of sympathetic arousal or activation can be sensed as perturbation in the fluids, especially cerebrospinal fluid. This is an expression of the discharge of autonomic energies into the system. It may also be a sign of the processing of these forces by the potency in the fluids. As the sympathetics discharge, the practitioner and client might sense an electric-like streaming through the body. It is not uncommon to sense this kind of discharge from the top of the body downward and from the center of the body to the periphery. An example of this might be a discharge of energy inferiorly through the sympathetic ganglia chain, through the sacrococcygeal ganglion, and down the legs. It not uncommon to sense this kind of discharge while holding the sacrum as the holistic shift deepens, or inertial forces are resolved.

Other signs of sympathetic activation may include tissue fibrillation or body trembling and shaking, skin color changes such as redness and red blotches, sweating, and increased breathing and cardiac rates. Also included in this kind of activation are states of emotional flooding and processes that suddenly and dramatically speed up. The person may be flooded with alternating memories, images, and related emotional couplings. Cranial approaches here classically include exhalation stillpoints and orientation to Long Tide and Dynamic Stillness. The practitioner must appreciate that emotional flooding is a manifestation of past traumatization and the use of appropriate verbal skills, as described in Chapter 22, may be pivotal in their resolution. Acknowledgment of the power of the emotional process, slowing the process so it can complete in resources, orienting the client to feeling-tone and body sensations, and helping to resource the client in the midst of the experience are key orientations here.

Alternatively, you may sense a more parasympathetic state in the body. There may be a sense of density, coldness, numbness, and fluid stagnation as you orient to a particular area. This indicates the presence of inertial potencies centering and containing some kind of force in the system. Clients commonly relate that they are cold, or that a part of their body is cold or numb. Experiences of numbed areas of the body, or even of immobilization and seeming paralysis, are possible. For instance, clients may report that their legs have gone numb and they cannot move them. This can be a frightening experience for both client and practitioner. The practitioner must understand that this is an opportunity to resolve the forces cycling in the system. A verbal acknowledgment of the power of the process and verbal reassurance to the client are very important here. Common cranial approaches to these more frozen states might include inhalation stillpoints, orientation to Long Tide, and the use of fluid skills such as lateral fluctuation and fluid drive processes. Again, appropriate verbal skills are of immense benefit when these kinds of processes are experienced.

Cranial Approaches to the Triune Nervous System and Its Hierarchy of Defensive Strategies

The following explorations orient to very specific work related to the triune nervous system and a restoration of its homeostasis as issues of traumatization, shock states, and autonomic activity emerge in session work. The clinical orientations described in Chapter 19 are also very relevant here, as is an awareness of the stress response and central nervous system motility (explored in Foundations Volume One).

The following two approaches owe much thanks to the influence of John Chitty RCST, who introduced me to Porges's work many years ago and created the first approach to the polyvagal paradigm in the cranial field, and to Katherine Ukleja DO, an old friend and colleague, for her input on a second clinical approach to this system. Both approaches are presented below, first my extrapolations of John's original process and then a description of the second approach, which I now use in clinical work and teach in classroom situations. I am including John's approach both to honor his original work and for historical completeness.

These are followed later in this chapter with a straightforward approach to the orienting response that includes practitioner orientation to the neck and brain stem areas.

John's work is described in three basic stages:

- First, resolution of parasympathetic activation

- Second, resolution of sympathetic activation

- Third, re-establishment of the social nervous system

In working with each of the three autonomic systems, session work will include palpation skills and client interaction.

Exploration 1:
Triune Nervous System _____

The process described here intentionally works with the hierarchy of nervous system response and activation in a structured fashion, and can be repeated a number of times in a session to help down-regulate the cycling stress cascade. In each phase, there is a particular hand position, an anatomical visualization, and a component of client participation. Getting the client's participation helps to clearly engage the particular system and empowers the client to experience his or her own process in present time. In the next clinical exploration, we will follow the hierarchy back up from the parasympathetic, to the sympathetic, and finally to the social nervous system response.

Parasympathetic Activation

After starting as usual, move to an occipital cradle hold, and establish your wide perceptual field. Be sure that the client has accessed a felt-sense of inner resource (see sections on resourcing processes in Foundations Volume One). Shift this hold more caudal (inferior) to place your index fingers on either side of the anterior-lateral aspect of the neck, over the pathway of the vagus nerve as it exits the jugular foramen on each side. Visualize the torso of the person as an elongated tube, banded in the middle by the diaphragm. This orients you to parasympathetic territory, a visceral tube and the ancient worm-like nature of a primitive digestive tube (Figure 20.5).

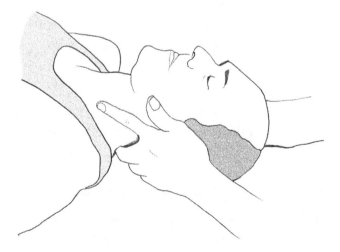

Figure 20.5. Parasympathetic nervous system hold.

Now visualize both visceral vagus nerves and, in your wide perceptual field, orient to their dual pathway from the jugular foramen, innervating the heart and lungs, through the diaphragm and over the organs below the diaphragm. This need not be an exact anatomical image. Simply visualize its branching, tree-like nature. Combine this with your visualization of the tube-like shape as one whole unit of primitive function. Maintain your wide perceptual field, orient to the physical and fluid bodies, and to this visceral tube and the vagus nerves within it as a whole.

When the relationship is well established, ask the client to actively participate in the process by bringing attention to the sensations generated in the belly by the movement of his or her breath. Let this continue as a focus of attention for a minute or so until the client seems to settle into breathing and a parasympathetic level of functioning. Some clients may have a hard time staying with this attention to the breath process, either falling asleep or spacing out as the parasympathetic state becomes established. If this happens, simply carry on with the work; it is not necessary to make clients try to stay focused for an extended time period.

Settle into your relationship. Orient to the fluid tide and then include tissue motility. See if you can allow the motility of this visceral tube-vagus unit of function to come into your awareness in the phases of primary respiration. As an inertial pattern or healing intention manifests, orient to states of equilibrium and to any level of healing process that emerges.

Also listen for signs of the processing and discharge of shock affects and a shift in the system. The client may cycle from numb, frozen, and immobilized states to more active sympathetic processes. The client may sense his or her body literally coming alive, or may sense reassociating and reembodying. You may notice bodily movements, perturbations in the fluids, discharges of energy, and so on. The client may sense trembling, streaming of sensations in arms and/or legs, tingling, feelings of fight-or-flight impulses like the urge to move, and emotions arising. He or she may also begin to move the head and neck in orienting types of motions. Allow this to settle. These are all indications that the system is shifting out of a frozen parasympathetic state to a wider autonomic repertoire. These are cues to move to the next phase of the process. All this can occur in a relatively short period of time, even after just a few minutes.

Some supplemental processes may also be of use in parasympathetic freeze states. It is not uncommon for clients to experience numbing sensations during sessions. They may even feel like a part of their body is frozen, commonly legs and pelvis, or arms, shoulders, and upper back. This is a sign of an incomplete fight-or-flight response, like a need to run or kick in some way. For instance, clients may sense that their legs have become numb or immobilized as the session progresses. This may occur in any session. One approach in this context is to ask where they feel OK in their body, where there is still a sense of warmth and movement. Have them rest their awareness in that area. After resourcing there, ask them to slowly move their awareness to the edge of where the numbness is experienced. Slowly have them shuttle back and forth between the more resourced sensations and the edge of where they sense the numbing. This, along with your presence, can begin to activate the frozen energies and shift to a more mobilized state.

Physical mobilization processes may also be useful in the resolution of parasympathetic frozen states. For instance, after making sure that clients are in touch with their felt-resources, have them bring awareness to the limbs that feel frozen or numb. Have them then slowly tense their arms and legs, making fists and pulling their toes back, holding for a short period, and then slowly relaxing the tension. This may need to be repeated once or twice and commonly helps mobilize the frozen energies and shift to a discharge and clearing of underlying sympathetic cycling. This must be done in the resources of the client, with appropriate pacing, and cranial and verbal skills.

Sympathetic Activation

When you sense the system expressing a more sympathetic nervous system response, shift your orientation from the parasympathetic nervous system to the sympathetic nervous system. The placement of your hands stays roughly the same, with your index fingers shifting slightly posterior over the superior cervical sympathetic ganglion at the superior aspect of the sympathetic chain on both sides. This ganglion is immediately adjoining the vagus nerve in the sides of the neck used in the previous part of the process. The fingers are pointing inferior from just below the head toward the feet.

Now visualize and sense the pathway of the sympathetic ganglion chain down either side of the vertebral column. See if you can orient to its overall form, including its connections to the spinal cord and its termination in a single ganglion just anterior to the coccyx (sacro-coccygeal ganglion). Each chain also has a filament supplying sympathetic innervation to the cranium. Orient to the whole of the sympathetic chain at once. Again hold this in a wide perceptual field with a holistic awareness of the body and biosphere. You are not tracking the chain top-to-bottom; rather, you are holding all of it at once in your wide perceptual

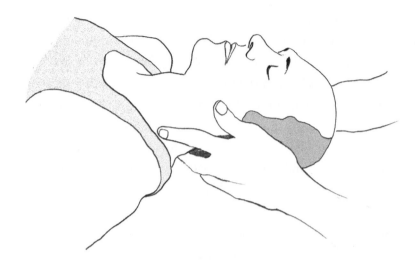

Figure 20.6. Sympathetic nervous system hold.

field. Review the anatomy of this area. When you can orient to the sympathetic chain in this way, you will have a sense of its continuity (Figure 20.6).

When your relationship to the sympathetics seems well established, enlist client participation again. As suggested above, ask the client to very slowly and briefly flex the arms and clench the fists. As he or she does this, ask the client to slowly tighten the pelvic and leg muscles, flex the feet back, and push through the heels of the feet. This engages the musculoskeletal echoes of the fight-or-flight response in the body. Have the client briefly do this and then instruct him or her to soften and relax, and then orient to the sensations that may arise in the body. You can have the client repeat this a number of times if appropriate.

As the client stays with sensations and feeling-tones that may have been elicited in the process, orient to the whole of the sympathetic pathway-ganglion chain. Again, as an inertial pattern or healing intention manifests, orient to states of balance and equilibrium, to any level of healing process that emerges, and to any sympathetic nervous system clearing. This may be sensed as a streaming of electric-like energies, as perturbations in the fluids, and as the clearing of the inertial forces and force vectors involved.

The cue to the transition to the social nervous system is a resolution of the sympathetic activation, a resolution of the inertial forces involved, and a settling of the sympathetic nervous system into stillness with a concomitant rise in the sense of potency in the system. You may even sense the orienting response being elicited as the person begins to rotate or move the head, or the face becomes animated. This sympathetic process seems to often take more time than the parasympathetic, and it can be more dramatic in terms of discharge. Again, trauma resolution verbal skills are especially relevant.

Social Nervous System Re-Establishment

In this next part of the process, we shift our orientation to the social nervous system. The visualization component is based on its anatomy. To access the social nervous system as a whole, change your hand position to a contact spreading across the sides of the face and upper sides of the throat. This position approximates the pharyngeal arch structure that contains the original fibers of cranial nerves V, VII, IX, and part of X. With your thumb lightly in the ear canal, spread your other fingers over the mandible and upper anterior neck.

Once you negotiate and settle into this new hold, visualize the inner-ear structures, especially the inner-ear muscles—the stapedius and tensor tympani—and cranial nerves V and VII. Visualize the relationship of these nerves to the inner ear. You can also include an awareness of the nucleus ambiguus in the brain stem at the level of the foramen magnum. Your main orientation will be to the petrous temporal bone and its inner-ear structures. Let these structures come to you. Do not narrow your perceptual field to do this. Once again, review your anatomy so that these structures are clear to you. Settle into a wide perceptual field with a mid-tide orientation (Figure 20.7).

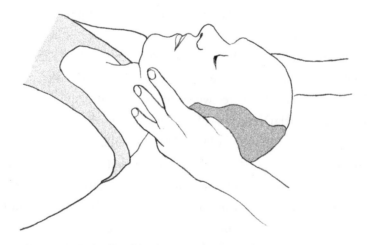

Figure 20.7. Social nervous system hold.

Again enlist the client's active participation in the process. Ask the client to visualize a person from early childhood whose "eyes would light up" in appreciative greeting when they met. This should be a person with whom the client had a simple, mutually warm and friendly relationship. Friends, pets, and relatives all qualify here, or even an archetypal image of some kind, such as a baby or spiritual image. Be creative and negotiate with the client to identify a good visualization of a truly nonthreatening person. The relationship with close family members (especially parents) is commonly too complex; an aunt or uncle, friend, or pet is more likely to be effective for invoking the appreciative, positive felt-sense experience. To encourage this access, it may be helpful to have the client imagine an encounter with this resourcing person/animal from early childhood, complete with recalling the likely setting of the encounter in some detail, including visual, auditory, and/or kinesthetic components. The key here is the ability to access the feeling-tone of the bright, affectionate, and smiling facial expression of that person/animal, to hear or see their warm greeting in the imagination. The intention of this is to generate the sense of an early nurturing encounter that elicits the social nervous system and its orienting processes.

Sometimes clients cannot relate to early childhood, or the question brings up upsetting memories. If this occurs, have them first orient to any person, pet, or relationship from any phase of their life, with whom they had a fully resourcing connection. Sometimes orienting to a place where they feel or felt safe, like a particular place in the natural world, can help.

Once this imagined encounter is established, orient to the pharyngeal arches and/or the inner structures of the temporal bone. Be especially aware of the fine inner muscles that relate to orienting to sound. Do not narrow your perceptual field as you do this; remember to hold an awareness of the whole and to let these inner structures come to you. If your anatomy knowledge is sufficient, include an awareness of the cranial nerves serving this area, especially cranial nerves V and VII and the brain stem area where the nucleus ambiguus resides.

Again, as an inertial issue or healing intention clarifies, orient to states of balance and equilibrium and to any level of healing process that emerges, and allow any processing of stress responses that may arise. It is common for the client to begin to express orienting motions, such as head rotation and eye movements. Similarly, warmth and tingling may spread through the face, and memories of loving contact may arise. Brief waves of feelings, positive and/or negative, may wash over the lower face, including the throat area. Allow these to occur, slowing the process if necessary. Acknowledge to the client anything that seems important.

These three phases of hierarchical work may cycle through relatively quickly, and the whole process can be repeated in a session to gradually arrive at a sense of real completion. It may also take a number of sessions to resolve a particular level of stress response in the system.

Another useful approach in this context relates to the orienting response mediated by the nucleus ambiguus. Have your client consciously enter present time by bringing his or her attention to hearing, seeing, and sensations in the body. Then orient him or her to hearing and seeing, and then to slowly look around the room, turning the neck while doing this. This helps shift the system to the prefrontal cortex and present-time processing, and helps down-regulate the stress response and reorient to the social nervous system. This can be coupled with the exercise of remembering a totally resourcing person or image. I commonly end sessions with this intention, even for a few moments, to ensure that a client leaves my office space oriented in present time. (A fuller orienting exercise is described in Chapter 22.)

As a final note for this exploration, some clients may manifest a more purely parasympathetic state, presenting immobilized and numbed states, coupled with dissociation. This is commonly an expression of very early childhood overwhelm, or of extreme, rapid overwhelming experiences. Resourcing work and inhalation stillpoints can be a very beneficial strategy in these cases. Inhalation stillpoints are excellent for clients who are set in dissociative and low-energy parasympathetic states without an underlying sympathetic response. As noted above, inhalation stillpoints gradually help clients re-associate and mobilize potency for healing processes. Mobilization processes described in Chapter 22 include useful verbal skills and clinical intentions in these circumstances.

Exploration 2:
Triune Nervous System

Here is another approach to restoring the triune nervous system—social, sympathetic, and parasympathetic—to homeostasis. It clearly takes advantage of the triune nature of the innervation to the cardio-respiratory system. In the context of the triune nervous system, this area receives input from all three levels of the autonomic nervous system, including the dorsal motor nucleus, the nucleus ambiguus, and the sympathetic nervous system. I find this exploration to be a straightforward and more spontaneous approach than the one above, as the triune nervous system will process its affects in a sequence appropriate to that person's particular needs in the resolution of traumatic cycling and activation.

The exploration begins with an occipital cradle hold to orient to the motility of the sensorimotor-brain stem area and its nuclei, and then moves to an occiput-cardio-respiratory hold that orients the session to all three triune relationships at once. The practitioner then finishes with a social nervous system hold similar to the one described above. Alternatively, the practitioner can start with a vault hold, which helps the practitioner relate to a more overall sense of CNS motility and to orient to any level of CNS function, cycling, or activation that may arise for resolution.

It is very important before using this approach that a safe holding environment has been established. It is also important for the practitioner to be aware of CNS motility, the motility of the heart and its embryology, and the process of heart ignition (see Chapter 20, Foundations Volume One). Finally, remember that if a person's system is very activated or inertial, it will be important to orient him or her to felt-resources and to work with deepening stillpoint processes so that a holistic shift can clarify.

Start as usual at the side of the table, then move to the client's feet and orient to primary respiration and the holistic shift. When the relational field and holistic shift have deepened, move to an occipital cradle hold at the head of the treatment table. In a wide perceptual field, orient to the motility of the CNS and brain stem. First orient to the fluid tide and then include the CNS and its ventricles in your awareness. Be patient and settle into a wide perceptual field and let the healing process emerge in its own time.

Orient to any inertial fulcrums that arise, the deepening of the state of balance, and allow any inertial forces to process and any CNS activation to complete and clear. Note any discharges or clearings from brain stem nuclei. These may be perceived as local electric-like vibrations, perturbations, and fluid fluctuations, and as wider streaming-clearing of electric-like sensations, commonly down the client's vertebral column and through his or her arms and legs.

Now shift your position to the right side of the treatment table with your chair close to the head of the table. Place your cephalad hand under the client's occiput with your arm or elbow on the table. Be sure to find a stable and centered place for the client's head and a comfortable position for yourself. Then, with appropriate negotiation, slowly place your caudal hand gently over the client's cardio-respiratory area (Figure 20.8).

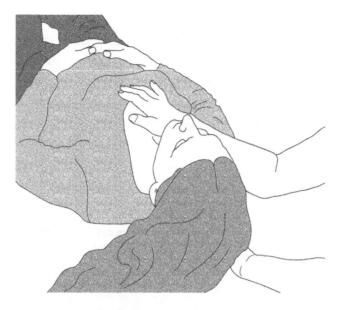

Figure 20.8. Polyvagal hold.

Settle into an awareness of the motility of the heart in the phases of primary respiration—in inhalation the heart spirals inferior top-down, from the right side of the body toward the left (this mirrors its embryological development). Orient to any healing processes that emerge in your receptive holding field. Once these processes complete, as you hold the occiput-brain stem and heart areas in awareness, orient to the triune innervation to the cardio-respiratory system. Include the vagus nerve and its nuclei—both the NA and the DMN—and the sympathetic innervation to the heart area in your awareness. You are now in relationship to all three levels of the triune hierarchy—social, sympathetic, and parasympathetic nervous systems. Settle into a still and receptive space. The intention here is to orient to stillness and states of equilibrium as the triune system expresses and resolves any cycling and returns to homeostasis.

As your contact and the client's system settle, you may sense a mutual expression of potency at both holds, with pulsation, vibration, and clearing. You may then sense a further deepening into equilibrium and stillness and one level of the triune system may begin to discharge and resolve its cycling. Commonly either the parasympathetic dorsal motor nucleus or sympathetic innervation to the heart will begin to clear.

As the sympathetic cycling clears, you will sense an electric-like clearing from the brain stem, through the sympathetic ganglion along the spine, and a general sense of clearing from the top down and center out—commonly with streaming down the client's legs and/or arms. When the dorsal motor nuclei begin to clear their cycling, you may sense a vibration or pulsation in the brain stem area around the fourth ventricle, and a clearing through the vagus nerve with a sense of wave-like streaming down through the client's chest area and lower viscera. When this occurs, the client's breath commonly deepens and he or she feels warmth in the chest and belly areas. This parasympathetic level of clearing has an embodied, visceral feel to it.

Allow these to complete and then move to a social nervous system hold. You may use the one explored above or use a simpler alternative hold. Here the practitioner places his or her palms over the client's ears and spreads the rest of the fingers over the facial area—zygomas, maxillae, and mandible (Figure 20.9).

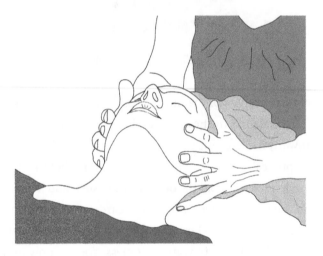

Figure 20.9. Alternative social nervous system hold.

With either hold, orient the client to the felt-resources and to a figure from childhood (person or pet) who was totally resourcing. If he or she cannot think of a person or animal in this context, then use a resourcing image to work with. This can be a place, activity, or spiritual image that is familiar and comforting to the client. Again allow the system to enter equilibrium and deepen into Long Tide and Dynamic Stillness. Again orient to any CNS clearing that arises, or to any other process that emerges, with appropriate relationship to any level of activation occurring. Issues around safety, intimacy, early experience, attachment issues, and even birth-related issues may emerge for healing purposes. Finish at the sacrum or sacrum-occiput with an orientation to the primal midline.

As a negotiated contact is made with the client's heart and heart center, and with the social nervous system hold, deep emotional and heart-centered feelings may arise and need to be acknowledged, developmental trauma may be accessed, and issues around intimacy and safety may clarify, along with pre- and perinatal and early childhood experiences of safety, caregiver attunement, breaches and inconsistencies in the holding field, and bonding and attachment issues. These early experiences set the tone for the development of our personality, defensive tendencies, and attachment system, and must be negotiated and held in a paced and resourced relational field. Appropriate verbal skills are also essential to maintain pacing and help process any emotional tones that may arise.

The Stress Cascade and the Triune Nervous System

The physiology of the stress cascade was introduced in Chapter 19, and it is now appropriate to fill out its basic physiology in the light of Porges's work. The above approaches, along with those described in Chapter 19, will help to down-regulate the stress cascade and its fight-or-flight response, integrate early childhood experience, and re-establish normal autonomic baselines. As described earlier, there are four basic stages to the stress cascade: (1) ideal state, (2) active-alert/orienting, (3) fight-or-flight, and (4) overwhelm-shock (Figure 20.10).

As the stress cascade unfolds in threatening or novel situations, the various parts of the triune autonomic nervous system act communally to meet the arising experience, and the dorsal motor nucleus (DMN) and nucleus ambiguus (NA) work cooperatively.

The ideal state is largely one of homeostasis with appropriate responses to present-time conditions and rest, repose, and vegetative functions. There is a fluid relationship in the functioning of all three levels of the autonomic nervous system, with rest, repose, and vegetative functions available. There is high NA vagal tone to the heart and bronchi, with relational needs being met via the social nervous system. There is also high DMN vagal tone, allowing for digestion, rest, and repose.

During the active-alert or orienting phase, the amygdala and hypothalamus signal the dorsal motor nucleus, the nucleus ambiguus, and the locus ceruleus that danger is present. The DMN momentarily surges to stop us so that we can orient to the environment. Along with this, the locus ceruleus acts to release norepinephrine, and we enter the active-alert state. During this state, the NA acts to coordinate the overall orienting response. Head and neck motions are co-coordinated with breathing, heart rate, and active attention to scan the environment for danger. Here the

Ideal State:

Fully resourced;
relaxed, resourced, and present

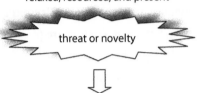

threat or novelty

Active-Alert State:

Freezing, orienting response; heightened alertness; orienting to danger.

Fight-or-Flight Response:

Highly aroused state, highly charged mobilization of defensive energies.

Overwhelm:

Resources overwhelmed.

Shock Response:

Freezing, immobilization, dissociation.

Figure 20.10. The stress cascade.

dorsal motor nucleus and the nucleus ambiguus act cooperatively. As we shall see, this cooperative process can break down.

In fight-or-flight, a present danger is sensed and physiology rapidly changes. The nucleus ambiguus and dorsal motor nucleus are down-regulated and the sympathetics surge. The system is flooded with epinephrine, norepinephrine, and cortisol, nonessential activities are down-regulated, energy reserves are accessed, and the musculoskeletal system is mobilized for action.

If this process is thwarted or overwhelmed in any way, the person may go into shock, immobilization, and dissociation. In overwhelm, a strong surge of the DMN generates a frozen and immobilized state. This is different from the surge that occurred during the orienting response. It is both more intense and of longer duration. There is a concurrent flooding of the system with endorphins and dopamine.

This places the person in a dissociated and euphoric state. This is why a client who manifests frozen and immobilized states generally also experiences dissociation.

Ideally, this shock state only lasts for ten minutes or so. As the person comes out of overwhelm, the sympathetic surge re-emerges, and the release of dopamine and endorphins subsides. The person may then tremble, shake, express anger, or even run to discharge the cycling sympathetic energies. If this happens, a resolution of cycling energies and a return to homeostatic balance is more likely to occur (Figure 20.11).

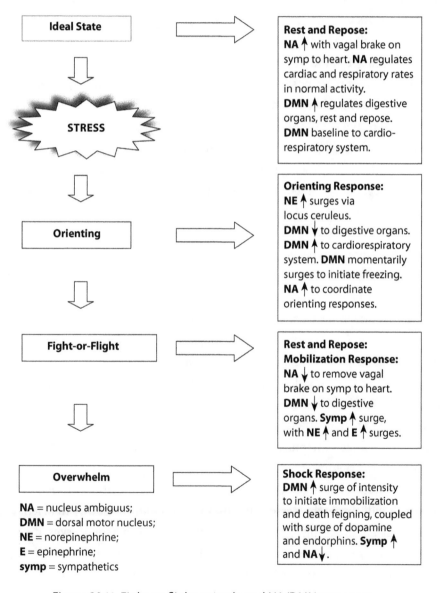

Figure 20.11. Fight-or-flight cascade and NA/DMN responses.

Repercussions of Unresolved Hypersensitization

A return to homeostatic balance after traumatic experiences may not go as smoothly as one would hope. As we saw in Chapter 19, cortical loops of memory and meaning can intercede and keep the process running. These can be memories of past trauma, psychological life statements, or even cultural injunctions such as "big boys don't cry" or "emotions shouldn't be shown in public." So cortical processing—thoughts, memory, and meaning—can signal the amygdala and hypothalamus either that the event is not yet over, or can literally get in the way of the discharge and clearing process. As we have seen, the amygdala also mediates emotional memory. The amygdala itself may be cycling implicit emotional memories of past trauma and these too can get in the way of resolving the present traumatic experience.

Due to all of these possibilities, confusion may set in and any of the stages of the stress cascade below the ideal homeostatic state may become locked in cycling unresolved responses to traumatic experience, through the states of active-alert or orienting response, fight-or-flight response, and dissociation, immobilization, and/ or freezing. In a free-flowing nontraumatized system, the individual would ideally be able to negotiate all stages as appropriate to current circumstances. However, if a person encounters trauma and is overwhelmed by its circumstances, he or she may become locked in cycling levels of the stress response in various ways: cycling the active-alert state as hypervigilance and/or the inability to orient to present conditions; the flight-or-flight response as anxiety and depression, with the possibility of inappropriate behaviors coupled with fear and anger; and the overwhelmed state as dissociation, depressive collapse, and immobilized/frozen states.

In overwhelming circumstances such as severe or repetitive trauma, the parasympathetic surge of the dorsal motor nucleus in the overwhelm state may become hypersensitized and not down-regulate, and the underlying sympathetic energies may not be fully cleared. The person is then left in a dissociative state, cycling *both* unresolved parasympathetic and sympathetic energies. The next time that person meets stress or feels threatened in any way, the DMN may not turn off when it fires as part of the orienting response. It may respond as though the current situation is totally overwhelming and may start to work in opposition to the NA. If this occurs, it will throw the person into dissociation and the ability to orient is then lost. Instead of orienting to present circumstances, the person freezes, dissociates, and can become confused or fearful. In these cases, the DMN and the NA are both surging and the person is left frozen, dissociated, and hypervigilant at the same time. This is common in PTSD. Likewise, the sympathetic nuclei that surge

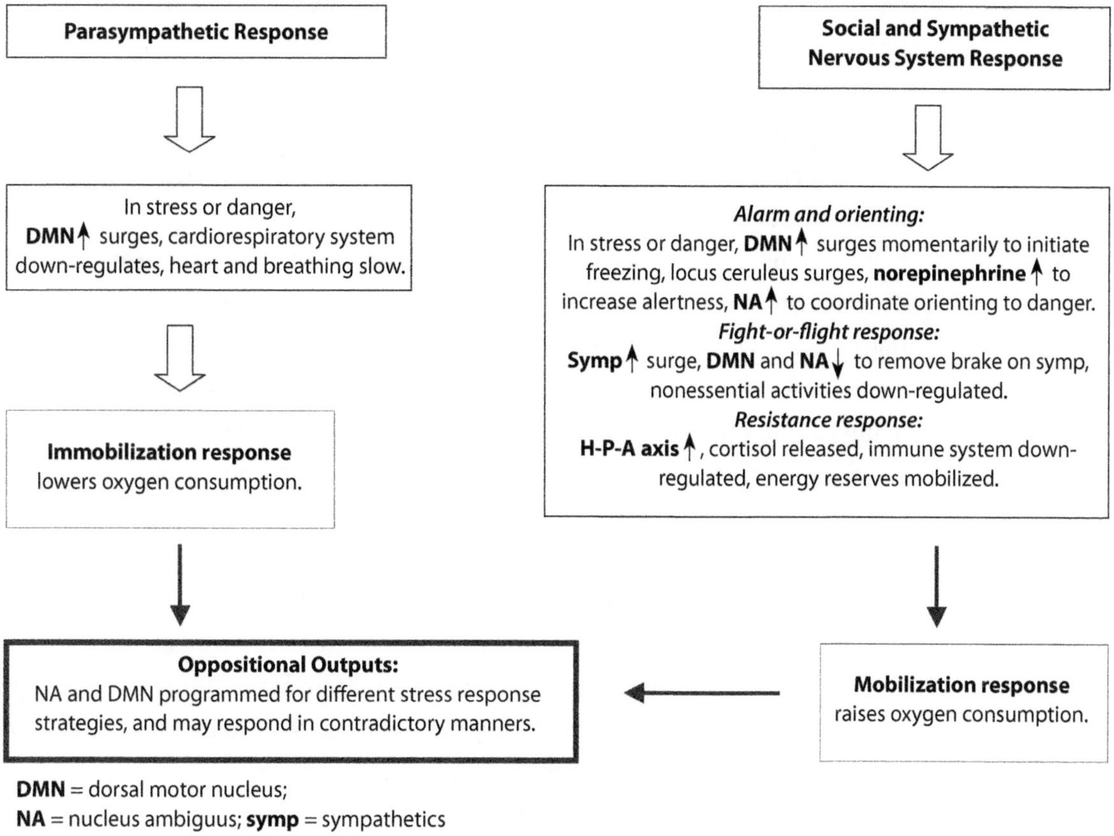

```
┌─────────────────────────────┐          ┌─────────────────────────────┐
│   Parasympathetic Response  │          │    Social and Sympathetic   │
│                             │          │   Nervous System Response   │
└─────────────────────────────┘          └─────────────────────────────┘
              ⇓                                          ⇓
┌─────────────────────────────┐          ┌─────────────────────────────┐
│   In stress or danger,      │          │   Alarm and orienting:      │
│ DMN↑ surges, cardiorespir-  │          │ In stress or danger, DMN↑   │
│ atory system down-regulates,│          │ surges momentarily to       │
│ heart and breathing slow.   │          │ initiate freezing, locus    │
└─────────────────────────────┘          │ ceruleus surges, norepine-  │
              ⇓                           │ phrine↑ to increase         │
┌─────────────────────────────┐          │ alertness, NA↑ to coordinate│
│  Immobilization response    │          │ orienting to danger.        │
│ lowers oxygen consumption.  │          │   Fight-or-flight response: │
└─────────────────────────────┘          │ Symp↑ surge, DMN and NA↓ to │
              ↓                           │ remove brake on symp,       │
┌─────────────────────────────┐          │ nonessential activities     │
│    Oppositional Outputs:    │          │ down-regulated.             │
│ NA and DMN programmed for   │          │   Resistance response:      │
│ different stress response   │ ←──────── │ H-P-A axis↑, cortisol       │
│ strategies, and may respond │          │ released, immune system     │
│ in contradictory manners.   │          │ down-regulated, energy      │
└─────────────────────────────┘          │ reserves mobilized.         │
                                          └─────────────────────────────┘
                                                        ↓
                                          ┌─────────────────────────────┐
                                          │    Mobilization response    │
                                          │ raises oxygen consumption.  │
                                          └─────────────────────────────┘
```

DMN = dorsal motor nucleus;
NA = nucleus ambiguus; **symp** = sympathetics

Figure 20.12. Polyvagal responses to stress and oppositional outputs.

in fight-or-flight response may become hypersensitized to stimuli and the individual may be locked in anxiety, tension, and inappropriate emotional responses and behaviors (Figure 20.12).

Early Childhood Trauma

It became obvious early in my clinical practice that the hypoarousal physiology at work in many young children is very different from the classic stress cascade. There seemed to be no underlying sympathetic cycling involved. This was also the case in some adult clients. Some discussions I had with William Emerson, one of the fathers of pre- and perinatal psychology, in the 1980s and 1990s were very helpful. In his huge experience with infants and their prenatal and birth patterning, he had clearly seen that a large proportion of infants and young children, if overwhelmed by their experience, default to the most primitive protective response, the parasympathetic.

Infants cannot protect themselves either by fighting or fleeing; hence, their primal defensive strategy is withdrawal and dissociation. You see this in even small ways in infants. If they do not like something—a sound, sight, or person—they simply turn away from it. In other words, they withdraw. The understanding that infants and young children tend to more readily default to a parasympathetic response has been borne out by research projects (Perry and Pollard 1998).

Porges's polyvagal concept has helped clarify some of what is happening in such cases and how to orient to it clinically. If an infant is rapidly overwhelmed, the DMN surges, coupled with a flooding of serotonin, endorphins, and dopamine, and the infant enters a frozen and dissociated state. This may occur before any sympathetic cycling can be generated. These infants are not generally seen to have problems. They sleep a lot, are "good" babies, and do not give the parents any trouble. They may have some feeding and attention difficulties, but these are not generally picked up or considered to be a problem.

There is evidence that this kind of early childhood experience can generate a parasympathetic set point. The person becomes set in a parasympathetic response to stress and cannot mobilize sympathetic energies. In later childhood, attention deficit states may occur, with an inability to concentrate or to mobilize to achieve success. In later life, the person may collapse into depressive states of listlessness, tiredness, oversleeping, poor motivation, and even immobility. Chronic fatigue syndrome may also have its roots here. It is a chronically exhausted, low-sympathetic, low-cortisol, low-norepinephrine state in which the person enters dissociation easily and has problems focusing attention and maintaining awareness. He or she may withdraw from stressful situations, avoid challenges, become very tired easily, collapse into sleep states, and so on.

The immune system is greatly affected by all this. The sympathetic supply to lymph nodes tends to generate a sympathetic brake on the immune system. It down-regulates immune responses and helps keep the immune system from eating us alive. Furthermore, cortisol also functions as a brake on the immune system. Because, in these cases, the system has shifted to a chronic parasympathetic state, the H-P-A axis is down-regulated and cortisol levels are lower than normal. As people set in parasympathetic mode have low sympathetic tonus and low cortisol levels, this brake on the immune system is compromised. These people are thus prone to autoimmune conditions, inflammatory responses, muscular and connective tissue pain, and breakdown. As well as chronic fatigue and autoimmune conditions, some arthritic and rheumatic conditions may also have their origins here (Figure 20.13).

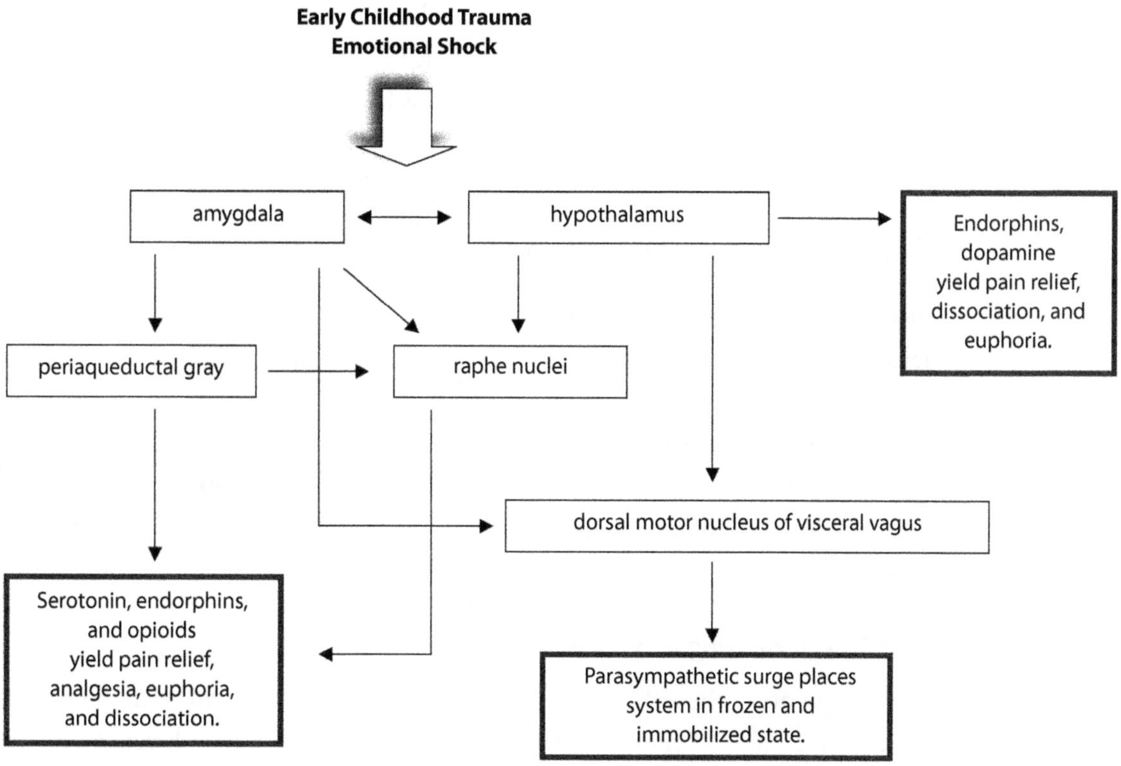

Figure 20.13. The physiology of early childhood trauma and the parasympathetic stress response.

Working with the Orienting Response

As we have seen, the orienting response is the initial stage of the stress response. In traumatization, this response can become hypersensitized, with the affected person stuck in hypervigilance, losing the ability to orient in present time. It is common, as part of this picture, that neck muscles become chronically tense. As discussed in Chapter 19, there is a neurological feedback loop between the neck area and brain stem. The locus ceruleus receives proprioceptive input from neck muscles. This gives the stress system feedback about danger through the orienting response. When neck muscles tense, the locus ceruleus reads this as possible environmental danger. The sympathetics are up-regulated, and the active-alert state intensifies. If the system is in a chronic hyperarousal state, a feedback loop can ensue in which the neck muscles are chronically signaled to tense and the tension is read by the locus ceruleus as an orienting response to danger. The person is caught in a chronic orienting-active-alert feedback loop. Thus neck tension is commonly a sign of unresolved stress in the system. The next exploration orients to this neck tension-orienting response feedback loop. We discuss verbal skills and include an important orienting exercise in Chapter 22 that also helps down-regulate neck tension and restore the orienting response. Please also read that section.

Cranial Hold for the Orienting Response and Neck Tension

Neck tension can be an indicator of a sensitized stress response. The locus ceruleus has connections to the neck area. It monitors for neck tension, which is read as an indication that there is a need to orient to possible danger. As discussed in Chapter 19, this can keep a hypersensitization of the locus ceruleus, amygdala, and hypothalamus/H-P-A axis running. The following clinical approach helps down-regulate neck tension and locus ceruleus activation. It is presented as a two-step process.

Step One: Orienting to Neck Tension

After negotiating the holistic shift, the practitioner moves to an occipital cradle hold oriented to CNS motility, especially to the brain stem, fourth ventricle, and locus ceruleus areas. He or she holds the brain stem area in awareness and allows any discharge or clearing from its nuclei to arise and complete.

The practitioner then shifts his or her contact and orients to the neck-cervical area. Shifting fingers footward, the fingers of both hands line up inferior under the occiput, over the cervical articular masses. The little finger of each hand is just below the occiput, while the other fingers spread vertically footward either side of midline (see Chapter 8). While making a firm yet negotiated contact, orient to cervical motility and to emergent states of balance and equilibrium.

As the inertial fulcrums and forces involved enter equilibrium, the feedback loop from the cervical area to the locus ceruleus is encouraged to down-regulate. This can also access the relationships of the orienting response and triune nervous system, helping integrate the interrelationships between social, sympathetic, and parasympathetic systems. The approaches to the triune nervous system, explored earlier, can also be combined with the above orienting exercise (Figure 20.14).

Step Two: Orienting to the Brain Stem and Neck Tension

The orientation to neck tension in step one can be followed up with a more specific orientation to the brain stem-locus ceruleus and neck muscles. After orienting to the occipital hold and brain stem motility, the practitioner shifts the hold to an

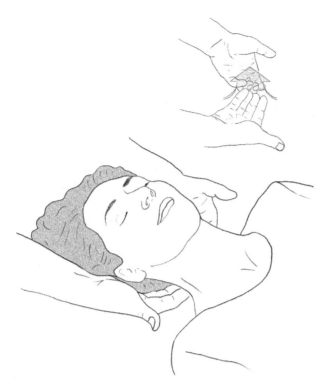

Figure 20.14. Cervical orienting hold.

occipital-neck hold. Sitting at the corner of the cephalad end of the treatment table, he or she places the cephalad hand under the occiput and the caudal hand cupped under the neck area (Figure 20.15).

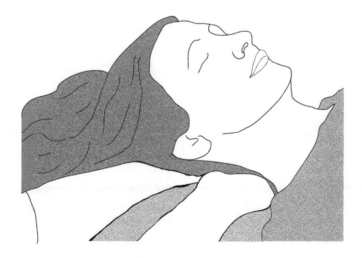

Figure 20.15. Brain stem and cervical hold.

The practitioner settles into an orientation to CNS and brain stem motility while holding the locus ceruleus and neck area in a wide perceptual field. He or she orients to a deepening equilibrium in the relationships, the action of potency, and any clearing sensed in CNS nuclei, the neck area, and the sympathetic nervous system. When the system enters equilibrium the practitioner may sense a reciprocal expression of potency in the brain stem and neck areas, and a related clearing in mid-brain hypothalamus areas. Then he or she waits for the system to express a clear fluid tide, and finishes with a sacral-occipital hold.

CHAPTER 21

Nociception and the Stress Response

As we discussed earlier, internal stressors can be just as powerful as external stressors in setting off the general adaptation response and its stress cascade, an important point often missed or overlooked by the trauma therapy community. This chapter focuses on internal stress response mechanisms and the underappreciated role of nociceptors. These ubiquitous nerve endings sense for danger, tissue damage, and toxicity in the body. Internal stressors, such as inflammatory processes, fluid congestion, tissue damage, and pathologies of various kinds can set off the stress cascade just like external stressors do. Indeed, many of the complaints we see in our practice can be traced to nociceptive activity, including chronic pain, injuries that don't get better, anxiety states, and ongoing disorders that have no apparent cause or external etiology. A cranial approach to these internal stressors can be direct, precise, and effective.

The Spinal Segment

Understanding spinal segments and the simple reflex arc forms a basis for our exploration of internal stress responses. A basic spinal segment is composed of (1) a sensory nerve, (2) a neuron in the dorsal horn area of the spinal cord, (3) a connecting intermediary or secondary neuron in the spinal cord, and (4) a motor nerve. The spinal segment also sends and receives information, via secondary neurons, to and from higher-level processors in the brain. Let's first review the interrelationships of a basic spinal segment.

Information is sent to the spinal cord by sensory (afferent) peripheral nerves. These are in contact with either visceral or somatic tissues and the fluids around these tissues. The neurons or cell bodies of these nerves are located in the dorsal root ganglia near the spinal cord. Both visceral and somatic sensory nerves travel in a peripheral spinal nerve and have their neurons located there. From here they enter the spinal cord and synapse with multiple dorsal horn neurons. The dorsal horn cells form what has been described as an *interneuronal pool*. This is a three-dimensional pool of connected dorsal horn neurons. These cells form a matrix that is more like the multiple nonlinear interconnections of servers on the Internet than like the linear connections of a telegraph or telephone system. Input to one neuron can take many routes and affect many others, and many neurons may be affected by incoming information.

Dorsal horn cells function as local processors of information. From here a reflex motor (efferent) response may be sent back to the particular somatic or visceral tissue from which the input originated, forming an inclusive information loop by which a peripheral area reports to the spine and the spine responds with command messages. This simple input-local processing-output loop is called a *reflex arc* (Figure 21.1). At this stage, no higher-level processing is needed, and homeostasis can be maintained without overwhelming the higher level processes with information.

The system is adaptable in that sensory input meets the interneuronal pool and is received in up to three spinal segments. The spine is not horizontally segmented

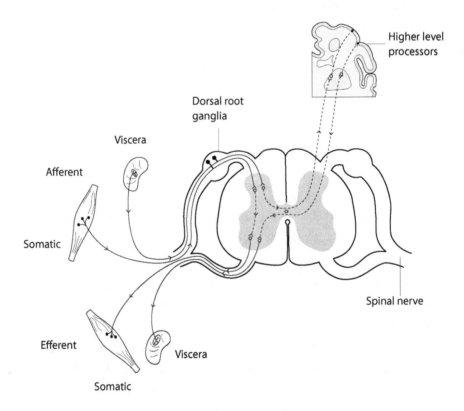

Figure 21.1. The spinal segment reflex arc.

for this purpose, but rather the dorsal horn cells directly interconnect to several vertebral levels. Information also travels up and down the spinal cord and can stimulate response in many areas. The spinal cord itself is thus vertically, not horizontally, oriented (Figure 21.2). Thus there is built-in redundancy, which means that responses can be multifaceted and rapid.

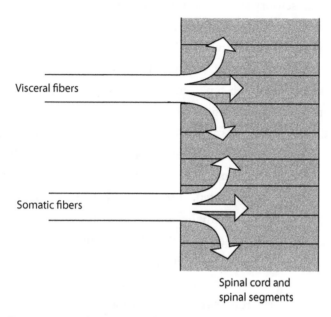

Spinal cord and
spinal segments

Figure 21.2. Multisegmental sensory input to the spinal cord.

In addition, signals may be sent to the brain via secondary neurons from the dorsal horn interneuronal pool to brain stem nuclei, the amygdala, the thalamus, the hypothalamus, and the cortex for higher-level processing. If the signals are intense enough, the dorsal horn cells tell these higher-level processors that something serious is happening below.

Composition of the Spinal Nonsegmented Neuronal Web

Visceral or somatic sensory afferent nerves with their neurons in the dorsal root ganglion

Multiple connections (up to three segments) from these nerves to the dorsal horn neurons

The dorsal horn neurons and the interneuronal pool they are part of

Efferent motor nerve or nerves

Facilitation and the Facilitated Segment

The term *facilitation* is a classic osteopathic term, which means that something has been made easier. In this case, it indicates that a nerve has become hypersensitive or hyperexcitable. The nerve's threshold of firing has been lowered and it fires with less-than-normal sensory stimulation. Facilitation commonly occurs when there is ongoing and chronic input to a nerve. The nerve becomes overwhelmed by the input and becomes hypersensitive, and its firing is made easier due to some chronic pathological process in the body. The spinal segment described above or its wider multisegmental neuronal web can become facilitated and hypersensitized.

This has important repercussions throughout the system. Spinal nerve segments that serve both the visceral and somatic components of the body may become hypersensitive and fire inappropriately, generating somatic and visceral pathologies. Tense or flaccid muscles, loss of joint mobility, joint pathologies, and visceral dysfunctions can all arise due to these facilitated, chronic nociceptive inputs. Most important, chronic nociceptive input to the higher-order nuclei of the brain stem, diencephalon, and cortex can set off the general adaptation response and its stress cascade.

In osteopathic practice, a sensitized spinal segment is called a *facilitated segment*, and it is seen to have a number of possible origins. One is a vertebral fixation that impinges on a nerve root leaving or entering the spinal cord, as nociceptive input floods the sensory nerves and spinal cord. Other common origins of facilitation are chronic inflammation in the musculoskeletal system and visceral inflammation and pathology.

Constant nociceptive input into sensory neurons can cause what is known as *transduction*. In transduction, the nature of the nucleus and cell membrane of neurons changes. The nerve becomes more easily stimulated, and the output from the cell nucleus may change. Nerves that normally produce particular hormones or proteins may begin to produce others in response to the ongoing nociceptive input and hypersensitivity. In some respects, it is a local version of what happens under constant stress in the body at large. Cells become overwhelmed and change physiology.

Transduction has major repercussions for sensory, nociceptive nerves. Nociceptors monitor for danger, tissue damage, and inflammation. They are sometimes called pain receptors. They are high-threshold, small-caliber nerves; it takes relatively intense inputs to set them off. Other sensory nerves, such as touch receptors, proprioceptors, and mechanoreceptors, are low-threshold, large-caliber nerves; they are faster nerves, and less stimulation is needed to set them off. This allows for sensitive feedback in relatively subtle processes like touch and pressure reception, and body position and motion. Under chronic sensory input, nociceptors can transduce and become sensitized to lower levels of input. They then begin to act as though they are low-threshold nerves, and ordinary stimuli, such as moving an arm or pressure against the skin, can then be erroneously interpreted as danger, with a resulting pain response (Willard and Patterson 1994).

Visceral-Somatic Convergence and the Spinal Segment

Another complication arises because the neurons of incoming sensory nerves are located in the dorsal root ganglia, where all of the nociceptors, proprioceptors, mechanoreceptors, chemoreceptors, and nerves from somatic and visceral sources are interconnected via dendrite synapses. When the neurons of nociceptors transduce and become sensitized, they can then signal other sensory neurons in the dorsal root ganglia that danger is present. This occurs even before input reaches the spinal cord. Other normally nonrelated areas of the body may then become involved in the sensitized nociceptive sensorimotor loop. Remote sensory nerve endings may then release a chemical called *substance P* into their areas, setting off inflammatory processes. Thus, even before input is sent to the dorsal horn cells in the spinal cord, whole-body referred inflammatory processes can be initiated. In the dorsal root ganglia a somatic-visceral convergence can also occur. Somatic sensory nerves can begin to signal visceral sensory nerves that danger is present, and likewise, visceral sensory nerves can signal somatic nerves.

There is also visceral-somatic convergence in the spinal cord itself. Both visceral and somatic nerves synapse with multiple spinal cord segments and multiple dorsal horn neurons. Their sensory inputs converge on the dorsal horn interneuronal pool, and multiple motor outputs result. Thus input from a visceral sensory nerve may stimulate somatic efferent output and vice versa. A sensitized spinal segment may therefore affect many areas of the body and many systems, both somatic and visceral. Here we are really talking about a facilitated nonsegmental neuronal web with wide repercussions in the body.

Last, there is also visceral-somatic convergence with the secondary neurons that carry information from the dorsal horn area to higher centers above. The convergence in the dorsal horn area can also lead to interlinked output to higher centers such as the hypothalamus, thalamus, amygdala, locus ceruleus, and autonomic nuclei (Figure 21.3).

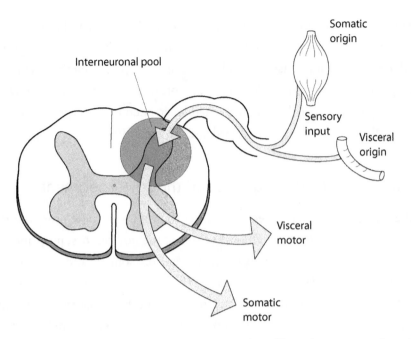

Figure 21.3. Visceral-somatic convergence in dorsal horn interneuronal pool.

Four Stages of Facilitation

The facilitation process can enter the deepest recesses of the nervous system. In this process, a disturbance of some kind generates a local cascade of pro-inflammatory, neuroendocrine-active and immune-active chemicals. The presence of tissue damage and inflammation will be registered by local nociceptive nerve endings, and these nerves will send input into the dorsal horn of the spinal cord. If the disturbance is chronic, the sensory nociceptive nerve will transduce and become sensitized to further input. This sensitized input goes to the dorsal horn neurons, and motor output is sent back to the area of disturbance. A sensitized spinal segment begins to form.

In the next stage, the dorsal horn neurons also transduce, and the sensitized reflex arc is even more intensified. The transduced dorsal horn cells, whose interneuronal pool receives input from all sorts of sensory processes, begins to read all sensory inputs as though they are nociceptive. Inputs that warn of danger flood the higher centers of the brain, and the stress cascade can be set off. The nuclei and neurons of higher-level processors, such as autonomic nuclei, the amygdala, and the hypothalamus, may also become overwhelmed by the amount of input arising, and become sensitized. A vicious circle results in which inputs and outputs keep the sensitized cycles running, in what I call the four stages of facilitation (Willard and Patterson 1994):

- The sensitization of a peripheral sensory nerve

- The sensitization of a spinal segment or segments

- The transduction of the dorsal horn neurons

- The sensitization and transduction of higher-level nuclei in the brain stem, diencephalon, and cortex, and the generation of a general adaptation stress response in the body that can enter the deepest recesses of the nervous system (Figure 21.4)

1. Sensitized peripheral nerve

Cell neuron

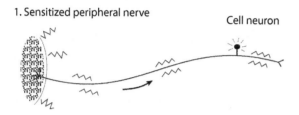

2. Hypersensitive spinal segment

Dorsal horn neuron

Sensory

Motor

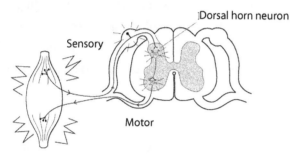

3. Transduction in dorsal horn cells

4. Higher level sensitization

Brain

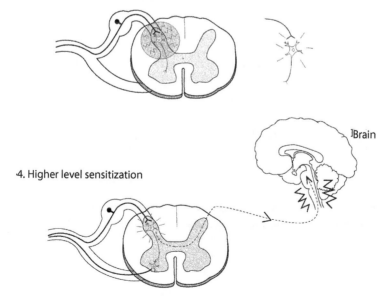

Figure 21.4. The four stages of facilitation.

Stage One

In the first stage, a disturbance of some kind, typically some kind of tissue fixation, pathology, or damage, generates a local inflammatory process. When cells are damaged, their cell membranes release a cascade of chemical messages. This includes neuroendocrine-active and immune-active chemicals. The intention of this cascade is both to warn the system that damage or danger is present and to initiate local healing responses. Sensory nociceptors respond to these pro-inflammatory chemicals by releasing substance P into the area that further stimulates the inflammatory response. Substance P stimulates a further cascade of histamines, prostaglandins, bradykinins, norepinephrine, serotonin, and cytokines, to name just a few. This becomes a sensitizing soup of neuroactive chemicals, which further stimulates nociceptive nerve endings. A vicious cycle can occur in which these chemicals stimulate the nerve endings of nociceptors to produce more substance P, thus initiating the release of more pro-inflammatory chemicals (Figure 21.5). The presence of tissue damage and inflammation is detected by local nociceptive nerve endings, and these nerves report the situation to the dorsal horn of the spinal cord.

If the disturbance continues and becomes chronic, the nociceptive nerve involved may become overwhelmed, its neuron may transduce and become

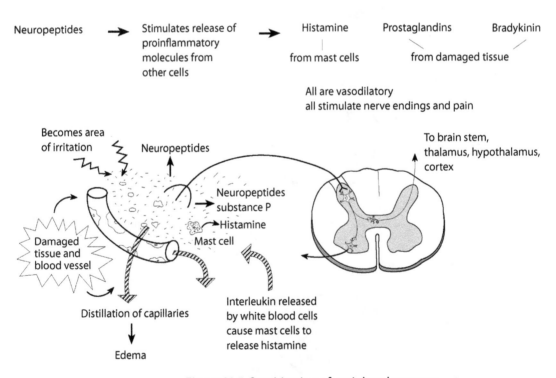

Figure 21.5. Sensitization of peripheral neurons.

sensitized, and the nerve—a high-threshold, small-caliber nerve—now acts as though it is a low-threshold, large-caliber nerve. Inputs that do not normally cause it to fire now will. Motion, pressure, and proprioceptive inputs will cause a firing of the nociceptor. Moving a knee, putting pressure on a leg, or just walking may all be registered as pain. What's more, if a nociceptor transduces, it may remain sensitized even when the initial disturbance has healed. Nociceptive input may still be sent to the spinal cord, even when the disturbance is over (Figure 21.6).

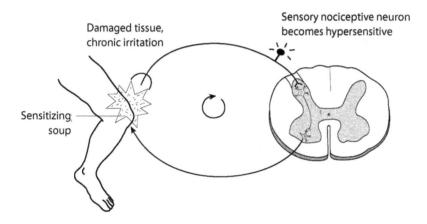

Figure 21.6. Sensitization of peripheral fibers.

Stage Two

In the second stage, a sensitized spinal segment begins to form. The transduced nociceptive nerves alert the dorsal horn cells in the spinal cord that something is up. These, in turn, trigger firing of motor neurons related to the area, initiating a sensorimotor reflex arc, intensifying the whole situation. As more input floods the dorsal horn area, more motor output is produced and more sensory input is stimulated. A vicious circle is set up.

Stage Three

In the third stage, the dorsal horn neurons, flooded with information, also transduce. The sensitized reflex arc is then even more intensified. The transduced dorsal horn cells, whose interneuronal pool receives input from all sorts of sensory processes, begins to read all sensory inputs as though they are nociceptive. The multilevel spinal segment will be kept cycling by this misinterpretation of sensory input. The somatic or visceral tissues that the reflex arc serves now also become sensitized, leading to joint dysfunction, muscle tension or spasms, and functional degeneration. There is some evidence that arthritis in joints may be generated by this process. Similarly, facilitation of nerves supplying viscera can produce increased sympathetic tonus, changes in organ function, changes in vasomotor tone, and changes in fluid balance (Figure 21.7).

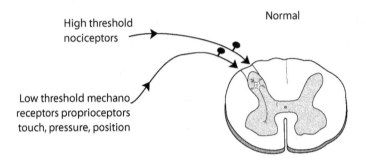

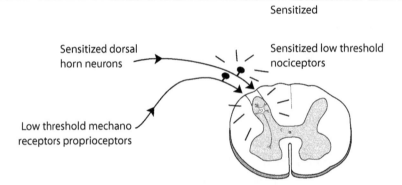

Figure 21.7. Sensitization of dorsal horn cells.

Stage Four

This leads to the fourth stage, in which inputs warning of danger floods higher brain centers, and the general adaptation response and its stress cascade is set off. The transduced dorsal horn cells, misinterpreting sensory information, begin to signal higher-order processors that there is danger below. These inputs to higher centers travel via secondary nerves in the spinothalamic tract, the spinohypothalamic tract, and the spinoreticular tract. When nociceptive inputs reach the cortex via the thalamus, they are registered as pain. However, low-level inflammatory processes may not be intense enough to initiate a cortex mediated perception of pain, yet may still impinge upon brain stem, limbic system, and diencephalon neurons. The nuclei and neurons of higher-level processors, including autonomic and brain stem nuclei, the amygdala, and the hypothalamus, may also be overwhelmed by the input arising and become sensitized to further input. A vicious circle results in which inputs and outputs keep the sensitized cycles running. It becomes self-perpetuating, beyond the original disturbance, which by this time may have already healed. This is a physical parallel to the amygdala's misinterpreting current-time events as threatening based on past history. What emerges is a systemwide alarm state that is internally generated, self-perpetuating, and perhaps unrelated to any continuing real threat. A state of anxiety comparable to PTSD symptoms may ensue that originates in a seemingly simple, low-grade inflammatory process (Figure 21.8).

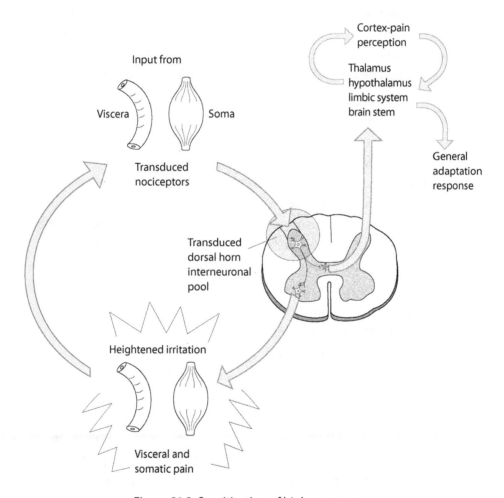

Figure 21.8. Sensitization of higher centers.

Higher-Level Facilitation

We can now understand facilitation in the higher processing centers more specifically as incoming nociceptive input converge on a number of important interrelated
nuclei. The nucleus paragigantocellularius (PGi) is a bilateral nucleus in the brain
stem with multiple afferent and efferent connections, including connections with
stress-related nuclei. It receives input from both visceral and somatic nociceptors,
the hypothalamus, the amygdala, the nucleus and tract of solitarius, and other
sources. It has important connections both to the sympathetic chain and to the
locus ceruleus. It receives direct visceral and somatic nociceptive input from the
dorsal horn interneuronal pool via secondary nerves. It also receives input from the
nucleus and tract of solitarius, the major nuclei in the brain stem receiving visceral
input from below. It is thus in an excellent position to monitor both visceral and
somatic inputs coming from the whole body. It becomes a real switch point for
autonomic activation and the general adaptation response.

The PGi has efferent connections to the amygdala, the sympathetic chain, and
to the locus ceruleus. Chronic ongoing nociceptive input to the PGi can set off the
general adaptation response via these connections. It can generate sympathetic
arousal and the release, via the locus ceruleus, of norepinephrine, placing the system in active-alert and signaling the hypothalamus to release CRH to activate the
H-P-A axis. The sympathetic stress response cascades, muscles tense for action,
epinephrine (adrenaline) is released into the system, and the person is now on a
mobilization road for no external reason, as the fight-or-flight response is generated
by internal danger signals mediated by facilitated nociceptive input.

This can be confusing for the practitioner and crazy-making for the client, who
feels aroused, tense, and anxious without any obvious reason. Symptoms can shift
around the body, and both practitioner and client need to be patient and resourced
to meet what is sometimes an onslaught of seemingly disconnected symptoms of
hyperarousal, visceral and somatic pain, and dysfunction. Here is an instance where
Sutherland's admonition to "trust the tide" is especially relevant.

Importantly, nociceptive input also travels directly to the hypothalamus via the
spinohypothalamic tract (Willard and Patterson 1994). This is a relatively newly
discovered tract that is diffused through the spinal cord, where incoming information does not have to first go to the thalamus on its way to the hypothalamus. It is
a direct, fast tract route through which danger signals can reach the hypothalamus
for immediate processing. As this fast route engages, the stress response may be
activated as direct, facilitated nociceptive input alerts the hypothalamus to internal

danger and signals the sympathetics and the locus ceruleus to place the system in active-alert and mobilization.

The amygdala also receives nociceptive input from below, further complicating the situation. Nociceptive input arrives at the amygdala via the PGi and other brain stem nuclei and causes the amygdala to set off the stress response. The amygdala can thus respond directly to internal danger in much the same way that it responds to external danger. High cortisol levels may also be cycling due to the heightened H-P-A axis, keeping the amygdala in its stress response. (Figure 21.9).

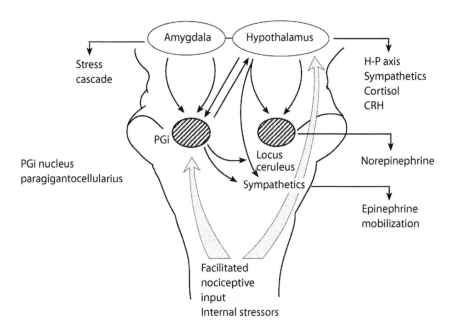

Figure 21.9. Facilitation of higher centers driven by sensitized input from below.

Explorations

The following explorations are meant to give a clear sense of internal stress response relationships; they are not intended to be treatment protocols. Once you have the knowledge, let the treatment plan unfold and respond appropriately to the conditions present. I have had good success with this approach in peripheral joint dysfunction and pain, and in visceral issues.

Let's assume that a client comes to see you with ongoing chronic pain, anxiety, and exhaustion. Pain shifts around the body, and there has been no clear diagnosis offered from either orthodox or complementary sources. I have encountered this scenario many times—haven't you?

The first thing to do is to form a supportive relationship with a person who may be oversensitized and in chronic pain and who may have lost hope in the situation. A relational field must be generated within which the client begins to feel resourced and held in his or her pain. This is a humbling experience for both client and practitioner. Promising results at this point would be foolhardy and unethical, but I do promise, however, to embark on a mutual journey that may help the client's situation. I can usually say from past experience that the work has helped in similar conditions, but sessions are presented as exploratory and open. From my experience, it can take anywhere from six to ten sessions to get through to a person's system at a level deeper than the physiology and pain that is cycling. My intention generally is to help initiate resources in the client's system, to access primary respiration, and to resource him or her in the session process. Resourcing the client, the holistic shift, states of balance, orienting to Long Tide and Dynamic Stillness, and holding a wide and open perceptual field are all important.

As sessions continue, the potency will move to process the stress responses cycling in the system. When potency begins to become available in a client's system, particular fulcrums will be highlighted and particular stress patterns will come to the forefront. Activation may occur, and related inertial and traumatic forces and patterns will clarify. Again, you must have the sensitivity to orient to all of this and to relate appropriately to the activation present. The following explorations break down the treatment process into stages for learning purposes. In real clinical situations, these will merge in organic ways as the inherent treatment plan unfolds.

Facilitation Stages One and Two:
The Sensitizing Soup and Peripheral Nerve Facilitation _____

In this exploration, we are working with peripheral fulcrums that can generate chronic nociceptive signals and nerve sensitization. Our focus is on somatic (muscular) or visceral (organ) fulcrums, to lower hypertonis of the peripheral nociceptors and help to reset the CNS. Here we will relate the peripheral area to its related spinal segments. In this exploration you will choose a particular joint or organ peripheral issue and will relate it to the appropriate spinal cord level.

Start as usual, first standing by the side of the table, orienting to primary respiration both in your own system and the client's. Then move to the foot of the table and negotiate contact at the client's feet. When your relational field has settled, choose one fulcrum of either visceral or somatic origin and place both hands there. For the sake of this clinical exercise, this may be a current issue, or something that your client knows is an issue from past history. This might be a somatic tissue area, such as a joint or connective tissue relationship, or a visceral structure such as the liver, pancreas, or kidney.

Settle into your orientation to the area in question, maintaining a wide perceptual awareness of the three bodies (physical, fluid, and tidal bodies). Sense that the local physical area—perhaps a joint—is literally suspended in the fluid and tidal bodies. Orient to mid-tide in a wider perceptual framework. As you relate to this particular area, such as a knee or hip joint, you may encounter the sensitizing soup discussed above for Stage One. This may have an activated quality with fluid perturbation and electric-like pulsations and discharge.

As you orient to the area in the phases of primary respiration, an inertial fulcrum and pattern may clarify. Listen for Becker's three-phase awareness, a deepening state of balance, the action of potency in the local area, and for resolution and reorganization and reorientation to midline.

Now connect that area to the related area of the spinal cord. Keep one hand on the peripheral area (organ, joint, etc.) and move your other hand to the spinal cord and dorsal horn area that relates to the somatic or visceral relationship. The general guide for finding the spinal cord area is based on embryology and spinal nerve pathways. For lower limbs and areas below the diaphragm, place your upper hand under T11–L2. For the upper limbs and areas above the diaphragm, orient to the C7–T4 area. When the matching spinal cord area is contacted it may seem to "light up" with a pulsatory recognition or felt-sense of energetic connectedness. The spinal contact spans multiple vertebrae, as the sensitized nerve or nerves involved communicate with a wider interneuronal pool in the spinal cord, and not just with narrow horizontal bands or single facilitated segments.

Holding both the spinal segment area (orienting to its dorsal horn) and the peripheral fulcrum, again orient to primary respiration and a mutual state of balance. When the interrelationships are fully accessed, you may perceive the whole sensorimotor loop clarify and, as the state of balance deepens, a resonant pulsation may be sensed at each contact. Listen for any release of neural charge such as the peripheral nerve or related sympathetic nerves discharging their cycling energies. This indicates that the sensitized peripheral nerve is clearing its facilitation. Wait for a settling of all of this into stillness. Listen for a reorganization and realignment of the tissue field from the spinal segment to the peripheral area. See how these tissues now orient to the primal midline.

In the explorations below, you will follow the above work by orienting to other levels of facilitation, including brain stem and mid-brain issues. As seen in our descriptions above, dorsal horn neurons can transduce and become hypersensitized. Although this facilitation may have been resolved, the different levels of facilitation can also be oriented to and followed through in session work. In the next exploration, you will first orient to the local spinal cord-dorsal horn area, and then to its relationship with the brain stem. This can all be oriented to as a continuation of the session work described in this exploration.

Facilitation Stage Three: Dorsal Horn Facilitation and Brain Stem Nuclei

After the work with the local peripheral area and related spinal cord level settles and completes, change your hand position to hold the dorsal horn area more specifically. Place your caudal hand under this area with the client's spine in the center of your hand as you comfortably spread your fingers. Let your hand relax and imagine it is settling under the treatment table. In a wide perceptual field, orient to the dorsal horn area of the spinal cord that relates to the nociceptive loop that you have just worked with. Again sense this local area to be suspended in the wider physical and fluid bodies, and orient to primary respiration and mid-tide.

Wait for the system to settle and deepen into equilibrium or balance, and for action of potency to be expressed in the dorsal horn area. Notice any discharge of neural energy and allow this to dissipate and resolve. It is common to sense a discharge or clearing from the dorsal horn area and some kind of change in its local dynamic when its facilitation-hypersensitization has been resolved. You may sense easier local motility, softening and reorganization of vertebral relationships, better fluid motion, and a down-regulation of the charge that seemed to be cycling from that area.

Once you sense a clearing from the dorsal horn area, place your other hand under the occiput and also orient to the brain stem area. Holding both the dorsal horn area and the brain stem in your awareness, again wait for the system to enter equilibrium and the state of balance to deepen. Again be aware of any neural clearing and dissipation of the facilitation. You may sense electric-like clearing or fluid perturbations. Commonly, when the state of balance has deepened, the two areas will then express a resonant and synchronous pulsation of potency and energy. Stillpoints facilitated from the sacrum or occiput may also help to restore equilibrium to dorsal horn cells. Becker wrote that repeated stillpoints can process the "memory traces" in the spinal cord (Becker 1997).

Stage Four: Brain Stem Nuclei

As we have seen, the brain stem is a major focus for sensorimotor processing, and for the body's protective responses. Its nuclei are switch points for information and responses to stress and traumatic situations. There are neural connections from below bringing information about visceral and somatic homeostasis to its nuclei, and from the hypothalamus and amygdala above. The brain stem then responds to this input as part of the stress cascade and the fight-or-flight response.

In this exploration we continue our orientation to levels of facilitation in the system by changing our hold and orienting to the brain stem via the occipital cradle hold. As the session progresses, again be aware of any electric-like discharge and resolution of neural energies from brain stem nuclei.

From the holds described above (one hand at the dorsal horn area and the other under the occiput-brain stem), move to the occipital cradle hold. In the occipital cradle, orient to the client's wider biosphere and again allow-sense your hands to be suspended in fluid with you and your client suspended in a wider fluid field. Imagine-sense that the client's brain is suspended in the fluid body, which is, in turn, suspended in the tidal body of the Long Tide. Orient to the fluid tide and then include the ventricle system and the motility of the brain and brain stem in your awareness. In inhalation, the brain stem may be sensed to rise toward the lamina terminalis and slightly widen. Follow this in the cycles of surge and settling in primary respiration.

As you orient to this, see if a fulcrum or inertial pattern clarifies. Orient to the state of balance and a deepening equilibrium in the system as a whole. As areas of hypersensitization in brain stem nuclei clarify, you may sense a palpable electric-like "buzz" or "hum" as the neural energies involved in the facilitated nuclei begin to clear. As these forces resolve you may also sense a streaming of electric-like discharges, perturbations in fluids, and/or tissue trembling and shaking. Allow these to occur and resolve; do not rush the process. Listen for the expression of potency as forces are processed. Remember that it is the potency that is doing the work, not your machinations. Wait for reorganization of tissues, fluids, and potency.

As clients' process unfolds, their traumatic cycling of the various stages of the stress response may also be expressed. This may manifest in emotional processes, freezing or immobilized states, and in dissociative states. In these cases, the use of appropriate verbal and cranial skills is essential.

Continuing Stage Four: The Brain Stem-Limbic-Hypothalamus-Adrenal Axis

In this exploration, you continue to orient to higher centers from the occipital cradle by including the brain stem-limbic axis and brain stem-hypothalamus-pituitary-adrenal axis in your field of awareness.

From the occipital cradle hold, move to the Sutherland vault hold, maintaining your wide perceptual field (holding the physical, fluid, and tidal bodies in awareness) and including the brain stem, the floor of the third ventricle (for the hypothalamus), and the floor of the lateral ventricle (for the hippocampus and amygdala) in your local orientation. Again, imagine-sense that the brain and its ventricles are suspended in the wider fluid and tidal bodies. Allow yourself to deepen into this wider orientation and visualize-sense this brain stem-limbic-hypothalamus axis, reviewing anatomy as needed. See what clarifies in the phases of the fluid tide and primary respiration.

Note any inertial fulcrums, patterns, and areas of facilitation that clarify. As a particular area clarifies for healing purposes, you may again sense electric-like discharges from the nuclei involved. For instance, you may sense the motility of the ventricles and brain begin to organize around the right amygdala as a healing process orients to clearing its sensitization.

Deepen into the state of balance and the wider equilibrium that emerges until a deeper stillness is sensed. Again, you may sense neural energy discharging as this occurs. This may take the form of a local discharge from particular nuclei, or a sympathetic nervous system clearing sensed as electric-like clearing down the spine and out the client's arms and legs. The client may become aware of this clearing as a sense of tingling and warmth in the extremities. Deepen into the stillness as this unfolds and see what healing processes continue to emerge. Complete with some integrative holds such as a sacral-occipital or sacral-ethmoid hold.

The Knee as an Example

Let's look at these stages in the context of a single session. To illustrate this intention, let's imagine that a client injured the knee playing football, and it has not resolved. After a few sessions, you sense the system organizing around the affected knee joint and that it is an organizing site for segmental and dorsal horn facilitation in the spinal cord.

Start as usual at the side of the treatment table and orient to primary respiration in yourself and in relationship to the client's system. Move to the feet and orient to the settling of the relational field and the deepening of the holistic shift. Then move to the knee in question. Hold the knee with both hands in any comfortable position that allows you to orient to its dynamics. Maintaining a wide perceptual field, again imagine-sense that the physical body is suspended in the fluid body, which is, in turn, suspended in the tidal body or the Long Tide.

Again also sense-imagine that your hands are suspended in fluid and you and your client are suspended in a wider fluid field. In the phases of primary respiration, orient to whatever inertial fulcrum or pattern clarifies. Deepen into the state of balance and equilibrium in the forces at work in the local area and body as a whole. As the state of balance deepens, orient to the stillness that clarifies. In the stillness, you may sense the processing of the sensitization in the area. Again, there may be electric-like discharges from nerve endings and fluid fluctuations as the potency acts in the state of balance to increase circulation and clear the sensitizing soup that may be present. Wait for a sense of settling and realignment to the midline.

When you sense a local resolution, connect the knee to the related dorsal horn-spinal cord level. One hand stays under or over the knee, and the other hand moves under the spinal cord at T11–L2. Orient to the whole fluid-tissue field as you hold both poles of the sensorimotor nerve loop. Orient to any fulcrum or pattern that clarifies and for a settling into a state of balance. As this deepens, and the potency begins to manifest in the facilitated sensorimotor circuit, you may sense a synchronous pulsation of potency at each contact. Be aware of the processing of neural cycling and the discharge of neural energy through the relationships being held. You may literally sense the whole sensitized nerve loop clearing.

If you sense that the facilitation extends to the higher centers, proceed up the body as above. One hand is placed under the spinal cord at T11–L2 while the other holds the occiput and brain stem area, again orienting to a deepening state of balance, a mutual expression of potency at both poles of the relationship, and for any neural clearing that occurs. Finally, moving to the head, use the occipital cradle and/or vault hold to orient to the higher centers as described above.

In all of these relationships and intentions, let the inherent treatment plan guide your sequence and pacing. You may feel called to repeat one step or omit a step, or to cycle back and forth between two hand positions.

CHAPTER 22

Trauma Resolution and Verbal Skills

The sections in this chapter outline important verbal skills that can, along with biodynamic session work, help resolve traumatic cycling in the nervous system. Helping your clients orient to felt-sensation and feeling-tones can empower them to moderate their own stress states as they learn mindfulness practices that engage the prefrontal cortex and present-time awareness. The first sections here orient to the nature of mindfulness practice as an important aspect of trauma resolution and healing. We will also orient to specific verbal skills that help down-regulate hyper- and hypoarousal states and help clients in dissociative states to re-embody.

Mindfulness-Based Verbal Skills for Trauma Resolution

Mindfulness is an ancient form of healing practice that was first brought into the world via the teachings of the Gautama Buddha, more than 2,500 years ago. It has become very much part of health systems, with much research into its effective use in healing trauma and down-regulating the stress response, and in the alleviation of suffering caused by overly defended self-systems, such as borderline personality disorder. Mindfulness-based stress reduction and mindfulness-based cognitive therapy are two forms commonly found in health systems and psychology trainings today.

Simply put, the Buddha stressed that present-time awareness of body and sensations, feeling states, states of mind and consciousness, and one's cognitive formations alleviate suffering. With growing mindfulness practice, the meditator learns to differentiate what interior states and interpersonal ways of being lead to continued suffering as opposed to greater ease and freedom in one's life. In terms of nervous system processing, present-time sensory awareness orients the client's system to the prefrontal cortex and social nervous system, and helps down-regulate the stress response. Mindfulness practice, over time, shifts the system from survival modes to greater ease and homeostasis.

The heart of mindfulness practice is derived from a discourse of the Buddha, the *Satipatthāna Sutta*—the Foundations of Mindfulness. The core of this meditative process is the state of *sati*, or presence. The Buddha, in the early discourses, used the term sati in a number of ways. Its Sanskrit root, *smrti*, has the connotation of recalling or remembering that is, at its depth, the recalling of a deeper truth and a remembering to be present in the here and now. The practitioner learns to rest in the truth of the present moment and orients to the client from this perspective. Likewise, the practitioner helps the client develop a mindful sensory orientation to inner states and relational processes. Sati, usually translated as mindfulness, has many nuances in meaning. In the widest sense, sati is a state of inclusive presence, a spacious state of wakefulness that allows a person to consciously hold the whole of an arising process and all of its particulars in awareness.

The Buddha gives clear instructions in the Satipatthāna Sutta as to the nature of sati and its prudent use in awareness and healing practice. The initial perceptual moment of object-orientation is also a moment of knowing. Each and every moment of perception has awareness enfolded within it. As the inquirer settles into a state of presence and develops witness consciousness, awareness expands to hold the whole of the present moment.

A common starting point in this process of inquiry is awareness of the body, with an orientation to breath, feeling-tone, and sensation. As awareness is brought to the arising of feeling-tone and the changing nature of sensation, the cycling of stress states are held in a wider perceptual field. This is then expanded to include all forms that arise in the field of awareness, body states, feeling-tones, emotions, sensations, cognitive processes, thoughts, qualities, and states of mind, along with the tonal quality of mind-body as a feeling form. This intention again brings the client into the prefrontal cortex and social nervous system, encouraging a down-regulation of defended states and the cycling of the stress response.

In session work, this kind of awareness can be actively encouraged as the practitioner orients the client to an awareness of inner states, feelings, intentionality, and emergent process as an embodied experience. A simple request by the practitioner, when appropriate, to notice what is emerging in present-time, to talk *from* the client's present-time embodied experience, rather than about it, initiates a witness consciousness that can hold activation without totally identifying with it or becoming it.

The Buddha, in the Foundations of Mindfulness, also encouraged the meditator to bring awareness to an arising process inwardly, outwardly, and as a whole. One is advised not just to be mindful of an arising internal process, be it a sensation, feeling-tone, thought, or state of consciousness, but also its *relationship* to the external world and relational interchange and, even more important, to sense the interrelated flux of experience as a whole. Thus mindfulness practice is eminently relational in nature. This fact is sometimes overlooked in mindfulness training, but is key to its use and usefulness in clinical practice.

The Buddha further encouraged inquirers to be aware of their inner processes by truly being *in* the process. For instance, he encouraged the meditator to be aware of the "body *in* the body," "the feeling *in* the feeling," or "the mind-state *in* the mind-state"—in other words, to be aware of inner processes in a nondissociative state (Nyānasatta 1979), The Buddha stressed that this kind of holistic nondissociative awareness can begin to open the intransigent cycling of suffering. These astounding insights into human nature and the possibility of true freedom were described more than 2,500 years ago!

The Foundations of Mindfulness also includes clear instructions as to what states and conditions lead to ease and the reduction of suffering, such as clear intention, energy, mindfulness, and so on, and what leads to further entanglement, such as sloth and torpor, confusion, automatic behavior, and attachment to the ego-system. Part of the meditative process was to be able to wisely discern between these states and conditions. In this vein, as awareness is brought to an arising process, two important qualities emerge: *sampajāna*, clear comprehension, and *yoniso manasikāra*, wise discernment. In a clinical context these qualities are of supreme importance. As session work unfolds over time, both practitioner and client learn to clearly comprehend and wisely discern the nature of the client's suffering and its dynamics. Over time, the practitioner learns to clearly comprehend the nature of the client's process and relational tendencies and to wisely discern what is helpful and what leads to further entanglement. This is then the ground for appropriate clinical responses to these conditions.

The Development of Practitioner Presence

A huge number of contemplative practices both encourage therapeutic presence and help anchor or ground the practitioner in the relational field. Formal training in presence and awareness practice is very helpful in training situations. It is not enough to simply ask someone to be present. Although presence is innate, due to the weight of our history and conditioning, our ability to enter a state of presence can be problematic and the capacity to be present must be developed and refined.

The first step in the practice of presence is to become aware of oneself. This may seem obvious, but how many of us really take the time to become aware of our innermost processes and their outer manifestations? This entails the development of a personal mindfulness practice—the ability to simply *be* with whatever is arising in terms of self-process, feeling-tone, thoughts, tendencies, and so on. Remembering the Foundations of Mindfulness, the practitioner senses the arising of his or her process inwardly, outwardly, and as a whole. This is, again, a process of awareness that includes self-other interchange, whose development can have huge repercussions in everyday life. The development of presence is largely about learning what gets in the way of simply being, our innate ability to be still and know. The following section is a contemplative exercise that may help to develop a simple state of presence. It is from this state that the practitioner learns to hold the client and the arising process in a wide and holistic listening field.

Exploration:
Contemplative Exercise _____

In this exploration, we use the natural motion and sensation of breathing to develop the ability to settle into a being-state. The breath is always present and is a useful reference point from which to explore one's ability to simply be present. In the tradition of Tibetan Buddhism, there is a saying that if one really "lives in the breath," insight and a serene life will ensue. We then orient to a felt-sensory awareness of our inner state.

Phase one: As you sit comfortably erect, orient to the sensations in your body and simply become aware of your breathing. Rest your awareness in the movement of your breath and the sensations in your body as you inhale and exhale. This first step creates an anchor for your awareness and attention. As you do this, notice the quality of your breath. Is it easier to inhale or exhale? Is one breathing phase fuller than the other? As you inhale, how far into your body can your attention go? Can you inhale and allow your attention to follow the movement of your breath right down into your pelvis? Are there areas of your body that are not available to your attention?

Phase two: Once you find that your awareness is fairly settled in breath, and your mind is relatively still, follow your breath into the body one more time, let it go on in its natural expression, and then shift your awareness to the general quality of sensations and feelings in your body. Simply rest in your body-space and orient to the quality of the sensations within it. Are there any areas of pain or distress, or of ease and OK-ness? Are there any emotional tones or feelings?

Phase three: Once your awareness can spaciously rest in sensation and allow its movements and qualities to simply be, let go of your orientation to sensation and see if you can simply sit with a spacious awareness of *anything* that arises in your perceptual field. As you orient to this, hold the *whole* of yourself in your field of awareness and extend your perceptual field to include your body and the local field around it.

You may notice feeling-tones, thoughts, images, sounds, and so on. Can you have an open relationship to these? Can you notice whatever arises and let it pass away? Can you not get caught up in it? Can you be like a vast sky of awareness and let whatever arises in your field of perception pass like clouds moving through? This has the felt-quality of holding a wide and soft field of awareness oriented to your body-space and local field, allowing whatever arises and passes to simply be.

Soften your attention and see if your mind settles into a simple space of listening. It may seem as though your mind settles into a state of balance, neither coming nor going, simply receiving. There is nothing you can *do* to make this happen. It is about allowing and letting go. What do you notice? Does your mind still? Is there more clarity?

If you find that your mind becomes caught up in thinking, or images, or feelings, simply notice that and return to the breath to settle your awareness. Then once again see if you can simply be aware first of sensation and feeling-tone, and then of whatever arises in your larger field of perception. Once again soften and widen your listening and see if your mind settles naturally into a still and receptive state. Do this exercise a number of times a day. Let the potential for inner awareness and space become part of your life. The intention is, in a soft and wide state of presence, to allow whatever emerges in your field of awareness to simply be, to not get caught up in cyclical thinking, images, fantasy, projections into the future, or memories, but rather to be able to attend to anything in the present moment that arises and passes in your perceptual field. Over time, this practice helps the mind to settle into a natural state of stillness and presence, and it is from this settled state of mind that the practitioner learns to orient to the client and the process.

Phase four: Incorporate the above practices directly into session work. Extend a wide perceptual field, settle into the state of presence outlined above, and then hold the client and the arising process in the same quality of awareness that you have been developing relative to your own. Now both the inner states and the client's unfolding process can be held in the wider state of sati, or presence, fulfilling the Satipatthāna Sutta's admonition to hold awareness of the arising process both inwardly and outwardly as a whole.

Orienting a Client to Mindful Inquiry

Let's bring the mindfulness phases explored above more directly into session work. These can help a client mindfully explore an arising process, and will aid in the down-regulation of the stress response. Clients can also be encouraged to practice these mindfulness exercises at home in order to help ameliorate or moderate their activation and experience of suffering, along with appropriate resourcing and trauma skills building. As above, these comprise various stages of practice, including breath awareness, awareness of sensation and feeling states, and a more open awareness of sensation, feelings, cognitive forms, emotional states, and behavior.

In terms of brain physiology, when clients settle into a state of presence oriented to sensory awareness, they are entering the territory of the medial prefrontal cortex. As we have seen, this area of the brain mediates present-time experience and has connections to all major brain centers. As one comes into present-time awareness and orients to sensations and sensory experiences, the prefrontal cortex tells the rest of the brain that there is no "tiger" out there and levels of the stress response and cycling depressive and anxiety states then also have the potential for down-regulation as a shift to more fluid homeostasis takes place over time. Likewise, when this occurs in a resourced and safe holding environment, the presence of a receptive and reflective other also helps engage the social nervous system, which, concurrent with the basic sate of presence, further helps to down-regulate states of autonomic activation.

Explorations: Basic Mindfulness Practices _____

Phase One: Breath

Encourage the client to sit comfortably erect. First bring the awareness to the sitting position and the sensations present and see if he or she can rest in the sitting position. Help orient the client to felt-resources if needed or appropriate. Then suggest simply becoming aware of the breathing. Suggest that the client rest the awareness in the movement of the breath.

When the client's mind becomes distracted or busy, encourage him or her to gently acknowledge that and return to resting in breath sensation.

Verbal suggestions to the client:

"See if you can rest your awareness in the movement of your breath and the sensations in your body as you inhale and exhale."

"Be aware of the experience of breathing in and out—notice the feelings and sensations in your body as they come into your awareness."

"If your mind becomes distracted by thoughts, feelings, memories, then gently acknowledge this and return to simply following the sensations of breathing in and out and/or resting in your breath."

These first steps help create an anchor for client awareness and attention.

Further related suggestions for inquiry:

"As you do this, notice the quality of your breath. Is it easier to inhale or exhale? Is one phase fuller than the other? As you inhale, how far into your body can your attention go? Can you inhale and allow your attention to follow the movement of your breath right down into your pelvis? Are there areas of your body that are not available to your attention?"

Phase Two: Sensation

Here, the intention is to help shift the client's orientation to the sensations and feeling-tones in the body—to bring an embodied awareness to the arising and passing of the sensations and feeling-tones present. In terms of brain physiology, it helps the client to deepen into present-time sensory awareness in the medial prefrontal cortex, helps down-regulate stress responses and states of anxiety and depression, and has the potential to create space in defensive personality tendencies.

Once you find that your client's awareness is fairly settled in breath, have him or her follow the breath into the body one more time, and suggest letting it go on in its natural expression. Have the client shift the awareness to a more open awareness of *sensation* in the body. Suggest that he or she place awareness in the body-space and orient to the quality of the sensations within it. Again, when the client's mind becomes distracted or busy, encourage him or her to gently acknowledge that and return to resting in breath and then to sensation.

Verbal suggestions to the client:

"We are going to orient to a more open exploration of the sensations and feelings present in your body. This will help you generate some space around what is uncomfortable or difficult, and to also develop sensations and feeling-tones that are more resourced and supportive."

"Follow your breath into your body one more time, and this time let go of your breath and keep your awareness in your body and its sensations."

"Bring awareness to the sensations and feelings present."

Further inquiries:

"Are there any areas of pain or distress, or of ease and OK-ness? Are there any emotional tones or feelings?"

"What sensations are associated with those feelings?"

"What is most prominent for you just now?"

Phase Three: Open Awareness

Once the client's awareness can spaciously rest in sensations, suggest that he or she let go of the orientation solely to sensations and widen the inquiry to whatever is present in his or her field of awareness. You might suggest that, while resting in the embodied awareness developed above, the client simply sit with a spacious awareness of *anything* that arises in the perceptual field. As the client orients to this, suggest that he or she hold the *whole* of him- or herself in the field of awareness, extending the field of awareness to include the body and the local field around it.

This fulfills the wider Foundations of Mindfulness as it now includes states, qualities, and content of consciousness and mind. This might embrace awareness of arising thoughts, repetitive thinking, images, dreams, and memories. As these arise in awareness, the intention is always then to orient to the embodied feeling-tone of what is present, or the felt-sense of the arising thought, image, or memory. That allows a more embodied inquiry and helps uncouple and create space in the thoughts, feelings, images, memories, and behaviors generated by traumatic experience. In terms of brain function, it brings the present-time awareness mediated by the prefrontal cortex into relationship to any aspect of an arising process with the psycho-neurological potential of down-regulation and a return to more homeostatic functioning.

Verbal suggestions to the client:

"As you settle your awareness into your body, notice any sensations, feelings, feeling-qualities, thoughts, images, or sounds present. Can you hold these in awareness? What is most prominent for you?"

"Can you notice whatever arises in your awareness and let it pass away? Can you not get caught up in what emerges?" (This has the felt-quality of holding a wide and soft field of awareness oriented to the body-space and local field, allowing whatever arises and passes to simply be.)

"Can you soften your attention and see if your mind settles into a simple space of listening?"

These same suggestions can be transferred to the treatment table as difficult feelings or sensations arise. For instance, if unpleasant feelings emerge, orient the client to the breath and then ask him or her to describe the sensations present. If a strong emotion arises, again have the client orient to the breath and describe the sensations coupled with the emotional process. For instance, if sadness emerges, you might ask, "Where do you sense the sadness in your body?" or "What sensations tell you that's sadness?" or "What sensations are present in that area where you feel sad?" These help the client shift from a cycling of the emotional state to inquiry and possible resolution and completion.

In more general table work, orienting clients to an awareness of sensation and feeling-tone can support a deeper exploration into their arising process. This is especially important when strong emotions or traumatic activation emerges. We explore this emotional territory more fully in the following sections.

Working with Traumatic Activation: The Zone of Resource

As we further explore verbal skills useful in clinical work, it is important for the clinician to be able to orient to the client's arising state, and to know what territories these are in (hyperarousal, hypoarousal, dissociation, and so on). Peter Levine outlines a straightforward framework for appropriately orienting to traumatic activation, illustrated in Figure 22.1. The illustration relates states of hyper- or hypoarousal to a resourced zone where clients can safely process their activation. Levine calls this zone the *zone of activation*, or the *warble zone*. I call it the *zone of resourced resolution,* or more briefly the *resourced zone*. It is a therapeutic space within which a client is resourced and has the opportunity to process and complete arising states of autonomic activation in present time. In this zone, the client can discharge trauma-bound energies and complete frozen defensive intentions, without the danger of retraumatization or entering dissociative states. If the client moves out of the resourced zone, he or she may discharge too rapidly and move into either hyperarousal states of emotional flooding and speeding up of process or hypoarousal states of immobilization, freezing, and numbness. The two poles of *overwhelm* outside the resourced zone are, therefore: (1) hyperarousal, in which the cycling fight-or-flight energies are rapidly expressed, and (2) hypoarousal states, in which the frozen and immobilized energy is experienced as stuckness, numbness, coldness, lack of sensation, and even as paralysis. Dissociation is commonly coupled with these states (Levine 1997, 2010).

Within the scope of either pole—hyperarousal or hypoarousal—powerful experiences of terror, fear, anger, rage, and anxiety may arise. In hyperarousal states the client may experience emotional flooding, rapid speeding up of process, physical states of trembling or shaking, heat or cold, and sweating. These are all signs of autonomic nervous system discharge. In freezing states, the client may experience states of immobilization, stuckness, numbness, and coldness. Clients may lose contact with all or part of their body. This can be a scary and even terrifying experience. In both cases, they are being flooded with the effects of previous traumatic experience. Dissociative states are commonly coupled with these states, as dissociation is a most fundamental response to being overwhelmed by an experience. It is important to recognize when a client is accessing any of these states and what states above or below the resourced zone are being activated. These states are commonly misinterpreted as emotional catharsis and emotional healing (Figure 22.1).

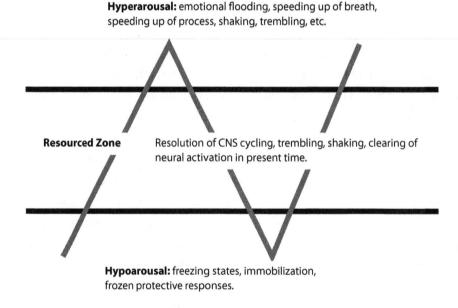

Figure 22.1. Zone of resourced resolution.

In the following sections, we explore mindfulness-based skills that relate more specifically to the arising of traumatic activation and overwhelming emotional states in session work. We orient to appropriate verbal skills that can help clients down-regulate emergent states of hyperarousal and emotional flooding, and states of hypoarousal, freezing, and dissociation. These interactive processes also help clients develop the important inner skills of presence and self-regulation.

Recognition, Acknowledgment, and Reassurance

When traumatic activation occurs in clinical sessions, the maintenance of a clear and receptive relational field is crucial. The practitioner's capacity to safely hold the arising process is a key relational resource that comes to the forefront in states of activation. Aspects of this include containment, acceptance, and reassurance. The practitioner's presence and appropriate interventions help clients contain the arising activation and stay in the resourced zone. The intention is to empower clients to hold and manage their own process.

Work in any therapy form is deeply relational in nature. When a client manifests states of activation and overwhelm, basic human needs are also always present. If we remember Lake's concepts of primal being and wellbeing needs, we will remember that the *basic needs of being* are also present throughout life. These are *recognition, acknowledgment,* and *unconditional acceptance.* These are also primary needs during the prenatal period and early childhood. When an infant and young child feels met at these levels by primary caregivers, a sense of basic trust is maintained, an inner sense of safety and security is experienced over time, and a continuity and cohesiveness of being are also experienced at the core of the developing self-system.

When clients enter a state of activation or overwhelm, one of the first steps is to meet these basic needs by speaking words of reassurance, recognition, acknowledgment, and acceptance. An initial verbal expression of acceptance and reassurance by the practitioner may be very important here. Clients may need to know that the practitioner is OK with the arising process and can hold the space for them. As clients manifest activation, the practitioner might use words like "There is something important arising here" or "Something important is emerging that is part of a healing or clearing process; let's see how to be with this." It is important that clients know that you unconditionally accept them as they are, and are willing and able to hold the space for healing to occur. It is also important to speak words of reassurance.

Likewise, clients may feel embarrassed by what is arising, be afraid of the feelings present, or concerned that the process may be overwhelming for the practitioner. Here clients may need to be reassured that their state is recognized, and that the practitioner can hold it and be with it. A simple reassurance that the process is an expression of a natural movement to health, that it is an attempt to resolve something from the past, and that the practitioner is OK with it and can be with it may be all clients need to hear. Sometimes clients' greatest fear is that their process is "too much" for the practitioner to hold, or will overwhelm the practitioner.

Speaking words like "I am familiar with this and can help you process it" can be very reassuring. The principles of recognition, acknowledgment, and unconditional acceptance move through our lives and are a basic ground for relational ease. We all seek to have these needs met in intimate relationships with friends, family, and partners. When they are met, and we sense ourselves to be received and seen at the level of our being, we can settle and "simply be" in the presence of another.

As we enter the territories in the following sections, it is important to remember the work presented in Volume One, where we described processes that help clients settle into a more resourced state, an essential starting point in session work. We will begin with a review of the importance of felt-resources and then continue with an exploration of dissociation and hyper- and hypoarousal states.

Summary of Initial Intentions

When traumatic hyperarousal or hypoarousal states arise:

- Help the client orient to resources

- Acknowledge that an important process is arising

- Reassure the client that you are present for what is arising and that it is OK to be with

- Reassure the client that it is a natural process with the potential for healing

- Maintain unconditional acceptance and appropriate response to the arising process

Helping Clients Access Felt-Resources

We discussed the importance of helping clients access a sense of felt-resource in Volume One, where we discussed practices and suggestions that help clients orient to and access a felt-sense of inner resource. This is crucially helpful when traumatic activation arises and is always a useful starting point in session work. If clients can access a sense of felt-resource as they settle onto your treatment table, then the relational field and holistic shift will more easily settle.

Accessing Resourced Sensations and Feeling-Tones

Help clients settle into an awareness of the body and sensations. Suggesting that they become aware of the breathing as in the mindfulness exercise above is a good starting point. Orient clients to the body and its feelings, floating a question like "In the midst of whatever is present for you, what tells you you're OK just now?" and "As you settle with that, notice the feeling-tones and sensations of that OK-ness, and try to find a few words that describe it."

Clients may describe sensations directly, or via metaphors and images that resonate with their experience of OK-ness. These words can become an important resource in oneself. In the midst of arising activation, like strong emotional states or overwhelming sensations, these words can be used to help remind clients of this resourced quality so that they can be with the state with more space and present-time awareness.

If it is not so easy to access a felt sense of OK-ness, we can extend this intention with the following process. Ask clients to imagine a person, place, activity, thing, or memory that they really like, which is totally resourcing to them. If it is a person, choose a person who truly represents a resource. The clients may find that relationships hold a lot of ambiguity and it may be better to use a place, an activity, resourcing memory, or an object the first time trying this exercise.

Have clients bring the image of this resource into the body. Then ask them to notice the quality of the feeling-tone and sensations that arise in the body while holding this image or memory in awareness. Questions like "Do you sense anything that tells you that you are OK?" and "Where in the body do you sense these?" or "What is the *felt sense* of this resource?" or "Are the sensations or feeling-tones familiar?" can be very helpful in this inquiry. When a felt-sense of resource is accessed, then the question "Again, can you find some words or phrases that describe them?" will help clients access the sense of resource later in session work. I might, as practitioner, remind clients of the word or image that connects them to the resource at times in the session. These can be used to access the sense of felt-resource when difficulty, stress, or emotional flooding is experienced during session work.

In a clinical setting, an awareness of resourced sensations can be a sanctuary. In times of overwhelming sensation and emotional tone, it is a godsend. Clients can learn to orient to resourced sensations and balance any overwhelming feelings and emotions that may arise in sessions. For instance, if a client experiences the arising of strong emotional processes, like a flooding of sadness, a perceptual shift to more resourced sensations can help contain, balance, and slow the process down. The client may then be able to stay with the arising emotions with more space and clarity. This can have extremely valuable clinical outcomes. Clients may be able to meet the shocked, frozen, and emotionally charged sensations with more space and some sense of control and containment.

Working with Dissociation

It is important that the practitioner is aware of the possibility of dissociative processes emerging in session work. Dissociation is a defensive response to overwhelming experience. As we introduced earlier, when the fight-or-flight response is thwarted, there is a parasympathetic and hormonal surge that generates dissociation and immobilization. This protects people from the overwhelming nature of the experience as they split off from arising sensations and feelings coupled to the trauma.

Dissociation may take many forms in the therapeutic setting. A client may manifest a dissociative personality, in which he or she may be hard to sense or meet in present time. There may be a sense of vacancy, as though no one is present and the person may seem distant, spacey, or disconnected from the present relationship. What the client shares or says may not be appropriate to present circumstances. The eyes may glaze over, or he or she may seem dreamy, far away, and easily distracted, or seem diffused in energies and attention. Likewise, the client may seem to live in a mental realm of thoughts and ideas, may tend to become lost in thought and mental processes, may be uncomfortable with feelings and sensations, may be overanalytical about his or her process and the process of others, and may be difficult to settle into a present-time orientation to feelings and sensations.

In dissociative processes it is common for a client to feel cold or contracted. Likewise, parts of the body may feel frozen, he or she may lose connection to a limb or area of the body, and may even experience what seems to be paralysis in a limb or limbs. These kinds of processes are all expressions of thwarted sympathetic nervous system fight-or-flight energies and must be negotiated in session work in appropriate ways.

A craniosacral practitioner may sense dissociative states arising in session work in a number of ways. As you orient to the system, you may sense a quality of "thinness" and lack of surge or depth in the fluid tide; likewise, you may lose orientation to the client's system and become unclear, dreamy, or disoriented as you resonate with the dissociative process. Alternatively, if anesthesia was coupled with the dissociative response, as may happen during the birth process or in surgery, you may sense a fog-like state emerging both perceptually and in the field around you.

You may also note other clues that orient you to the presence or emergence of a client's dissociation or dissociative processes. A traumatized client may have difficulty in being present and in orienting to current experience. He or she may seem disconnected, uncommunicative, and/or disoriented.

Let's begin to explore some useful responses to dissociative process as they may arise in sessions.

Containment

When strong activation arises it is important to help clients contain their process. Containment occurs via the quality of the practitioner's presence and by verbal reassurance and suggestions. If clients' process speeds up uncontrollably and manifests hyperarousal states, then it is initially important to help them slow things down. If clients are aware of present sensations and feeling-tones, and are resourced in present time, the resolution of shock affect in the system becomes more likely. The practitioner's role is to contain and support the process and to slow things down if clients become overwhelmed by their arising experience. We will look at specific hyperarousal skills in session work later in this chapter.

Helping Generate Present-Time Awareness and Initiate Inquiry

If dissociative states arise in a session, it is important to orient clients to present time as best as possible. This is to ensure that they are not lost in their dissociation or activation as though the trauma is happening again. The generation of present-time awareness is crucial; it is very much a factor of the practitioner's ability to maintain his or her presence and to encourage clients' own presence or ability to be in present time. It is most important to help clients stay in contact with their experience and in relationship to the practitioner. One way to do this is to maintain verbal contact with clients and to initiate an inquiry into what is being experienced. Try to get clients curious about their state. See if you can initiate an inquiry into the felt nature of the present experience.

If clients experience dissociation, one way of helping them come into the present is to initiate an inquiry into the dissociative state itself. The process of inquiry generates an inner witness who has a more spacious relationship to the arising experience. In physiological terms, it begins to orient a person to the prefrontal cortex and social nervous system. As dissociative processes emerge, questions like "Where do you sense yourself to be just now?" or "How far away are you?" or "Can you describe that foggy state?" or "What is the quality of that for you?" or "What is happening just now?" may help bring clients into relationship to the felt experience of their dissociation. Initiating an inquiry takes time and patience. It is an open process in which the practitioner must offer suggestions slowly in relationship to the nature of the dissociative state being experienced. It may take many sessions for clients to shift from dissociation to inquiry and present-time awareness of their felt-experience.

Once clients have some relationship to their present experience, it can be very useful to initiate an inquiry into the nature of the sensations and feeling-tones present in their body. Questions like "Can you sense that in your body?" or "What do you sense in your body right now?" or "Where do your sense that in your body just now?" or "What is prominent in your body right now?" can initiate a present-time inquiry into the felt nature of their experience. When people can begin to orient to their present sensations and feeling-tones, a re-associative process usually ensues.

Orienting to Resources

One intention of the practitioner is to help clients establish a felt-sense of resource in their body-mind experience. At the start of session work, help orient clients to the felt bodily sensation of these resources. Again, it is very helpful to orient clients to resourced sensations and feeling-tones in the midst of what may seem overwhelming. Questions like "What tells you that you are OK just now?" or "Can you remember an image or memory of something that is totally resourcing, totally OK, and as you do that, what sensations arise in your body?" may be helpful. Once clients learn what their dissociation feels like, and have a handle on the sensations that signal this state, they can explore dissociation in present time. They then may be able to start to connect to related sensations and feeling-tones and have a witness to the present nature of the experience. Doing this, they may begin to feel what it is like to be embodied, and then even dissociation itself can become a resource. For instance, if they sense that they are dissociating as a present-time felt experience, this can become a signal that "something important is happening." They can then skillfully choose not to dissociate, reorient to the present experience, and meet the current situation with more clarity. We present an exercise at the end of this chapter that helps clients work with the orienting response and can also aid in re-association and re-embodiment.

Summary of Therapeutic Intentions in Dissociation

When an emotional process arises, or a process speeds up, or frozen, numbed qualities arise, listen for dissociative states. Explore the dissociative state. In highly dissociative states it is important to offer contact by the quality of your presence and voice and to orient clients to present time as a process of inquiry.

Questions like the following can be useful entry points into inquiry:
"Where are you right now?"

"Where are you viewing from?"

"How far away are you?"

"What is the quality of that?" or "Can you describe the imagery/feelings/sensations/sense of ... for that state?"

"Can you describe sensations or feeling-tones in the body from where you are?"

Explore the feeling-sense, imagery, and so on of the dissociative state. Can the client find the way back into contact with the sensations, body, or feeling-tones? Can he or she find the way into *contact* with you in present time?

Hyperarousal States

As we have seen, traumatic activations may take the form of hyperarousal states. These are sympathetic nervous system states in which clients' process speeds up in an overwhelming fashion. Clients may manifest various kinds of activation. Their breathing may speed up or intensify, or their body may tremble and shake. They may become very hot or very cold or alternate in these sensations. They may sweat, their skin tone or color may change, and their eyes may alternately dilate and contract. Emotions may flood the system and they may experience a whole range of affect from fear and terror, to anger and rage. They will commonly experience dissociation along with these processes and may be difficult to contact or may have difficultly orienting to you in present time.

Pacing and Slowing Things Down

In states of hyperarousal it is important to slow the process down—help clients reconnect to their resources and lower the hypertonis of the system so that they settle into the resourced zone. Containment and appropriate pacing is essential. Helping clients settle into present time is essential. Simple verbal contact and the initiation of inquiry is the ground of this intention. If emotional flooding arises, clients may totally identify with the state and will then be carried away by the flood and will lose sense of present time. As far as their nervous system is concerned, they are having a new trauma. Levine cautions practitioners to be aware of the potential for retraumatization in these circumstances (Levine 2010).

Slowing the process down is not about stopping the process, but appropriately pacing its arising and containing it in resources and grounding. Phrases like "Can you be with this?" may help clients sense both the nature of their state and orient to their resources. Words like "Can you let that wave pass through?" can help give clients a sense that the process is not endless, that it can move on, and they are not stuck in it. One way to help slow the process down is to suggest to clients that they slow their breath down; words like "Can you take a deep breath with that?" are helpful. Basically, you are trying to help clients pace their experience in a way that it becomes manageable and the potential for resolution and completion comes to the forefront.

Orienting to Resources

As introduced in sections above, once the hyperarousal process has slowed down and been contained, it is important to reorient clients to their resources. Orient clients to sensations and feeling-tones, floating a question like "What tells you, in the midst of this, that you are OK?" You can also use images and memories that are totally resourcing, as described earlier, such as "Are there any memories, places, images, things, or activities that are totally resourcing to you? Can you bring that into your body and become aware of the sensations and feeling-tones that relate to that resource?" Beginning an inquiry helps to establish a witness consciousness and is the starting point in the healing process.

Hyperarousal and Emotional Flooding

During clinical sessions, activation in the form of emotional flooding is not uncommon. If emotional flooding arises, it is important to slow things down, help establish present-time awareness, and initiate an inquiry. As introduced above, one way to slow down emotional flooding is to suggest that clients take a deeper breath and, as they do this, slow their breath. As they start to do this, you can then help them come into present-time awareness of the emotional state by starting an inquiry.

One way to begin a process of inquiry is to ask clients where they sense the emotional state in their body. Phrases like "Where do you sense that (naming the particular emotion they are experiencing) in your body?" can initiate an inquiry into the state, helps generate a present-time orientation to sensory awareness, enlists their curiosity, and may begin to ground them in present time. Help clients orient to that area of the body and then have them shift their attention to sensations and feeling-tones by using such phrases as "What sensations tell you that is … (naming the emotion they are experiencing)?"

For instance, if sadness is emerging, you might ask, "Where do you sense that sadness in your body?" After some exploration of that you might continue with the inquiry by asking, "What tells you that's sadness?" or "What sensations tell you that's sadness?" This can help bring clients into present time and direct sensory awareness as they begin to form a relationship to the felt-arising process. Orienting to the actual felt-sensations in the experience of emotional flooding can help uncouple the emotion from bodily sensations. It is generally less overwhelming to stay with the sensations and felt-sense of the experience, rather than with the emotional state, and is potentially more transformative. If clients can access the felt-sense level of the experience, they may uncover deeper meaning. This may shift the arising state to a more profound exploration of traumatization and self-nature. The intention is to help clients settle into a therapeutic zone where resources are accessed, shock affects dissipate without overwhelm, and an orientation to felt meaning is possible.

Summary of Basic Intentions in Emotional Flooding and Hyperarousal

When an emotion floods clients' experience, help slow the process down. See what helps to do that. An awareness of breath, slowing breath down, allowing the wave of the emotion to pass through, awareness of sensations, and so on will all help to mediate the intensity of the process. Presence, contact, and containment are essential. Help clients find their way back into contact in present time. Once the emotional process is appropriately paced and contained in present time, start an exploration of its felt-quality in the body. Get clients curious about their emotional state by starting a process of inquiry. Help generate a witness who is exploring that state.

To help slow the process down and re-establish resources and space:

Bring attention to the body: "Where do you sense that … (naming the particular emotion they are experiencing) in your body?"

Bring attention to the sensation and felt-sense of that in the body: "What sensations tell you that is … (naming the emotion they are experiencing)?"

Help clients track the sensations and felt-sense of it in the body. The felt-sense may also uncover deeper meanings and move the process along into a depth exploration of the traumatization.

Allow any processes of discharge, such as trembling or shaking, to complete. Reassure, slow things down, and resource the client if an autonomic discharge becomes overwhelming.

Hypoarousal States, Freezing, and Immobilization

As past traumatic impacts emerge in therapy sessions, clients may also experience parasympathetic hypoarousal states. These may emerge as experiences of numbness, coldness, and even as freezing states and immobilization. Clients may even experience temporary paralysis as these states are activated in their system. These kinds of freezing states can be thought of as a dissociation of a body part from the whole and are commonly coupled with dissociative processes. For instance, clients may experience one leg becoming cold and numb and seemingly paralyzed. These kinds of states are all manifestations of unresolved fight-or-flight intentions, and are expressions of overwhelm and shock responses to traumatic experience. At some time in their life, their fight-or-flight response was thwarted, an intention to protect was overwhelmed, and a parasympathetic defensive surge was initiated. This unresolved defensive intention was then locked into their body-mind system as an undercurrent of autonomic nervous system cycling.

Basic Clinical Approaches

It is important to remember that frozen states commonly have a huge amount of energy bound up within them, yielding great potential for mobilization and resolution. As practitioner, you can help clients mobilize the cycling energies and resolve the coupled defensive intentions. Encouraging present awareness in the body will help clients move from a frozen state to a state where trauma-bound energies can be accessed, mobilized, and resolved. The intention is to mobilize frozen energies in present time, so that a shift from parasympathetic freeze to sympathetic mobilization can occur in a paced and resourced manner, and the shock affects and nervous system cycling can then more fully resolve.

One approach is to help clients mobilize the frozen defensive intentions in order to complete the unresolved defensive need. When there are frozen energies and processes of immobilization present, there is always an unresolved *intention* to defend or protect locked into the system. These commonly manifest in the joints, connective tissues, and muscles of the body as tension and restriction. The following sections outline some approaches to working with frozen, trauma-bound energies and unresolved defensive intentions.

Acknowledgment and Reassurance

Hypoarousal states can be very alarming. The experience of frozen states, and in the extreme temporary paralysis, can be very frightening. If clients lose a sense of present time, it may feel like the trauma is occurring again and this alone may be fear-provoking. The experience in the treatment session may then just serve to reinforce the trauma or to send it deeper into the system. Again, verbal acknowledgment and reassurance by the practitioner are crucial. The frozen state, and any coupled emotional affects, are verbally acknowledged and clients are reassured that the arising process is an important part of the healing and completion of past experience. Again, it may also be important for clients to hear that you, as practitioner, are OK with the process and can hold the space for them.

Shuttling: Awareness of Sensations and the Edges of the Frozen State

If clients encounter freezing states, it is helpful to bring their awareness to the sensations and feeling-tones of the arising experience in present time. This has to be done in a paced and appropriately resourced manner. Frozen or immobilized states are commonly sensed in the shoulders, pelvis, and limbs—indeed, any parts of the body that manifest fight-or-flight intentions. These are expressions of unresolved trauma and incomplete responses to perceived danger.

As frozen states arise in session work, the first step is to help clients orient to areas of their body that are more resourced. Let's say that the experience is a sense of numbing and coldness below the navel with numbness in the legs. As this arises, remind these clients of their felt-resources and see if they can access a present-time experience of resource. Ask clients to notice where there *is* movement, or a sense of resource in their body. This might be a sense of warmth, tingling, or any sensation that is experienced as moving. Help them bring their attention to that part of the body. Let them settle into this area of the body and deepen into the experience of motion and resource. In this example, let's imagine that a client finds a sense of resource in the chest and heart area.

From there, see if they can gently bring their attention to the edge of the frozen area, in this case to the navel area where numbness is sensed. You might suggest, "See if you can slowly move your awareness from your heart area to the edge of where things feel frozen." This may initiate an activation of sensation in the frozen area. Clients may experience some movement of sensation at the edges of the frozen area, and can then be encouraged to track these sensations as they manifest in their body. This can encourage a dissipation and clearing of the frozen intentions and its autonomic energies.

Once this ground of awareness is established, clients can be encouraged to slowly shuttle back and forth from their resourced area and sensations to the edge of the frozen area. Have clients move their awareness to the edge of the frozen area, stay with this for a while, and then shuttle back to the more resourced area in the body. Have them stay with this area of resource for a while and then again slowly shuttle back to the edge of the frozen or immobilized area. Help clients shuttle back and forth, giving time to experience the sensations generated by the process.

Again, help clients track the sensations or feelings that arise as they do this. Do they sense anything changing? Are there sensations of movement from the area of immobilization? Are there any tremblings or sensations of energy moving? Stay with this shuttling process for a while and finish by again acknowledging the resourced sensations, or any other perception of resources that arise.

As they hold awareness at the edge of the frozen area, the energies will gradually shift to a more sympathetic nervous system level and they may find that the underlying sympathetic cycling begins to discharge and clear. Let's imagine that you have been holding their sacrum and they have experienced their legs becoming cold and immobilized. As they work with the shuttling process, the underlying intention to protect—such as a need to run, push, or kick—may begin to emerge and the sympathetic nervous system will begin to discharge. As this occurs, both you and your client may experience tingling, electric-like streaming, and warmth returning to the area.

Some people are more comfortable to work with this process in other ways. For instance, they may find that they can take the resources into the frozen area rather than stay on the edge of it. See what works for individual clients and keep exploring these ideas.

Mobilization Processes

Mobilization is another approach to working with frozen limbs and parasympathetic states on the treatment table. Let's again imagine that a client begins to experience a frozen, cold, and/or immobilized state. The first step is to again establish such clients' sense of felt-resource and also see if there is an area in their body that is not frozen and is sensed to be more alive. Have them orient to the sense of resource and area of the body that feels more alive, warm, moving, and so on, and ask them to settle or deepen into the experience of OK-ness there.

Once this is established, have clients work with the following mobilization process, in which they will slowly tense and relax their body. Explain that they will be working with an exercise that helps the frozen areas of their body come alive and processes the frozen state. Have them become aware of their arms and legs and body in general. As they do this, orient them to present-time sensory awareness by simply having them notice what sensations are present in their body. Then ask them to slowly pull their toes back and begin to let their hands form fists and then to also very slowly begin to tense their feet, hands, arms, and legs, along with pelvis, shoulders, and whole body, until they are holding a strong tension throughout their body. After just a few seconds of holding the height of the tension, ask them to very,

very slowly release the tension. As this occurs, the nervous system will commonly shift from the parasympathetic freeze, to a more sympathetic state of mobilization.

This may have to be slowly repeated, but no more than two or three times. It is important that clients are settled into resources before engaging their muscles and joints in this way, and that they stay connected with this sense of resource as they slowly mobilize. As the sympathetic defensive intentions emerge, the sympathetic nervous system will commonly begin to discharge and their frozen areas, such as legs or arms, will begin to feel warm and tingling. As practitioner, you may sense their sympathetics clearing via electric-like discharges, commonly from the head down and center out. This will feel good to the client and will again commonly clear in waves of discharge interspersed with sensations of space and warmth.

Unconscious Intentions and Frozen Sensations in the Body

You may notice, as a session progresses, that a client's hand, arm, foot, or leg is moving in some way, or more evident jerking or shaking may manifest. Or, as above, a client may feel numb, frozen, or even paralyzed in his or her arms or legs. All of these possibilities may indicate that a frozen defensive *intention* is beginning to manifest and that a need to fight or flee was not able to complete at the time of a traumatic experience. This is an expression of an incomplete defensive process still cycling in the body. These intentions are commonly held in arms or legs, as it is our arms and legs that we use to flee or protect ourselves in some way. For instance, the client may have been attacked in the street and could not complete a protective motion with the arms or legs, or was hit by a car and could not run away, or may have experienced repetitive physical or psychological abuse and could not respond. The following sections outline further therapeutic approaches that help mobilize and complete these frozen intentions. Following Levine's wording, in the sections below, we call the cycling energies of the autonomic nervous system *trauma-bound energies*.

Scenario one: movements emerge: Let's say that you are in session work and you notice that a client's arms begin to express a particular motion, or take on a particular form. This may be an expression of some need to protect, to reach out, or to be received by another in some way. One way to orient to this is to ask the client to become aware of the motion or shape that the arms are taking. Have the client also notice the sensations and qualities of intention that may be present. A question like "What do your arms want or need to do?" can help clarify the intention that is being expressed. As he or she deepens into this sensory awareness, ask the client to slowly explore the motion or form and see what process or felt-meaning clarifies. As a frozen protective intention clarifies you may also want to explore the next scenario below, where we help the client more actively resolve the cycling autonomic energies.

Scenario two: frozen areas, arms, or legs emerge: Imagine that, as the session progresses, a client experiences a quality of numbness and immobility in the pelvis and legs. The first step, as we have seen, is to ensure that the client is resourced. Asking him or her where in the body does it feel OK, warm or not frozen, may help the client settle into a resourced zone. Then simply ask the client to bring awareness to the area involved and notice the sensations present. As he or she settles into that awareness, ask if he or she senses an intention beginning to come through. As above, a question like "What do your legs want or need to do?" can be helpful.

Again, the client is most likely experiencing some kind of frozen defensive intention. If it manifests in the hands and arms, it may be about hitting, blocking, or pushing away; if it is in the feet and legs, it may be about kicking or running. Let the client explore the sensations and allow the intention to simply surface. When the intention begins to make itself known, you can use a simple process to help the client pace the experience and discharge the frozen intention. This can also be used in the scenario above where subtle motions or forms begin to clarify in the arms or legs. The idea in all of these processes is to help mobilize the trauma-bound energy in a resourced and contained space. This pacing process is summarized below.

Once the client has a felt-sense of the frozen intention in the limb:

- Step one is to have the client *imagine* that he or she is doing something (e.g., completing the intention). Most clients can usually imagine doing something without going into overwhelm. Once the client imagines doing it, say, in this case, pushing out with the legs, then have the client relax and hold the sensations that arise in awareness. Go slowly here.

- If the client's trauma bound energy is still unresolved, then a second step is useful. In this step, ask the client to prepare to do whatever it is that the limb seems to want to do. Here it is about the legs pushing out. Ask the client to engage and tense all the muscles and joints necessary to *prepare to do* the pushing. He or she may be surprised at what parts of the body need to be engaged to help in the preparation. Have the client *prepare to do* without actually doing it. Then have him or her relax and orient to the arising sensations. This may set off a cycle of discharge and clearing.

- If the client's process is still unresolved, a third step is useful. Again, as above, have the client *prepare to do* by engaging all the joints and muscles that are needed in the preparation. In this case, ask the client to slowly tense and engage all the muscles and joints needed in order to feel prepared to push out with the legs. This time, also ask the client to *slowly do* the action, whatever it is, in this case, to slowly push out with the legs. By first *preparing to do*, and then *slowly doing*, no piece of the trauma-bound energy is left out of the process. If the discharge occurs too rapidly, the energy may just recycle. Again, if emotional flooding occurs, or if the system goes into hyperarousal of any kind, slow the process down. Have the client come into the breath and his or her resources. Then have the client relax and again orient to the arising sensations. This may then set off a cycle of discharge and clearing.

- A final step may be needed to complete the cycle of discharge and to help the trauma-bound energy find completion in its intention. Again have the client *prepare to do*. Again ask him or her to slowly do it. This time, as the client expresses the motion, give the pelvis and legs a firm yet yielding resistance for them to push against. Using a large pillow or cushion to slowly push against is a good approach. This generally will help to mobilize any energies still bound in the system. Go slowly and track the arising process.

Summary of Working with Frozen Fight-or-Flight Intentions

Shuttling:

If your client is experiencing freezing states, start an inquiry into it: "Where do you sense the numbness, coldness, etc., in your body?" or "Where do you sense movement?" or "Where is it OK?" Ask your client to place awareness on the edge of the frozen state in the body after first having established some resources. See if the energies begin to move. Ask him or her to shuttle from a place where there is resource and movement to the edge of the frozen place/state in the body. Ask the client to orient to any sensations that emerge. Slowly help the client explore the shuttling process—staying with resourced sensations for a while, then shuttling to the edge of the frozen state, staying with that for a while, slowly shuttling back and forth as needed. See if the frozen state begins to shift and mobilize. Help the client stay with the emergent sensations.

Progressively explore the intention to defend:

Frozen states are expressions of frozen intentions. Again, first establish a place or quality of resource and OK-ness in the body. Help the client explore the withheld defensive intention. If the person senses frozen states, or numbness in the body, especially shoulders, arms, pelvis, or legs, start an inquiry into intentions.

Place awareness in the frozen or numb shoulder, arm, leg, etc., and ask the client, "Can you sense what that arm wants or needs to do?" Let the person stay with this exploration for a while. See if any autonomic and limbic affects need to discharge (such as trembling, shaking, or emotional tones).

Next in the progression, if appropriate, is an exploration into imagery. "Can you imagine that you are doing that?" See if the person can imagine that he or she is defending him- or herself, or doing the "intention" in some way. It is usually OK for a person to first imagine doing the intention as actually doing it may put him or her into overwhelm. Let any autonomic affects emerge and resolve. Help the person orient to any clearing or releases that manifest in the body.

Then, if energies are still running, the next step in the progression is "Can you prepare to do that?" See if the person can prepare to do the discovered intention (like pushing, defending) by slowly getting the body ready to do it in present time. "What parts of your body need to prepare or tense or tighten to prepare to do this?" "Can you slowly tense/tighten your body to prepare to do that?" It is surprising to notice how much and what parts of the body need to prepare to defend. Then orient the client to any arising sensations and feelings that emerge.

If the frozen state does not mobilize and the intention begins to resolve, have the client actually do it, but slowly. "Can you prepare to do that and then slowly do it?" Again, after the person slowly expresses the intention to push, defend, run, and so on, see if any autonomic affects resolve.

Finally, if there are still unresolved energies running, then have the person again "prepare to do" and then slowly do it against resistance. Holding a cushion for the client to push against is a useful approach. Initiate this slowly in resources and help process the release of any traumatic affect or sensations that arise. Does a sense of groundedness and empowerment come through?

Orienting

Traumatized people may have difficulty orienting to present experience. They may be caught in the active-alert state of the stress response, startle easily, and lose the ability to orient to present-time experience. This final section outlines an approach based on Levine's work and on core process psychotherapy that may help clients return to present time, re-establish the orienting response, and complete any unresolved orienting issues. It also helps relieve neck tension based on the cycling of the stress response and helps dissociative clients reorient to present time and re-embody. As we have seen, the orienting response is an important stage of the fight-or-flight hierarchy. It is commonly compromised due to traumatic cycling of unresolved autonomic energies. A particular set of nuclei in the brain stem coordinate the orienting response, and when these are re-engaged in resourced, present-time awareness, the stress response has a chance to down-regulate and the autonomic nervous system will then reset to a more homeostatic baseline.

In the exploration below, we take advantage of a further physiological process. As described in Chapters 19 and 20, there is a feedback loop between the neck area, brain stem, and prefrontal cortex. Neck motions and muscle tension gives the stress system feedback about danger through neural connections. When neck muscles tense, the brain stem reads this as possible environmental danger. The active-alert state of the stress response intensifies. If the system is in a chronic hyperarousal state, a feedback loop can ensue in which the neck muscles are signaled to tense and the tension is read by brain stem nuclei as an orienting response to danger. The person is caught in a chronic orienting-active-alert feedback loop. As we have seen, the prefrontal cortex mediates present-time awareness and has feedback loops to brain stem stress nuclei and to the nuclei that mediate the orienting response. When a person begins to orient via sight, sound, and neck-head motions in present time, the prefrontal cortex sends signals to the brain stem indicating that there is no present danger, and the system has a chance to down-regulate its stress response.

In this process, we will work with these orienting issues and ask our clients to really come into present time via the senses of seeing and hearing. We will then have them very slowly rotate their head from one side to the other as they scan the environment, actively listening and seeing as they scan the space they are sitting in. As they do this, we will also ask them to be aware of the sensations and feeling-tones that arise in their body, and help them track those sensations and work appropriately with them.

As clients enter present time, their cortex conveys information about the current nature of experience to stress nuclei. If the relationship with the practitioner is sensed as a resource, and there is trust present, then this will be communicated to the deepest recesses of the mind-body system.

Exploration:
Orienting _____

This exploration assumes that the client has developed sufficient resources and skills to orient to sensations and feeling-tones in the body without immediately dissociating. It also assumes that a safe therapeutic environment has been established. There must be a sense of trust and safety, both in the environment and in the relationship for any of this to be helpful.

Have the client sit comfortably in a chair or on a cushion. Sit in a position that the client feels comfortable with. He or she may want you to sit a certain distance away, or in a certain position, such as diagonally instead of directly opposite. Find an appropriate viewing distance and location.

First help the client orient to the embodied space. Help him or her form a relationship to sensations and feeling-tones in the body. Sometimes following the breath into the inner body space can help. Do not, however, force a person to be in sensation or in the body, but rather to simply orient to sensation and feeling-tones. Respect where the client needs to be.

Remind the client of felt resources, which have ideally been worked with in past sessions. He or she may bring in a totally resourcing memory or image to help access this territory. Find a word or phrase that helps the client connect with these resourced feeling-tones.

Then instruct the client to really pay attention to the seeing and hearing experiences. Help him or her to look at the objects in the room—the light, colors, forms—and help him or her to hear the sounds, the tones, the pitches in the environment. Then ask the client to very, very slowly and gently rotate the head, first in the direction it seems to want to go and then in the other direction. As he or she does this, again help him or her to perceive the sensations and feeling-tones in the body.

As the client slowly rotates the head, he or she may find a subtle barrier to the rotation—this may be a sense of tension in the neck muscles, or a sense of strain. Have the client stay near this edge and explore the sensations and feeling-tones that arise. This subtle boundary indicates the "edges" of the field of orientation in everyday life. Traumatization tends to literally narrow this field. This is physically expressed by subtle or gross restriction to allowable head motions, by neck tension and strain. These edges may even be expressions of unresolved birth trauma and must be sensitively negotiated. This is the time to remind the client to orient to felt resources and to seeing, hearing, and the outer environment. As the client stays at the edge of the tensions experienced, have him or her explore the sensations and feeling-tones that arise in the body. This helps the client enter present-time, right-brain/prefrontal cortex sensory awareness, which, in turn, helps down-regulate the stress response and encourages the re-establishment of appropriate affect regulation.

When the edge of tension softens, ask the client to continue to rotate the head in that direction until another barrier or tension edge is sensed. Again encourage an exploration of the arising process, sensations, and feeling-tones that emerge. Continue the exploration until there is a sense of resolution or completion, or until it seems that enough has been accomplished in the session.

Also help orient the client to the felt-sense of what arises—the overall feeling-sense of what is present—which also brings the felt meaning of the activation into play and may help down-regulate cortical involvement. Suggest that the client orient to the deeper holistic sense of what he or she is feeling and see if there is a word or phrase that describes what is being sensed. For instance, the client may sense contraction, feelings of fear, and an unclear deeper sense of "something." As he or she finds words that describe this "something," it may help him or her to let go of coupled meanings and memories and generate space in these mental-emotional couplings. Simply explore and see what arises without any need for anything particular to happen.

Gently work with these intentions and notice any activation that arises. Help the client work with any quality of activation that emerges. This may occur in any pole of the sympathetic-parasympathetic spectrum. It may even rapidly shift from one to the other. Slow things down and help the client be with one process at a time and, when appropriate, have him or her slowly shuttle between the felt-resource and the experience of the activation.

This simple process can be very powerful. It is something that might be worked with when clients have built resources and trust, and can be with their arising process. In my experience it does help people reorient and come into present time. It allows the parasympathetic-sympathetic poles of cycling to arise in their own time and to process and resolve in resources. I commonly use a simplified version of this process as clients sit up after a table session. This helps them make the transition from table work to a present-time orientation to completion and leaving my office space.

Reviewing and Grounding Concepts and Considerations

It is important to appropriately pace session work and to help clients be spaciously present and maintain a quality of witness consciousness and present-time awareness. The safety of the therapeutic environment is essential and the quality of the therapeutic relationship is the important foundation for healing to occur. The practitioner has to be able to hold the therapeutic space by being fully present and accepting what arises in the session with receptivity and without judgment.

If an arising process overwhelms clients, they may experience the present release of traumatic cycling as though a new trauma is happening. For instance, they may dissociate from the reality of the present as strong emotions flood their system. In this context, it is the role of the practitioner to help clients contain their process and to bring them back to the present by slowing things down and encouraging an awareness of the sensations in their body. Sometimes, a simple thing like having clients slow their breath and remember their ability to be in the body with awareness of sensation is all that is needed. Sometimes, simple phrases like "Can you let that move through you?" or "Can you let that wave through you?" are helpful when strong emotions arise. The expression and release of strong emotional charge may be an essential part of the healing process, but containment in resources is essential if it is to be an empowering experience.

It is important that clients have the inner resources to be with these strong emotions with space, with a clear sense of their witness. Remind clients of their resources and of their resourced sensations. It may take any number of sessions for clients to begin to be able to be with their process with space. Once they can do this, it becomes a life skill that they can bring to their everyday situations. The most important thing during session time is to work slowly and help clients pace their work so that trauma states can be processed without retraumatizing their system.

Basic intentions when working with trauma-bound states:

- Acceptance and reassurance

- Present-time mindfulness—help clients explore their present sensory experience and find the "present-time-ness" of it

- Resources—help clients find and explore their resources and resourced sensations and/or feeling-tones

- Tracking skills—help clients orient to their experience in present time. These include sensations, feeling-tone, emotional states, images, cognitive states, meaning, and so on. As any aspect of Levine's SIBAM—sensation, images (including cognitive processes), behavioral tendencies, affect and emotion, and meaning— arises, have clients initiate a felt sensory awareness in present time.

- Shuttling skills—help clients learn to "shuttle" from a resourced place in the body to the area of difficulty, or from the resource generally, like resourced images, feeling-tones, etc. to the state that expresses overwhelm/freezing

- Dissociative process—help clients explore their dissociative state in present-time awareness

- Emotional flooding—slow down or contain emotional processes with a focus on body awareness

- Frozen states and movement tendencies—help clients mobilize the frozen energies in their resources

The heart of these skills is presence and relational resonance. The core of the work is a deep trust in the human condition and awareness as a healing tool.

REFERENCES

Alberts, B., Bray, D., Lewis, J., et al. (1994) *Molecular Biology of the Cell,* 3rd edition. Garland Science.

Ankerberg, J., and Weldon, J. (1989) *When Does Life Begin? And 39 Other Tough Questions about Abortion.* Welgemuth & Hyatt.

Audette, J. R. (1982) Historical Perspectives on Near-Death Episodes and Experiences. In C. R. Lundahl (ed.), *A Collection of Near-Death Research Readings: Scientific Inquiries into the Experiences of Persons Near Physical Death* (pp. 21–43). Nelson-Hall.

Babic, Z. (1993) Towards a Linguistic Framework of Prenatal Language Stimulation. In T. Blum (ed.), *Prenatal Perception Learning and Bonding* (pp. 361–386). Leonardo.

Bauer, P. J. (2006) Remembering the Times of Our Lives: Memory in Infancy and Beyond (Developing Mind Series). Lawrence Erlbaum Associates.

BBC News (2005) Poor Cell Memory Is Key to Cancer, http://news.bbc.co.uk/go/pr/fr/-/1/hi/health/3955719.stm.

BBC News (2010) NE Scotland, Orkney, & Shetland, 20 July.

Becker, R. (1963, 1964, 1965) *Diagnostic Touch: Its Principles and Applications,* Vols. I, II, III, IV. Academy of Applied Osteopathy Yearbooks.

———(1988) Mechanism to Mechanism, How to Get Started (a recorded lecture).

———(1997) *Life In Motion.* Rudra Press.

———(2000) *The Stillness of Life.* Stillness Press.

Bergman, K., Sarkar, P., Glover, V., and O'Connor, T. G. (2010) Maternal Prenatal Cortisol and Infant Cognitive Development: Moderation by Infant-Mother Attachment, *Biol Psychiatry,* Jun 1;67(11):1026–1032. Epub 2010 Feb 25.

Blechschmidt, E. (2004) *The Ontological Basis of Human Anatomy.* North Atlantic Books.

Blechschmidt, E., and Gasser, R. F. (1978) *Biokinetics and Biodynamics of Human Differentiation.* Charles C. Thomas.

Bowman, C. (1997) *Children's Past Lives: How Past Life Memories Affect Your Child.* Bantam.

Buchheimer, A. (1987) Memory: Preverbal and Verbal. In T. R. Verny (ed.). *Pre- and Perinatal Psychology: An Introduction* (pp. 52–65). Human Sciences.

Castellino, R. (1995) How Babies Heal, paper given to F. Sills by Castellino.

———(1996) *Being with Newborns: An Introduction to Somatotropic Therapy; Attention to the Newborn; Healing Betrayal, New Hope for the Prevention of Violence.* (Available from Castellino Prenatal and Birth Therapy, 1105 N. Ontare Road, Santa Barbara, CA 93105.)

———(1998) Somatotropic Facilitation of Prenatal and Birth Trauma, draft of class notes and text for forthcoming book given to F. Sills by Castellino.

———(2000) The Stress Matrix: Implications for Prenatal and Birth Therapy. *Journal of Prenatal and Perinatal Psychology and Health,* 15(1):31–62.

Chamberlain, D. B. (1990) The Expanding Boundaries of Memory, *Pre- and Perinatal Psychology Journal,* 4(3):171–189.

———(1992) Is There Intelligence Before Birth? *Pre- and Peri-Natal Psychology Journal,* 6(3):217–237.

———(1994) The Sentient Prenate: What Every Parent Should Know. *Pre- and Perinatal Psychology Journal,* 9(1):9–31.

———(1996) Life in the Womb: Dangers and Opportunities. Paper presented to the International Congress Apprendizaje y Comunicacion Pre- and Postnatal, Valencia, Spain (in Spanish). (Also in Selected Works: *Journal of* Prenatal and Perinatal Psychology and Health, 1999, 14(1–2):31–43.

———(1998) *The Mind of Your Newborn Baby.* North Atlantic Books.

———(1999a) Prenatal Body Language: A New Perspective on Ourselves. *Journal of* Prenatal and Perinatal Psychology and Health, 14(1–2):169–185.

———(1999b) Life in the Womb: Dangers and Opportunities. *Journal of* Prenatal and Perinatal Psychology and Health, 14(1–2):31–43.

———(1999c) Foundations of Sex, Love and Relationships: From Conception to Birth. *Journal of Prenatal and Perinatal Psychology and Health,* 14(1–2):45–64.

———(1999d) The Significance of Birth Memories. *Journal of Prenatal and Perinatal Psychology and Health,* 14(1–2):65–83.

———(1999e) Transpersonal Adventures in Prenatal and Perinatal Hypnotherapy. *Journal of Prenatal and Perinatal Psychology and Health,* 14(1–2):85–95.

———(1999i) Prenatal Body Language: A New Perspective on Ourselves. *Journal of Prenatal and Perinatal Psychology and Health,* 14(1–2):169–185.

———(2011) The Sentient Prenate: What Every Parent Should Know, *Journal of Prenatal and Perinatal Psychology and Health,* 26(1):37–59.

Chamberlain, D. B., and Arms, S. (1999) Obstetrics and the Prenatal Psyche, *Journal of Prenatal and Perinatal Psychology and Health,* 14(1–2):97–118.

Cheek, D. B. (1986) Prenatal and Perinatal Imprints: Apparent Prenatal Consciousness as Revealed by Hypnosis. *Pre- and Perinatal Psychology Journal,* 1(2):97–110.

———(1992) Are Telepathy, Clairvoyance and "Hearing" Possible in Utero? Suggestive Evidence as Revealed During Hypnotic Age-Regression Studies of Prenatal Memory. *Pre- and Perinatal Psychology Journal,* 7(2):125–137.

Childre, D., and Martin, H. (1999) *The Heartmath Solution.* HarperCollins.

Childs, M. R. (1998) Prenatal Language Learning. *Journal of Prenatal and Perinatal Psychology and Health,* 13(2):99–121.

Clemente C. (2001) *Anatomy: A Regional Atlas of the Human Body,* 4th ed., plate 768. Williams & Wilkins.

Condon, W. S., and Sander, L. W. (1974) Neonate Movement Is Synchronized with Adult Speech: Interactional Participation and Language Acquisition. *Science,* 183:99–101.

Courage, M. L., and Howe, M. L. (2004) Advances in Early Memory Development Research: Insights about the Dark Side of the Moon. *Developmental Review,* 24:6–32.

Cozolino, L. (2002) *The Neuroscience of Psychotherapy.* W. W. Norton.

David, H. P., Dytrych, Z., Matejcek, Z., and Schuller, V. (1988) *Born Unwanted: Developmental Effects of Denied Abortion.* Springer.

Davis-Floyd, R. E. (1992) *Birth as an American Rite of Passage.* University of California Press.

DeCasper, A., & Fifer, W. (1980) Of Human Bonding: Newborns Prefer Their Mother's Voices. *Science,* 208:1174–1176.

DeMause, L. (1982) *Foundations of Psychohistory.* Creative Roots.

De Vries, J. I. P. (1992) The First Trimester. In J. G. Nijhauis (ed.), *Fetal Behaviour: Developmental and Perinatal Aspects* (pp. 3–16). Oxford University Press.

Doughty, F. M. (2007) Sending and Receiving: Biochemical Communication of Emotions between Prenate and Mother: A Call for Early Intervention, *Journal of Prenatal and Perinatal Psychology and Health,* 21(3):281–304.

Emerson, W. R. (1989) Psychotherapy with Infants and Children, *Journal of Pre- and Perinatal Psychology,* 3(3), 190–217.

⸺ (1995) Lecture notes from The Evaluation of Trauma and Shock, course conducted in Denver, CO, August, 4–7.

⸺ (1996) The Vulnerable Prenate. *Pre- and Perinatal Psychology Journal* 10(3):125–141.

⸺ (1998) Birth Trauma: The Psychological Effects of Obstetrical Interventions, *Journal of Prenatal and Perinatal Psychology and Health,* 13(1):11–44.

Emerson, W. R., and Schorr-Kon, S. (1993) Somatotropic Therapy: The Work of Dr. William R. Emerson. Unpublished manuscript.

Emoto, M., translated by Thayne, D. A. (2004) *The Hidden Messages in Water.* Beyond Words Publishing.

Emoto, M. (1999) *Messages from Water.* Hado Kyoikusha.

Fairbairn, R. (1994a) in E. Birtles and D. Sharff (eds.), *Clinical and Theoretical Papers.* Vol. I of *From Instinct to Self: Selected Papers of W. R. D. Fairbairn.* Jason Aronson.

⸺ (1994b) in E. Birtles and D. Sharff (eds.), *Applications and Early Contributions.* Vol. II of *From Instinct to Self: Selected Papers of W. R. D. Fairbairn.* Jason Aronson.

⸺ (1994c) The Screber Case and In Defense of Object Relations Theory, in E. Birtles and D. Sharff (eds.), *Clinical and Theoretical Papers.* Vol. I of *From Instinct to Self: Selected Papers of W. R. D. Fairbairn.* Jason Aronson.

⸺ (1994d) The Nature of Hysterical States, in E. Birtles and D. Sharff (eds.), *Clinical and Theoretical Papers.* Vol. I of *From Instinct to Self: Selected Papers of W. R. D. Fairbairn.* Jason Aronson.

Farrant, G. (1986) Cellular Consciousness, *Aesthema,* 7:28–39.

Farrant, G., and Larimore, T. (1995). Six Universal Body Movements Expressed in Cellular Consciousness and Their Meanings, *Primal Renaissance: The Journal of Primal Psychology,* 1(1):17–24.

Feldman, R., Weller, A., Sirota, L., and Eidelman, A. I. (2003). Testing a Family Intervention Hypothesis: The Contribution of Mother-Infant Skin-to-Skin Contact (Kangaroo Care) to Family Interaction, Proximity, and Touch. *Journal of Family Psychology,* 17(1):94–107.

Field, T., Diego, M., and Hernandez-Reif , M. (2006). Prenatal Depression Effects on the Fetus and Newborn: A Review. *Infant Behavior and Development,* 29:445–455.

Field, T., Hernandez-Rief, M., Diego, M., Figueiredo, B., Schanberg, S., and Kuhn, C. (2004) Prenatal Cortisol, Prematurity and Low Birthweight, *Infant Behavior and Development,* 27(2), May:216–229.

Finkelstein, Y., Koffler, B., Rabey, J., and Gilad, G. (1985) Dynamics of Cholinergic Synaptic Mechanisms in Rat Hippocampus After Stress, *Brain Research*, September:314–319.

Fodor, N. (1949) *The Search for the Beloved: A Clinical Investigation of the Trauma of Birth and Pre-Natal Conditioning.* Hermitage Press.

Forray, A., Mayes, L. C., Magriples, U., and Epperson, C. N. (2009) Prevalence of Post-Traumatic Stress Disorder in Pregnant Women with Prior Pregnancy Complications, *Journal of Maternal-Fetal and Neonatal Medicine, 22*(6):522–527.

Foster, S. M. (2007) The Development of Sensory Systems During the Prenatal Period, *Journal of Prenatal and Perinatal Psychology and Health, 21*(3).

Freud, W. E. (1987) Prenatal Attachment and Bonding. In T. R. Verny (ed.), *Pre- and Perinatal Psychology: An Introduction* (pp. 90–106). Human Sciences Press.

Fuller, B. (1975, 1979) *Synergetics, Explorations in the Geometry of Thinking.* Macmillan.

Garfield, C. A. (1982) The Dying Patient's Concern with Life After Death. In C. R. Lundahl (ed.), *A Collection of Near-Death Research Readings: Scientific Inquiries into the Experiences of Persons Near Physical Death* (pp. 160–164). Nelson-Hall.

Gaskin, I. M. (2003) *Ina May's Guide to Childbirth.* Bantam.

Gellrich, M. (1993) Development of Musicality before Birth and in Early Childhood. In T. Blum (ed.), *Prenatal Perception Learning and Bonding* (pp. 279–306). Leonardo.

Gendlin, E. (1978, 1981, 2003) *Focusing.* Rider.

Giesler, G. J. (1994). Nociception and the Neuroendocrine-Immune Connection: Studies of Spinal Cord Neurons that Project Directly to the Hypothalamus. In H. Willard and M. M. Patterson (eds.), *Nociception and the Neuroendocrine-Immune Connection..* American Academy of Osteopathy.

Ginsburg, S., and Jablonka, E. (2009) Epigenetic Learning in Non-Neural Organisms, *J. Biosci. 34*(4):633–646..

Glover, V. (2011) The Effects of Prenatal Stress on Child Behavioural and Cognitive Outcomes Start at the Beginning, *Encyclopedia on Early Childhood Development.* Published online, January 17, 2011, London: Centre for Excellence for Early Childhood Development.

Goldberg, H. (2007) The Potential Risks of Ultrasound Examinations on Fetal Development, *Journal of Prenatal and Perinatal Psychology and Health, 21*(3):261–270.

Grof, S. (1993) *The Holotropic Mind.* Harper's San Francisco.

Grosso, M. (1982) Toward an Explanation of Near-Death Phenomena. In C. R. Lundahl (ed.), *A Collection of Near-Death Research Readings: Scientific Inquiries into the Experiences of Persons Near Physical Death* (pp. 205–230). Nelson-Hall.

Gudrais, E. (2001) Modern Myelinization: The Brain at Midline, *Harvard Magazine*, http://harvardmagazine.com, May–June.

Hallett, E. (1995). *Soul Trek: Meeting Our Children on the Way to Birth.* Light Hearts.

Hatch, F. W., and Maietta, L. (1991) The Role of Kinesthesia in Pre- and Perinatal Bonding. *Pre- and Perinatal Psychology Journal, 5*(3):253–270.

Hendricks, G., and Hendricks, K. (1991) *Radiance! Breathwork, Movement and Body-Centered Psychotherapy.* Wingbow.

Henshaw, S. K. (1998) Unintended Pregnancy in the United States, *Family Planning Perspectives, 30*(1):24-29, 46.

Ho, M. W. (1998) *The Rainbow and the Worm: The Physics of Organisms.* World Scientific.

Ho, M. W., and Knight, D. (2000) The Acupuncture System and the Liquid Crystalline Collagen Fibres of the Connective Tissues and Liquid Crystalline Meridians, paper, Institute Bioelectrodynamics Laboratory, Open University, Walton Hall, Milton Keynes and Dept. of Biological Sciences, King Alfred's College, Winchester U.K. and Institute of Science in Society, *American Journal of Complementary Medicine.*

Iacoboni, M. (2008) *Mirroring People.* Farrar, Straus and Giroux.

Janov, A. (1983) *Imprints: The Lifelong Effects of the Birth Experience.* Coward McCann.

Jibu, M., and Yasue, K. (1995) *Quantum Brain Dynamics and Consciousness: An Introduction.* John Benjamins.

Johnson, C. (2010) Impact of Kangaroo Care (Skin-to-Skin Contact) on Attachment Formation between Preterm Infants and Their Caregivers, *Pediatrics CATs.* Paper 9.

Jonathan M. (2011) The Face of a Frog: Time-Lapse Video Reveals Never-Before-Seen Bioelectric Pattern, *Science News,* December 13, http://www.evolutionnews.org/2011/12/the_face_of_a_f054131.html.

Kang, R. (1978) Parent-Infant Attachment. In M. L. Duxbury and P. Carroll (eds.), *The First Six Hours of Life: Early Parent-Infant Relationships: A Staff Development Program in Prenatal Nursing Care,* Series 1, Module 3 (pp. 70–73). National Foundation/March of Dimes.

Kapanji, I. A. (1974) *The Physiology of the Joints.* Churchill Livingston.

Karen, R. (1994) *Becoming Attached: First Relationships and How They Shape Our Capacity to Love.* Oxford University Press.

Karr-Morse, R., and Wiley, M. S. (1997) *Ghosts from the Nursery: Tracing the Roots of Violence.* The Atlantic Monthly Press.

Keleman, S. (1986) *Bonding: A Somatic-Emotional Approach to Transference.* Center Press.

Kestenberg, J. S. (1987) Empathy for the Fetus: Fetal Movements and Dreams. In T. R. Verny (ed.), *Pre- and Perinatal Psychology: An Introduction* (pp. 138–150). Human Sciences Press.

Kirschvink J. L., Winklhofer, M., and Walker, M. M. (2010) Biophysics of magnetic orientation: strengthening the interface between theory and experimental design. *J R Soc Interface.* 2010 Apr 6;7 Suppl 2:S179–191. Epub 2010 Jan 13.

Klaus, M. H., and Kennell, J. H. (1976) *Maternal-Infant Bonding: The Impact of Early Separation or Loss on Family Development.* C. V. Mosby.

Klaus, M. H., Klaus, P. H., and Kennell, J. H. (1995) *Bonding: Building the Foundations for Secure Attachment and Independence.* Addison-Wesley.

Kovacevic, M. (1993) A New Perspective of Psycholinguistics: Prenatal Language Development. In T. Blum (ed.), *Prenatal Perception Learning and Bonding* (pp. 331–360). Leonardo.

Lake, F. (1979) *Studies in Constricted Confusion: Exploration of a Pre- and Peri-natal Paradigm.* Clinical Theology Association.

———— (1986a) *Charts.* Clinical Theology Association.

———— (1986b) *The Dynamic Cycle.* Clinical Theology Association.

LeDoux, J. (1998) *The Emotional Brain.* Simon & Schuster.

Levine, P. (1997) *Waking the Tiger*. North Atlantic Books.

———(2008) *Healing Trauma*. Sounds True.

———(2010) *In an Unspoken Voice: How the Body Releases Trauma and Restores Goodness.* North Atlantic Books.

Liedloff, J. (1977) *The Continuum Concept: Allowing Human Nature to Work Successfully.* Addison-Wesley.

Lifton, B. J. (1992) The Adopted Self: Toward a Theory of Cumulative Trauma. Unpublished doctoral dissertation, The Union Institute.

Lipton, B. H. (1998) Nature, Nurture and the Poser of Love, *Journal of Prenatal and Perinatal Psychology and Health,* 13(1):3–10.

Llinás, R. R. (2001) *i of the Vortex: From Neurons to Self.* MIT Press.

Ludington-Hoe, S. M., and Swinth, J. Y. (1996) Developmental Aspects of Kangaroo Care. *Journal of Obstetric, Gynecologic, and Neonatal Nursing,* 25:691–703. doi: 10.1111/j.1552-6909.1996.tb01483.x.

Luminare-Rosen, C. (2000) *Parenting Begins Before Conception: A Guide to Preparing Body, Mind, and Spirit for You and Your Future Child.* Healing Arts Press.

Lundahl, C. R. (1982) Near-Death Experiences of Mormons, in C. R. Lundahl (ed.), *A Collection of Near-Death Research Readings: Scientific Inquiries into the Experiences of Persons Near Physical Death* (pp. 165–179). Nelson-Hall.

Maroney, D. I. (2003) Recognizing the Potential Effect of Stress and Trauma on Premature Infants in the NICU: How Outcomes Are Affected, *Journal of Perinatology,* Dec., 23:679–683.

McCraty, R. (2002) Influence of Cardiac Afferent Input on Heart-Brain Synchronization and Cognitive Performance, *International Journal of Psychophysiology,* 45(1–2):72–73.

Milne, H. (1995) *The Heart of Listening.* North Atlantic Books.

Moody, R. (1982) The Experience of Dying, in C. R. Lundahl (ed.), *A Collection of Near-Death Research Readings: Scientific Inquiries into the Experiences of Persons Near Physical Death* (pp. 89–109). Nelson-Hall.

Nathanielsz, P. W. (1999) *Life in the Womb: The Origin of Health and Disease,* Promethean.

Nyānasatta (1979) *The Foundations of Mindfulness.* Buddhist Publication Society:Wheel Publication No. 19.

Ogden, P. (2006) *Trauma and the Body: A Sensorimotor Approach to Psychotherapy.* W. W. Norton.

Osis, K., and Haraldsson, E. (1982) Deathbed Observations by Physicians and Nurses: A Cross-Cultural Survey, in C. R. Lundahl (ed.), *A Collection of Near-Death Research Readings: Scientific Inquiries into the Experiences of Persons Near Physical Death* (pp. 65–88). Nelson-Hall.

Oxorn, H. (1986) *Human Labor and Birth,* 5th ed. McGraw-Hill.

Parvati Baker, J., and Baker, F. (1974, 1986) *Conscious Conception: Elemental Journey through the Labyrinth of Sexuality.* North Atlantic Books and Freestone Publishing.

Paus, T., Zijdenbos, A., Worsley, K., Collins, D. L., Blumental, J., Giedd, J. N., Rapoport, J. L., and Evans, A. C. (1999). Structural Maturation of Neural Pathways in Children and Adolescents: In Vivo Study. *Science,* 283 (19 March):1908.

Pearce, J. C. (speaker) (1991). *Biological Connections of the Heart-Mind System. The Pre-and Peri-Natal Psychology Association of North America Fifth International Congress.* (Cassette Recording No. F001, Tape 1.) Sounds True.

Perry, B. and Pollard, R. (1998) Homeostasis, Stress, Trauma, and Adaptation: A Neuro-Developmental View of Childhood Trauma, *Child and Adolescent Psychiatric Clinics of North America,* 7(1), January:31–51.

Pert, C. B. (1997). *Molecules of Emotion: Why You Feel the Way You Feel.* Scribner.

Piontelli, A. (1992). *From Fetus to Child: An Observational and Psychoanalytic Study.* Routledge.

Porges, S. (1995) Orienting in a Defensive World: Mammalian Modifications of Our Evolutionary Heritage. A Polyvagal Theory, *Psychophysiology,* 32.

——— (2001) The Polyvagal Theory: Phylogenetic Substrates of a Social Nervous System, *International Journal of Psychophysiology,* 42:123–146.

——— (2007). The Polyvagal Perspective. *Biological Psychology,* 74(2):116–143.

——— (2011) *The Polyvagal Theory.* W.W. Norton.

Righard, R. and Franz, K. (1995) *Delivery Self-Attachment.* Geddes Productions.

Ring, K., and Cooper, S. (1997) Near-Death and Out-of-Body Experiences in the Blind: A Study of Apparent Eyeless Vision, *Journal of Near-Death Studies,* 16(2):101–147.

Rizzolatti, G., and Arbib, M. A. (1998) Language within Our Grasp. *Trends in Neurosciences,* 21(5):188–194.

Rizzolatti, G., and Craighero, L. (2004) The Mirror-Neuron System. *Annual Review of Neuroscience* 27:169–192.

Rizzolatti, G., and Sinigaglia, C. (2008) *Mirrors in Our Brain: How Our Minds Share Actions and Emotions.* Oxford University Press.

Rizzolatti, G., Fadiga, L., Fogas, L., and Gallese, V. (1996) Premotor Cortex and the Recognition of Motor Actions, *Cognitive Brain Research,* 3:131–141.

Robinson, M., Mattes, E., Oddy, W. H., Pennell, C. E., van Eekelen, A., McLean, N. J., Jacoby, P., Li, J., De Klerk, N. H., Zubrick, S. R., Stanley, F. J., and Newnham, J. P. (2011) Prenatal Stress and Risk of Behavioral Morbidity from Age 2 to 14 years: The Influence of the Number, Type, and Timing of Stressful Life Events. *Development and Psychopathology,* 23:507–520.

Rothschild, B. (2000) *The Body Remembers.* W. W. Norton.

Sabom, M. B., and Kreutziger, S. S. (1982). Physicians Evaluate the Near-Death Experience. In C. R. Lundahl (ed.), *A Collection of Near-Death Research Readings: Scientific Inquiries into the Experiences of Persons Near Physical Death* (pp. 148–159). Nelson-Hall.

Sapolsky, R., et al. (1989) Hippocampal Damage Associated with Prolonged and Fatal Stress in Primates, *Journal of Neuroscience,* May, g(5):1705–1711.

Schore, A. (2001a) Effects of a Secure Attachment Relationship on Right Brain Development and Infant Mental Health, *Infant Mental Health Journal,* 22:1–2, 7–66.

——— (2001b) The Effects of Early Relational Trauma on Right Brain Development: Affect Regulation and Infant Mental Health, *Infant Mental Health Journal,* 22(1–2):201–269.

——— (2003) *Affect Regulation and the Repair of the Self.* W.W. Norton.

Schneier, M., and Burns, R. (1991) Atlanto-Occipital Hypermobility in Sudden Infant Death Syndrome, *Chiropractic: the Journal of Chiropractic Research and Clinical Investigation,* July, 7(2):33ff.

Shea, M. J. (2010) *Biodynamic Craniosacral Therapy,* Vol. 3. North Atlantic Books.

Sheldrake, R. (2012). BBC interview, Joan Bakewell, Belief, BBC Radio 3, 9:30 PM, Monday, 2 January.

Siegel, D. (2007) *The Mindful Brain.* W.W. Norton.

_____ (2010) *The Mindful Therapist.* W. W. Norton.

Sills, F. (2008) *Being and Becoming.* North Atlantic Books.

Solter, A. J. (1984). *The Aware Baby: A New Approach to Parenting.* Shining Star Press.

Stern, D. (1985) *The Interpersonal World of the Infant: A View from Psychoanalysis and Developmental Psychology.* Karnac Books.

_____ (1995) *The Motherhood Constellation: A Unified View of Parent-Infant Psychotherapy.* Basic Books.

Stone, C. (2007) *Visceral and Obstetric Osteopathy.* Churchill Livingstone.

Stone, R. (1986, 1999) *Polarity Therapy,* Vol. 1, Book 2. Book Publishing Company.

Sutherland, W. G. (1990) *Teachings in the Science of Osteopathy.* Rudra Press.

_____ (1998) *Contributions of Thought.* Rudra Press.

Talbot, M. (1991) *The Holographic Universe.* HarperCollins.

Tiller, W. A., Dibble, Jr., W. E., and Kohane, M. J. (2001) *Conscious Acts of Creation: The Emergence of a New Physics.* Pavior.

Tufts University (2011) Bioelectric Fields and the Frog Embryo, *Tufts Now,* 80 George St., Medford, Massachusetts 02155.

Van de Carr, F. R., and Lehrer, M. (1997) *While You Are Expecting: Creating Your Own Prenatal Classroom.* Humanics Trade.

Van der Wal, J. (2005) Workshop lecture notes, Boulder, CO.

_____ (2007) Human Conception: How to Overcome Reproduction? in M. J. Shea, *Biodynamic Craniosacral Therapy,* Vol. 1 (pp. 137–155). North Atlantic Books.

Verny, T., and Kelly, J. (1981) *The Secret Life of the Unborn Child.* Summit Books.

Verny, T. (ed.) (1987) *Pre- and Perinatal Psychology: An Introduction.* Human Sciences.

Verrier, N. (1993) *The Primal Wound: Understanding the Adopted Child.* Gateway Press.

Wade, J. (1996) *Changes of Mind: A Holonomic Theory of the Evolution of Consciousness.* State University of New York Press.

Wadhwa, P. D. (2005) Psychoneuroendocrine Processes in Human Pregnancy Influence Fetal Development and Health, *Psychoneuroendocrinology,* 30(8):724–743.

Weil, A. (1996) *Spontaneous Healing: How to Discover and Enhance Your Body's Natural Ability to Maintain and Heal Itself,* Chap. 2. Ballentine Books.

Willard, F. H. (1995) The Anatomy of the Lumbosacral Connection, *Spine: State of the Art Reviews,* 9(2):333–335.

Willard, F. H., and Patterson, M. M., eds. (1994) *Nociception and the Neuroendocrine-Immune Connection.* American Academy of Osteopathy.

Winnicott, D. W. (1965a) *The Maturational Environment and the Facilitating Environment.* Hogarth.

_____ (1965b) *The Family and Individual Development.* Tavistock.

_____ (1987) *Babies and Their Mothers.* Free Association Press.

Wirth, F. (2001) *Prenatal Parenting.* Regan Books.

INDEX

A

abortion
  behavior of survivors, 57–58
  prenatal responses to planning
    or attempting, 35–37
  acceptance and reassurance
  See recognition
acetylcholine (ACh), 506
acknowledgment and
    reassurance. *See* recognition
activation
  of condensed experience and
    unresolved forces, 319–20
  heart area work may bring up
    early trauma, 35
  need to understand nature of
    traumatic, 297–98
  parasympathetic, 537–39
  signs of autonomic, 535–36
  sympathetic, 517–18, 539–41
  transitions and unresolved
    birth trauma, 47
  and trigeminal nuclei, 405
  use of stillpoints in states of,
    523–26
active-alert/orienting level stage
    of stress response, 489
adaptation. *See* general
    adaptation response; stress;
    stress response
adoption
  adoptees' reports of prenatal
    experiences, 45
  grief over loss of birth mother,
    60
  prenatal responses to planning
    or attempting, 35–37

adrenal glands
  connection with sympathetic
    nervous system, 508
  increase adrenaline production
    in stress response, 493–94
  See also H-P-A axis
adrenocorticotropic hormone
    (ACTH), 502
alar ligaments, 277
amniocentesis, baby's experience
    of, 56–57
amygdala
  initiates stress cascade, 515
  and limbic emotions, 85, 486
  role in stress response, 497,
    503, 505–7, 508, 511, 512, 569
android pelvic shape, 106, 158–
    60, *159*
anesthesia
  and attachment issues, 65–67
  in birth process, 63–64, 84, 155
  coupled with dissociative
    response, 87, 177, 178–79, 590
  and partial ignition, 154
angle of descent, 106–8
ankle joint, clinical highlight,
    449–50
anterior sacroiliac ligament,
    243–44
anterior-posterior forces, *142, 145*
anthropoid pelvic shape, 106,
    156–57
apical ligament, 277
Aqueduct of Sylvius, 102, 180
arachnoid granulations, *322*
arteries affected by occipital triad
    compression, 279

articular motions, of TMJ,
    407–11
asynclitic births, 108
atlanto-axial ligament, anterior
    and posterior, 275
atlanto-occipital membrane,
    anterior and posterior,
    274–75
atlas
  in compression of occipital
    triad, 281–82
  exploration of occiput-atlas
    relationships, 284–87
  locating via spinal landmarks,
    218
  relationships to occiput and
    axis, 273–77
attachment
  attachment theory, 41–43,
    52–54
  postnatal bonding and
    attachment issues, 65–67,
    84–86, 155
attention affects, as trauma
    indicator, 90
attention deficit disorders, early
    trauma as root of, 86, 474
attitudes and presentations at
    birth, 111–12
attunement
  with caregivers, 75–79, 453–55
  with clients, 2
  prenatal, 48–51, 56
  when holding environment
    lacks, 46
augmentation of fluid drive. *See*
    fluid drive, augmentation of

ABOUT THE CONTRIBUTORS

Franklyn Sills has pioneered the development of a biodynamic approach to craniosacral therapy and was the early innovator in the field. He has been teaching for twenty-eight years and has influenced many current teachers of biodynamic craniosacral therapy in North America and Europe. His books, *Craniosacral Biodynamics,* Volumes One and Two, were seminal texts in the field. Sills was also one of the early teachers of the work of Randolph Stone and has written a book on his work, *The Polarity Process.*

Sills is the co-director of the Karuna Institute, a retreat and teaching center that offers trainings in craniosacral therapy as well as a master's degree in core process psychotherapy, a Buddhist-influenced mindfulness therapy form. In the core process psychotherapy trainings, Sills offers his expertise through lecturing on Buddhist psychology, trauma and trauma resolution skills, and prenatal and birth psychology. He has also studied and collaborated with Dr. William Emerson, one of the prime developers of pre- and perinatal psychology. Buddhist teachings are the foundation of Sills's approach; he was a Buddhist monk under the most Venerable Taungpulu Kaba-Aye Sayadaw of Northern Burma, and has studied in the Zen and Taoist traditions. His experience in the cranial field has convinced him that the body must be included in any form of therapy. He offers teachings internationally, including in the United States, Germany, Italy, Holland, and Switzerland. His original texts on craniosacral biodynamics were written in 1995 and he is now writing and publishing new texts to reflect current thinking and practice.

Cherionna Menzam-Sills has been a practitioner since 1978. She is accredited by the Biodynamic Craniosacral Therapy Association of North America as a teacher and has a PhD in pre- and perinatal psychology. She is also an authorized Continuum Movement instructor, and has training and experience as an occupational therapist, massage therapist, dance/movement therapist, bodymind psychotherapist, and prenatal and birth therapist. Her background includes extensive training with William Emerson and Ray Castellino, with whom she worked for four years in his clinic for babies, children, and families in Santa Barbara. Cherionna teaches biodynamics and Continuum Movement across North America and Europe. She lives with her husband, Franklyn Sills, in Devon, England, where she has a private practice.

Dominique Degranges directs the Da-Sein Institut of Biodynamic Craniosacral Therapy in Winterthur, Switzerland. Having studied painting at L'École des Beaux Arts in Paris, he worked for many years at a psychiatric practice where he did therapeutic art with patients. He is a teacher of craniosacral therapy and therapy for pre- and perinatal trauma and leads classes at the Da-Sein Institut and at trainings in many European countries. He received his own training from Franklyn Sills in craniosacral therapy and pre- and perinatal therapy with Ray Castellino, and he has worked on trauma with Peter Levine. He has illustrated several books.